Procedures and Techniques in Intensive Care Medicine

Third Edition

Procedures and Techniques in Intensive Care Medicine

Third Edition

Editors

Richard S. Irwin, M.D.
Professor of Medicine and Nursing
University of Massachusetts Medical School
and Graduate School of Nursing
Chief, Division of Pulmonary, Allergy, and
Critical Care Medicine
UMass Memorial Health Care
Worcester, Massachusetts

James M. Rippe, M.D.
Associate Professor of Medicine (Cardiology)
Tufts University School of Medicine
Boston, Massachusetts
Founder and Director
Rippe Lifestyle Institute
Shrewsbury, Massachusetts
Founder and Director
Rippe Health Assessment at Florida Hospital
Celebration Health
Orlando, Florida

Frederick J. Curley, M.D.
Associate Professor of Medicine
University of Massachusetts Medical School
Worcester, Massachusetts
Director of Pulmonary and Critical Care Services
Milford-Whitinsville Regional Hospital
Milford, Massachusetts

Stephen O. Heard, M.D.
Interim Chair
Professor of Anesthesiology and Surgery
Co-Director, Surgical Intensive Care Units
Department of Anesthesiology
UMass Memorial Medical Center
Worcester, Massachusetts

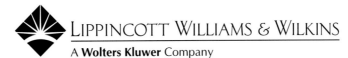
LIPPINCOTT WILLIAMS & WILKINS
A **Wolters Kluwer** Company
Philadelphia · Baltimore · New York · London
Buenos Aires · Hong Kong · Sydney · Tokyo

Executive Editor: R. Craig Percy
Developmental Editor: Keith Donnellan
Supervising Editor: Mary Ann McLaughlin
Production Editor: Erica Broennle Nelson, Silverchair Science + Communications
Manufacturing Manager: Colin Warnock
Cover Designer: Christine Jenny
Compositor: Silverchair Science + Communications
Printer: Maple Press

ISBN: 0-7817-4334-6

Care has been taken to confirm the accuracy of the information presented and to describe generally accepted practices. However, the authors, editors, and publisher are not responsible for errors or omissions or for any consequences from application of the information in this book and make no warranty, expressed or implied, with respect to the currency, completeness, or accuracy of the contents of the publication. Application of this information in a particular situation remains the professional responsibility of the practitioner.

The authors, editors, and publisher have exerted every effort to ensure that drug selection and dosage set forth in this text are in accordance with current recommendations and practice at the time of publication. However, in view of ongoing research, changes in government regulations, and the constant flow of information relating to drug therapy and drug reactions, the reader is urged to check the package insert for each drug for any change in indications and dosage and for added warnings and precautions. This is particularly important when the recommended agent is a new or infrequently employed drug.

Some drugs and medical devices presented in this publication have Food and Drug Administration (FDA) clearance for limited use in restricted research settings. It is the responsibility of health care providers to ascertain the FDA status of each drug or device planned for use in their clinical practice.

10 9 8 7 6 5 4 3 2 1

Contents

Contributing Authors

Maria E. Abruzzo, M.D.
Fellow in Rheumatology
Department of Medicine
Division of Rheumatology
UMass Memorial Health Care
Worcester, Massachusetts
Chapter 24

Harry L. Anderson III, M.D., F.A.C.S., F.C.C.M.
Clinical Associate Professor of Surgery
University of Pennsylvania School of Medicine
Philadelphia, Pennsylvania
Attending Surgeon
Division of Trauma and Surgical Critical Care
St. Luke's Hospital
Bethlehem, Pennsylvania
Chapter 10

Gerard P. Aurigemma, M.D.
Professor of Medicine
Division of Cardiology
UMass Memorial Health Care
Worcester, Massachusetts
Chapter 7

Philip J. Ayvazian, M.D.
Assistant Professor of Urology
University of Massachusetts Medical Center
Worcester, Massachusetts
Chapter 23

Richard C. Becker, M.D.
Professor of Medicine
Division of Cardiology
University of Massachusetts Medical School
Worcester, Massachusetts
Chapter 8

Eric A. Bedell, M.D.
Associate Professor of Anesthesiology
University of Texas Medical Branch at Galveston
Galveston, Texas
Chapter 22

Bernard D. Clifford, M.D.
Holyoke, Massachusetts
Chapter 16

Joseph A. Coladonato, M.D.
Duke Institute of Renal Outcomes
Research and Health Policy
Duke University Medical Center
Durham, North Carolina
Chapter 30

A. Alan Conlan, M.B., B.C.H., F.R.C.S. (C.), F.R.C.S. (E.)
Professor of Surgery
Department of Thoracic Surgery
UMass Memorial Health Care
Worcester, Massachusetts
Chapters 15, 29

Frederick J. Curley, M.D.
Associate Professor of Medicine
University of Massachusetts Medical School
Worcester, Massachusetts
Director of Pulmonary and Critical Care Services
Milford-Whitinsville Regional Hospital
Milford, Massachusetts
Chapters 26, 27

Bruce S. Cutler, M.D.
Professor and Chairman
Division of Vascular Surgery
UMass Memorial Health Care
Worcester, Massachusetts
Chapter 9

Seth T. Dahlberg, M.D.
Assistant Professor of Medicine and
    Radiology
Division of Cardiology
University of Massachusetts Medical Center
Worcester, Massachusetts
Chapter 5

Ashley Davidoff, M.D.
Associate Professor of Radiology
Co-Director of Abdominal Imaging
UMass Memorial Health Care
Worcester, Massachusetts
Chapter 28

**Robin I. Davidson, M.D., F.A.C.S., Capt., M.C.,
    U.S.N.R.**
Assistant Head and Staff Neurosurgeon
Department of Neurosurgery
Naval Medical Center Portsmouth
Charette Health Care Center
Portsmouth, Virginia
Chapter 21

Mark Dershwitz, M.D., Ph.D.
Professor of Anesthesiology and Biochemistry and Molecular
    Pharmacology
University of Massachusetts Medical School
Worcester, Massachusetts
Chapter 25

Donald J. Deyo, M.D.
Department of Anesthesiology
University of Texas Medical Branch at
    Galveston
Galveston, Texas
Chapter 22

Glenn D. Focht, M.D.
Instructor
Department of Internal Medicine
Milford-Whitinsville Regional Hospital
Milford, Massachusetts
Chapter 8

Todd F. Griffith, M.D.
Fellow
Department of Medicine
Division of Nephrology
Duke University Medical Center
Durham, North Carolina
Chapter 30

Stephen O. Heard, M.D.
Interim Chair
Professor of Anesthesiology and Surgery
Co-Director, Surgical Intensive Care Units
Department of Anesthesiology
UMass Memorial Medical Center
Worcester, Massachusetts
Chapter 1

Richard S. Irwin, M.D.
Professor of Medicine and Nursing
University of Massachusetts Medical School and Graduate
    School of Nursing
Chief, Division of Pulmonary, Allergy, and Critical Care
    Medicine
UMass Memorial Health Care
Worcester, Massachusetts
Chapters 12, 13, 14, 29

Eric W. Jacobson, M.D.
Associate Professor of Medicine
Division of Rheumatology
UMass Memorial Health Care
Worcester, Massachusetts
Chapter 24

Wandana Joshi-Ryzewicz, D.O.
Department of Anesthesiology
Tufts University School of Medicine
Boston, Massachusetts
Director, Clinical Affairs
Baystate Medical Center
Springfield, Massachusetts
Chapter 25

Shubjeet Kaur, M.D.
Assistant Professor
Clinical Director of Anesthesia Services
Co-Medical Director, Operative Services
Department of Anesthesiology
UMass Memorial Health Care
Worcester, Massachusetts
Chapter 1

Scott E. Kopec, M.D.
Assistant Professor of Medicine
Division of Pulmonary, Allergy, and Critical Care
    Medicine
University of Massachusetts Medical School
UMass Memorial Health Care
Worcester, Massachusetts
Chapters 15, 29

Peter E. Krims, M.D.
Associate Professor of Medicine
Division of Digestive Disease and Nutrition
UMass Memorial Health Care
Worcester, Massachusetts
Chapter 16

Stephen J. Krinzman, M.D.
Assistant Professor of Medicine
Division of Pulmonary, Allergy, and Critical Care
    Medicine
University of Massachusetts Medical Center
Worcester, Massachusetts
Chapter 12

Robert A. Lancey, M.D.
Director, Division of Cardiac Surgery
Bassett Healthcare
Cooperstown, New York
Chapters 10, 11

Laurence Landow, M.D.
Medical Officer
Department of Hematology
Office of Blood Research and Review
Center for Biologic Evaluation and Research
U.S. Food and Drug Administration
Rockville, Maryland
Chapter 25

Deborah H. Markowitz, M.D.
Assistant Professor of Medicine
Division of Pulmonary, Allergy, and Critical Care
    Medicine
University of Massachusetts Medical
    School
Worcester, Massachusetts
Chapter 14

D. Robert McCaffree, M.D., M.S.H.A.
Professor of Medicine
Department of Internal Medicine
Pulmonary Disease and Critical Care Section
University of Oklahoma College of Medicine
Veterans Administration Medical Center
Oklahoma City, Oklahoma
Chapter 4

Michael G. Mooradd, M.D.
Attending Cardiologist
Director of Nuclear Cardiology
Doylestown Hospital
Central Bucks Cardiology
Doylestown, Pennsylvania
Chapter 5

Brian E. Moore, M.D.
Research Fellow
Department of Research
Roger Williams Medical Center
Providence, Rhode Island
Chapter 20

Lena M. Napolitano, M.D.
Professor of Surgery
University of Maryland School of Medicine
VA Maryland Health Care System
Baltimore, Maryland
Chapters 17, 19

William F. Owen, Jr., M.D.
Brigham and Women's Hospital
Boston, Massachusetts
Chapter 30

Marie T. Pavini, M.D.
Assistant Professor of Anesthesiology
Division of Critical Care Medicine
UMass Memorial Health Care
Worcester, Massachusetts
Chapter 18

Donald S. Prough, M.D.
Professor and Chair
Department of Anesthesiology
University of Texas Medical Branch at
    Galveston
John Sealy Hospital
Galveston, Texas
Chapter 22

Juan Carlos Puyana, M.D.
Associate Professor of Surgery and Critical Care
    Medicine
University of Pittsburgh Medical Center
Pittsburgh, Pennsylvania
Chapter 18

Michael G. Seneff, M.D.
Associate Professor of Anesthesiology and Critical Care
    Medicine
George Washington University Medical Center
Washington, D.C.
Chapters 2, 3

Wayne E. Silva, M.D.
Professor and Vice Chairman
Department of Surgery
UMass Memorial Health Care
Worcester, Massachusetts
Chapter 15

Michael J. Singh, M.D.
Assistant Professor of Surgery
University of Massachusetts Medical School
Vascular Surgeon
UMass Memorial Health Care
Worcester, Massachusetts
Chapter 9

Nicholas A. Smyrnios, M.D.
Associate Professor of Medicine
Director, Medical Intensive Care Unit
Division of Pulmonary, Allergy, and Critical Care
    Medicine
University of Massachusetts Medical
    School
Worcester, Massachusetts
Chapters 26, 27

Michael O. Sweeney, M.D.
Assistant Professor of Medicine
Harvard Medical School
Cardiac Arrhythmia Service
Brigham and Women's Hospital
Boston, Massachusetts
Chapter 6

Irma O. Szymanski, M.D.
Professor
Department of Pathology
Director of Transfusion Services
Department of Hospital Laboratories
UMass Memorial Health Care
Worcester, Massachusetts
Chapter 20

Viviane Tabar, M.D.
Assistant Professor
Department of Neurosurgery
Memorial Sloan-Kettering Cancer Center
New York, New York
Chapter 21

Dennis A. Tighe, M.D., F.A.C.C., F.A.C.P.
Director, Echocardiography Laboratory
Associate Director, Noninvasive Cardiology
Associate Professor of Medicine
University of Massachusetts Medical School
Worcester, Massachusetts
Chapter 7

Stephen J. Voyce, M.D.
Assistant Clinical Professor of Medicine
Allegheny University-Hahnemann/HCP School of Medicine
Philadelphia, Pennsylvania
Director, Clinical Cardiology
Community Medical Center
Scranton, Pennsylvania
Chapter 4

John P. Weaver, M.D.
Associate Professor of Neurosurgery
Department of Surgery
Division of Neurosurgery
University of Massachusetts Medical Center
Worcester, Massachusetts
Chapter 21

Mark M. Wilson, M.D.
Associate Professor of Medicine
University of Massachusetts Medical School
Worcester, Massachusetts
Chapter 13

Preface

Rapid advances continue to occur in every area of critical care medicine. Since the publication in 1985 of the first edition of our comprehensive textbook, *Irwin and Rippe's Intensive Care Medicine* (now in its fifth edition), important breakthroughs have occurred in every branch of medicine, surgery, and anesthesiology, revolutionizing the management of critically ill patients. Procedures and techniques used to treat such desperately ill patients have also witnessed significant advances. Since the second edition of our book, *Procedures and Techniques in Intensive Care Medicine*, advances have occurred in virtually every interventional procedure and technique used in the intensive care unit.

Procedures and Techniques in Intensive Care Medicine (third edition) is an outgrowth of our textbook, *Irwin and Rippe's Intensive Care Medicine*, in which procedures and techniques have come to occupy increasingly prominent roles. Please note that all chapter cross-references in this volume are to corresponding chapters in the larger text. We have chosen to publish this vitally important information on modern procedures and techniques both as the first section of the current edition of *Irwin and Rippe's Intensive Care Medicine* and in this separate, smaller text. We are convinced that this smaller, more portable book will continue to be useful not only to the critical care specialist but also to emergency department physicians; surgeons; critical care nurses; medical, surgical, and anesthesia residents; and medical students.

The third edition of *Procedures and Techniques in Intensive Care Medicine* is a completely updated monograph. Comprehensive, evidence-based, updated information is included on virtually every technique and procedure used in the field of adult critical care. Detailed illustrations regarding how to perform each procedure, along with step-by-step instructions, are also included. Thorough, evidence-based discussions address indications, contraindications, complications, equipment, and ongoing equipment maintenance for common procedures used in critical care. *The procedures and techniques required for certification in critical care or tested in internal medicine, surgical, or anesthesiology critical care board examinations are presented and discussed in depth.*

In the current edition, the reader will find comprehensive guides to most techniques and procedures performed in intensive care. Techniques such as endotracheal intubation and pulmonary artery catheterization should be mastered by all critical care physicians. Other procedures, such as percutaneous tracheotomy and percutaneous cystotomy, which were once only performed by consulting specialists, are now increasingly performed by critical care practitioners and are included, along with detailed instructions. Other techniques that are still performed by consulting specialists are also included, because the intensivist must understand the indications, contraindications, likely results, and complications of these procedures.

Publication of medical textbooks is a team effort. The completion of *Procedures and Techniques in Intensive Care Medicine* would not have been possible without the combined efforts, talent, and hard work of many fine individuals. We have been blessed over the years with wonderful friends, colleagues, and staff members who have played crucial roles at every stage of the preparation of this text. Special gratitude and thanks are due Elizabeth Porcaro, Editorial Director of Dr. Rippe's laboratory, as well as of this text and our larger textbook, *Irwin and Rippe's Intensive Care Medicine*. Beth possesses superb organizational skills, a solid background in medical publishing, and the work ethic and good humor required to bring a textbook to completion. Karen Barrell, Administrative Assistant to Dr. Irwin, continued to organize a very busy schedule, allowing time to complete this and many other editorial tasks. Susan St. Martin, Administrative Assistant to Dr. Heard, helped facilitate every aspect of this project from start to finish. We also appreciate the continued help of our friend and Editor at Lippincott Williams & Wilkins, Craig Percy, who always provides encouragement, guidance, and great skill throughout the editorial process.

Finally, we wish to thank our colleagues, students, and families, who continue to inspire, teach, and support us. We hope that this third edition of *Procedures and Techniques in Intensive Care Medicine* will continue to serve as a useful guide to the dedicated physicians who practice critical care and will also advance the field of critical care medicine.

Richard S. Irwin, M.D.
James M. Rippe, M.D.
Frederick J. Curley, M.D.
Stephen O. Heard, M.D.

Procedures and Techniques in Intensive Care Medicine

Third Edition

1. Airway Management and Endotracheal Intubation

Shubjeet Kaur and Stephen O. Heard

In the emergency room and critical care environment, management of the airway to ensure optimal ventilation and oxygenation is of prime importance. Although initial efforts should be directed toward improving oxygenation and ventilation without intubating the patient, any prolonged efforts eventually require the placement of an endotracheal tube. Although endotracheal intubation is best left to the trained specialist, emergencies often require that the procedure be performed before a specialist arrives. Because intubated patients are commonly seen in the intensive care unit (ICU) and coronary care unit, all physicians who work in these environments should be skilled in the techniques of airway management, endotracheal intubation, and management of intubated patients.

Anatomy

An understanding of the techniques of endotracheal intubation and potential complications is based on knowledge of the anatomy of the respiratory passages [1]. Although a detailed anatomic description is beyond the scope of this book, an understanding of some features and relationships is essential to performing intubation.

NOSE. The roof of the nose is partially formed by the cribriform plate. The anatomic proximity of the roof to intracranial structures dictates that special caution be exercised during nasotracheal intubations. This is particularly true in patients with significant maxillofacial injuries.

The mucosa of the nose is provided with a rich blood supply from branches of the ophthalmic and maxillary arteries, which allow air to be warmed and humidified. Because the conchae provide an irregular, highly vascularized surface, they are particularly susceptible to trauma and subsequent hemorrhage. The orifices from the paranasal sinuses and nasolacrimal duct open onto the lateral wall. Blockage of these orifices by prolonged nasotracheal intubation may result in sinusitis [2].

MOUTH AND JAW. The mouth is formed inferiorly by the tongue, alveolar ridge, and mandible. The hard and soft palates compose the superior surface, and the oropharynx forms the posterior surface. Assessment of the anatomic features of the mouth and jaw is essential before orotracheal intubation. A clear understanding of the anatomy is also essential when dealing with a patient who has a difficult airway and learning how to insert newer airway devices such as the laryngeal mask airway (LMA; discussed in the section Management of the Difficult Airway).

NASOPHARYNX. The base of the skull forms the roof of the nasopharynx, and the soft palate forms the floor. The roof and the posterior walls of the nasopharynx contain lymphoid tissue (adenoids), which may become enlarged and compromise nasal airflow or become injured during nasal intubation, particularly in children. The eustachian tubes enter the nasopharynx on the lateral walls and may become blocked secondary to swelling during prolonged nasotracheal intubation.

OROPHARYNX. The soft palate defines the beginning of the oropharynx, which extends inferiorly to the epiglottis. The palatine tonsils protrude from the lateral walls and in children occasionally become so enlarged that exposure of the larynx for intubation becomes difficult. A large tongue can also cause oropharyngeal obstruction. Contraction of the genioglossus muscle normally moves the tongue forward to open the oropharyngeal passage during inspiration. Decreased tone of this muscle (e.g., in the anesthetized state) can cause obstruction. The oropharynx connects the posterior portion of the oral cavity to the hypopharynx.

HYPOPHARYNX. The epiglottis defines the superior border of the hypopharynx, and the beginning of the esophagus forms the inferior boundary. The larynx is anterior to the hypopharynx. The pyriform sinuses that extend around both sides of the larynx are part of the hypopharynx.

LARYNX. The larynx (Fig. 1-1) is a complex, highly integrated area that houses the vocal cords. It allows the passage of air into the trachea, prevents aspiration, and provides support and protection to the apparatus of voice production. The larynx is bounded by the hypopharynx superiorly and is continuous with the trachea inferiorly. The thyroid, cricoid, epiglottic, cuneiform, corniculate, and arytenoid cartilages compose the laryngeal skeleton. The thyroid and cricoid cartilages are readily palpated in the anterior neck. The cricoid cartilage articulates with the thyroid cartilage and is joined to it by the cricothyroid ligament. When the patient's head is extended, the cricothyroid ligament can be pierced with a scalpel or large needle to provide an emergency airway (see Chapter 15). The cricoid cartilage completely encircles the airway. It is attached to the first cartilage ring of the trachea by the cricotracheal ligament. The anterior wall of the larynx is formed by the epiglottic cartilage, to which the arytenoid cartilages are attached. Fine muscles span the arytenoid and thyroid cartilages, as do the vocal cords. The true vocal cords and space between them are collectively termed the *glottis* (Fig. 1-2). The glottis is the narrowest space in the adult upper airway. In children, the cricoid cartilage defines the narrowest portion of the airway. Because normal voice production relies on the precise apposition of the true vocal cords, even a small lesion can cause hoarseness. The fact that lymphatic drainage to the true vocal cords is sparse indicates that inflammation or swelling caused by tube irritation or trauma may take considerable time to resolve. The structures of the larynx are innervated by the superior and recurrent laryngeal nerve branches of the vagus nerve. The superior laryngeal nerve supplies sensory innervation from the inferior surface of the epiglottis to the superior surface of the vocal cords. From its takeoff from the vagus nerve, it passes deep to

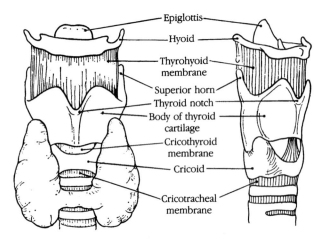

Fig. 1-1. Anatomy of the larynx, anterior and lateral aspects. (From Ellis H: *Anatomy for Anaesthetists.* Oxford, Blackwell Scientific, 1963, with permission.)

both branches of the carotid artery. A large internal branch pierces the thyrohyoid membrane just inferior to the greater cornu of the hyoid. This branch can be blocked with local anesthetics for oral or nasal intubations in awake patients. The recurrent laryngeal branch of the vagus nerve provides sensory innervation below the cords. It also supplies all the muscles of the larynx except the cricothyroid, which is innervated by the external branch of the superior laryngeal nerve.

TRACHEA. The adult trachea averages 15 cm long. Its external skeleton is composed of a series of C-shaped cartilages. It is bounded in the rear by the esophagus and in front for the first few cartilage rings by the thyroid gland. The trachea is lined with ciliated cells that secrete mucus; through the beating action of the cilia, foreign substances are propelled toward the larynx. The carina is located at the fourth thoracic vertebral level (of relevance when judging proper endotracheal tube positioning on chest radiograph). The right main bronchus takes off at a less acute angle than the left, making right main bronchial intubation more common if the endotracheal tube is in too far.

Emergency Airway Management

In an emergency situation, establishing adequate ventilation and oxygenation assumes primary importance [3]. Too fre-

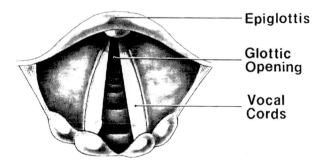

Fig. 1-2. Superior view of the larynx (inspiration). (From Stoelting RH, Miller RD: *Basics of Anesthesia.* 2nd ed. New York, Churchill Livingstone, 1989, with permission.)

quently, inexperienced personnel believe that this requires immediate intubation; however, attempts at intubation may delay establishment of an adequate airway. Such efforts are time consuming, can induce arrhythmias, and may induce bleeding and regurgitation, making subsequent attempts to intubate significantly more difficult. Some simple techniques and principles of emergency airway management can play an important role until the arrival of an individual who is skilled at intubation.

AIRWAY OBSTRUCTION. Compromised ventilation often results from upper airway obstruction by the tongue, by substances retained in the mouth, or by laryngospasm. Relaxation of the tongue and jaw leading to a reduction in the space between the base of the tongue and the posterior pharyngeal wall is the most common cause of upper airway obstruction. Obstruction may be partial or complete. The latter is characterized by total lack of air exchange. The former is recognized by inspiratory stridor and retraction of neck and intercostal muscles. If respiration is inadequate, the head-tilt–chin-lift or jaw-thrust maneuver should be performed. In patients with suspected cervical spine injuries, the jaw-thrust maneuver (without the head tilt) may result in the least movement of the cervical spine. The head-tilt maneuver is accomplished by placing a palm on the patient's forehead and applying pressure to extend the head about the atlantooccipital joint. The chin lift is performed by placing several fingers of the other hand in the submental area and lifting the mandible. Care must be taken to avoid airway obstruction by pressing too firmly on the soft tissues in the submental area. The jaw thrust is performed by lifting up on the angles of the mandible [3] (Fig. 1-3). Both of these maneuvers open up the oropharyngeal passage. Laryngospasm can be treated by maintaining positive airway pressure using a face mask and bag valve device (see the following section). If the patient resumes spontaneous breathing, establishing this head position may constitute sufficient treatment. If obstruction persists, a check for foreign bodies, emesis, or secretions should be performed [4].

USE OF FACE MASK AND BAG VALVE DEVICE. If an adequate airway has been established and the patient is not breathing spontaneously, oxygen can be delivered via a face mask and a bag valve device. It is important to establish a tight

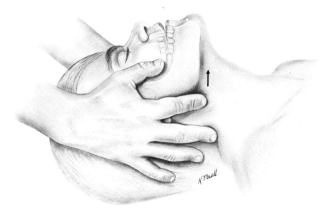

Fig. 1-3. In an obtunded or comatose patient, the soft tissues of the oropharynx become relaxed and may obstruct the upper airway. Obstruction can be alleviated by placing the thumbs on the maxilla with the index fingers under the ramus of the mandible and rotating the mandible forward with pressure from the index fingers *(arrow)*. This maneuver brings the soft tissues forward and, therefore, frequently reduces the airway obstruction.

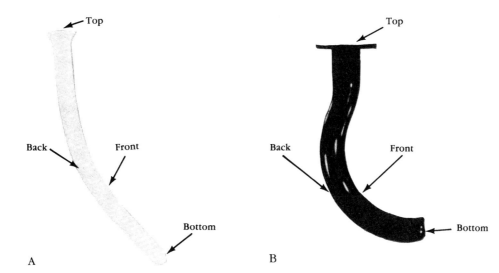

Fig. 1-4. Nasopharyngeal **(A)** or oropharyngeal **(B)** airways can be used to relieve soft tissue obstruction if elevating the mandible proves ineffective.

fit with the face mask, covering the patient's mouth and nose. This is accomplished by applying the mask initially to the bridge of the nose and drawing it downward toward the mouth, using both hands. The operator stands at the patient's head and presses the mask onto the patient's face with the left hand. The thumb should be on the nasal portion of the mask, the index finger near the oral portion, and the rest of the fingers spread on the left side of the patient's mandible so as to pull it slightly forward. The bag is then alternately compressed and released with the right hand. A good airway is indicated by the rise and fall of the chest; moreover, lung-chest wall compliance can be estimated from the amount of pressure required to compress the bag. The minimum effective insufflation pressure should be used to decrease the risk of aspiration.

AIRWAY ADJUNCTS. If proper positioning of the head and neck or clearance of foreign bodies and secretions fails to establish an adequate airway, several airway adjuncts may be helpful if an individual who is skilled in intubation is not immediately available. An oropharyngeal or nasopharyngeal airway occasionally helps to establish an adequate airway when proper head positioning alone is insufficient (Figs. 1-4 and 1-5). The oropharyngeal airway is semicircular and made of plastic or hard rubber. The two types are the Guedel airway, with a hollow tubular design, and the Berman airway, with airway channels along the sides. Both types are most easily inserted by turning the curved portion toward the palate as it enters the mouth. It is then advanced beyond the posterior portion of the tongue and rotated downward into the proper position (Fig. 1-5). Often, depressing the tongue or moving it laterally with a tongue blade helps to position the oropharyngeal airway. Care must be exercised not to push the tongue into the posterior pharynx, causing or exacerbating obstruction. Because insertion of the oropharyngeal airway can cause gagging or vomiting, or both, it should be used only in unconscious patients.

The nasopharyngeal airway is a soft tube approximately 15 cm long that is made of rubber or plastic (Figs. 1-4 and 1-6). It

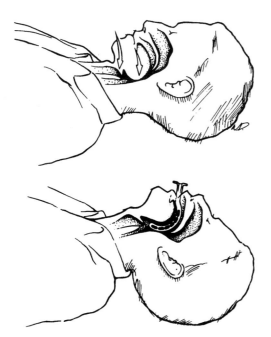

Fig. 1-5. The mechanism of upper airway obstruction and the proper position of the oropharyngeal airway. (From *Textbook of Advanced Cardiac Life Support.* Dallas, American Heart Association, 1997, with permission.)

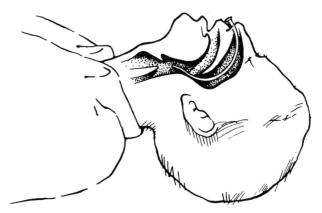

Fig. 1-6. The proper position of the nasopharyngeal airway. (From *Textbook of Advanced Cardiac Life Support.* Dallas, American Heart Association, 1997, with permission.)

is inserted via the nostril into the posterior pharynx. Before insertion, the airway should be lubricated with an anesthetic gel, and, preferably, a vasoconstrictor should be administered into the nostril. The nasopharyngeal airway should not be used in patients with extensive facial trauma or cerebrospinal rhinorrhea, as it could be inserted through the cribriform plate into the brain.

Indications for Intubation

The indications for endotracheal intubation can be divided into four broad categories: (a) acute airway obstruction, (b) excessive pulmonary secretions or inability to clear secretions adequately, (c) loss of protective reflexes, and (d) respiratory failure (Table 1-1).

Preintubation Evaluation

Even in the most urgent situation, a rapid assessment of the patient's airway anatomy can expedite the choice of the proper route for intubation, the appropriate equipment, and the most useful precautions to be taken. In the less emergent situation, several minutes of preintubation evaluation can decrease the likelihood of complications and increase the probability of successful intubation with minimal trauma.

Table 1-1. Indications for Endotracheal Intubation

Acute airway obstruction
  Trauma
    Mandible
    Larynx (direct or indirect injury)
  Inhalation
    Smoke
    Noxious chemicals
    Foreign bodies
  Infection
    Acute epiglottitis
    Croup
    Retropharyngeal abscess
  Hematoma
  Tumor
  Congenital anomalies
    Laryngeal web
    Supraglottic fusion
  Laryngeal edema
  Laryngeal spasm (anaphylactic response)
Access for suctioning
  Debilitated patients
  Copious secretions
Loss of protective reflexes
  Head injury
  Drug overdose
  Cerebrovascular accident
Respiratory failure
  Hypoxemia
    Acute respiratory distress syndrome
    Hypoventilation
    Atelectasis
    Secretions
    Pulmonary edema
  Hypercapnia
    Hypoventilation
    Neuromuscular failure
    Drug overdose

Anatomic structures of the upper airway, head, and neck must be examined, with particular attention to abnormalities that might preclude a particular route of intubation. Evaluation of cervical spine mobility, temporomandibular joint function, and dentition is important. Any abnormalities that might prohibit alignment of the oral, pharyngeal, and laryngeal axes should be noted.

Cervical spine mobility is assessed by flexion and extension of the neck (performed only after ascertaining that no cervical spine injury exists). The normal range of neck flexion-extension varies from 165 to 90 degrees, with the range decreasing approximately 20% by age 75 years. Conditions associated with decreased range of motion include any cause of degenerative disk disease (e.g., rheumatoid arthritis, osteoarthritis, ankylosing spondylitis), previous trauma, or age older than 70 years. Temporomandibular joint dysfunction can occur in any form of degenerative arthritis (particularly rheumatoid arthritis), in any condition that causes a receding mandible, and in rare conditions such as acromegaly.

Examination of the oral cavity is mandatory. Loose, missing, or chipped teeth and permanent bridgework are noted, and removable bridgework and dentures should be taken out. Mallampati et al. [5] developed a clinical indicator based on the size of the posterior aspect of the tongue relative to the size of the oral pharynx (Fig. 1-7). The patient should be sitting, with the head fully extended, protruding the tongue and phonating [6]. When the faucial pillars, the uvula, the soft palate, and the posterior pharyngeal wall are well visualized, the airway is classified as class I, and a relatively easy intubation can be anticipated. When the faucial pillars and soft palate (class II) or soft palate only (class III) are visible, there is a greater chance of problems visualizing the glottis during direct laryngoscopy. Difficulties in orotracheal intubation may also be anticipated if (a) the patient is an adult and cannot open his or her mouth more than 40 mm (two finger breadths), (b) the distance from the thyroid notch to the mandible is less than three finger breadths (less than or equal to 7 cm), (c) the patient has a high arched palate, or (d) the normal range of flexion-extension of the neck is decreased (less than or equal to 80 degrees) [7]. The positive predictive values of these tests alone or in combination are not particularly high; however, a straightforward intubation can be anticipated if the test results are negative [8].

Equipment for Intubation

Assembly of all appropriate equipment before attempted intubation can prevent potentially serious delays in the event of an unforeseen complication. Most equipment and supplies are readily available in the ICU but must be gathered so that they are immediately at hand. A supply of 100% oxygen and a well-fitting mask with attached bag valve device are mandatory, as is suctioning equipment, including a large-bore tonsil suction attachment (Yankauer) and suction catheters. Adequate lighting facilitates airway visualization. The bed should be at the proper height, with the headboard removed and the wheels locked. Other necessary supplies include gloves, Magill forceps, oral and nasal airways, laryngoscope handle and blades (straight and curved), endotracheal tubes of various sizes, stylet, tongue depressors, a syringe for cuff inflation, and tape for securing the endotracheal tube in position. Table 1-2 is a checklist of supplies needed.

It is particularly important that an adequate number of personnel be available to assist the operator. Endotracheal intubation and emergency airway management are not one-person jobs. While the operator is performing a rapid preintubation assessment, ICU personnel should be gathering equipment. During and before intubation, a respiratory therapist should be

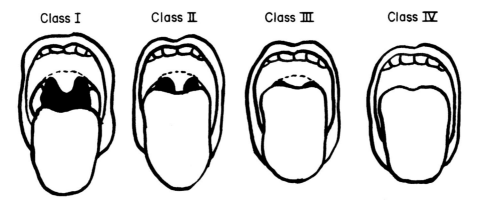

Fig. 1-7. Samsoon and Young modification of the Mallampati classification. Class I: Tonsillar pillars are easily visualized. Class II: The entire uvula is visualized. Class III: Only the base of the uvula is visualized. Class IV: Only the hard palate is seen. (From Samsoon GL, Young JR: Difficult tracheal intubation: a retrospective study. *Anaesthesia* 42:487–490, 1987, with permission.)

present, whose sole concerns should be assisting in airway control before intubation and providing adequate oxygenation. It is helpful to have another assistant present who is familiar with the procedure and equipment and who should be ready to hand items to the operator on request.

LARYNGOSCOPES. The two-piece laryngoscope has a handle containing batteries that power the bulb in the blade. The blade snaps securely into the top of the handle, making the electrical connection. Failure of the bulb to illuminate suggests improper blade positioning, bulb failure, a loose bulb, or dead batteries. Modern laryngoscope blades with fiberoptic lights obviate the problem of bulb failure. Many blade shapes and sizes are available. The two most commonly used blades are the curved (MacIntosh) and straight (Miller) blades (Fig. 1-8). Although pediatric blades are available for use with the adult-sized handle, most anesthesiologists prefer a smaller handle for better control in the pediatric population. The choice of blade shape is a matter of personal preference and experience; however, one study has suggested that less force and head extension are required when performing direct laryngoscopy with a straight blade [9].

ENDOTRACHEAL TUBES. The internal diameter of the endotracheal tube is measured using both millimeters and

Table 1-2. Equipment Needed for Intubation

Supply of 100% oxygen
Face mask
Bag valve device
Suction equipment
   Suction catheters
   Large-bore tonsil suction apparatus (Yankauer)
Stylet
Magill forceps
Oral airways
Nasal airways
Laryngoscope handle and blades (curved, straight; various sizes)
Endotracheal tubes (various sizes)
Tongue depressors
Syringe for cuff inflation
Headrest
Supplies for vasoconstriction and local anesthesia
Tape
Tincture of benzoin

French units (the former being most commonly used in the United States). This number is stamped on the tube. Tubes are available in 0.5-mm increments, starting at 2.5 mm. Lengthwise dimensions are also marked on the tube in centimeters, beginning at the distal tracheal end.

Selection of the proper tube diameter is of utmost importance and is a frequently underemphasized consideration. The resistance to airflow varies with the fourth power of the radius of the endotracheal tube. Thus, selection of an inappropriately small tube can significantly increase the work of breathing [10]. Moreover, certain diagnostic procedures (e.g., bronchoscopy) done through endotracheal tubes require appropriately large tubes (see Chapter 12).

In general, the larger the patient, the larger the endotracheal tube that should be used. Approximate guidelines for tube sizes and lengths by age are summarized in Table 1-3. Most adults should be intubated with an endotracheal tube with an inner diameter of at least 8.0 mm, although occasionally nasal intubation in a small adult requires a 7.0-mm tube.

ENDOTRACHEAL TUBE CUFF. Endotracheal tubes have low-pressure, high-volume cuffs to reduce the incidence of ischemia-related complications. Tracheal ischemia can occur any time cuff pressure exceeds capillary pressure (approximately 32 mm Hg), thereby causing inflammation, ulceration, infection, and dissolution of cartilaginous rings. Failure to recognize this progressive degeneration sometimes results in erosion through the tracheal wall (into the innominate artery if the erosion was anterior or the esophagus if the erosion was posterior) or long-term sequelae of tracheomalacia or tracheal stenosis. With cuff pressures of 15 to 30 mm Hg, the low-pressure, high-volume cuffs conform well to the tracheal wall and provide an adequate seal during positive-pressure ventilation. Although low cuff pressures can cause some damage (primarily ciliary denudation), major complications are rare. Nevertheless, it is important to realize that a low-pressure, high-volume cuff can be converted to a high-pressure cuff if sufficient quantities of air are injected into the cuff.

Anesthesia before Intubation

Because patients who require intubation often have a depressed level of consciousness, anesthesia is usually not required. If intubation must be performed on the alert, respon-

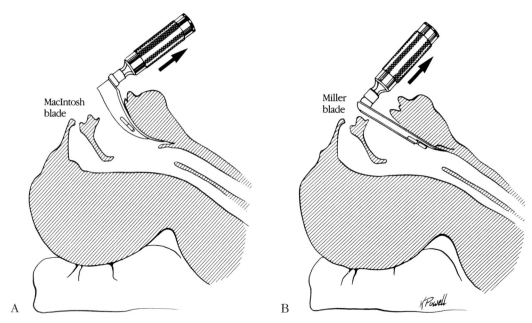

Fig. 1-8. The two basic types of laryngoscope blades, MacIntosh **(A)** and Miller **(B)**. The MacIntosh blade is curved. The blade tip is placed in the vallecula and the handle of the laryngoscope pulled forward at a 45-degree angle. This allows visualization of the epiglottis. The Miller blade is straight. The tip is placed posterior to the epiglottis, pinning the epiglottis between the base of the tongue and the straight laryngoscope blade. The motion on the laryngoscope handle is the same as that used with the MacIntosh blade.

sive patient, sedation or general anesthesia exposes the individual to potential pulmonary aspiration of gastric contents because protective reflexes are lost. This risk is a particularly important consideration if the patient has recently eaten and must be weighed against the risk of various hemodynamic derangements that may occur secondary to tracheal intubation and initiation of positive-pressure ventilation. Laryngoscopy in an inadequately anesthetized patient can result in tachycardia and an increase in blood pressure. This may be well tolerated in younger patients but may be detrimental in a patient with coronary artery disease or raised intracranial pressure. Sometimes laryngoscopy and intubation may result in a vasovagal response, leading to bradycardia and hypotension. Initiation of positive-pressure ventilation in a hypovolemic patient can lead to hypotension from diminished venous return.

Some of these responses can be attenuated by providing local anesthesia to the nares, mouth, and posterior pharynx

Table 1-3. Dimensions of Endotracheal Tubes Based on Patient Age

Age	Internal diameter (mm)	French unit	Distance between lips and location in midtrachea of distal end (cm)[a]
Premature	2.5	10–12	10
Full term	3.0	12–14	11
1–6 mo	3.5	16	11
6–12 mo	4.0	18	12
2 yr	4.5	20	13
4 yr	5.0	22	14
6 yr	5.5	24	15–16
8 yr	6.5	26	16–17
10 yr	7.0	28	17–18
12 yr	7.5	30	18–20
≥14 yr	8.0–9.0	32–36	20–24

[a]Add 2 to 3 cm for nasal tubes.
From Stoelting RK: Endotracheal intubation, in Miller RD (ed): *Anesthesia.* 2nd ed. New York, Churchill Livingstone, 1986, p 531, with permission.

before intubation. Topical lidocaine (1% to 4%) with phenylephrine (0.25%) or cocaine (4%, 200 mg total dose) can be used to anesthetize the nasal passages and provide local vasoconstriction. This allows the passage of a larger endotracheal tube with less likelihood of bleeding. Aqueous lidocaine-phenylephrine or cocaine can be administered via atomizer, nose dropper, or long cotton-tipped swabs inserted into the nares. Alternatively, viscous 2% lidocaine can be applied via a 3.5-mm endotracheal tube or small nasopharyngeal airway inserted into the nose. Anesthesia of the tongue and posterior pharynx can be accomplished with lidocaine spray (4% to 10%) administered via an atomizer or an eutectic mixture of local anesthetics (EMLA) cream applied on a tongue blade and oral airway [11]. Alternatively, the glossopharyngeal nerve can be blocked bilaterally with an injection of a local anesthetic, but this should be performed by experienced personnel.

Anesthetizing the larynx below the vocal cords before intubation is controversial. The cough reflex can be compromised, increasing the risk of aspiration. However, tracheal anesthesia may decrease the incidence of arrhythmias or untoward circulatory responses to intubation and improve patient tolerance of the endotracheal tube. Clinical judgment in this situation is necessary. Several methods can be used to anesthetize these structures. Transtracheal lidocaine (4%, 160 mg) is administered by cricothyroid membrane puncture with a small needle and anesthetizes the trachea and larynx below the vocal cords. Alternatively, after exposure of the vocal cords with the laryngoscope, the cords can be sprayed with lidocaine via an atomizer. Aerosolized lidocaine (4%, 6 mL) provides excellent anesthesia to the mouth, pharynx, larynx, and trachea [12]. The superior laryngeal nerve can be blocked with 2 mL of 1.0% to 1.5% lidocaine injected just inferior to the greater cornu of the hyoid bone. The rate of absorption of lidocaine differs by method, being greater with the aerosol and transtracheal techniques. The patient should be observed for signs of lidocaine toxicity (circumoral paresthesia, agitation, and seizures).

If adequate topical anesthesia cannot be achieved or if the patient is not cooperative, general anesthesia may be required

Table 1-4. Drugs Used to Facilitate Intubation

Drug	IV dose (mg/kg)	Onset of action (sec)	Side effects
Induction drugs			
Thiopental	2.5–4.5	20–50	Hypotension
Propofol	1.0–2.5	<60	Pain on injection
			Hypotension
Midazolam	0.02–0.20	30–60	Hypotension
Ketamine	0.5–2.0	30–60	Increases in intra-cranial pressure
			Increase in secretions
			Emergence reactions
Etomidate	0.2–0.3	20–50	Adrenal insufficiency
			Pain on injection
Muscle relaxants			
Succinyl-choline	1–2	45–60	Hyperkalemia
			Increased intragastric pressure
			Increased intracranial pressure
Mivacurium	0.20–0.25	90–120	Mild hypotension
Rocuronium	0.6–1.0	60–90	—

for intubation. Table 1-4 lists common drugs and doses that are used to facilitate intubation. Ketamine and etomidate are two drugs that are used commonly because cardiovascular stability is maintained. Use of opioids such as morphine, fentanyl, sufentanil, alfentanil, or remifentanil allow the dose of the induction drugs to be reduced and may attenuate the hemodynamic response to laryngoscopy and intubation. Muscle relaxants can be used to facilitate intubation, but unless the practitioner has extensive experience with these drugs and airway management, alternative means of airway control and oxygenation should be used until an anesthesiologist arrives to administer the anesthetic and perform the intubation.

Techniques of Intubation

In a true emergency, some of the preintubation evaluation is necessarily neglected in favor of rapid control of the airway. Attempts at tracheal intubation should not cause or exacerbate hypoxia. Whenever possible, an oxygen saturation monitor should be used. The risk of hypoxemia during intubation can be minimized with preoxygenation and by limiting the duration of the attempt to 30 seconds or less [13].

Preoxygenation (denitrogenation), which replaces the nitrogen in the patient's functional residual capacity with oxygen, can maximize the time available for intubation. During laryngoscopy, apneic oxygenation can occur from this reservoir. Preoxygenation is achieved by providing 100% oxygen at a high flow rate via a tight-fitting face mask for 3.5 to 4.0 minutes. Just before intubation, the physician should assess the likelihood of success of each route of intubation, the urgency of the clinical situation, the likelihood that intubation will be prolonged, and the prospect of whether diagnostic or therapeutic procedures such as bronchoscopy will eventually be required. Factors that can affect patient comfort should also be weighed. In the unconscious patient in whom a secure airway must be established immediately, orotracheal intubation with direct visualization of the vocal cords is generally the preferred technique. In the conscious patient, blind nasotracheal intubation is often favored because it affords greater patient comfort. Nasotracheal intubation should be avoided in patients with coagulopathies or those who are anticoagulated

for medical indications. In the trauma victim with extensive maxillary and mandibular fractures and inadequate ventilation or oxygenation, cricothyrotomy may be mandatory (see Chapter 15). In the patient with cervical spine injury or decreased neck mobility, intubation using the fiberoptic bronchoscope may be necessary. Many of these techniques require considerable skill and should be performed only by those who are experienced in airway management [14].

Specific Techniques and Routes of Endotracheal Intubation

OROTRACHEAL INTUBATION. Orotracheal intubation is the technique most easily learned and most often used for emergency intubations in the ICU. Traditional teaching dictates that successful orotracheal intubation requires alignment of the oral, pharyngeal, and laryngeal axes by putting the patient in the "sniffing position," in which the neck is flexed and the head is slightly extended about the atlantooccipital joint. However, a magnetic resonance imaging study has called this concept into question, as the alignment of these three axes could not be achieved in any of the three positions tested: neutral, simple extension, and the "sniffing position" [15]. In addition, a randomized study in elective surgery patients examining the utility of the sniffing position as a means to facilitate orotracheal intubation failed to demonstrate that such positioning was superior to simple head extension [16]. In a patient with a full stomach, the esophagus can be occluded by compressing the cricoid cartilage posteriorly against the vertebral body. This technique, known as *Sellick's maneuver*, can prevent passive regurgitation of stomach contents into the trachea during intubation [17].

The laryngoscope handle is grasped in the left hand while the patient's mouth is opened with the gloved right hand. Often, when the head is extended in the unconscious patient, the mouth opens; if not, the thumb and index finger of the right hand are placed on the lower and upper incisors, respectively, and moved past each other in a scissor-like motion. The laryngoscope blade is inserted on the right side of the mouth and advanced to the base of the tongue, pushing it toward the left. If the straight blade is used, it should be extended below the epiglottis. If the curved blade is used, it is inserted in the vallecula.

With the blade in place, the operator should lift forward in a plane 45 degrees from the horizontal to expose the vocal cords (Figs. 1-2 and 1-8). It is essential to keep the left wrist stiff and to do all lifting from the arm and shoulder, to avoid turning the patient's teeth into a fulcrum. The endotracheal tube is then held in the right hand and inserted at the right corner of the patient's mouth in a plane that intersects with the laryngoscope blade at the level of the glottis. This prevents the endotracheal tube from obscuring the view of the vocal cords. The endotracheal tube is advanced through the vocal cords until the cuff just disappears from sight. The cuff is then inflated with enough air to prevent a leak during positive-pressure ventilation with a bag valve device.

A classification grading the view of the laryngeal aperture during direct laryngoscopy has been described [18] and is depicted in Figure 1-9. Occasionally, the vocal cords cannot be seen entirely; only the corniculate and cuneiform tubercles, interarytenoid incisure, and posterior portion of the vocal cords or only the epiglottis is visualized (grades II to IV view, Fig. 1-9). In this situation, it is helpful to insert the

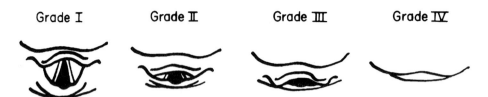

Fig. 1-9. The four grades of laryngeal view during direct laryngoscopy. Grade I: The entire glottis is seen. Grade II: Only the posterior aspect of the glottis is seen. Grade III: Only the epiglottis is seen. Grade IV: The epiglottis is not visualized. (From Cormack RS, Lehane J: Difficult tracheal intubation in obstetrics. *Anaesthesia* 39:1105–1111, 1984, with permission.)

soft metal stylet into the endotracheal tube and bend it into a hockey-stick configuration. The stylet should be bent or coiled at the proximal end to prevent the distal end from extending beyond the endotracheal tube and causing tissue damage. The stylet should be lubricated to ensure easy removal. The BURP maneuver (backward-upward-rightward pressure on the larynx) improves the view of the laryngeal aperture [19]. Alternatively, a control-tip endotracheal tube can be used. This tube has a nylon cord running the length of the tube attached to a ring at the proximal end, which allows the operator to direct the tip of the tube anteriorly. Another aid is a stylet with a light (light wand). With the room lights dimmed, the endotracheal tube containing the lighted stylet is inserted into the oropharynx and advanced in the midline. When it is just superior to the larynx, a glow is seen over the anterior neck. The stylet is advanced into the trachea, and the tube is threaded over it. The light intensity is diminished if the wand enters the esophagus [20]. Endotracheal tubes are now available that have a fiberoptic bundle intrinsic to the tube that can be attached to a video monitor. If the attempt to intubate is still unsuccessful, the algorithm as detailed in the section Management of the Difficult Airway should be followed.

Proper depth of tube placement is clinically ascertained by observing symmetric expansion of both sides of the chest and auscultating equal breath sounds in both lungs. The stomach should also be auscultated to ensure that the esophagus has not been entered. If the tube has been advanced too far, it will lodge in one of the main bronchi (particularly the right bronchus), and only one lung will be ventilated. If this error goes unnoticed, the nonventilated lung may collapse. A useful rule of thumb for tube placement in adults of average size is that the incisors should be at the 23-cm mark in men and the 21-cm mark in women [21]. Palpation of the anterior trachea in the neck may detect cuff inflation as air is injected into the pilot tube and can serve as a means to ascertain correct tube position [22]. Placement can also be confirmed by measurement of end-tidal carbon dioxide by standard capnography if available or by means of a calorimetric chemical detector of end-tidal carbon dioxide (e.g., Easy Cap II, Nellcor, Inc., Pleasanton, CA), which can be used to verify correct endotracheal tube placement or detect esophageal intubation. This device is attached to the proximal end of the endotracheal tube and changes color on exposure to carbon dioxide. An additional method to detect esophageal intubation uses a bulb that attaches to the proximal end of the endotracheal tube [23]. The bulb is squeezed: If the tube is in the trachea, the bulb reexpands, and if the tube is in the esophagus, the bulb remains collapsed. It must be remembered that none of these techniques is foolproof. Bronchoscopy is the only method to be absolutely sure the tube is in the trachea. After estimating proper tube placement clinically, it should be confirmed by chest radiograph

or bronchoscopy because the tube may be malpositioned. The tip of the endotracheal tube should be several centimeters above the carina (T-4 level). It must be remembered that flexion or extension of the head can advance or withdraw the tube 2 to 5 cm, respectively.

NASOTRACHEAL INTUBATION. Many of the considerations concerning patient preparation and positioning outlined for orotracheal intubation apply to nasal intubation as well. Blind nasal intubation is more difficult to perform than oral intubation, because the tube cannot be observed directly as it passes between the vocal cords. However, nasal intubation is usually more comfortable for the patient and is generally preferable in the awake, conscious patient. Nasal intubation should not be attempted in patients with abnormal bleeding parameters, nasal polyps, extensive facial trauma, cerebrospinal rhinorrhea, sinusitis, or any anatomic abnormality that would inhibit atraumatic passage of the tube.

As discussed in the section Airway Adjuncts, after the operator has alternately occluded each nostril to ascertain that both are patent, the nostril to be intubated is anesthetized. The patient should be monitored with a pulse oximeter, and supplemental oxygen should be given as necessary. The patient may be either supine or sitting with the head extended in the sniffing position. The tube is guided slowly but firmly through the nostril to the posterior pharynx. Here the tube operator must continually monitor for the presence of air movement through the tube by listening for breath sounds with the ear near the open end of the tube. The tube must never be forced or pushed forward if breath sounds are lost, because damage to the retropharyngeal mucosa can result. If resistance is met, the tube should be withdrawn 1 to 2 cm and the patient's head repositioned (extended further or turned to either side). If the turn still cannot be negotiated, the other nostril or a smaller tube should be tried. Attempts at nasal intubation should be abandoned and oral intubation performed if these methods fail.

Once positioned in the oropharynx, the tube should be advanced to the glottis while listening for breath sounds through the tube. If breath sounds cease, the tube is withdrawn several centimeters until breath sounds resume, and the plane of entry is adjusted slightly. Passage through the vocal cords should be timed to coincide with inspiration. This is often signaled by a paroxysm of coughing and an inability to speak. The cuff should be inflated and proper positioning of the tube ascertained as previously outlined.

Occasionally, blind nasal intubation cannot be accomplished. In this case, after adequate topical anesthesia, laryngoscopy can be used to visualize the vocal cords directly and Magill forceps used to grasp the distal end of the tube and guide it through the vocal cords (Fig. 1-10). Assistance in pushing the tube forward is essential during this maneuver, so

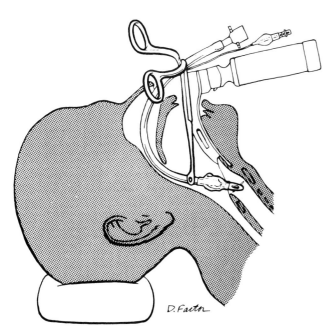

Fig. 1-10. Magill forceps may be required to guide the endotracheal tube into the larynx during nasotracheal intubation. (From Barash PG, Cullen BF, Stoelting RK: *Clinical Anesthesia.* 2nd ed. Philadelphia, JB Lippincott Co, 1992, with permission.)

that the operator merely guides the tube. The balloon on the tube should not be grasped with the Magill forceps.

Occasionally, one may not be able to successfully place the endotracheal tube in the trachea. The technique of managing a difficult airway is detailed below.

Management of the Difficult Airway

A difficult airway may be recognized (anticipated) or unrecognized at the time of the initial preintubation airway evaluation. Difficulty managing the airway may be the result of abnormalities such as congenital hypoplasia, hyperplasia of the mandible or maxilla, or prominent incisors; injuries to the face or neck; acromegaly; tumors; and previous head and neck surgery. Difficulties ventilating the patient with a mask can be anticipated if two of the following factors are present: age older than 55 years, body mass index greater than 26 kg per m^2, beard, lack of teeth, and a history of snoring [24]. When a difficult airway is encountered, the algorithm as detailed in Figure 1-11 should be followed [25].

When a difficult airway is recognized before the patient is anesthetized, an awake tracheal intubation is usually the best option. Multiple techniques can be used and include (after adequate topical or local anesthesia) direct laryngoscopy, LMA (or variants), blind or bronchoscopic oral or nasal intubation, retrograde technique, rigid bronchoscopy, lighted stylet, or a surgical airway.

FIBEROPTIC BRONCHOSCOPIC INTUBATION. Fiberoptic bronchoscopy is an efficacious method of intubating the trachea in difficult cases. It may be particularly useful when

the upper airway anatomy has been distorted by tumors, trauma, endocrinopathies, or congenital anomalies. This technique is sometimes valuable in accident victims in whom a question of cervical spine injury exists and the patient's neck cannot be manipulated [26]. An analogous situation exists in patients with severe degenerative disk disease of the neck or rheumatoid arthritis with markedly impaired neck mobility. After adequate topical anesthesia is obtained as described in the section Anesthesia before Intubation, the bronchoscope can be used to intubate the trachea via either the nasal or oral route. An appropriately sized endotracheal tube is positioned over the bronchoscope, which is inserted into the mouth or nose and advanced through the vocal cords into the trachea. The endotracheal tube is moved over the bronchoscope and positioned above the carina under direct vision. The fiberoptic bronchoscope has also been used as a stent over which endotracheal tubes are exchanged and as a means to assess tracheal damage periodically during prolonged intubations. (A detailed discussion of bronchoscopy is found in Chapter 12.) Intubation by this technique requires skill and experience and is best performed by a fully trained operator.

If the operator is able to maintain mask ventilation in a patient with an unrecognized difficult airway, a call for experienced help should be initiated (Fig. 1-11). If mask ventilation cannot be maintained, a cannot ventilate–cannot intubate situation exists and immediate lifesaving rescue maneuvers are required. Options include an emergency cricothyrotomy or insertion of specialized airway devices [LMA or Combitube (Sheridan Catheter, Argyle, NY)].

OTHER AIRWAY ADJUNCTS. The LMA is composed of a plastic tube attached to a shallow mask with an inflatable rim (Fig. 1-12). When properly inserted, it fits over the laryngeal inlet and allows positive-pressure ventilation of the lungs. Although aspiration can occur around the mask, the LMA can be lifesaving in a cannot ventilate–cannot intubate situation. A new intubating LMA (LMA-Fastrach, LMA North America, Inc., San Diego, CA) has been developed [27] that has a shorter plastic tube and can be used to provide ventilation as well as to intubate the trachea with or without the aid of a fiberoptic bronchoscope (Fig. 1-13). The esophageal tracheal Combitube (Tyco-Healthcare-Kendall USA, Mansfield, MA; Fig. 1-14) combines the features of an endotracheal tube and an esophageal obturator airway and reduces the risk of aspiration [28]. Use of the LMA and the Combitube together can be easily learned by personnel who are unskilled in airway management [29].

Special rigid fiberoptic laryngoscopes [Bullard Elite Laryngoscope, ACMI Circon, Stamford, CT (Fig. 1-15) or the Upsher Laryngoscope, Mercury Medical, Clearwater, FL] are useful in patients with difficult airways [30]. In addition, cervical spine extension appears to be reduced with their use [31]. The use of these laryngoscopes requires much more training and skill than the use of the LMA or Combitube.

CRICOTHYROTOMY. In a truly emergent situation, when intubation is unsuccessful, a cricothyrotomy may be required. The technique is described in detail in Chapter 15. The quickest method, needle cricothyrotomy, is accomplished by introducing a large-bore (i.e., 14-gauge) catheter into the airway through the cricothyroid membrane while aspirating on a syringe attached to the needle of the catheter. When air is aspirated the needle is in the airway, and the catheter is passed over the needle into the trachea. The

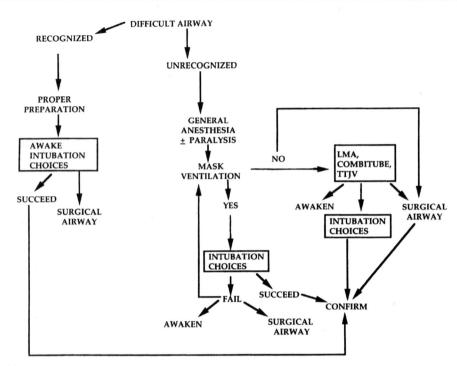

Fig. 1-11. Modification of the difficult airway algorithm. Awake intubation choices include direct laryngoscopy with topical or local anesthesia, blind nasal intubation, fiberoptic-assisted oral or nasal intubation, intubation through a laryngeal mask airway (LMA), or the retrograde technique. TTJV, transtracheal jet ventilation. (Adapted from Benumof JL: Laryngeal mask airway and the ASA difficult airway algorithm. *Anesthesiology* 84:686–699, 1996, with permission.)

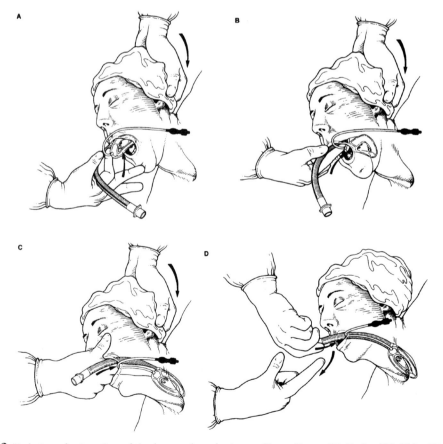

Fig. 1-12. Technique for insertion of the laryngeal mask airway. (From Civetta JM, Taylor RW, Kirby RR: *Critical Care.* 3rd ed. Philadelphia, Lippincott–Raven Publishers, 1997, with permission.)

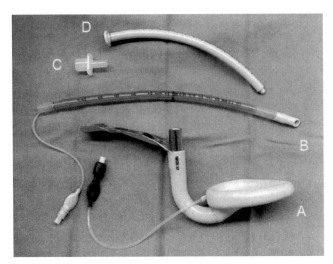

Fig. 1-13. The laryngeal mask airway (LMA)-Fastrach (A) has a shorter tube than a conventional LMA. A special endotracheal tube (B) [without the adapter (C)] is advanced through the LMA-Fastrach into the trachea. The extender (D) is attached to the endotracheal tube, and the LMA-Fastrach is removed. After the extender is removed, the adapter is placed back on the tube.

needle is attached to a high-frequency jet ventilation apparatus. Alternatively, a 3-mL syringe barrel can be connected to the catheter. A 7-mm inside diameter endotracheal tube adapter fits into the syringe and can be connected to a high-pressure gas source or a high-frequency jet ventilator (Fig. 1-16).

MANAGEMENT OF AIRWAY IN PATIENT WITH SUSPECTED CERVICAL SPINE INJURY. Any patient with multiple trauma who requires intubation should be treated as if cervical spine injury is present. In the absence of severe maxillofacial trauma or cerebrospinal rhinorrhea, nasal intubation can be considered. However, in the profoundly hypoxemic or apneic patient, the orotracheal approach should be used. If oral intubation is required, an assistant should maintain the neck in the neutral position by ensuring axial stabili-

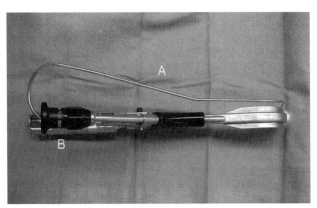

Fig. 1-14. The proper placement of the Combitube. (Sheridan Catheter, Argyle, NY, with permission.)

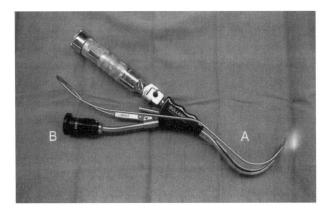

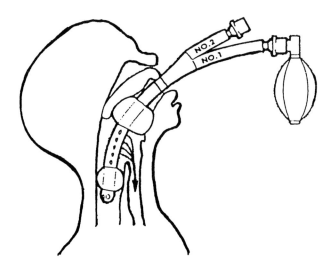

Fig. 1-15. The Bullard laryngoscope. The endotracheal tube is loaded onto the stylet (A) and advanced into the trachea under visualization via the eyepiece (B).

zation of the head and neck as the patient is intubated [32]. A cervical collar also assists in immobilizing the cervical spine. In a patient with maxillofacial trauma and suspected cervical spine injury, retrograde intubation can be performed by puncturing the cricothyroid membrane with an 18-gauge catheter and threading a 125-cm Teflon-coated (0.025-cm diameter) guidewire through the catheter. The wire is advanced into the oral cavity, and the endotracheal tube is then advanced over the wire into the trachea. Alternatively, the wire can be threaded through the suction port of a 3.9-mm bronchoscope.

Airway Management in the Intubated Patient

Once the endotracheal tube is in position, proper management assumes the utmost importance. From a pulmonary standpoint, an intubated patient is a compromised host, robbed of normal upper airway defenses that protect the lungs from bacteria, other foreign bodies, and the aspiration of secretions. Some simple precautions and a careful approach to airway management can minimize complications.

SECURING THE TUBE. Properly securing the endotracheal tube in the desired position is important for three reasons: (a) to prevent accidental extubation, (b) to prevent advancement into one of the main bronchi, and (c) to minimize fric-

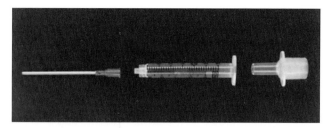

Fig. 1-16. A needle cricothyrotomy set. A large-bore (14-gauge) catheter is inserted through the cricothyroid membrane. The needle is removed, and the catheter is attached to a 3-mL syringe barrel. A 7-mm endotracheal tube adapter is then attached to the syringe barrel. Alternatively, a 3-mm endotracheal tube adapter can be attached directly to the catheter.

tional damage to the upper airway, larynx, and trachea caused by patient motion. The endotracheal tube is usually secured in place with adhesive tape wrapped around the tube and applied to the patient's cheeks. Tincture of benzoin sprayed on the skin provides greater fixation. Alternatively, tape, intravenous (IV) tubing, or umbilical tape can be tied to the endotracheal tube and brought around the patient's neck to secure the tube. Care must be taken to prevent occlusion of neck veins. Other products (e.g., Velcro straps) to secure the tube are available. A bite block can be positioned in patients who are orally intubated to prevent them from biting down on the tube and occluding it. Once the tube has been secured and its proper position verified, it should be plainly marked on the portion protruding from the patient's mouth or nose so that advancement can be noted.

CUFF MANAGEMENT. Although low-pressure cuffs have markedly reduced the incidence of complications related to tracheal ischemia, monitoring cuff pressures remains important. The cuff should be inflated just beyond the point where an audible air leak occurs. Maintenance of intracuff pressures between 17 and 23 mm Hg should allow an adequate seal to permit mechanical ventilation under most circumstances while not compromising blood flow to the tracheal mucosa. The intracuff pressure should be checked periodically by attaching a pressure gauge and syringe to the cuff port via a three-way stopcock. The need to add air continually to the cuff to maintain its seal with the tracheal wall indicates that (a) the cuff or pilot tube has a hole in it, (b) the pilot tube valve is broken or cracked, or (c) the tube is positioned incorrectly, and the cuff is between the vocal cords. The tube position should be reevaluated to exclude the latter possibility. If the valve is broken, attaching a three-way stopcock to it will solve the problem. If the valve housing is cracked, cutting the pilot tube and inserting a blunt needle with a stopcock into the lumen of the pilot tube can maintain a competent system. A hole in the cuff necessitates a change of tubes.

TUBE SUCTIONING. A complete discussion of tube suctioning can be found in Chapter 62. Routine suctioning should not be performed in patients in whom secretions are not a problem. Suctioning can produce a variety of complications, including hypoxemia, elevations in intracranial pressure, and serious ventricular arrhythmias. Preoxygenation should reduce the likelihood of arrhythmias. Closed ventilation suction systems (Stericath) may reduce the risk of hypoxemia and infection.

HUMIDIFICATION. Intubation of the trachea bypasses the normal upper airway structures responsible for heating and humidifying inspired air. It is thus essential that inspired air be heated and humidified (see Chapter 62).

Tube Replacement

At times, endotracheal tubes may need to be replaced because of an air leak, obstruction, or other problem. Before attempting to change an endotracheal tube, one should assess how difficult it will be. After obtaining appropriate topical anesthesia or IV sedation and achieving muscle relaxation, direct laryngoscopy can be performed to ascertain whether there will be difficulties in visualizing the vocal cords. If the cords can be seen, the defective tube is removed under direct visualization and reintubation performed using the new tube. If the cords cannot be seen on direct laryngoscopy, the tube can be changed over a long, plastic stylet (Eschmann stylet), an airway exchange catheter, or fiberoptic bronchoscope. The airway exchange catheter (Cook Critical Care, Bloomington, IN) allows insufflation of oxygen via either standard oxygen tubing or a bag valve device [33]. The disadvantage to using the bronchoscope is that the old tube must be cut away with a scalpel before the new tube can be advanced into the trachea. In a patient with a large intrapulmonary shunt, severe hypoxemia might develop while the old tube is being replaced. Alternatively, the bronchoscope (with the new tube on it) can be advanced into the trachea next to (rather than through) the old endotracheal tube after deflating the cuff. The old tube is then withdrawn and the new tube positioned over the bronchoscope.

Complications of Endotracheal Intubation

Complications associated with endotracheal intubation may occur (a) during intubation, (b) while the endotracheal tube is in place, or (c) after extubation. Table 1-5 is a partial listing of these complications. The exact incidence of complications is difficult to determine, varying widely in published reports and depending to some extent on the vigor of efforts to identify them. Factors implicated in the etiology of complications include tube size, characteristics of the tube and cuff, trauma during intubation, duration and route of intubation, metabolic or nutritional status of the patient, tube motion, and laryngeal motor activity.

COMPLICATIONS DURING INTUBATION. During endotracheal intubation, traumatic injury can occur to any anatomic structure from the lips to the trachea. Possible complications include (a) aspiration, (b) damage to teeth and dental work, (c) corneal abrasions, (d) perforation or laceration of the pharynx, larynx, or trachea, (e) dislocation of an arytenoid cartilage, (f) retropharyngeal perforation, (g) epistaxis, (h) hypoxemia, (i) myocardial ischemia, (j) laryngospasm with noncardiogenic pulmonary edema, and (k) death [34]. Many of these complications can be avoided by paying careful attention to technique and ensuring that personnel with the greatest skill and experience perform the intubation.

Table 1-5. Complications of Endotracheal Intubation

Complications during intubation
  Spinal cord injury
  Excessive delay of cardiopulmonary resuscitation
  Aspiration
  Damage to teeth and dental work
  Corneal abrasions
  Perforation or laceration of
    Pharynx
    Larynx
    Trachea
  Dislocation of an arytenoid cartilage
  Passage of endotracheal tube into cranial vault
  Epistaxis
  Cardiovascular problems
    Ventricular premature contractions
    Ventricular tachycardia
    Bradyarrhythmias
    Hypotension
    Hypertension
    Hypoxemia
Complications while tube is in place
  Blockage or kinking of tube
  Dislodgment of tube
  Advancement of tube into a bronchus
  Mechanical damage to any upper airway structure
  Problems related to mechanical ventilation (see Chapter 58)
Complications following extubation
  Immediate complications
    Laryngospasm
    Aspiration
  Intermediate and long-term complications
    Sore throat
    Ulcerations of lips, mouth, pharynx, or vocal cords
    Tongue numbness (hypoglossal nerve compression)
    Laryngitis
    Vocal cord paralysis (unilateral or bilateral)
    Laryngeal edema
    Laryngeal ulcerations
    Laryngeal granuloma
    Vocal cord synechiae
    Tracheal stenosis

A variety of cardiovascular complications can accompany intubation. Ventricular arrhythmias have been reported in 5% to 10% of intubations. Ventricular tachycardia and ventricular fibrillation are uncommon but have been reported. Patients with myocardial ischemia are susceptible to ventricular arrhythmias, and lidocaine prophylaxis (100 mg IV bolus) before intubation may be warranted in such individuals. Bradyarrhythmias can also be observed and are probably caused by stimulation of the laryngeal branches of the vagus nerve. They may not require therapy but usually respond to IV atropine (1 mg IV bolus). Hypotension and hypertension can occur during intubation. In the patient with myocardial ischemia, short-acting agents to control blood pressure (nitroprusside) and heart rate (esmolol) during intubation may be needed.

COMPLICATIONS WHILE TUBE IS IN PLACE. Despite adherence to guidelines designed to minimize damage from endotracheal intubation, the tube can damage local structures. Microscopic alterations to the surface of the vocal cords can occur within 2 hours after intubation. Evidence of macroscopic damage can occur within 6 hours. As might be expected, clinically significant damage typically occurs when intubation is prolonged. The sudden appearance of blood in tracheal secretions suggests anterior erosion into overlying vascular structures, and the appearance of gastric contents suggests posterior erosion into the esophagus. Both situations require urgent bronchoscopy, and it is imperative that the mucosa underlying the cuff be examined. Other complications include tracheomalacia and stenosis and damage to the larynx. Failure to secure the endotracheal tube properly or patient agitation can contribute to mechanical damage.

Another complication is blockage or kinking of the tube, resulting in compromised ventilation. Occlusion of the tube caused by the patient biting down on it can be minimized by placing a bite block in the patient's mouth. Blockage from secretions can usually be solved by suctioning, although changing the tube may be necessary.

Unplanned extubation and endobronchial intubation are potentially life threatening. Appropriately securing and marking the tube should minimize these problems. Daily chest radiographs with the head always in the same position can be used to assess the position of the tube. Other complications that occur while the tube is in position relate to mechanical ventilation (e.g., pneumothorax) and are discussed in detail in Chapter 58.

COMPLICATIONS AFTER EXTUBATION. Sore throat occurs after 40% to 100% of intubations. The incidence of postextubation sore throat and hoarseness may be decreased by using a smaller endotracheal tube [35]. Ulcerations of the lips, mouth, or pharynx can occur, being more common if the initial intubation was traumatic. Pressure from the endotracheal tube can traumatize the hypoglossal nerve, resulting in numbness of the tongue that can persist for 1 to 2 weeks. Irritation of the larynx appears to be due to local mucosal damage and occurs in as many as 45% of individuals after extubation. Unilateral or bilateral vocal cord paralysis is an uncommon but serious complication following extubation. Recurrent laryngeal nerve damage can be caused by inflation of the cuff in the larynx, which compresses and damages the recurrent laryngeal nerve as it passes between the arytenoid cartilage and thyroid lamina [36].

Some degree of laryngeal edema accompanies almost all endotracheal intubations. In adults, this is usually clinically insignificant. In children, however, even a small amount of edema can compromise the already small subglottic opening. In a newborn, 1 mm of laryngeal edema results in a 65% narrowing of the airway. Laryngeal ulcerations are commonly observed after extubation. They are more commonly located at the posterior portion of the vocal cords, where the endotracheal tube tends to rub. Ulcerations become increasingly common the longer the tube is left in place. The incidence of ulceration is decreased by the use of endotracheal tubes that conform to the anatomic shape of the larynx [37]. Laryngeal granulomas and synechiae of the vocal cords are extremely rare, but these complications can seriously compromise airway patency. Surgical treatment is often required to treat these problems.

A feared late complication of endotracheal intubation is tracheal stenosis. This occurs much less frequently now that high-volume, low-pressure cuffs are routinely used. Symptoms can occur weeks to months after extubation. In mild cases, the patient may experience dyspnea or ineffective cough. If the airway is narrowed to less than 5 mm, the patient presents with stridor. Dilation may provide effective treatment, but in some instances surgical intervention is necessary.

Extubation

The decision to extubate a patient is based on (a) a favorable clinical response to a carefully planned regimen of weaning from mechanical ventilation (see Chapter 60), (b) recovery of consciousness following anesthesia, or (c) sufficient resolution of the initial indications for intubation.

TECHNIQUE OF EXTUBATION. The patient should be alert, lying with the head of the bed elevated to at least a 45-degree angle. The posterior pharynx must be thoroughly suctioned. The procedure is explained to the patient. The cuff is deflated, and positive pressure is applied to expel any foreign material that has collected above the cuff as the tube is withdrawn. Supplemental oxygen is then provided.

In situations in which postextubation difficulties are anticipated, equipment for emergency reintubation should be assembled at the bedside. Some clinicians have advocated the "leak test" as a means to ensure that no significant subglottic edema is present that could compromise the airway after extubation; however, the utility of this procedure appears to be limited [38]. Probably the safest means to extubate the patient if there are concerns about airway edema or the potential need to reintubate a patient with a difficult airway is to use an airway exchange catheter (Cook Critical Care, Bloomington, IN) [33]. This device is inserted through the endotracheal tube, and then the tube is removed over the catheter. Supplemental oxygen can be provided via the catheter to the patient, and the catheter can be used as a stent for reintubation if necessary.

One of the most serious complications of extubation is laryngospasm, which is much more likely to occur if the patient is not fully conscious. The application of positive pressure can sometimes relieve laryngospasm. If this maneuver is not successful, succinylcholine (by the IV or intramuscular route) can be administered. Succinylcholine can cause severe hyperkalemia in a variety of clinical settings; therefore, only clinicians who are experienced with its use should administer it. Mechanical ventilation is needed until the patient has recovered from the succinylcholine.

TRACHEOSTOMY. In the past it was common to perform a tracheostomy to replace the endotracheal tube as soon as the need for prolonged airway control became apparent. Improvements in cuff design have permitted progressively longer periods of translaryngeal intubation. The optimal time of conversion from an endotracheal tube to a tracheostomy remains controversial, and decisions regarding the timing of tracheostomy should be based on the overall clinical situation. The reader is referred to Chapter 15 for details on tracheostomy.

References

1. Snell RS, Katz J: *Clinical Anatomy for Anesthesiologists.* Norwalk, CT, Appleton & Lange, 1988.
2. Fassoulaki A, Pamouktsoglou P: Prolonged nasotracheal intubation and its association with inflammation of paranasal sinuses. *Anesth Analg* 69:50–52, 1989.
3. Natanson C, Shelhamer JH, Parrillo JE: Intubation of the trachea in the critical care setting. *JAMA* 253:1160–1165, 1985.
4. Guidelines 2000 for cardiopulmonary resuscitation and emer-
   gency cardiovascular care. Part 3: adult basic life support. The American Heart Association in collaboration with the International Liaison Committee on Resuscitation. *Circulation* 102:I-22–I-59, 2000.
5. Mallampati SR, Gatt SP, Gugino LD, et al: A clinical sign to predict difficult tracheal intubation: a prospective study. *Can Anaesth Soc J* 32:429–434, 1985.
6. Lewis M, Keramati S, Benumof JL, et al: What is the best way to determine oropharyngeal classification and mandibular space length to predict difficult laryngoscopy? *Anesthesiology* 81:69–75, 1994.
7. Stone DJ, Gal TJ: Airway management, in Miller RD (ed): *Anesthesia.* 5th ed. Philadelphia, Churchill Livingstone, 2000, pp 1414–1451.
8. Tse JC, Rimm EB, Hussain A: Predicting difficult endotracheal intubation in surgical patients scheduled for general anesthesia: a prospective blind study. *Anesth Analg* 81:254–258, 1995.
9. Hastings RH, Hon ED, Nghiem C, et al: Force, torque, and stress relaxation with direct laryngoscopy. *Anesth Analg* 82:456–461, 1996.
10. Wright PE, Marini JJ, Bernard GR: *In vitro* versus *in vivo* comparison of endotracheal tube airflow resistance. *Am Rev Respir Dis* 140:10–16, 1989.
11. Larijani GE, Cypel D, Gratz I, et al: The efficacy and safety of EMLA cream for awake fiberoptic endotracheal intubation. *Anesth Analg* 91:1024–1026, 2000.
12. Venus B, Polassani V, Pham CG: Effects of aerosolized lidocaine on circulatory responses to laryngoscopy and tracheal intubation. *Crit Care Med* 12:391–394, 1984.
13. Hee MK, Plevak DJ, Peters SG: Intubation of critically ill patients. *Mayo Clin Proc* 67:569–576, 1992.
14. Hastings RH, Marks JD: Airway management for trauma patients with potential cervical spine injuries. *Anesth Analg* 73:471–482, 1991.
15. Adnet F, Borron SW, Dumas JL, et al: Study of the "sniffing position" by magnetic resonance imaging. *Anesthesiology* 94:83–86, 2001.
16. Adnet F, Baillard C, Borron SW, et al: Randomized study comparing the "sniffing position" with simple head extension for laryngoscopic view in elective surgery patients. *Anesthesiology* 95:836–841, 2001.
17. Sellick BA: Cricoid pressure to control regurgitation of stomach contents during induction of anesthesia. *Lancet* 2:404, 1961.
18. Cormack RS, Lehane J: Difficult tracheal intubation in obstetrics. *Anaesthesia* 39:1105–1111, 1984.
19. Ulrich B, Listyo R, Gerig HJ, et al: The difficult intubation. The value of BURP and 3 predictive tests of difficult intubation. *Anaesthetist* 47:45–50, 1998.
20. Agro F, Hung OR, Cataldo R, et al: Lightwand intubation using the Trachlight: a brief review of current knowledge. *Can J Anaesth* 48:592–599, 2001.
21. Owen RL, Cheney FW: Endobronchial intubation: a preventable complication. *Anesthesiology* 67:255–257, 1987.
22. Chander S, Feldman E: Correct placement of endotracheal tubes. *N Y State J Med* 79:1843–1844, 1979.
23. Kasper CL, Deem S: The self-inflating bulb to detect esophageal intubation during emergency airway management. *Anesthesiology* 88:898–902, 1998.
24. Langeron O, Masso E, Huraux C, et al: Prediction of difficult mask ventilation. *Anesthesiology* 92:1229–1236, 2000.
25. Benumof JL: Laryngeal mask airway and the ASA difficult airway algorithm. *Anesthesiology* 84:686–699, 1996.
26. Fuchs G, Schwarz G, Baumgartner A, et al: Fiberoptic intubation in 327 neurosurgical patients with lesions of the cervical spine. *J Neurosurg Anesthesiol* 11:11–16, 1999.
27. Brain AI, Verghese C, Addy EV, et al: The intubating laryngeal mask. I. Development of a new device for intubation of the trachea. *Br J Anaesth* 79:699–703, 1997.
28. Urtubia RM, Aguila CM, Cumsille MA: Combitube: a study for proper use. *Anesth Analg* 90:958–962, 2000.
29. Yardy N, Hancox D, Strang T: A comparison of two airway aids for emergency use by unskilled personnel. The Combitube and laryngeal mask. *Anaesthesia* 54:181–183, 1999.
30. MacQuarrie K, Hung OR, Law JA: Tracheal intubation using Bullard

laryngoscope for patients with a simulated difficult airway. *Can J Anaesth* 46:760–765, 1999.

31. Watts AD, Gelb AW, Bach DB, et al: Comparison of the Bullard and Macintosh laryngoscopes for endotracheal intubation of patients with a potential cervical spine injury. *Anesthesiology* 87:1335–1342, 1997.

32. Criswell JC, Parr MJ, Nolan JP: Emergency airway management in patients with cervical spine injuries. *Anaesthesia* 49:900–903, 1994.

33. Loudermilk EP, Hartmannsgruber M, Stoltzfus DP, et al: A prospective study of the safety of tracheal extubation using a pediatric airway exchange catheter for patients with a known difficult airway. *Chest* 111:1660–1665, 1997.

34. Schwartz DE, Matthay MA, Cohen NH: Death and other complications of emergency airway management in critically ill adults.

A prospective investigation of 297 tracheal intubations. *Anesthesiology* 82:367–376, 1995.

35. Stout DM, Bishop MJ, Dwersteg JF, et al: Correlation of endotracheal tube size with sore throat and hoarseness following general anesthesia. *Anesthesiology* 67:419–421, 1987.

36. Brandwein M, Abramson AL, Shikowitz MJ: Bilateral vocal cord paralysis following endotracheal intubation. *Arch Otolaryngol Head Neck Surg* 112:877–882, 1986.

37. Eckerbom B, Lindholm CE, Alexopoulos C: Airway lesions caused by prolonged intubation with standard and with anatomically shaped tracheal tubes. A post-mortem study. *Acta Anaesthesiol Scand* 30:366–373, 1986.

38. Engoren M: Evaluation of the cuff-leak test in a cardiac surgery population. *Chest* 116:1029–1031, 1999.

2. Central Venous Catheters

Michael G. Seneff

Central venous catheter–related complications, especially infection, are a major cause of morbidity in the critically ill. For example, vascular catheters are the most common source for methicillin-resistant *Staphylococcus aureus* and vancomycin-resistant enterococcal bloodstream infection, one of the most important problems facing intensivists today [1]. Fortunately, our knowledge of catheter-related complications and how to prevent them has been greatly expanded through better catheter technology and an increased number of scientifically conducted clinical trials. This chapter reviews the techniques and complications of the various routes of cannulation and presents an overall strategy for catheter management that incorporates many of the recent advances. The guidelines presented should be used by every hospital to develop intensive care unit (ICU)-specific catheter management protocols and continuous quality improvement efforts that definitively reduce catheter-related complications, especially infection [2].

Historical Perspective

Aubaniac [3] is credited with the first description of infraclavicular subclavian venipuncture in humans in 1952. A major advance in intravenous catheter technique came the following year, when Seldinger [4] described the replacement of a catheter needle using a guidewire, a technique that now bears his name. During the mid-1950s, percutaneous catheterization of the inferior vena cava via a femoral vein (FV) approach became popular until reports of a high incidence of complications were published [5,6].

An important development occurred in 1959, when Hughes and Magovern [7] described the clinical use of central venous pressure (CVP) measurements in humans undergoing thoracotomy. In 1962, Wilson et al. [8] extended the practicality of CVP monitoring by using percutaneous infraclavicular subclavian vein (SV) catheterization. This technique achieved wide clinical acceptance, but enthusiasm was tempered when various, sometimes fatal, complications were reported. Subsequently, Yoffa [9] reported his experience with supraclavicular subclavian venipuncture, claiming a lower incidence of complications, but his results were not uniformly reproduced.

Motivated by the search for a "golden route" [10], Nordlund and Thoren [11] and then Rams et al. [12] performed external jugular vein (EJV) catheterization and advocated more extensive use of this approach. Although EJV catheterization met the goal of causing fewer complications during venipuncture, positioning of the catheter tip in a central venous location was sometimes impossible.

The first large series on internal jugular vein (IJV) catheterization appeared in 1969, when English et al. [13] reported on 500 percutaneous IJV catheterizations. Reports confirming this route's efficiency and low complication rate followed, and it has remained a popular site for central venous access. Finally, the antecubital veins have once again become a viable option for central venous access because of the increased use of peripherally inserted central catheters (PICCs) and midline catheters in the critically ill [14–16].

Indications and Site Selection

Technical advances and a better understanding of anatomy have made insertion of central venous catheters easier and safer, but there still is an underappreciation of the inherent risks. Like any medical procedure, central venous catheterization (CVC) has specific indications and should be reserved for the patient who has the potential to benefit from it. After determining that CVC is necessary, physicians often proceed with catheterization at the site with which they are most experienced, which might not be the most appropriate route in that particular patient. Table 2-1 lists general priorities in site selection for different indications of CVC; the actual site cho-

Table 2-1. Indications for Central Venous Catheterization

Indication	Site selection		
	First	Second	Third
Pulmonary artery catheterization	RIJV	LSV	LIJV or RSV
With coagulopathy	EJV	IJV	FV
With pulmonary compromise or high-level positive end-expiratory pressure	RIJV	LIJV	EJV
Total parenteral nutrition	SV	IJV	
Long term	SV (surgically implanted)	PICC	
Acute hemodialysis/plasmapheresis	IJV	FV	SV
Cardiopulmonary arrest	FV	SV	IJV
Emergency transvenous pacemaker	RIJV	SV	FV
Hypovolemia, inability to perform peripheral catheterization	SV or FV	IJV	
Preoperative preparation	IJV	SV	
Neurosurgical procedure	AV/PICC	SV	
General purpose venous access, vasoactive agents, caustic medications, radiologic procedures	IJV or SV	FV	EJV
With coagulopathy	EJV	IJV	FV
Emergency airway management	FV	SV	IJV
Inability to lie supine	FV	EJV	AV/PICC

AV, antecubital vein; EJV, external jugular vein; FV, femoral vein; IJV, internal jugular vein; L, left; PICC, peripherally inserted central venous catheter; R, right; SV, subclavian vein.

sen in a particular patient should vary based on individual institutional and operator experiences.

Volume resuscitation alone is not an indication for CVC. A 2.5-in., 16-gauge catheter used to cannulate a peripheral vein can infuse two times the amount of fluid as an 8-in., 16-gauge central venous catheter [17]. However, peripheral vein cannulation can be impossible in the hypovolemic, shocked individual. In this instance, the SV is the most reliable central site because it remains patent as a result of its fibrous attachments to the clavicle. Depending on the clinical situation, the FV is a reasonable alternative, but multiple reports have increased the long-standing concern of deep venous thrombosis associated with this route [18–21].

Central venous access is often required for the infusion of irritant medications (concentrated potassium chloride) or vasoactive agents and certain diagnostic or therapeutic radiologic procedures and in any patient in whom peripheral access is not possible. For these indications, the IJV is a reasonable choice because of its reliability and low rate of major complications with insertion. However, the risk for infection is probably higher with IJV insertions, and for experienced operators, the SV is an excellent alternative.

Long-term total parenteral nutrition is best administered through SV catheters, which should be surgically implanted if appropriate. The IJV is now the preferred site for acute hemodialysis because of the relatively high incidence of subclavian stenosis following temporary dialysis using the SV [22–25]. The FV is also suitable for acute short-term hemodialysis or plasmapheresis in nonambulatory patients [26].

Emergency transvenous pacemakers and flow-directed pulmonary artery catheters are best inserted through the right IJV because of the direct path to the right ventricle. This route is associated with the fewest catheter tip malpositions. For patients with coagulopathy, the EJV, if part of the surface anatomy, is an acceptable alternative, but we rarely find it necessary. The SV is an alternative second choice for pulmonary artery catheterization, even in many patients with coagulopathy [27], but the left SV is preferred to the right SV [28]. The reader is referred to Chapter 4 for additional information on the insertion and care of pulmonary artery catheters.

Preoperative CVC is desirable in a wide variety of clinical situations. If fluid status requires close monitoring, a pulmonary artery catheter should be inserted, because CVP can be an unreliable predictor of left heart filling pressures [29]. In most preoperative patients, the IJV is the best route, because pneumothorax is very rare, and even a small pneumothorax is at risk of expanding under general anesthesia [30]. One specific indication for preoperative right ventricular catheterization is the patient undergoing a posterior craniotomy or cervical laminectomy in the sitting position. These patients are at risk for air embolism, and the catheter can be used to aspirate air from the right ventricle [31]. Neurosurgery is the only common indication for an antecubital approach, as IJV catheters are in the operative field and theoretically can obstruct blood return from the cranial vault and increase intracranial pressure. Subclavian catheters are an excellent alternative for preoperative neurosurgical patients if pneumothorax is ruled out before induction of general anesthesia.

Venous access during cardiopulmonary resuscitation warrants special comment. Peripheral vein cannulation in circulatory arrest may prove impossible, and circulation times of drugs administered peripherally are prolonged when compared to central injection [32]. Drugs injected through femoral catheters also have a prolonged circulation time unless the catheter tip is advanced beyond the diaphragm, although the clinical significance of this is controversial. Effective drug administration is an extremely important element of successful cardiopulmonary resuscitation, and all physicians should understand the appropriate techniques for establishing venous access. It is logical to establish venous access as quickly as possible, either peripherally or centrally, if qualified personnel are present. Prolonged attempts at arm vein cannulation are not warranted, and under these circumstances the FV is a good alternative. If circulation is not restored after administration of appropriate drugs and defibrillation, central access should be obtained by the most experienced operator available with a minimum interruption of cardiopulmonary resuscitation [33].

General Considerations and Complications

General considerations for CVC independent of the site of insertion are catheter tip location, vascular erosions, catheter-associated thrombosis, air and catheter embolism, and coagulopathy, which are discussed below. Catheter-associated infection is discussed separately.

CATHETER TIP LOCATION. Catheter tip location is a very important consideration in CVC. The ideal location for the catheter tip is the distal innominate or proximal SVC, 3 to 5 cm proximal to the caval-atrial junction. Positioning of the catheter tip within the right atrium or right ventricle must be avoided. Cardiac tamponade secondary to catheter tip perforation of the cardiac wall is not rare, and two-thirds of patients who experience this complication die [34]. Perforation results from catheter tip migration that occurs from the motion of the beating heart as well as patient arm and neck movements. Migration of catheter tips can be impressive: 5 to 10 cm with antecubital catheters and 1 to 5 cm with IJV or SV catheters [35,36]. Other complications from intracardiac catheter tip position include provocation of arrhythmias from mechanical irritation and infusion of caustic medications or unwarmed blood [37].

Correct placement of the catheter tip is relatively simple, beginning with an appreciation of anatomy. The caval-atrial junction is approximately 16 to 18 cm from right-sided skin punctures and 19 to 21 cm from left-sided insertions and is relatively independent of patient gender and body habitus [38,39]. Insertion of a standard triple-lumen catheter to its full 20 cm frequently places the tip within the heart, especially after right-sided insertions. A chest radiograph should be obtained following every initial central venous catheter insertion to ascertain catheter tip location and to detect complications. The right tracheobronchial angle is the most reliable landmark on plain film chest x-ray for the upper margin of the SVC, which averages 6 to 7 cm in length. The catheter tip should lie 2 to 3 cm below this landmark and above the right upper cardiac silhouette [40].

VASCULAR EROSIONS. Large-vessel perforations secondary to central venous catheters are uncommon and often not immediately recognized. Vessel perforation typically occurs 1 to 7 days after catheter insertion. Patients usually present with sudden onset of dyspnea and often with new pleural effusions on chest radiography [41]. Catheter stiffness, position of the tip within the vessel, and the site of insertion are important factors causing vessel perforation. The relative importance of these variables is unknown. Repeated irritation of the vessel wall by a stiff catheter tip or infusion of hyperosmolar solutions may be the initiating event. Vascular erosions are commoner with left IJV and EJV catheters, because for anatomic reasons the catheter tip is more likely to be positioned laterally under tension against the SVC wall [42]. Positioning of the catheter tip within the vein parallel to the vessel wall must be confirmed on chest radiograph. Free aspiration of blood from the catheter is not always sufficient to rule out a vascular perforation.

AIR AND CATHETER EMBOLISM. Significant air and catheter embolism are rare and preventable complications of CVC. Catheter embolism can occur at the time of insertion when a catheter-through- or over-needle technique is used and the operator withdraws the catheter without simultaneously retracting the needle. It more commonly occurs with antecubital or femoral catheters after insertion, because they are prone to breakage when the agitated patient vigorously bends an arm or leg. Prevention, recognition, and management of catheter embolism are covered in detail elsewhere [43].

Air embolism is of greater clinical importance, often goes undiagnosed, and may prove fatal [44–47]. Theoretically, it is totally preventable with compulsive attention to proper catheter insertion and maintenance. Factors resulting in air embolism during insertion are well known, and methods to increase venous pressure, such as the use of Trendelenburg's position, should not be forgotten. Catheter disconnect or passage of air through a patent tract after catheter removal is a more common cause of catheter-associated air embolism. An air embolus should be suspected in any patient with an indwelling or recently discontinued CVC in whom sudden unexplained hypoxemia or cardiovascular collapse develops, often after being moved out of bed or to another stretcher. A characteristic mill wheel sound may be auscultated over the precordium. Treatment involves placing the patient in the left lateral decubitus position and using the catheter to aspirate air from the right ventricle. Hyperbaric oxygen therapy to reduce bubble size has a controversial role in treatment [44]. The best treatment is prevention, and prevention can be most effectively achieved through comprehensive physician-in-training educational modules and proper supervision of inexperienced operators [45].

COAGULOPATHY. Central venous access in the patient with a bleeding diathesis is problematic. The SV and IJV routes have increased risks in the presence of coagulopathy, but it is not known at what degree of abnormality the risk becomes unacceptable. A coagulopathy is generally defined as a prothrombin time greater than 15 seconds, platelet count less than 50,000, or bleeding time greater than 10 minutes. Although it is clear that safe venipuncture is possible with greater degrees of coagulopathy [27], the literature is also fraught with case reports of serious hemorrhagic complications. In patients with severe coagulopathy, the EJV is an alternative for central venous access, especially pulmonary artery catheterization, whereas the FV offers a safe alternative for general purpose venous access. In appropriate patients, PICC catheters are useful. If these sites cannot be used, the IJV is the best alternative, because it is a compressible site and there is positive experience with this route in patients with coagulopathy [51].

THROMBOSIS. Catheter-related thrombosis is very common but usually of little clinical significance. The spectrum of thrombotic complications ranges from a sleeve of fibrin that surrounds the catheter from its point of entry into the vein distal to the tip; to mural thrombus, a clot that forms on the wall of the vein secondary to mechanical or chemical irritation; or occlusive thrombus, which occludes flow and may result in collateral formation [49]. All of these lesions are usually clinically silent; therefore, studies that do not use venography or color flow Doppler imaging to confirm the diagnosis underestimate its incidence. Using venography, fibrin sleeve formation can be documented in a majority of catheters, mural thrombi in 10% to 30%, and occlusive thrombi in 0% to 10% [49–56]. In contrast, clinical symptoms of thrombosis occur in only 0% to 3% of patients [21,49,52]. The incidence of thrombosis probably increases with duration of catheterization but does not appear reliably related to the site of insertion [21,49–57]. However, FV catheter-associated thrombosis in the lower extremity is almost certainly more clinically important than upper extremity thrombosis caused by IJ and SV catheters [18–20]. The presence of catheter-associated thrombosis is also associated with a higher incidence of infection [56,58].

Catheter design and composition have an impact on the frequency of thrombotic complications. The ideal catheter material is nonthrombogenic and relatively stiff at room temperature to facilitate percutaneous insertion, yet soft and pliable at body temperature to minimize intravascular mechanical trauma. Not all studies are consistent, but polyurethane, especially when coated with hydromer, appears to be the best material available for bedside catheter insertions [59,60]. Silastic catheters have low thrombogenicity but must be surgically implanted, and pressure monitoring may not be possible. Heparin bonding of catheters decreases thrombogenicity, but the clinical importance of this remains uncertain [61–63]. Low-dose heparin infused through the catheter or administered subcutaneously and very-low-dose warfarin therapy also decrease the incidence of venogram-proven and clinically apparent thrombosis [64–66]. This approach holds promise, but heparin and warfarin have several relevant drug interactions and complications in the critically ill patient, and further study is warranted.

Routes of Central Venous Cannulation

ANTECUBITAL APPROACH. The antecubital veins are increasingly used in the ICU for CVC with PICC and midline catheters. Use of PICC catheters in critically ill adults is limited by lack of surface anatomy in obese and edematous patients, lack of technological versatility (i.e., limited pressure monitoring [67], small lumens, and no triple-lumen capability), and increased time and decreased predictability of bedside insertion. PICC catheters are potentially useful in highly selected ICU patients undergoing neurosurgery, with coagulopathy, or in the rehabilitative phase of critical illness for which general purpose central venous access is required for parenteral nutrition or long-term medication access [14–16,68] (Table 2-1). The technique of percutaneous insertion of these catheters using the basilic, cephalic, or brachial vein is described below.

Anatomy. The basilic vein is formed in the ulnar part of the dorsal venous network of the hand (Fig. 2-1). It may be found in the medial part of the antecubital fossa, where it is usually joined by the median basilic vein. It then ascends in the groove between the biceps brachii and pronator teres on the medial aspect of the arm to perforate the deep fascia distal to the midportion of the arm, where it joins the brachial vein to become the axillary vein. The basilic vein is almost always of substantial size, and the anatomy is predictable; because the axillary vein is a direct continuation of it, the basilic vein provides an unimpeded path to the central venous circulation [69,70].

The cephalic vein begins in the radial part of the dorsal venous network of the hand and ascends around the radial border of the forearm (Fig. 2-1). In the lateral aspect of the antecubital fossa, it forms an anastomosis with the median basilic vein and then ascends the lateral part of the arm in the groove along the lateral border of the biceps brachii. It pierces the clavipectoral fascia in the deltopectoral triangle and empties into the proximal part of the axillary vein caudal to the clavicle. The variability of the cephalic vein anatomy renders it less suitable than the basilic vein for CVC. It joins the axillary vein at nearly a right angle, which can be difficult for a catheter to traverse. Instead of passing beneath the clavicle, the cephalic vein may pass through the clavicle, compressing the vein and making catheter passage impossible. Furthermore, in a significant percentage of cases, the cephalic does not empty into the axillary vein but divides into smaller branches or a venous plexus, which empties into the ipsilateral EJV. The cephalic vein may also simply terminate or become attenuated just proximal to the antecubital fossa [69,70].

Technique of Cannulation. Several kits are available for antecubital CVC. The PICC and midline catheters are made of silicone or polyurethane and, depending on catheter stiffness and size, are usually placed through an introducer. The method

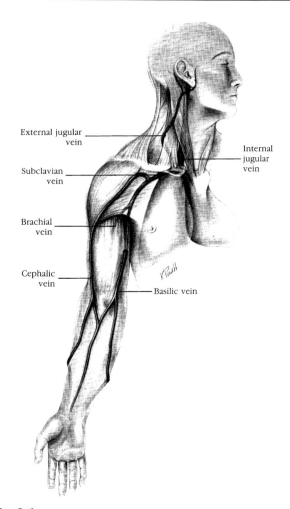

Fig. 2-1. Venous anatomy of the upper extremity. The internal jugular, external jugular, and subclavian veins are also shown.

described below is for a PICC catheter inserted through a tearaway introducer.

The right basilic vein should be selected for the initial attempt at CVC because of anatomic considerations and clinical studies that confirm a higher success rate with the basilic than the cephalic vein [71,72]. The success rates from either arm are comparable, although the catheter must traverse a greater distance from the left. With the patient's arm at his or her side, the antecubital fossa is prepared and draped, adhering to strict aseptic technique. A tourniquet is placed proximally, and if an appropriate vein is not part of the surface anatomy, we use a bedside ultrasound device (SiteRite, DyMAX Corp., Pittsburgh, PA) to identify the basilic or its main branches. After local anesthesia, venipuncture is performed with the thin-wall entry needle proximal to the antecubital crease to avoid catheter breakage and embolism. When free back flow of venous blood is confirmed, the tourniquet is released and the guidewire carefully threaded into the vein for a distance of 15 to 20 cm. Leaving the guidewire in place, the thin-wall needle is withdrawn and the puncture site enlarged with a scalpel blade. The sheath-introducer assembly is then threaded over the guidewire with a twisting motion, and the guidewire is removed. Next, leaving the sheath in place, the dilator is removed, and the introducer is now ready for PICC insertion. The PICC is supplied with an inner obturator that provides stiffness for insertion and must be inserted into the PICC after it has been flushed and before insertion. The length of insertion is estimated by measuring the distance along the predicted vein path from the venipuncture site to the manubriosternal junction. Once the PICC has been trimmed to the desired length, the obturator is inserted into the PICC and advanced until the tips are equal. The PICC/obturator is then inserted through the introducer to the appropriate distance, the introducer peeled away, and the obturator removed. The PICC is then secured in place and a chest x-ray obtained to determine tip position.

If resistance to advancing the PICC is met, options are limited. Techniques such as abducting the arm are of limited value. If a catheter-through- or over-needle device has been used, the catheter must never be withdrawn without simultaneously retracting the needle to avoid catheter embolism. If the catheter cannot be advanced easily, another site should be chosen.

Success Rate and Complications. Using the above technique, PICC catheters have a 75% to 95% successful placement rate, and success is increased with operator experience, identification of a large vein, or the use of fluoroscopy [14–16,68,73]. Overall, PICCs appear to be at least as safe as CVCs, but important complications include sterile phlebitis, thrombosis (especially of the SV and IJV), infection, limb edema, and pericardial tamponade. Phlebitis may be commoner with antecubital central venous catheters, probably due to less blood flow in these veins as well as the proximity of the venipuncture site to the skin [74,75]. The risk of pericardial tamponade may also be increased because of greater catheter tip migration occurring with arm movements [76]. Complications are minimized by strict adherence to recommended techniques for catheter placement and care.

INTERNAL-EXTERNAL JUGULAR APPROACH. The IJV provides one of the most favorable sites for access to the great thoracic veins. IJV cannulation offers a high success rate with few complications. Pediatricians used the IJV for venous access long before Hermosura et al. [77] described the technique and advocated its use in adults in 1966. In 1969, English et al. [13] reported the first large series of IJV cannulations; subsequently, the procedure became commonplace and in many centers the preferred method of CVC. In 1974, Blitt et al. [78] described a technique of CVC via the EJV employing a J wire. Although the success rate of this route is lower than with the IJV, a "central" venipuncture is avoided, and in selected cases catheterization via the EJV is an excellent alternative.

Anatomy. The IJV emerges from the base of the skull through the jugular foramen and enters the carotid sheath dorsally with the internal carotid artery (ICA) (Fig. 2-1). It then courses posterolaterally to the artery and runs beneath the sternocleidomastoid (SCM) muscle. The vein lies medial to the anterior portion of the SCM muscle in its upper part and then runs beneath the triangle formed by the two heads of the muscle in its medial portion before entering the SV near the medial border of the anterior scalene muscle beneath the sternal border of the clavicle. The junction of the right IJV (which averages 2 to 3 cm in diameter) with the right SV and then the innominate vein forms a straight path to the SVC. As a result, malpositions and looping of a catheter inserted through the right IJV are unusual. In contrast, a catheter passed through the left IJV must negotiate a sharp turn at the left jugulosubclavian junction, which results in a greater percentage of catheter malpositions [79]. This sharp turn may also produce tension and torque at the catheter tip, resulting in a higher incidence of vessel erosion [41,42].

Knowledge of the structures neighboring the IJV is essential, as they may be compromised by a misdirected needle. The ICA runs medial to the IJV but, rarely, may lie directly posteriorly. Behind the ICA, just outside the sheath, lie the stellate

ganglion and the cervical sympathetic trunk. The dome of the pleura, which is higher on the left, lies caudal to the junction of the IJV and SV. Posteriorly, at the root of the neck, course the phrenic and vagus nerves [69,70]. The thoracic duct lies behind the left IJV and enters the superior margin of the SV near the jugulosubclavian junction. The right lymphatic duct has the same anatomic relationship but is much smaller, and chylous effusions typically occur only with left-sided IJV cannulations.

Techniques of Cannulation. Internal jugular venipuncture can be accomplished by a variety of methods; all methods use the same landmarks but differ in the site of venipuncture or orientation of the needle. Defalque [80] grouped the methods into three general approaches: anterior, central, and posterior (Fig. 2-2). The author prefers the central approach for the initial attempt, but the method chosen varies with the institution and operator's experience. All approaches require identical equipment, and the operator may choose from many different catheters and prepackaged kits.

Standard triple-lumen catheter kits include the equivalent of a 7-French (Fr) triple-lumen catheter with 20 (recommended) or 30 cm of usable length, a 0.032-in. diameter guidewire with straight and J tip, an 18-gauge thin-wall needle, an 18-gauge catheter-over-needle, a 7-Fr vessel dilator, a 22-gauge "finder" needle, and appropriate syringes and suture material. Preparation of the guidewire and catheter before insertion is important; all lumens should be flushed with saline and the cap to the distal lumen removed. The patient is placed in a 15-degree Trendelenburg's position to distend the vein and minimize the risk of air embolism, with the head turned gently to the contralateral side. The surface anatomy is identified, especially the angle of the mandible, the two heads of the SCM, the clavicle, the EJV, and the trachea (Fig. 2-2). The neck is then prepared with an appropriate antiseptic solution and fully draped, following full triple barrier protection.

For the central approach [80–82], skin puncture is at the apex of the triangle formed by the two muscle bellies of the SCM and the clavicle. The ICA pulsation is usually felt 1 to 2 cm medial to this point, beneath or just medial to the sternal head of the SCM. The skin at the apex of the triangle is infiltrated with 1% lidocaine using the 22-gauge needle, which is then used to locate the IJV. Use of a small-bore finder needle to locate the IJV should prevent inadvertent ICA puncture and unnecessary probing with a larger-bore needle. The operator should maintain slight or no pressure on the ICA with the left hand and insert the finder needle with the right hand at the apex of the triangle (or slightly more caudal) at a 30- to 45-degree angle with the frontal plane, directed at the ipsilateral nipple. After expulsion of any skin plug, the needle is advanced steadily with constant back pressure, and venipuncture occurs within 3 to 5 cm. If venipuncture does not occur on the initial thrust, back pressure should be maintained and the needle slowly withdrawn, as venipuncture frequently occurs on withdrawal. If the first attempt is unsuccessful, the operator should reassess patient position, landmarks, and techniques to ensure that he or she is not doing anything to decrease IJV lumen size (see below). Subsequent attempts can be directed slightly laterally or medially to the initial thrust, as long as the plane of the ICA is not violated. If venipuncture does not occur after three to five attempts, further attempts are unlikely to be successful and only increase complications [48,83,84].

When venipuncture has occurred with the finder needle, the operator can either withdraw the finder needle and introduce the large-bore needle in the identical plane or leave the finder needle in place and introduce the larger needle directly above it. If using the latter technique, the operator or assistant must be careful not to exert tension on the finder needle, as

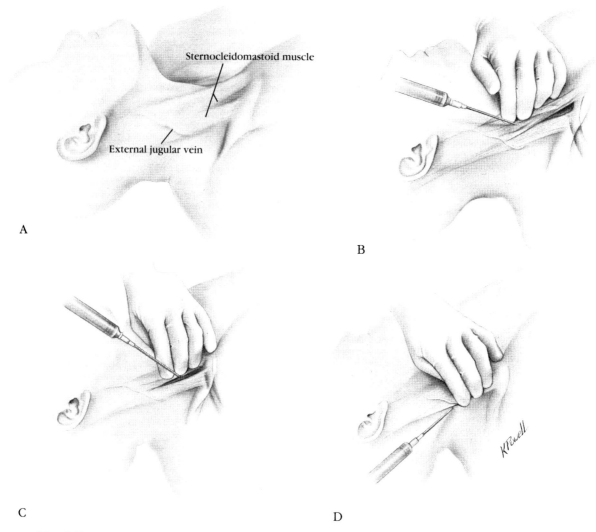

Fig. 2-2. Surface anatomy and various approaches to cannulation of the internal jugular vein. **A:** Surface anatomy. **B:** Anterior approach. **C:** Central approach. **D:** Posterior approach.

this may decrease the lumen size of the IJV and make catheterization more difficult. Many kits provide an 18-gauge thin-wall needle through which a guidewire can be directly introduced and a 16-gauge catheter-over-needle device. With the latter apparatus, the catheter is threaded over the needle into the vein, the needle withdrawn, and the guidewire inserted through the catheter. Both techniques are effective; the choice is strictly a matter of operator preference. Regardless of which large-bore needle is used, once venipuncture has occurred the syringe is removed during expiration or Valsalva maneuver and the hub occluded with a finger after ensuring that the back flow of blood is not pulsatile. The J tip of the guidewire is then inserted and should pass freely up to 20 cm, at which point the thin-wall needle or catheter is withdrawn. The tendency to insert the guidewire deeper than 15 to 20 cm should be avoided, as it is the most common cause of ventricular arrhythmias during insertion and also poses a risk for cardiac perforation. Occasionally, the guidewire does not pass easily beyond the tip of the thin-wall needle. The guidewire should then be withdrawn, the syringe attached, and free back flow of blood reestablished and maintained while the syringe and needle are brought to a more parallel plane with the vein. The guidewire should then pass easily. If

resistance is still encountered, rotation of the guidewire during insertion often allows passage, but extensive manipulation and force only lead to complications.

With the guidewire in place, a scalpel is used to make two generous 90-degree stab incisions at the skin entry site to facilitate passage of the 7-Fr vessel dilator. The dilator is inserted down the wire to the hub, ensuring that control and sterility of the guidewire are not compromised. The dilator is then withdrawn and gauze used at the puncture site to control oozing and prevent air embolism down the needle tract. The triple-lumen catheter is then inserted over the guidewire, ensuring that the guidewire protrudes from the distal lumen hub before the catheter tip penetrates the skin. The catheter is then advanced 15 to 17 cm (17 to 19 cm for left IJV) into the vein, the guidewire withdrawn, and the distal lumen capped. The catheter is sutured securely to limit tip migration and is bandaged in a standard manner. A chest radiograph should be obtained to detect complications and tip location.

Alternative Approaches. The anterior and posterior approaches are identical in technique, differing only in venipuncture site and plane of insertion. For the anterior approach [80,85–87] (Fig. 2-2) the important landmark is the midpoint of the sternal head of the SCM, approximately 5 cm from the angle of the mandible and the sternum. At this point, the carotid artery can be palpated 1 cm inside the lateral border of the sternal head. The index and middle fingers of the left hand gently palpate the artery, and the needle is introduced 0.5 to 1.0 cm lateral to the pulsation. The needle should form a 30- to 45-degree angle with the frontal plane and be directed caudally parallel to the carotid artery toward the ipsilateral nipple. Venipuncture occurs within 2 to 4 cm, sometimes only while the needle is slowly withdrawn. If the initial thrust is unsuccessful, the next attempt should be at a 5-degree lateral angle, followed by a cautious attempt more medially, never crossing the plane of the carotid artery.

The posterior approach [80,88–90] (Fig. 2-2) uses the EJV as a surface landmark. The needle is introduced 1 cm dorsally to the point where the EJV crosses the posterior border of the SCM or 5 cm cephalad from the clavicle along the clavicular head of the SCM. The needle is directed caudally and ventrally toward the suprasternal notch at an angle of 45 degrees to the sagittal plane, with a 15-degree upward angulation. Venipuncture occurs within 5 to 7 cm. If this attempt is unsuccessful, the needle should be aimed slightly more cephalad on the next attempt.

Success Rates and Complications. IJV catheterization is associated with a high rate of successful catheter placement regardless of the approach used. Elective procedures are successful more than 90% of the time, generally within the first three attempts, and catheter malposition is rare [79–81,83,85,86]. Operator experience does not appear to be as important a factor in altering the success rate of venipuncture as it is in increasing the number of complications [83,91]. Emergent IJV catheterization is less successful and is not the preferred technique during airway emergencies or other situations that may make it difficult to identify landmarks in the neck. The use of ultrasound localization to aid in IJV catheterization improves success rate and decreases the need for multiple attempts [92], but it has not been widely adapted, probably because of cost and training issues. In special circumstances, ultrasound or Doppler localization is helpful in performing difficult or previously unsuccessful IJV catheterization [93].

Ultrasound studies have been useful in delineating factors that improve the efficiency of IJV cannulation. The ability to perform IJV venipuncture is directly proportional to its cross-sectional lumen area (CSLA); thus, maneuvers that increase or decrease the vein's caliber have an impact on the success rate [94,95]. Maneuvers that decrease the CSLA include hypovolemia, carotid artery palpation, and excessive tension on a finder needle. Predictably, Valsalva maneuver and Trendelenburg's position increase CSLA, as does high-level positive end-expiratory pressure. As the IJV nears the SV, there is also a progressive increase in CSLA. Overrotation of the neck may place the vein beneath the SCM muscle belly [94].

Often, a difficult IJV cannulation is successful on the first attempt by optimizing CLSA through attention to the above measures. If the IJV is still not punctured after one or two attempts, it is usually because of anatomic variation, not because of the absence of jugular flow [95,96]. In this situation, the author uses an ultrasound device to locate the IJV because of its portability, overall convenience, and need for less operator expertise [97]. Whatever technique is used, prolonged attempts at catheterization after optimization of IJV CSLA are only likely to increase complications.

Complications. The incidence and types of complications are similar regardless of the approach. Operator inexperience appears to increase the number of complications, but to an undefined extent, and probably does not have as great an impact as it does on the incidence of pneumothorax in subclavian venipuncture [80,98,99].

The overall incidence of complications in IJV catheterization is 0.1% to 4.2% [13,80,88,98], with a few studies reporting higher rates [48,83,100]. Important complications include ICA puncture, pneumothorax, vessel erosion, thrombosis, and infection. By far the most common complication is ICA puncture, which constitutes 80% to 90% of all complications. In the absence of a bleeding diathesis, arterial punctures are benign and are managed conservatively without sequelae by applying local pressure for 10 minutes. Even in the absence of clotting abnormalities, a sizable hematoma may form, frequently preventing further catheterization attempts or, rarely, exerting pressure on vital neck structures [101,102]. Unrecognized arterial puncture can lead to catheterization of the ICA with a large-bore catheter or introducer and can have disastrous consequences, especially when heparin is administered [103]. Management of carotid cannulation with a large-bore catheter, such as a 7-Fr introducer, is controversial. Some experts advise administration of anticoagulants to prevent thromboembolic complications, whereas others advise the opposite. The author's approach is to remove the catheter and avoid heparinization if possible, as hemorrhage appears to be a greater risk than thromboembolism [103]. Chronic complications, which rarely result from ICA puncture, include hematomas that require surgical excision, arteriovenous fistula, and pseudoaneurysm [104].

Coagulopathy is a relative contraindication to IJV catheterization, but extensive experience suggests that it is generally safe [48]. In patients with clinical bleeding abnormalities, it is prudent to proceed first with EJV or FV catheterization, but if the IJV is considered most appropriate, a finder needle should always be used to try to avoid ICA puncture with a larger needle.

Pneumothorax is an unusual adverse consequence of IJV cannulation, with an average incidence of 0% to 0.2% [13,83,89,98]. It usually results from a skin puncture too close to the clavicle or, rarely, from other causes [48]. Pneumothorax may be complicated by heme, infusion of intravenous fluid, or tension.

An extraordinary number of case reports indicate that any complication from IJV catheterization is possible, even the intrathecal insertion of a Swan-Ganz catheter [105]. In reality, this route is reliable, with a low incidence of major complications. Operator experience is not as important a factor as in SV catheterization; the incidence of catheter tip malposition is low, and patient acceptance is high. It is best suited for acute, short-term hemodialysis and for elective or urgent catheterizations in volume-repleted patients, especially pulmonary artery catheterizations and insertion of temporary transvenous pacemakers. It is not the preferred site during airway emergencies, for parenteral nutrition, or for long-term catheterization because infectious complications are higher with IJV compared to SCV catheterizations.

EXTERNAL JUGULAR VEIN APPROACH. The main advantages to the EJV route for CVC are that it is part of the surface anatomy, it can be cannulated in the presence of clotting abnormalities, and the risk of pneumothorax is avoided. The main disadvantage is the unpredictability of passage of the catheter to the central compartment. We rarely use this approach anymore, primarily because of greater experience with the IJ and SV in patients with coagulopathy.

Anatomy. The EJV is formed anterior and caudal to the ear at the angle of the mandible by the union of the posterior auricular and retromandibular veins (Fig. 2-3). It courses obliquely across the anterior surface of the SCM, then pierces the deep

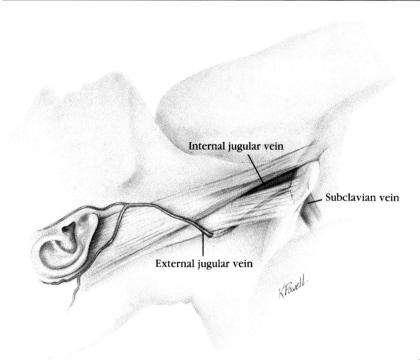

Fig. 2-3. External jugular vein.

fascia just posterior to the SCM, and joins the SV behind the medial third of the clavicle. In 5% to 15% of patients, the EJV is not a distinct structure but a venous plexus, in which case it may receive the ipsilateral cephalic vein. The EJV varies in size and contains valves throughout its course. Its junction with the SV may be at a severe, narrow angle that can be difficult for a catheter to traverse.

Technique. The EJV should be cannulated using the 16-gauge catheter-over-needle, because guidewire manipulations are often necessary and secure venous access with a catheter is preferable. The patient is placed in a slight Trendelenburg's position, with arms to the side and head turned gently to the contralateral side. The right EJV should be chosen for the initial attempt and can be identified where it courses over the anterior portion of the clavicular belly of the SCM. After sterile preparation, venipuncture is performed with the 16-gauge catheter-over-needle using the left index finger and thumb to distend and anchor the vein. Skin puncture should be well above the clavicle and the needle advanced in the axis of the vein at 20 degrees to the frontal plane. The EJV may be more difficult to cannulate than expected because of its propensity to roll and displace rather than puncture in response to the advancing needle. A firm, quick thrust is often required to effect venipuncture. When free back flow of blood is established, the needle tip is advanced a few millimeters further into the vein and the catheter is threaded over the needle. The catheter may not thread its entire length because of valves, tortuosity, or the SV junction but should be advanced at least 3 to 5 cm to secure venous access. The syringe and needle can then be removed and the guidewire, J tip first, threaded up to 20 cm and the catheter removed. Manipulation and rotation of the guidewire, especially when it reaches the SV junction, may be necessary but should not be excessive. On insertion, the J is usually directed medially to facilitate central passage rather than out to the arm. Various arm and head movements are advocated to facilitate guidewire passage; abduction of the ipsilateral arm and anterior-posterior pressure exerted on the clavicle may be helpful. Once the guidewire has advanced 20 cm, two 90-degree skin stabs are made with a scalpel and the vein dilator

inserted to its hub, maintaining control of the guidewire. The triple-lumen catheter is then inserted an appropriate length (16–17 cm on the right, 18–20 cm on the left). The guidewire is withdrawn, the catheter bandaged, and a chest radiograph obtained to screen for complications.

Success Rates and Complications. CVC via the EJV is successful in 80% of patients (range 75% to 95%) [78,106,107]. Inability to perform venipuncture accounts for up to 10% of failures [106,108,109], and the remainder are a result of catheter tip malpositioning. Failure to position the catheter tip is usually due to inability to negotiate the EJV-SV junction, loop formation, or retrograde passage down the ipsilateral arm.

Serious complications arising from the EJV approach are rare and almost always associated with catheter maintenance rather than venipuncture. A local hematoma forms in 1% to 5% of patients at the time of venipuncture [106,109,110] but has little consequence unless it distorts the anatomy, leading to catheterization failure. External jugular venipuncture is safe in the presence of coagulopathy. Infectious, thrombotic, and other mechanical complications are no more frequent than with other central routes.

FEMORAL VEIN APPROACH. The FV has many practical advantages for CVC; it is directly compressible, it is remote from the airway and pleura, the technique is relatively simple, and Trendelenburg's position is not required during insertion. FV catheterization was a common site for CVC in the 1950s but was largely abandoned after 1959, when Moncrief [5] and Bansmer et al. [6] reported a high incidence of complications, especially infection and thrombosis. In the subsequent two decades, FV cannulation was restricted to specialized clinical situations. Interest in short-term (less than 48 hours) FV catheterization was renewed by positive experiences during the Vietnam Conflict and with patients in the emergency department [111,112]. Reports on long-term FV catheterization [21,57,113–115] suggest an overall complication rate that is no higher than that with other routes, although deep vein thrombosis remains a legitimate concern.

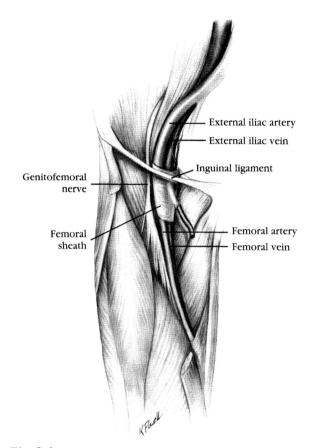

Fig. 2-4. Anatomy of the femoral vein.

Anatomy. The FV (Fig. 2-4) is a direct continuation of the popliteal vein and becomes the external iliac vein at the inguinal ligament. At the inguinal ligament the FV lies within the femoral sheath a few centimeters from the skin surface. Within the intermediate compartment of the sheath, the FV lies medial to the femoral artery, which in turn lies medial to the femoral branch of the genitofemoral nerve. The medial compartment contains lymphatic channels and Cloquet's node. The external iliac vein courses cephalad from the inguinal ligament along the anterior surface of the iliopsoas muscle to join its counterpart from the other leg and form the interior vena cava anterior to and to the right of the fifth lumbar vertebra [69,70].

Technique. FV cannulation is the easiest of all central venous procedures to learn and perform. Either side is suitable, and the side chosen is based on operator convenience. The patient is placed in the supine position (if tolerated) with the leg extended and slightly abducted at the hip. Excessive hair should be clipped with scissors and the skin prepped in standard fashion. The FV lies 1.0 to 1.5 cm medial to the arterial pulsation, and the overlying skin is infiltrated with 1% lidocaine. In a patient without femoral artery pulsations, the FV can be located by dividing the distance between the anterior superior iliac spine and the pubic tubercle is divided into three equal segments [111]. The femoral artery is usually found where the medial segment meets the two lateral ones, and the FV lies 1.0 to 1.5 cm medial. An 18-gauge thin-wall needle is inserted at this point, 2 to 3 cm inferior to the inguinal ligament, ensuring that venipuncture occurs caudal to the inguinal ligament and minimizing the risk of retroperitoneal hematoma in the event of arterial puncture. While maintaining constant back pressure on the syringe, the needle, tip pointed cephalad,

is advanced at a 45- to 60-degree angle to the frontal plane. Insertion of the needle to its hub is sometimes required in obese patients. Venipuncture may not occur until slow withdrawal. If the initial attempt is unsuccessful, landmarks should be reevaluated and subsequent thrusts oriented slightly more medial or lateral. A common error is to direct the needle tip too medially, toward the umbilicus. The femoral vessels lie in the sagittal plane at the inguinal ligament (Fig. 2-4), and the needle should be directed accordingly. If inadvertent arterial puncture occurs, pressure is applied for 5 to 10 minutes.

When venous blood return is established, the syringe is depressed to skin level and free aspiration of blood reconfirmed. The syringe is removed, ensuring that blood return is not pulsatile. The guidewire should pass easily and never forced, although rotation and minor manipulation are sometimes required. The needle is then withdrawn, two scalpel blade stab incisions made at 90 degrees above the guidewire insertion site, and the vein dilator inserted over the wire to the hub. The dilator is then withdrawn and a catheter appropriate to clinical requirements inserted, taking care never to lose control of the guidewire. The catheter is secured with a suture, and antiseptic ointment and a bandage are applied.

Success Rate and Complications. FV catheterization is successful in 90% to 95% of patients, including those in shock or cardiopulmonary arrest [111,113,115–117]. Unsuccessful catheterizations are usually a result of venipuncture failure, hematoma formation, or inability to advance the guidewire into the vein. Operator inexperience may increase the number of attempts and complication rate but does not significantly decrease the overall success rate [113].

Only three complications occur regularly with FV catheterization: arterial puncture with or without local bleeding, infection, and thromboembolic events. Other reported complications are rare and include scrotal hemorrhage, right lower quadrant bowel perforation, retroperitoneal hemorrhage, puncture of the kidney, and perforation of inferior vena cava tributaries. These complications occur when skin puncture sites are cephalad to the inguinal ligament or when long catheters are threaded into the FV.

Femoral artery puncture occurs in 5% to 10% of adults [111,113,116]. Most arterial punctures are uncomplicated, but major hematomas may form in 1% of patients [111,113]. Even in the presence of coagulopathy, arterial puncture with the 18-gauge thin-wall needle is usually of no consequence, with only rare reports of life-threatening thigh or retroperitoneal hemorrhage [117,118]. Arteriovenous fistula and pseudoaneurysm are rare chronic complications of arterial puncture; the former is more likely to occur when both femoral vessels on the same side are cannulated concurrently [119].

Infectious complications probably occur more frequently with FV catheters than with SV catheters but are comparable to those with IJV catheters [18,120,121]. Series involving short- and long-term FV catheterization in adults and children have reported significant catheter-related infection (CRI) rates of approximately 5% or less [111,113,115,122]. Further evidence that the inguinal site is not inherently "dirty" is provided by experience with femoral artery catheters, which have an infection rate comparable to that with radial artery catheters [123].

The most feared complication of FV catheterization is deep venous thrombosis of the lower extremity. Two reports in 1958 [5,6] highlighted the high incidence of FV catheter-associated deep vein thrombosis, but these studies were primarily autopsy based and before modern technological advances. Catheter-associated thrombosis is a risk of all central venous catheters, regardless of the site of insertion, and comparative studies using contrast venography, impedance plethysmography, or Doppler ultrasound suggest that FV cath-

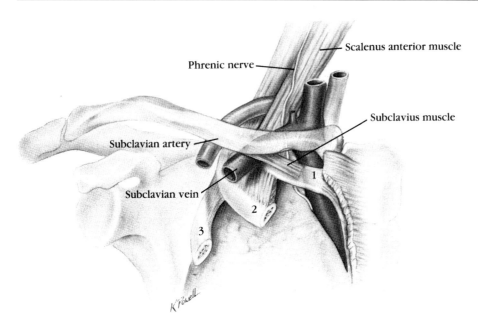

Fig. 2-5. Anatomy of the subclavian vein and adjacent structures.

eters are no more prone to thrombosis than upper extremity catheters [21,50,52,53,55,57]. Pulmonary emboli have been reported following CVC-associated upper extremity thrombosis [55,124], and the relative risk of femoral catheter-related thrombosis is unknown. Clearly, the potential thromboembolic complications of FV catheters cannot be discounted [125], but they do not warrant total abandonment of this approach. In patients at high risk for thrombotic complications, serial impedance plethysmography can be used to screen for femoral catheter-associated thrombosis [57,126].

In summary, available evidence supports the view that the FV can be cannulated safely in critically ill adults. It is particularly useful for inexperienced operators because of the high rate of success and lower incidence of major complications. FV catheterizations can be performed during airway emergencies and cardiopulmonary arrest, in patients with coagulopathy, and in patients who are unable to lie flat. The only major complication during venipuncture is arterial puncture, which is usually easily managed. Infection is no more common than with IJV catheters. Catheter-associated thrombosis occurs with similar frequency as with IJ and SV catheters but is likely more clinically relevant. Additional, well-controlled studies are needed.

SUBCLAVIAN VEIN APPROACH. Since Aubaniac [3] described the use of subclavian venipuncture in humans, controversy has surrounded this route of access to the central circulation. The 1962 report by Wilson et al. [8] generated much enthusiasm for SV catheterization, but soon the large number of serious complications, some fatal, resulted in some investigators urging a moratorium on the procedure [127]. A 1994 report indicated that little changed over 30 years [128,129]. The controversy involving SV catheterization derives from the significant impact of operator experience on the incidence of complications. Experienced operators have a pneumothorax rate of 1% or less and can justify use of the SV as primary central venous access in almost all patients. Inexperienced operators have a far greater rate of pneumothorax; therefore, in settings in which relatively inexperienced physicians perform the majority of CVCs, the SV should be used selectively [128]. The advantages of this route include consistent identifiable landmarks, easier long-term catheter maintenance with a comparably lower rate of infection, and relatively high patient comfort. Assuming that an experienced operator is available, the SV is the preferred site for CVC in patients with hypovolemia, for long-term total parenteral nutrition, and in patients with elevated intracranial pressure who require hemodynamic monitoring.

Anatomy. The SV is a direct continuation of the axillary vein, beginning at the lateral border of the first rib, extending 3 to 4 cm along the undersurface of the clavicle and becoming the brachiocephalic vein where it joins the ipsilateral IJV at Pirogoff's confluence behind the sternoclavicular articulation [69,70] (Fig. 2-5). The vein is 1 to 2 cm in diameter, contains a single set of valves just distal to the EJV junction, and is fixed in position directly beneath the clavicle by its fibrous attachments. These attachments prevent collapse of the vein, even with severe volume depletion. Anterior to the vein throughout its course lies the subclavius muscle, clavicle, costoclavicular ligament, pectoralis muscles, and epidermis. Posteriorly, the SV is separated from the subclavian artery and brachial plexus by the anterior scalenus muscle, which is 10 to 15 mm thick in the adult. Posterior to the medial portion of the SV are the phrenic nerve and internal mammary artery as they pass into the thorax. Superiorly, the relationships are the skin, platysma, and superficial aponeurosis. Inferiorly, the vein rests on the first rib, Sibson's fascia, the cupola of the pleura (0.5 cm behind the vein), and the pulmonary apex [130]. The thoracic ducts on the left and right lymphatic duct cross the anterior scalene muscle to join the superior aspect of the SV near its union with the IJV.

Technique. Although there are many variations, the SV can be cannulated by two basic techniques: the infraclavicular [3,8,10,130,131] or supraclavicular [132–134] approach (Fig. 2-6). The differences in success rate, catheter tip malposition, and complications between the two approaches are negligible, although catheter tip malposition and pneumothorax may be less likely to occur with supraclavicular cannulation [135,136]. In general, when discussing the success rate and incidence of complications of SV catheterization, there is no need to specify the approach used.

The 18-gauge thin-wall needle is preferable for SV cannulation [104]. The patient is placed in a 15- to 30-degree Trendelenburg's position, with a small bedroll between the shoulder blades. The head is turned gently to the contralateral side, and the arms are kept to the side. The pertinent landmarks are the clavicle, the two muscle bellies of the SCM, the suprasternal notch, and the manubriosternal junc-

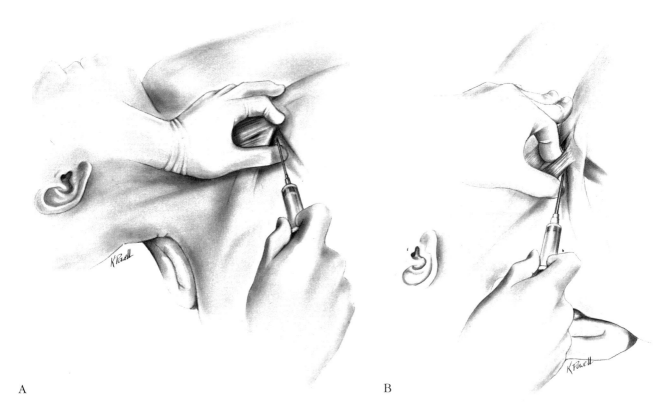

Fig. 2-6. A: Patient positioning for subclavian cannulation. **B:** Cannulation technique for supraclavicular approach.

tion. For the infraclavicular approach (Fig. 2-6), the operator is positioned next to the patient's shoulder on the side to be cannulated. For reasons cited earlier, the left SV should be chosen for pulmonary artery catheterization; otherwise, the success rate appears to be equivalent regardless of the side chosen. Skin puncture is 2 to 3 cm caudal to the midpoint of the clavicle, corresponding to the area where the clavicle turns from the shoulder to the manubrium. Skin puncture should be distant enough from the clavicle to avoid a downward angle of the needle in clearing the inferior surface of the clavicle, which also obviates the need to bend the needle. The path of the needle is toward the suprasternal notch or the medial end of the contralateral clavicle. After skin infiltration and liberal injection of the clavicular periosteum with 1% lidocaine, the 18-gauge thin-wall needle is mounted on a 10-mL syringe filled with saline. Skin puncture is accomplished with the needle bevel up, and a small amount of saline is expressed to eliminate any possible skin plug. The needle is advanced in the plane described above until the tip abuts the clavicle. The needle is then "walked" down the clavicle until the inferior edge is cleared.

As the needle is advanced further, the inferior surface of the clavicle should be felt hugging the needle. This ensures that the needle tip is as superior as possible to the pleura. The needle is advanced toward the suprasternal notch during breath holding or expiration, and venipuncture occurs when the needle tip lies beneath the medial end of the clavicle. This may require insertion of the needle to its hub. Venipuncture may not occur until slow withdrawal of the needle. If venipuncture is not accomplished on the initial thrust, the next attempt should be directed slightly more cephalad. If venipuncture does not occur by the third or fourth attempt, another site should be chosen, as additional attempts are unlikely to be successful and may result in complications [128].

When blood return is established, the bevel of the needle is rotated 90 degrees toward the heart. The needle is anchored firmly with the left hand while the syringe is detached with the right. Blood return should not be pulsatile, and air embolism prophylaxis is necessary at all times. The guidewire is then advanced through the needle to 15 cm and the needle withdrawn. The remainder of the procedure is as previously described. Triple-lumen catheters should be sutured at 16 to 17 cm on the right and 18 to 19 cm on the left to avoid intracardiac tip placement [38–40,137].

For the supraclavicular approach (Fig. 2-6), the important landmarks are the clavicular insertion of the SCM muscle and the sternoclavicular joint. The operator is positioned at the head of the patient on the side to be cannulated. The site of skin puncture is the claviculosternocleidomastoid angle, just above the clavicle and lateral to the insertion of the clavicular head of the SCM. The needle is advanced toward or just caudal to the contralateral nipple just under the clavicle. This corresponds to a 45-degree angle to the sagittal plane, bisecting a line between the sternoclavicular joint and clavicular insertion of the SCM [134]. The depth of insertion is from just beneath the SCM clavicular head at a 10- to 15-degree angle below the coronal plane. The needle should enter the jugulosubclavian venous bulb after 1 to 4 cm, and the operator can then proceed with catheterization.

Success and Complication Rates. SV catheterization is successful in 90% to 95% of cases, generally on the first attempt [128,131,138]. The presence of shock does not alter the success rate as significantly as it does during IJV catheterization [138]. Unsuccessful catheterizations are a result of venipuncture failure or inability to advance the guidewire or catheter [79,131]. Catheter tip malposition occurs in 5% to 20% of cases [79,131,135,138] and tends to be more frequent with the infraclavicular approach [79,131]. Malposition occurs most commonly to the ipsilateral IJV and contralateral SV and is usually correctable without repeat venipuncture.

The overall incidence of noninfectious complications varies depending on the operator's experience and the circumstances under which the catheter is inserted. Large series involving several thousand SV catheters have reported an incidence of major complications of 1% to 3%, with an overall rate of 5% [130,131]. In smaller, probably more clinically relevant studies, the major complication rate has ranged from 1% to 10% [79,111,128,138–140]. Factors resulting in a higher complication rate are operator inexperience, multiple attempts at venipuncture, emergency conditions, variance from standardized technique, and body mass index [128]. Major noninfectious complications include pneumothorax, arterial puncture, and thromboembolism. Many cases of isolated major complications involving neck structures or the brachial plexus have been reported; the reader is referred elsewhere for a complete listing of reported complications [141].

Pneumothorax accounts for one-fourth to one-half of reported complications, with an incidence of 1% to 5% [111,128,131,138,142,143]. The incidence varies inversely with the operator's experience and the number of "breaks" in technique [91,128,135,136,138–140]. No magic figure has been ascertained whereby an operator matures from inexperienced to experienced. Fifty catheterizations is cited frequently as a cutoff number, but it is reasonable to expect an operator to be satisfactorily experienced after having performed fewer. For the experienced operator, a pneumothorax incidence of less than 1% is expected. Most pneumothoraces are a result of lung puncture at the time of the procedure, but late-appearing pneumothoraces have been reported, and it is good practice to obtain a chest radiograph the day after the procedure.

Most pneumothoraces require thoracostomy tube drainage with a small chest tube and a Heimlich valve, but some can be managed conservatively with needle aspiration only [131,138,144]. Rarely, a pneumothorax is complicated by tension, heme, infusion of intravenous fluid (immediately or days to weeks after catheter placement), chyle, and massive subcutaneous emphysema. Bilateral pneumothoraces can occur from unilateral attempts at venipuncture. Pneumothorax, especially when it goes unrecognized, can result in death [145].

Subclavian artery puncture occurs in 0.5% to 1.0% of cases, constituting one-fourth to one-third of all complications [79,111,131,140]. Arterial puncture is usually managed easily by applying pressure above and below the clavicle. Bleeding can be catastrophic in patients with coagulopathy. As with other routes, arterial puncture may result in arteriovenous fistula or pseudoaneurysm.

Clinical evidence of central venous thrombosis, including SVC syndrome, development of collaterals around the shoulder girdle, and pulmonary embolism, occurs in 0% to 3% of SV catheterizations [21,49,50,52,53,55,146], but routine phlebography performed at catheter removal reveals a much higher incidence of thrombotic phenomena. The importance of the discrepancy between clinical symptoms and radiologic findings is unknown, but it exists for all routes of CVC. Duration of catheterization, catheter material, and patient condition may have an impact on the frequency of thrombosis, but to an uncertain degree.

In summary, the SV is an extremely reliable and useful route for CVC, but it has significant limitations. It should not be the primary choice in patients at high risk for bronchopleural fistula after lung puncture, in individuals who cannot tolerate a pneumothorax (severe lung disease, one lung), or in patients with severe coagulopathy. Inexperienced operators should be closely supervised and not be allowed to perform SV catheterization independently.

Infectious Complications

Tremendous advances in the understanding of the pathophysiology, causes, and prevention of CRI have occurred in recent years and have led to corresponding dramatic improvements in catheter technology, insertion, and management. In our ICU, we have achieved a dramatic reduction in CRIs by implementing an annual comprehensive standardized catheter educational seminar designed for the housestaff and other interested physicians [147], as well as incorporating some of the newer technological advances. Table 2-2 summarizes current recommendations or interventions that have been shown to reduce the risk of CRI. This section reviews these recommendations, focusing on the epidemiology, pathogenesis, diagnosis, management, and prevention of central CRI. A review is available for the reader who is interested in a more comprehensive discussion of intravascular device-related infections [148].

DEFINITIONS AND EPIDEMIOLOGY. Consensus regarding the definition and diagnosis of CRI is a necessary initial step in discussing catheter-related infectious complications. The semiquantitative culture method described by Maki et al. [149] for culturing catheter segments is the most accepted technique for diagnosing CRI. Which catheter segment to culture (the tip or intradermal segment) is still controversial; most centers routinely culture the catheter tip. Alternative methods to diagnose CRI include quantitative culture [149] and direct Gram's [150] or acridine-orange staining [151] of catheters. If semiquantitative methods are used, catheter contamination (probably occurring at time of withdrawal) is defined as less than 15 colony-forming units per culture plate. CRI is defined as greater than 15 colony-forming units and is identified as colonization (all other cultures negative and no clinical symptoms), local or exit-site infection (skin site with erythema, cellulitis, or purulence), catheter-related bacteremia (systemic blood cultures positive for identical organism on catheter segment and no other source), and catheter-related sepsis or septic shock.

The morbidity and mortality associated with CRI are truly impressive. Estimates vary, but overall more than 5 million CVCs are inserted annually in the United States, with 850,000 total episodes of CRI [152], of which at least 60,000 to 80,000 are associated with bacteremia [148,153,154]. The National Nosocomial Infection Surveillance System reports rates of CVC-related bloodstream infection averaging 5.3 per 1,000 catheter day [155]. The attributable mortality of catheter-

Table 2-2. Steps to Minimize Central Venous Catheterization (CVC)–Related Infection

Institution-supported standardized education of all physicians involved in CVC insertion and care

Strict protocols for catheter maintenance (including bandage and tubing changes), preferably by dedicated IV catheter team

Site preparation with approved chlorhexidine-based preparation

Appropriate site selection, avoiding heavily colonized or anatomically abnormal areas; use subclavian vein for anticipated CVC of >4 d

Maximal barrier precautions during catheter insertion

For anticipated duration of catheterization exceeding 96 h, use of silver-impregnated cuff, sustained-release chlorhexidine gluconate patch, and/or antibiotic-/antiseptic-impregnated catheters

Remove pulmonary artery catheters and introducers after 5 d

Use multilumen catheters only when indicated; remove when no longer needed

Avoid "routine" guidewire exchanges

Use surgically implanted catheters or peripherally inserted central catheters for long-term (i.e., >3 wk) or permanent CVC

related bloodstream infection is approximately 14% to 28% [156–159], and the added cost is as high as $40,000 per survivor [158]. These figures are a powerful impetus for critical care physicians to do everything possible to minimize CRI.

PATHOPHYSIOLOGY OF CATHETER INFECTION.
Assuming that they are not contaminated during insertion (see below), catheters can become infected from four potential sources: the skin insertion site, the catheter hub(s), hematogenous seeding, and infusate contamination. Animal and human studies have shown that catheters are most commonly infected by bacteria colonizing the skin site, followed by invasion of the intradermal catheter tract. Once the external surface of the intradermal catheter is infected, bacteria can quickly traverse the entire length and infect the catheter tip, sometimes encasing the catheter in a slime layer known as a *biofilm* (coagulase-negative staphyococcus). From the catheter tip, bacteria may shed into the bloodstream, potentially creating metastatic foci of infection [153,160,161]. The pathophysiology of most catheter infections explains why guidewire exchanges are not effective in preventing or treating CRI: The colonized tract and, in many cases, biofilm, remain intact and quickly reinfect the new catheter [162].

The catheter hub(s) also become(s) colonized but contribute(s) to catheter-related infectious complications less frequently than the insertion site [163–165]. Hub contamination may be relatively more important as a source of infection the longer the catheter remains in place [166]. Hematogenous seeding of catheters from bacteremia is an infrequent cause of CRI.

SITE PREPARATION AND CATHETER MAINTENANCE.
That the majority of CRIs are caused by skin flora highlights the importance of site sterility during insertion and catheter maintenance. Organisms that colonize the insertion site originate from the patient's own skin flora or the hands of operators. Catheters are frequently contaminated at the time of insertion, and scrupulous attention to aseptic technique is mandatory. Thorough hand-washing and wearing sterile gloves are mandatory for persons involved in catheter insertion or care. A prospective study proved that a nonsterile cap and mask, sterile gown, and a large drape covering the patient's head and body (maximal sterile barriers, compared to sterile gloves and small drape) reduced the catheter-related bloodstream infection rate sixfold and were highly cost effective [167]. If a break in sterile technique occurs during insertion, termination of the procedure and replacement of contaminated equipment are mandatory.

Iodine-containing disinfectants, such as 10% povidone-iodine, are the most commonly used skin disinfectants, but comparative studies have demonstrated the superiority of chlorhexidine preparations [168,169]. Chlorhexidine is now available for use in the United States and is the disinfectant of choice. Proper application includes liberally scrubbing the site using expanding concentric circles. Excessive hair should be clipped with scissors before application of the antiseptic, as shaving can cause minor skin lacerations and disruption of the epidermal barrier to infection.

Care of the catheter after insertion is extremely important in minimizing infection, and all medical personnel should follow standardized protocols [170,171]. The number of piggyback infusions and medical personnel handling tubing changes and manipulation of the catheter site should be minimized. Replacement of administration sets every 72 to 96 hours is safe and cost efficient [172], unless there are specific recommendations for the infusate (e.g., propofol). The use of transparent, semiocclusive dressings is prevalent, but these may actually increase the risk of site colonization because of moisture trapping, and no dressing has been proved to be superior to gauze and tape

[173]. Application of iodophor or polymicrobial ointments to the skin site at the time of insertion or during dressing changes does not convincingly reduce the overall incidence of catheter infection, and certain polymicrobial ointments may increase the proportion of *Candida* infections [174,175].

FREQUENCY OF CATHETER-ASSOCIATED INFECTION.
Observing the above recommendations for catheter insertion and maintenance will minimize but not eliminate catheter-associated infection. Colonization of the insertion site can begin within 24 hours and increases with duration of catheterization; 10% to 40% of catheters eventually become colonized [163,165,167,168,176]. Catheter-associated bacteremia and sepsis occur in 3% to 8% of catheters [2,18,120,163,165,167,168,176,177–179], although some studies incorporating newer catheter technologies and procedures have demonstrated rates of catheter-associated bacteremia of 2% or less [163,167,180–183]. Bacteremia is a significant complication, extending hospitalization, adding to cost, and resulting in metastatic infection and death in a significant percentage of patients [156–158,177,184]. Gram-positive organisms, especially coagulase-negative *Staphylococcus* species, are the most common infecting agents, but gram-negative enteric organisms are not rare. *Candida* species are more likely in certain clinical situations, such as the diabetic patient with prolonged catheterization on broad-spectrum antibiotics.

TYPE OF CATHETER.
The data presented above are derived from large studies and are not necessarily applicable to any given catheter because of variations in definitions, types of catheters, site of insertion, duration of catheterization, types of fluid infused, and policies regarding routine guidewire changes, all of which have been implicated at some point as important factors in the incidence of catheter-associated infection. The duration of catheterization in combination with the type of catheter are major factors; the site of insertion is less important. Guidewire changes have an important role in evaluation of the febrile catheterized patient, but routine guidewire changes do not prevent infection. Under ideal conditions, all of these factors are less important. Long-term total parenteral nutrition catheters can be maintained for months with low rates of infection, and there is no cutoff time at which colonization and clinical infection accelerate. Today, when the need for long-term catheterization is anticipated, surgically implanted catheters should be used. These catheters have low infection rates and are never changed routinely [185]. PICCs also appear to be an acceptable option for patients who require long-term CVC [73–75].

Catheters inserted percutaneously in the critical care unit, however, are not subject to ideal conditions and have a finite lifespan. For practical purposes, multilumen catheters have replaced single-lumen catheters for many indications for central venous access. Because catheter hubs are a potential source of infection and triple-lumen catheters can require three times the number of tubing changes, it was widely believed that they would have a higher infection rate. Studies have presented conflicting results, but overall the data support the view that triple-lumen catheters have a modestly higher rate of infection [176,186–189]. If used efficiently, however, they provide greater intravascular access per device and can decrease the total number of catheter days and exposure to central venipuncture. A slight increase in infection rate per catheter is therefore justifiable from an overall risk-benefit analysis if multilumen catheters are used only when multiple infusion ports are truly indicated.

Finally, it was hoped that routine subcutaneous tunneling of short-term central venous catheters, similar to long-term catheters, might be an effective way to minimize CRI. This approach is rational because the long subcutaneous tract acts to stabilize the catheter and perhaps act as a barrier to bacterial invasion, and great technical skill is not required. A meta-analysis did not support the routine practice of tunneling all percutaneously inserted CVCs [190], and it is not a common practice. However, further studies of the tunneling of short-term IJV and FV catheters is warranted, because these sites have a higher infection rate and past studies have generally favored this approach [190].

DURATION OF CATHETERIZATION. How long to leave catheters in place remains somewhat controversial, but evidence is mounting that multilumen catheters, especially if they are antiseptic coated or antibiotic impregnated, should remain in place routinely longer than 96 hours. Although changing triple-lumen catheters to a new site every 72 to 96 hours minimizes infection, it also increases mechanical complications associated with insertion. Data suggest that the daily risk of infection remains relatively constant and routine replacement of CVCs without a clinical indication does not reduce the rate of CRI [2,191,192]. Multiple clinical and experimental studies have also demonstrated that guidewire exchanges are not an effective method of infection control [2,162,191–194]. Every ICU should have its own protocol governing duration of catheterization that is based on its unique patient population and practice environment. Until additional data are available, many intensivists remain uncomfortable leaving multilumen catheters in place indefinitely, especially in critically ill patients with multiorgan dysfunction. Based on current information, it is reasonable to leave triple-lumen catheters in place for at least 6 to 7 days before changing to a new site. For selected patients, especially those at increased risk for complications from central venipuncture, triple-lumen catheters can be left in place for longer than a week, especially in the subclavian position.

The above recommendations do not necessarily apply to other special-use catheters, which can be exposed to different clinical situations and risk. Pulmonary artery catheters and the introducer should be removed after 96 to 120 hours because of the increased risk of infection after this time [176,195–198]. These catheters are at greater risk for infection because patients are sicker, the introducer used for insertion is shorter, and catheter manipulations are frequent [198].

Catheters inserted for acute temporary hemodialysis historically have had a higher rate of infection than other percutaneously placed catheters. Factors contributing to the increased rate have not been completely elucidated, but logically patient factors probably influence the incidence of infection more than the type of catheter or site of insertion. For acutely ill, hospitalized patients, temporary dialysis catheters should be managed similarly to other multilumen catheters. For ambulatory outpatients, long-term experience with double-lumen, Dacron-cuffed, silicone CVCs inserted in the IJV has been positive [199].

SITE OF INSERTION. The condition of the site is more important than the location. Whenever possible, sites involved by infection, burns, or other dermatologic processes, or in close proximity to a heavily colonized area (e.g., tracheostomy), should not be used as primary access. Data tend to support the fact that PICC and SV catheters are associated with the lowest rate of CRI, and IJV and FV catheters with the highest rate [18,120,148,153,200].

GUIDEWIRE EXCHANGES. Guidewire exchanges have always been theoretically flawed as a form of infection control, because, although a new catheter is placed, the site, specifically the intradermal tract, remains the same. Studies have shown that when the tract and old catheter are colonized, the new catheter invariably also becomes infected [162,195]. Alternatively, if the initial catheter is not colonized, there is no reason that the new catheter will be more resistant to subsequent infection than the original one. In neither situation does a guidewire change prevent infection [191,192]. However, guidewire changes continue to have a valuable role for replacing defective catheters, exchanging one type of catheter for another, and evaluating a febrile patient with an existing central catheter. In the latter situation, the physician can assess the sterility of the catheter tract without subjecting the patient to a new venipuncture, as detailed below. However one decides to use guidewire exchanges, they must be performed properly. Using maximal barriers, the catheter should be withdrawn until an intravascular segment is exposed, transected sterilely, and the guidewire inserted through the distal lumen. The catheter fragment can then be removed (always culture the tip) and a new catheter threaded over the guidewire. To ensure sterility, most operators should reprep the site and change gloves before inserting the new catheter or introducer over the guidewire. Insertion of the guidewire through the distal hub of the existing catheter is not appropriate.

New Catheter Technologies

Improvements in catheter technology continue to play an important role in minimizing catheter complications. Catheter material is an important factor in promoting thrombogenesis and adherence of organisms. Most catheters used for CVC are composed of flexible silicone (for surgical implantation) and polyurethane (for percutaneous insertion), because research has shown that these materials are less thrombogenic. Knowledge of the pathogenesis of most CRIs has stimulated improvements designed to interrupt bacterial colonization of the skin site, catheter, and intradermal tract and migration to the catheter tip. Two principal developments have resulted: the Vita-Cuff and antiseptic bonding or antibiotic impregnation of catheters. The Vita-Cuff has been effective in clinical trials [163,181] but has not gained widespread acceptance. On the other hand, antibiotic- and antiseptic-coated and impregnated catheters represent a major advance in catheter management. The catheters differ from one another in that one is coated with the antiseptics silver sulfadiazine and chlorhexidine (Arrowguard Blue, Arrow International, Reading, PA), whereas the other is impregnated with the antibiotics minocycline and rifampin (Cook Spectrum, Cook Critical Care, Bloomington, IN), which also protect the inner lumens. Clinical results with these commercially available catheters have been impressive, with a significant reduction in colonization and bacteremia [63,120,148,178–180,182,183,201–204]. Direct comparisons of the two catheter types have generally favored the minocycline-rifampin combination [205,206], but the silver sulfadiazine-chlorhexidine catheter is now also available in an impregnated form, and further studies are needed. When used appropriately, these catheters are cost effective and prolong the duration of safe catheterization [63,120,178], The emergence of resistant organisms and allergic reactions has not yet been a problem, but ongoing surveillance is needed. Likewise, other

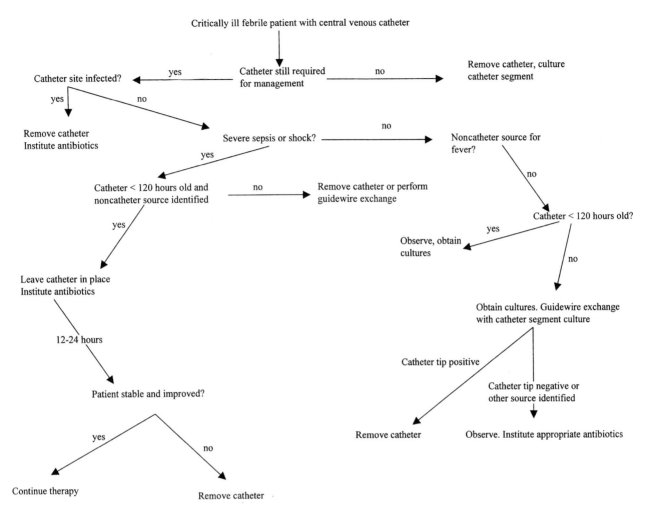

Fig. 2-7. Recommended approach to the catheterized patient with fever. Assumes use of antiseptic-coated or antibiotic-impregnated catheters.

catheter technologies currently being developed will require clinical validation before their impact is known.

Management of the Febrile Patient

Fever frequently develops in patients with a central venous catheter. Removal of the catheter in every febrile patient is neither feasible nor clinically indicated, because the fever is often unrelated to the catheter. Management must be individualized (Fig. 2-7) and depends on type of catheter, duration of catheterization, anticipated need for continued central venous access, risk of establishing new central venous access, and underlying medical condition and prognosis. All critical care units must have protocols for managing the febrile, catheterized patient. Decisions to withdraw, change over a guidewire, or leave catheters in place must be based on a fundamental knowledge of risks and benefits for catheters inserted at each site.

Catheter sites in the febrile patient should always be examined. Clinical infection of the site mandates removal of the catheter and institution of antibiotics. Surgically implanted catheters are not easily removed or replaced and can often be left in place while the infection is cleared with antibiotics, unless tunnel infec-

tion is present [185]. Percutaneously inserted central venous catheters are relatively easily removed, and the risks of leaving a catheter in place through an infected site outweigh the risk of replacement at a new site, except in very unusual circumstances.

In patients with severe sepsis or septic shock, central venous catheters should be considered a possible source. If all catheter sites appear normal and a noncatheter site can be implicated as the source for infection, appropriate antibiotics are initiated and the catheters left in place. The usual guidelines for subsequent catheter management should be followed, and this rarely results in treatment failure. In contrast, if a noncatheter source cannot be identified, central catheters that are in place for more than a few days should be managed individually, with attention to duration of catheterization (Fig. 2-7). For patients with excessive risks for new catheter placement (i.e., severe coagulopathy), guidewire exchange of the catheter is justifiable after obtaining blood cultures through the catheter and a peripheral site and semiquantitative culture of a catheter segment. If, within the next 24 hours, an alternative source for sepsis is found, or if the catheter segment culture is negative and the patient's condition improves and stabilizes, the guidewire catheter can be left in place and a risky procedure avoided. Alternatively, if the catheter culture becomes positive, especially if the same organism is identified on peripheral blood cultures, the cutaneous tract is also infected and the guidewire catheter should be removed and alternative access achieved.

The most common situation is the stable febrile patient with a central venous catheter in place. As above, if a noncatheter source for fever is identified, appropriate antibiotics are given and the catheter is left in place, assuming that it is still needed and the site is clinically uninvolved. In the patient with no obvious source of fever, indications for the central venous catheters should be reviewed and the catheter withdrawn if it is no longer required. Otherwise, the physician must decide between observation, potential premature withdrawal, or a guidewire change of the catheter. If the catheter is less than 120 hours old, observation is reasonable, as it is very unlikely that the catheter is already infected unless breaks in sterile technique occurred during insertion [2]. For catheters that are at least 120 hours old, guidewire exchanges are rational. An appropriately performed guidewire change allows comparison of catheter segment cultures to other clinical cultures without subjecting the patient to repeat venipuncture. If, within the next 24 hours, an alternative source for fever is identified or the initial catheter segment culture is negative, or both, the guidewire catheter can be left in place. Further management decisions regarding the catheter are complicated, but multiple guidewire changes of the same insertion site are not advisable.

When catheter-related bacteremia does develop, antibiotic therapy is necessary for a period of 7 to 14 days. Even in patients who are treated for 14 days, metastatic infection can develop. Catheter-related fever, infection, and septicemia are complicated diseases, and the expertise of an infectious disease consultant may be required to assist with the decision on how long to continue antibiotic therapy [184].

References

1. Vergis EN, Hayden MK, Chow JW, et al: Determinants of vancomycin resistance and mortality rates in enterococcal bacteremia. *Ann Intern Med* 135:484, 2001.
2. Civetta JM, Hudson-Civetta J, Ball S: Decreasing catheter-related infection and hospital costs by continuous quality improvement. *Crit Care Med* 24:1660, 1996.
3. Aubaniac R: L'injection intraveneuse sousclaviculare advantage et technique. *Presse Med* 60:1456, 1952.
4. Seldinger SI: Catheter replacement of the needle in percutaneous arteriography: a new technique. *Acta Radiol* 39:368, 1953.
5. Moncrief JA: Femoral catheters. *Ann Surg* 147:166, 1958.
6. Bansmer G, Keith D, Tesluk H: Complications following use of indwelling catheters of inferior vena cava. *JAMA* 167:1606, 1958.
7. Hughes RE, Magovern GJ: The relationship between right atrial pressure and blood volume. *Arch Surg* 79:238, 1959.
8. Wilson JN, Grow JB, Demong CV, et al: Central venous pressure in optimal blood volume maintenance. *Arch Surg* 85:55, 1962.
9. Yoffa D: Supraclavicular subclavian venipuncture and catheterization. *Lancet* 2:614, 1965.
10. Linos DA, Mucha P, Van Heerden JA: Subclavian vein: a golden route. *Mayo Clin Proc* 55:315, 1980.
11. Nordlund S, Thoren L: Catheter in the superior vena cava for parenteral feeding. *Acta Chir Scand* 127:39, 1964.
12. Rams JJ, Dalcoff GR, Moulder PV: A simple method for central venous pressure measurements. *Arch Surg* 92:886, 1966.
13. English ICW, Frew RM, Pigott JF, et al: Percutaneous cannulation of the internal jugular vein. *Thorax* 24:496, 1969.
14. Merrell SW, Peatross BG, Grossman MD, et al: Peripherally inserted central venous catheters: low-risk alternatives for ongoing venous access. *West J Med* 160:25, 1994.
15. Ng PK, Ault NU, Maldonado LS: Peripherally inserted central catheters in the intensive care unit. *J Intensive Care Med* 11:49,1996.
16. Lam S, Scannell R, Roessler D, et al: Peripherally inserted central catheters in an acute-care hospital. *Arch Intern Med* 154:1833, 1994.
17. Graber D, Dailey RH: Catheter flow rates updated. *JACEP* 6:518, 1977.
18. Merrer J, De Jonghe B, Golliot F, et. al: Complications of femoral and subclavian venous catheterization in critically ill patients. *JAMA* 286:700, 2001.
19. Trottier SJ, Veramakis C, O'Brien J, et al: Femoral deep vein thrombosis associated with central venous catheterization. *Crit Care Med* 23:52, 1995.
20. Joynt GM, Kew J, Gomersall CD, et al: Deep venous thrombosis caused by femoral venous catheters in critically ill adult patients. *Chest* 117:178, 2000.
21. Durbec O, Viviand X, Potie F, et al: A prospective, randomized, controlled trial in comatose or sedated patients undergoing femoral vein catheterization. *Crit Care Med* 25:1982, 1997.
22. Schwab SJ, Quarles D, Middleton JP, et al: Hemodialysis-associated subclavian vein stenosis. *Kidney Int* 38:1156, 1988.
23. Cimochowski G, Sartain J, Worley E, et al: Clear superiority of internal jugular access over the subclavian vein for temporary dialysis. *Kidney Int* 33:230, 1987.
24. Khanna S, Sniderman K, Simons M, et al: Superior vena cava stenosis associated with hemodialysis catheters. *Am J Kidney Dis* 21:278, 1993.
25. Surratt RS, Picus D, Hicks ME, et al: The importance of preoperative evaluation of the subclavian vein in dialysis access planning. *AJR Am J Roentgenol* 156:623, 1991.
26. Firek AF, Cutler RE, St. John Hammond PG: Reappraisal of femoral vein cannulation for temporary hemodialysis vascular access. *Nephron* 47:227, 1987.
27. Doerfler ME, Kaufman B, Goldenberg AS: Central venous catheter placement in patients with disorders of hemostasis. *Chest* 110:185, 1996.
28. Landow L: Complications of pulmonary artery catheter insertion. *Crit Care Med* 17:845, 1989.
29. Knobel E, Akamine N, Fernandes CJ, Jr, et al: Reliability of right atrial pressure monitoring to assess left ventricular preload in critically ill septic patients. *Crit Care Med* 17:1344, 1989.
30. Martin JT, Patrick RT: Pneumothorax: its significance to the anesthesiologist. *Anesth Analg* 39:420, 1960.
31. Dripps RD, Eckenhoff JE, Vandam LD: *Introduction to Anesthesia: The Principles of Safe Practice.* 6th ed. Philadelphia, WB Saunders, 1982.
32. Emerman CL, Pinchak AC, Hancock D, et al: Effect of injection site on circulation times during cardiac arrest. *Crit Care Med* 16:1138, 1988.
33. Kaye W, Bircher NG: Access for drug administration during cardiopulmonary resuscitation. *Crit Care Med* 16:179, 1988.
34. Long R, Kassum D, Donen N, et al: Cardiac tamponade complicating central venous catheterization for total parenteral nutrition: a review. *J Crit Care* 2:39, 1987.
35. Curelaru I, Linder LE, Gustavsson B: Displacement of catheters inserted through internal jugular veins with neck flexion and extension. *Intensive Care Med* 6:179, 1980.
36. Wojciechowski J, Curelaru I, Gustavsson B, et al: "Half way" venous catheters, III: Tip displacements with upper extremity movements. *Acta Anesth Scand* 81[Suppl]:36, 1985.
37. Marx GF: Clinical anesthesia conference: hazards associated with venous pressure monitoring. *N Y State J Med* 69:955, 1969.
38. Andrews RT, Bova DA, Venbrux AC: How much guidewire is too much? Direct measurement of the distance from subclavian and internal jugular vein access sites to the superior vena cava-atrial junction during central venous catheter placement. *Crit Care Med* 28:138, 2000.
39. Czepiak CA, O'Callaghan JM, Venus B: Evaluation of formulas for optimal positioning of central venous catheters. *Chest* 107:1662, 1995.
40. Adlany Z, Dewald CL, Heffner JE: MRI of central venous anatomy. Implications for central venous catheter insertion. *Chest* 114:820, 1998.
41. Robinson JF, Robinson WA, Cohn A, et al: Perforation of the great vessels during central venous line placement. *Arch Intern Med* 155:1225, 1995.
42. Duntley P, Siever J, Korwes ML, et al: Vascular erosion by central venous catheters. *Chest* 101:1633, 1992.
43. Doering RB, Stemmer EA, Connolly JE: Complications of indwelling venous catheters with particular reference to catheter embolism. *Am J Surg* 114:259, 1967.
44. Orebaugh SL: Venous air embolism: clinical and experimental considerations. *Crit Care Med* 20:1169, 1992.

45. Ely EW, Hite RD, Baker AM, et al: Venous air embolism from central venous catheterization: a need for increased physician awareness. *Crit Care Med* 27:2113, 1999.
46. Heckmann JG, Lang CJG, Kindler K, et al: Neurologic manifestations of cerebral air embolism as a complication of central venous catheterization. *Crit Care Med* 28:1621, 2000.
47. Kimura BJ, Chaux GE, Maisel AS: Delayed air embolism simulating pulmonary thromboembolism in the intensive care unit: role of echocardiography. *Crit Care Med* 22:1884, 1994.
48. Goldfarb G, Lebrec D: Percutaneous cannulation of the internal jugular vein in patients with coagulopathies: an experience based on 1000 attempts. *Anesthesiology* 56:321, 1982.
49. Ahmed N, Payne RF: Thrombosis after central venous cannulation. *Med J Aust* 1:217, 1976.
50. Brismar B, Hardstedt C, Jacobson S: Diagnosis of thrombosis by catheter phlebography after prolonged central venous catheterization. *Ann Surg* 194:729, 1981.
51. Wanscher M, Frifelt JJ, Smith-Sivertsen C, et al: Thrombosis caused by polyurethane double-lumen subclavian superior vena cava catheter and hemodialysis. *Crit Care Med* 16:624, 1988.
52. Efsing HO, Lindblad B, Mark J, et al: Thromboembolic complications from central venous catheters: a comparison of three catheter materials. *World J Surg* 7:419, 1983.
53. Axelsson K, Efsen F: Phlebography in long-term catheterization of the subclavian vein. *Scand J Gastroenterol* 13:933, 1978.
54. Bonnet F, Loriferne JG, Texier JP, et al: Evaluation of Doppler examination for diagnosis of catheter-related deep vein thrombosis. *Intensive Care Med* 15:238, 1989.
55. Prandoni P, Polistena P, Bernardi E, et al: Upper-extremity deep vein thrombosis. Risk factors, diagnosis, and complications. *Arch Intern Med* 157:57, 1997.
56. Raad II, Luna M, Khalil SAM, et al: The relationship between the thrombotic and infectious complications of central venous catheters. *JAMA* 271:1014, 1994.
57. Friedman B, Akers S, Gerber D, et al: The risk in ICU patients of deep venous thrombosis due to femoral vein catheterization. *Chest* 102:119S, 1992.
58. Tinsit JF, Farkas JC, Boyer JM, et al: Central vein catheter-related thrombosis in intensive care patients: incidence, risk factors, and relationship with catheter-related sepsis. *Chest* 114:207, 1998.
59. Linder LE, Curelaru I, Gustavsson B, et al: Material thrombogenicity in central venous catheterization: a comparison between soft, antebrachial catheters of silicone elastomer and polyurethane. *J Parenter Enteral Nutr* 8:399, 1984.
60. Madan M, Alexander DJ, McMahon MJ: Influence of catheter type on occurrence of thrombophlebitis during peripheral intravenous nutrition. *Lancet* 339:101, 1992.
61. Hoar PF, Wilson RM, Mangano DT, et al: Heparin bonding reduces thrombogenicity of pulmonary artery catheters. *N Engl J Med* 305:992, 1981.
62. Mangano DT: Heparin bonding and long-term protection against thrombogenesis. *N Engl J Med* 307:894, 1982.
63. Marin MG, Lee JC, Skurnick JH: Prevention of nosocomial bloodstream infections: effectiveness of antimicrobial-impregnated and heparin-bonded central venous catheters. *Crit Care Med* 28:3332, 2000.
64. Bern MM, Lukich JJ, Wallach SR, et al: Very low doses of warfarin can prevent thrombosis in central venous catheters: a randomized prospective trial. *Ann Intern Med* 112:423, 1990.
65. Borales P, Seale J, Prue J, et al: Prevention of central venous catheter associated thrombosis using minidose warfarin in patients with haematological malignancies. *Br J Haematol* 101:483, 1998.
66. Randolph AG, Cook DJ, Gonzales CA, et al: Benefit of heparin in central venous and pulmonary artery catheters: a meta analysis of randomized controlled studies. *Chest* 113:165, 1998.
67. Black IH, Blosser SA, Murray WB: Central venous pressure measurements: peripherally inserted catheters versus centrally inserted catheters. *Crit Care Med* 28:3833, 2000.
68. Heffner JE: A guide to the management of peripherally inserted central catheters. *J Crit Illness* 15:165, 2000.
69. Williams PL, Warwick R (eds): *Gray's Anatomy*. 8th ed. Philadelphia, WB Saunders, 1980.
70. Netter FH: *Atlas of Human Anatomy*. Summit, NJ, Ciba-GEIGY, 1989.
71. Lumley J, Russell WJ: Insertion of central venous catheters through arm veins. *Anesth Intensive Care* 3:101, 1975.
72. Webre DR, Arens JF: Use of cephalic and basilic veins for introduction of central venous catheters. *Anesthesiology* 38:389, 1973.
73. Cardella JF, Cardella K, Bacci N, et al: Cumulative experience with 1,273 peripherally inserted central catheters at a single institution. *JVIR* 7:5, 1996.
74. Raad I, Davis S, Becker M, et al: Low infection rate and long durability of nontunneled Silastic catheters. *Arch Intern Med* 153:1791, 1993.
75. Duerkson DR, Papineau N, Siemens J, et al: Peripherally inserted central catheters for parenteral nutrition: a comparison with centrally inserted catheters. *J Parenter Enteral Nutr* 23:85, 1999.
76. Gustavsson B, Curelaru I, Hultman E, et al: Displacements of the soft, polyurethane central venous catheters inserted by basilic and cephalic veins with arm in maximal adduction and elevation. *Acta Anaesthesiol Scand* 27:102, 1983.
77. Hermosura B, Vanags L, Dickey NW: Measurement of pressure during intravenous therapy. *JAMA* 195:321, 1966.
78. Blitt CD, Wright WA, Petty WC, et al: Central venous catheterization via the external jugular vein: a technique employing the J-wire. *JAMA* 229:817, 1974.
79. Malatinsky J, Faybik M, Griffith M, et al: Venipuncture, catheterization, and failure to position correctly during central venous circulation. *Resuscitation* 10:259, 1983.
80. Defalque RJ: Percutaneous catheterization of the internal jugular vein. *Anesth Analg* 53:1, 1974.
81. Daily PO, Griepp RB, Shumway NE: Percutaneous internal jugular vein cannulation. *Arch Surg* 101:534, 1970.
82. Morgan RNW, Morrell DF: Internal jugular catheterization. *Anaesthesia* 36:512, 1981.
83. Johnson FE: Internal jugular vein catheterization. *N Y State J Med* 78:2168, 1978.
84. Sznajder J, Zveibil FR, Bitterman H, et al: Central venous catheterization failure and complication rates by 3 percutaneous approaches. *Arch Intern Med* 146:259, 1986.
85. Mostert JW, Kenny GM, Murphy GP: Safe placement of central venous catheters into internal jugular veins. *Arch Surg* 101:431, 1970.
86. Civetta JM, Gabel JC, Geiner M: Internal jugular vein puncture with a margin of safety. *Anesthesiology* 36:622, 1972.
87. Petty C: An alternative method for internal jugular venipuncture for monitoring central venous pressure. *Anesth Analg* 54:157, 1975.
88. Jernigan WR, Gardner WC, Mahr NM, et al: Use of the internal jugular vein for placement of central venous catheter. *Surg Gynecol Obstet* 130:520, 1970.
89. Brinkman AJ, Costley DO: Internal jugular venipuncture. *JAMA* 223:182, 1973.
90. Kaiser CW, Koornick AR, Smith N, et al: Choice of route for central venous cannulation: subclavian or internal jugular vein? A prospective randomized study. *J Surg Oncol* 17:345, 1981.
91. Bo-Linn GW, Anderson DJ, Anderson KC, et al: Percutaneous central venous catheterization performed by medical house officers. *Cathet Cardiovasc Diagn* 8:23, 1982.
92. Randolph AG, Cook DJ, Gonzales CA, et al: Ultrasound guidance for placement of central venous catheters: a meta-analysis of the literature. *Crit Care Med* 24:2053, 1996.
93. Denys BG, Uretsky BF, Reddy PS: Ultrasound-assisted cannulation of the internal jugular vein. *Circulation* 87:1557, 1993.
94. Bazaral M, Harlan S: Ultrasonographic anatomy of the internal jugular vein relevant to percutaneous cannulation. *Crit Care Med* 9:307, 1981.
95. Mallory DL, Shawker T, Evans G, et al: Effects of clinical maneuvers on sonographically determined internal jugular vein size during venous cannulation. *Crit Care Med* 18:1269, 1990.
96. Denys BG, Uretsky BF: Anatomical variations of internal jugular vein location: impact on central venous access. *Crit Care Med* 19:1516, 1991.
97. Gilbert TB, Seneff M, Becker RB: Facilitation of internal jugular venous cannulation using an audio-guided Doppler ultrasound vascular access device: results from a prospective, dual-center, randomized, crossover clinical study. *Crit Care Med* 23:60, 1995.
98. Tyden H: Cannulation of the internal jugular vein: 500 cases. *Acta Anaesthesiol Scand* 26:485, 1982.
99. Eisenhauer ED, Derveloy RJ, Hastings PR: Prospective evaluation of central venous pressure (CVP) catheters in a large city-county hospital. *Ann Surg* 196:560, 1982.

100. Belani KG, Buckley JJ, Gordon JR, et al: Percutaneous cervical central venous line placement: a comparison of the internal and external jugular vein routes. *Anesth Analg* 59:40, 1980.
101. Klineberg PL, Greenhow DE, Ellison N: Hematoma following internal jugular vein cannulation. *Anesth Intensive Care* 8:94, 1980.
102. Briscoe CE, Brishman JA, McDonald WI: Extensive neurological damage after cannulation of internal jugular vein. *BMJ* 1:314, 1974.
103. Schwartz AJ, Jobes CR, Greenhow DE, et al: Carotid artery puncture with internal jugular cannulation. *Anesthesiology* 51:S160, 1980.
104. Seneff MG: Central venous catheterization: a comprehensive review, Pt II. *J Intensive Care Med* 2:218, 1987.
105. Nagai K, Kemmotsu O: An inadvertent insertion of a Swan-Ganz catheter into the intrathecal space. *Anesthesiology* 62:848, 1985.
106. Schwartz AJ, Jobes DR, Levy WJ, et al: Intrathoracic vascular catheterization via the external jugular vein. *Anesthesiology* 56:400, 1982.
107. Blitt CD, Carlson GL, Wright WA, et al: J-wire versus straight wire for central venous system cannulation via the external jugular vein. *Anesth Analg* 61:536, 1982.
108. Giesy J: External jugular vein access to central venous system. *JAMA* 219:216, 1972.
109. Riddell GS, Latto IP, Ng WS: External jugular vein access to the central venous system: a trial of two types of catheters. *Br J Anaesth* 54:535, 1982.
110. Jobes DR, Schwartz AJ, Greenhow DE: Safer jugular vein cannulation. Recognition of arterial puncture and preferential use of the external jugular route. *Anesthesiology* 59:353, 1983.
111. Getzen LC, Pollak EW: Short-term femoral vein catheterization. *Am J Surg* 138:875, 1979.
112. Dailey RH: "Code red" protocol for resuscitation of the exsanguinated patient. *J Emerg Med* 2:373, 1985.
113. Williams JF, Friedman BC, McGrath BJ, et al: The use of femoral venous catheters in critically ill adults: a prospective study. *Crit Care Med* 17:584, 1989.
114. Kruse JA, Carlson RW: Infectious complications of femoral vs internal jugular and subclavian vein central venous catheterization. *Crit Care Med* 19:843, 1991.
115. Murr MM, Rosenquist MD, Lewis RW, et al: A prospective safety study of femoral vein versus nonfemoral vein catheterization in patients with burns. *J Burn Care Rehabil* 12:576, 1991.
116. Dailey RH: Femoral vein cannulation: a review. *J Emerg Med* 2:367, 1985.
117. Gilston A: Cannulation of the femoral vessels. *Br J Anaesth* 48:500, 1976.
118. Sharp KW, Spees EK, Selby LR, et al: Diagnosis and management of retroperitoneal hematomas after femoral vein cannulation for hemodialysis. *Surgery* 95:90, 1984.
119. Fuller TJ, Mahoney JJ, Juncos LI, et al: Arteriovenous fistula after femoral vein catheterization. *JAMA* 236:2943, 1976.
120. Norwood S, Wilkins HE, Vallina VL, et al: The safety of prolonging the use of central venous catheters: a prospective analysis of the effects of using antiseptic-bonded catheters with daily care. *Crit Care Med* 28:1376, 2000.
121. Goetz AM, Wagener MM, Miller JM, et al: Risk of infection due to central venous catheters: effect of site of placement and catheter type. *Infect Control Hosp Epidemiol* 19:842, 1998.
122. Stenzel JP, Green TP, Fuhrman BP, et al: Percutaneous femoral venous catheterizations: a prospective study of complications. *J Pediatr* 114:411, 1989.
123. Russell JA, Joel M, Hudson RJ, et al: Prospective evaluation of radial and femoral artery catheterization sites in critically ill adults. *Crit Care Med* 11:936, 1983.
124. Jimenez CA, Huaringa AJ, Darwish AA, et al: Does upper limb deep venous thrombosis have the same significance than lower limb deep venous thrombosis? *Chest* 110:54S, 1996.
125. Lynn KL, Maling TMJ: A major pulmonary embolus as a complication of femoral vein catheterization. *Br J Radiol* 50:667, 1977.
126. Healy B, Seneff M, Massarin E, et al: Thrombotic complications following femoral vein catheterization. *Crit Care Med* 23:A30, 1995.
127. Shapira M, Stern WZ: Hazards of subclavian vein cannulation for central venous pressure monitoring. *JAMA* 201:327, 1967.
128. Mansfield PF, Hohn DC, Fornage BD, et al: Complications and failures of subclavian-vein catheterization. *N Engl J Med* 331:1735, 1994.
129. Haire WD, Lieberman RP: Defining the risks of subclavian-vein catheterization. *N Engl J Med* 331:1769, 1994.
130. Moosman DA: The anatomy of infraclavicular subclavian vein catheterization and its complications. *Surg Gynecol Obstet* 136:71, 1973.
131. Eerola R, Kaukinen L, Kaukinen S: Analysis of 13,800 subclavian catheterizations. *Acta Anaesthesiol Scand* 29:293, 1985.
132. James PM, Myers RT: Central venous pressure monitoring: misinterpretation, abuses, indications, and a new technique. *Ann Surg* 175:693, 1972.
133. Brahos GJ: Central venous catheterization via the supraclavicular approach. *J Trauma* 17:872, 1977.
134. MacDonnell JE, Perez H, Pitts SR, et al: Supraclavicular subclavian vein catheterization: modified landmarks for needle insertion. *Ann Emerg Med* 21:421, 1992.
135. Dronen S, Thompson B, Nowak R, et al: Subclavian vein catheterization during cardiopulmonary resuscitation: comparison of supra- and infraclavicular percutaneous approaches. *JAMA* 247:3227, 1982.
136. Sterner S: A comparison of the supraclavicular approach and the infraclavicular approach for subclavian vein catheterization. *Ann Emerg Med* 15:421, 1986.
137. McGee WT, Ackerman BL, Rouben LR, et al: Accurate placement of central venous catheters: a prospective, randomized, multicenter trial. *Crit Care Med* 21:1118, 1993.
138. Simpson ET, Aitchison JM: Percutaneous infraclavicular subclavian vein catheterization in shocked patients: a prospective study in 172 patients. *J Trauma* 22:781, 1982.
139. Herbst CA Jr: Indications, management, and complications of percutaneous subclavian catheters: an audit. *Arch Surg* 113:1421, 1978.
140. Bernard RW, Stahl WM: Subclavian vein catheterization: a prospective study; 1: Non-infectious complications. *Ann Surg* 173:184, 1971.
141. McGoon MD, Benedetto PW, Greene BM: Complications of percutaneous central venous catheterization: a report of two cases and review of the literature. *Johns Hopkins Med* 145:1, 1979.
142. Defalque RJ: Subclavian venipuncture: a review. *Anesth Analg* 47:677, 1968.
143. Ryan JA, Abel RM, Abbott WM, et al: Catheter complications in total parenteral nutrition: a prospective study of 200 consecutive patients. *N Engl J Med* 270:757, 1974.
144. Despars JA, Sassoon CSH, Light RW: Significance of iatrogenic pneumothoraces. *Chest* 105:1147, 1994.
145. Matz R: Complications of determining the central venous pressure. *N Engl J Med* 273:703, 1965.
146. Warden GD, Wilmore DW, Pruitt BA: Central venous thrombosis: a hazard of medical progress. *J Trauma* 13:620, 1973.
147. Sherertz RJ, Ely EW, Westbrook DM, et al: Education of physicians-in-training can decrease the risk for vascular catheter infection. *Ann Intern Med* 132:641, 2000.
148. Mermel LA: Prevention of intravascular catheter-related infections. *Ann Intern Med* 132:391, 2000.
149. Maki DG, Weise CE, Sarafin HW: A semiquantitative culture method for identifying intravenous catheter related infection. *N Engl J Med* 296:1305, 1977.
150. Cooper GL, Hopkins CC: Rapid diagnosis of intravascular catheter-associated infection by direct Gram staining of catheter segments. *N Engl J Med* 312:1142, 1985.
151. Zufferey J, Rime B, Francioli P, et al: Simple method for rapid diagnosis of catheter-associated infection by direct acridine orange staining of catheter tips. *J Clin Microbiol* 26:175, 1988.
152. Sitges-Serra A, Pi-Suner T, Garces JM, et al: Pathogenesis and prevention of catheter-related septicemia. *Am J Infect Control* 23:310, 1995.
153. Raad II: Intravascular catheter-related infections. *Lancet* 351:893, 1998.
154. Heiselman D: Nosocomial bloodstream infections in the critically ill. *JAMA* 272:1819, 1994.
155. National Nosocomial Infection Surveillance (NNIS) system report. *Am J Infect Control* 26:522, 1998.
156. Martin MA, Pfaller MA, Wenzel RP: Coagulase-negative staphylococcal bacteremia. Impact on mortality and hospital stay. *Ann Intern Med* 110:9, 1989.
157. Smith RL, Meixler SM, Simberkoff MS: Excess mortality in critically ill patients with nosocomial bloodstream infections. *Chest* 100:164, 1991.
158. Pittet D, Tarara D, Wenzel RP: Nosocomial bloodstream infection in critically ill patients: excess length of stay, extra costs, and attributable mortality. *JAMA* 162:1598, 1994.

159. Byers K, Adal K, Anglim A, et al: Case fatality rate for catheter-related bloodstream infections (CRBSI): a meta-analysis. *Infect Control Hosp Epidemiol* 16:23, 1995.

160. Passerini L, Lam K, Costerton JW, et al: Biofilms on indwelling vascular catheters. *Crit Care Med* 20:665, 1992.

161. Cooper GL, Schiller AL, Hopkins CC: Possible role of capillary action in pathogenesis of experimental catheter-associated dermal tunnel infections. *J Clin Microbiol* 26:8, 1988.

162. Olson ME, Lam K, Bodey GP, et al: Evaluation of strategies for central venous catheter replacement. *Crit Care Med* 20:797, 1992.

163. Maki DG, Cobb L, Garman JK, et al: An attachable silver-impregnated cuff for prevention of infection with central venous catheters: a prospective randomized multi-center trial. *Am J Med* 85:307, 1988.

164. Sitges-Serra A, Linares J, Garau J, et al: Catheter sepsis: the clue is the hub. *Surgery* 97:355, 1985.

165. Moro ML, Vigano EF, Lepri AC, et al: Risk factors for central venous catheter-related infections in surgical and intensive care units. *Infect Control Hosp Epidemiol* 15:253, 1994.

166. Raad II, Costerton W, Sabharwal U, et al: Ultrastructural analysis of indwelling vascular catheters: a quantitative relationship between luminal colonization and duration of placement. *J Infect Dis* 168:400, 1993.

167. Raad II, Hohn DC, Gilbreath J, et al: Prevention of central venous catheter-related infections by using maximal sterile barrier precautions during insertion. *Infect Control Hosp Epidemiol* 15:231, 1994.

168. Mimoz O, Pieroni L, Lawrence C, et al: Prospective, randomized trial of two antiseptic solutions for prevention of central venous or arterial catheter colonization and infection in intensive care unit patients. *Crit Care Med* 24:1818, 1996.

169. Maki DG, Ringer M, Alvarado CJ: Prospective randomized trial of povidone-iodine, alcohol, and chlorhexidine for prevention of infection associated with central venous and arterial catheters. *Lancet* 338:339, 1991.

170. Maki DG: Yes, Virginia, aseptic technique is very important: maximal barrier precautions during insertion reduce the risk of central venous catheter-related bacteremia. *Infect Control Hosp Epidemiol* 15:227, 1994.

171. Parras F, Ena J, Bouza E, et al: Impact of an educational program for the prevention of colonization of intravascular catheters. *Infect Control Hosp Epidemiol* 15:239, 1994.

172. Maki DG, Botticelli JT, LeRoy ML, et al: Prospective study of replacing administration sets for intravenous therapy at 48- vs 72-hour intervals. 72 hours is safe and cost effective. *JAMA* 258:1777, 1987.

173. Hoffman KK, Weber DJ, Samsa GP, et al: Transparent polyurethane film as an intravenous catheter dressing: a meta-analysis of the infection risks. *JAMA* 267:2072, 1992.

174. Maki DG, Band JD: A comparative study of polyantibiotic and iodophor ointments in prevention of vascular catheter-related infection. *Am J Med* 70:739, 1981.

175. Hill RL, Fisher AP, Ware RJ, et al: Mupirocin for the reduction of colonization of internal jugular cannulae—a randomized controlled trial. *J Hosp Infect* 15:311, 1990.

176. Miller JJ, Venus B, Mathru M: Comparison of the sterility of long term central venous catheterization using single lumen, triple lumen, and pulmonary artery catheters. *Crit Care Med* 2:634, 1984.

177. Arnow PM, Quimosing EM, Beach M: Consequences of intravascular catheter sepsis. *Clin Infect Dis* 16:778, 1993.

178. Veenstra DL, Saint S, Sullivan SD: Cost-effectiveness of antiseptic impregnated central venous catheters for the prevention of catheter-related bloodstream infection. *JAMA* 282:554, 1999.

179. Hanley EM, Veeder A, Smith T, et al: Evaluation of an antiseptic triple-lumen catheter in an intensive care unit. *Crit Care Med* 28:366, 2000.

180. Maki DG, Wheller SJ, Stolz SM, et al: Clinical trial of a novel antiseptic-coated central venous catheter, Abstract No. 461, in *Program and Abstracts of the 31st Interscience Conference on Antimicrobial Agents and Chemotherapy*. Washington, DC, American Society for Microbiology, 1991.

181. Flowers RH III, Schwenzer KJ, Kopel RF, et al: Efficacy of an attachable subcutaneous cuff for the prevention of intravascular catheter-related infection. *JAMA* 261:878, 1989.

182. Kamal GD, Pfaller MA, Rempe LE, et al: Reduced intravascular catheter infection by antibiotic bonding: a prospective, randomized controlled trial. *JAMA* 265:2364, 1991.

183. Collin GR: Decreasing catheter colonization through the use of an antiseptic impregnated catheter. A continuous quality improvement project. *Chest* 115:1632, 1999.

184. Mermel LA, Farr BM, Sheretz RJ, et al: Guidelines for the management of intravascular catheter-related infections. *Infect Control Hosp Epidemiol* 22:222, 2001.

185. Clarke DE, Raffin TA: Infectious complications of indwelling long-term central venous catheters. *Chest* 97:966, 1990.

186. McCarthy MC, Shives JK, Robison RJ, et al: Prospective evaluation of single and triple lumen catheters in total parenteral nutrition. *JPEN J Parenter Enteral Nutr* 11:259, 1987.

187. Christoff-Clark N, Watters VA, Sparks W, et al: Use of triple-lumen subclavian catheters for administration of total parenteral nutrition. *JPEN J Parenter Enteral Nutr* 16:403, 1992.

188. Farkas JC, Liu N, Bleriot JP, et al: Single- versus triple-lumen central catheter-related sepsis: a prospective randomized study in a critically ill population. *Am J Med* 93:277, 1992.

189. Hilton E, Haslett TM, Borenstein MT, et al: Central catheter infections: single- versus triple-lumen catheters. *Am J Med* 84:667, 1988.

190. Randolph AG, Cook DJ, Gonzales CA, et al: Tunneling short-term central venous catheters to prevent catheter-related infection: a meta-analysis of randomized, controlled trials. *Crit Care Med* 26:1452, 1998.

191. Eyer S, Brummitt C, Crossley K, et al: Catheter-related sepsis: prospective, randomized study of three methods of long-term catheter maintenance. *Crit Care Med* 18:1073, 1990.

192. Cobb DK, High KP, Sawyer RG, et al: A controlled trial of scheduled replacement of central venous and pulmonary artery catheters. *N Engl J Med* 327:1062, 1992.

193. Hagley MT, Martin B, Gast P, et al: Infectious and mechanical complications of central venous catheters placed by percutaneous venipuncture and over guidewires. *Crit Care Med* 20:1426, 1992.

194. Badley AD, Steckelberg JM, Wollan PC, et al: Infectious rates of central venous pressure catheters: comparison between newly placed catheters and those that have been changed. *Mayo Clin Proc* 71:838, 1996.

195. Mermel LA, McCormick RD, Springman SR, et al: The pathogenesis and epidemiology of catheter-related infection with pulmonary artery Swan-Ganz catheters: a prospective study utilizing molecular subtyping. *Am J Med* 91[Suppl 3B]:197S, 1991.

196. Rello J, Coll P, Net A, et al: Infection of pulmonary artery catheters. Epidemiologic characteristics and multivariate analysis of risk factors. *Chest* 103:132, 1993.

197. Raad II, Umphrey J, Khan A, et al: The duration of placement as a predictor of peripheral and pulmonary arterial catheter infections. *J Hosp Infect* 23:17, 1993.

198. Mermel LA, Maki DG: Infectious complications of Swan-Ganz pulmonary artery catheters. *Am J Respir Crit Care Med* 149:1020, 1994.

199. Mass AH, Vasilakis C, Holley JL, et al: Use of a silicone dual-lumen catheter with a Dacron cuff as a long-term vascular access for hemodialysis patients. *Am J Kidney Dis* 16:211, 1990.

200. Heard SO, Wagle M, Vijayakumar E, et al: Influence of triple lumen central venous catheters coated with chlorhexidine and silver sulfadiazine on the incidence of catheter-related bacteremia. *Arch Intern Med* 158:81, 1998.

201. Mermel LA, Stolz SM, Maki DG: Surface antimicrobial activity of heparin-bonded and antiseptic-impregnated vascular catheters. *J Infect Dis* 167:920, 1993.

202. Sheretz RJ, Carruth WA, Hampton AA, et al: Efficacy of antibiotic-coated catheters in preventing subcutaneous *Staphylococcal aureus* infections in rabbits. *J Infect Dis* 167:98, 1993.

203. Modak SM, Samputh L: Development and evaluation of a new polyurethane central venous antiseptic catheter: reducing central venous catheter infections. *Infect Med* 10:23, 1992.

204. Veenstra DL, Saint S, Saha S, et al: Efficacy of antiseptic impregnated central venous catheters in preventing catheter-related bloodstream infection. A meta-analysis. *JAMA* 281:261, 1999.

205. Darouiche RO, Raad II, Heard SO, et al: A comparison of two antimicrobial-impregnated central venous catheters. *N Engl J Med* 340:1, 1999.

206. Marik PE, Abraham G, Careau P, et al: The *ex vivo* antimicrobial activity and colonization rate of two antimicrobial-bonded central venous catheters. *Crit Care Med* 27:1128, 1999.

3. Arterial Line Placement and Care

Michael G. Seneff

Arterial catheterization is the second most frequently performed invasive procedure in the intensive care unit (ICU). In many centers, nonphysician personnel routinely insert, maintain, calibrate, and troubleshoot arterial catheters and pressure-monitoring equipment [1]. Although this has standardized care, many physicians no longer possess an adequate working knowledge of these important systems. This chapter reviews the indications, techniques, equipment, and complications of arterial cannulation. An overview of the principles governing pressure monitoring and equipment calibration is also presented, with the intent that every physician who cares for critically ill patients will be able to troubleshoot measurement errors when they arise.

Historical Perspective

Physicians have achieved access to the arterial circulation for many years, but early methods were comparatively crude and accompanied by a substantial risk of morbidity. The modern age of arterial monitoring was initiated by Farinas [2] in 1941, when he described cannulation of the aorta with a urethral catheter introduced through a surgically exposed femoral artery. Cannulation techniques, catheters, and monitoring equipment have since improved. The strain gauge manometer, introduced in 1947, consisted of a wheatstone bridge with four strain-sensitive wire elements [3]. Displacement of a bellows attached to the bridge caused a change in resistance of the wires, altering current output and converting a mechanical stimulus into a proportional electrical signal. Peterson et al. [4] described online arterial monitoring in 1949, using specially adapted intraarterial plastic cannulas, capacitance manometer, amplifier, and ink recorder. These authors were among the first to appreciate and describe the various factors that can result in over- or underdamping of pressure tracings.

Two important advances in arterial cannulation technique followed. In 1950, Massa et al. [5] reported the development of a cannula through which a needle protruded at the tip. Barr [6] described use of this device for radial artery cannulation in 1961. In 1953, Seldinger [7] described percutaneous placement of a catheter using a guidewire, a technique now used extensively for central venous and large artery cannulation.

The technological explosion of the past few decades has resulted in improvements to each component of the monitoring system. Catheters are more uniform and less thrombogenic. Disposable pressure transducers incorporate semiconductor technology and are very small, yet rugged and reliable [8]. Monitors are more user friendly, with internal calibration, better filtering capabilities, and pleasing color visual displays. Additional technological improvements will undoubtedly follow, but it is likely that future systems will continue to be plagued by certain physical and manmade restraints.

Indications for Arterial Cannulation

Arterial catheters should be inserted only when they are specifically required and removed immediately when they are no longer needed. Too often, they are left in place for convenience and to allow for easy access to blood sampling. Many studies have documented that arterial catheters are associated with an increased number of laboratory blood tests, leading to greater costs and excessive diagnostic blood loss (DBL) [9–11]. Protocols incorporating guidelines for arterial catheterization and alternative noninvasive monitoring, such as pulse oximetry and end-tidal carbon dioxide monitoring, have realized significant improvements in resource use and cost savings, without impacting the quality of care [12,13].

The indications for arterial cannulation can be grouped into four broad categories (Table 3-1). These include (a) hemodynamic monitoring; (b) frequent arterial blood gas sampling; (c) arterial administration of drugs, such as thrombolytics; and (d) intraaortic balloon pump use.

Noninvasive, indirect blood pressure measurements determined by auscultation of Korotkoff sounds distal to an occluding cuff (Riva-Rocci method) are generally accurate, although systolic readings are consistently lower compared to a simultaneous direct measurement. In hemodynamically unstable patients, however, indirect techniques may significantly underestimate blood pressure [14]. Automated noninvasive blood pressure measurement devices can also be inaccurate, particularly in rapidly changing situations, at the extremes of blood pressure, and in patients with dysrhythmias [15]. For these reasons, direct blood pressure monitoring is usually required for unstable patients. Rapid beat-to-beat changes can easily be monitored and appropriate therapeutic modalities initiated, and variations in individual pressure waveforms may prove diagnostic. Waveform inspection can rapidly diagnose electrocardiogram lead disconnect, indicate the presence of aortic valve disease, help determine the effect of dysrhythmias on perfusion, and reveal the impact of the respiratory cycle on blood pressure (pulsus paradoxus).

Management of patients in critical care units typically requires multiple laboratory determinations. Patients on mechanical ventilators or in whom intubation is contemplated need frequent monitoring of arterial blood gases. In these situations, arterial cannulation prevents repeated trauma by frequent arterial punctures and permits routine laboratory tests without multiple needle sticks. Typically, an arterial line for blood gas determination should be placed when a patient will require three or more measurements per day.

Equipment, Monitoring Techniques, and Sources of Error

The equipment necessary to display and measure an arterial waveform includes (a) an appropriate intravascular catheter, (b) fluid-filled noncompliant tubing with stopcocks, (c) transducer, (d) constant flush device, and (e) electronic monitoring equipment, consisting of a connecting cable, monitor with amplifier, oscilloscope display screen, and recorder. Using this equipment, intravascular pressure changes are transmitted through the hydraulic (fluid-filled) elements to the transducer, which converts mechanical displacement into a proportional electrical signal. The signal is amplified and processed by the monitor, and the waveform is displayed on the oscilloscope

Table 3-1. Indications for Arterial Cannulation

Hemodynamic monitoring
    Acutely hypertensive or hypotensive patients
        With use of vasoactive drugs
Multiple blood sampling
    Ventilated patients
    Limited venous access
Arterial administration of drugs
Intraaortic balloon pump use

screen, accompanied by a digital readout. Undistorted presentation of the arterial waveform is dependent on the performance of each component. A detailed discussion of relevant pressure monitoring principles is beyond the scope of this chapter, but consideration of a few basic concepts is adequate to understand the genesis of most monitoring inaccuracies.

The major problems inherent to pressure monitoring with a catheter system are inadequate dynamic response, improper zeroing and zero drift, and improper transducer/monitor calibration [16]. Most physicians are aware of zeroing and calibration techniques but underappreciate the importance of dynamic response in ensuring system fidelity. Catheter-tubing-transducer systems used for pressure monitoring can best be characterized as underdamped second-order dynamic systems with mechanical parameters of elasticity, mass, and friction [16]. Overall, the dynamic response of such a system is determined by its resonant frequency and damping coefficient (zeta). The resonant or natural frequency of a system is the frequency at which it oscillates when stimulated. When the frequency content of an input signal (i.e., pressure waveform) approaches the resonant frequency of a system, progressive amplification of the output signal occurs, a phenomenon known as *ringing* [17]. To ensure a flat frequency response (accurate recording across a spectrum of frequencies), the resonant frequency of a monitoring system should be at least five times higher than the highest frequency in the input signal [16]. Physiologic peripheral arterial waveforms have a fundamental frequency of 3 to 5 Hz, and, therefore, the resonant frequency of a system used to monitor arterial pressure should ideally be greater than 20 Hz to avoid ringing and systolic overshoot.

The system components that are most likely to cause amplification of a pressure waveform are the hydraulic elements. A good hydraulic system has a resonant frequency between 10 and 20 Hz, which may overlap with arterial pressure frequencies. Thus, amplification can occur, which may require damping to reproduce the waveform accurately [18].

The damping coefficient is a measure of how quickly an oscillating system comes to rest. A system with a high damping coefficient absorbs mechanical energy well (i.e., compliant tubing), causing a diminution in the transmitted waveform. Conversely, a system with a low damping coefficient results in underdamping and systolic overshoot. Damping coefficient and resonant frequency together determine the dynamic response of a recording system. If the system's resonant frequency is less than 7.5 Hz, the pressure waveform will be distorted no matter what the damping coefficient. On the other hand, a resonant frequency of 24 Hz allows a range in the damping coefficient of 0.15 to 1.1 without resultant distortion of the pressure waveform [16,19].

Although there are other techniques [20], the easiest method to test the damping coefficient and resonant frequency of a monitoring system is the fast-flush test, performed at the bedside by briefly opening and closing the continuous flush device, which produces a square wave displacement on the monitor followed by a return to baseline, usually after a few smaller oscillations (Fig. 3-1). Values for the damping coefficient and resonant frequency can be computed by printing the wave on graph paper [16], but visual inspection is usually adequate to ensure a proper frequency response. An optimum fast-flush test results in one undershoot followed by a small overshoot, then settles to the patient's waveform (Fig. 3-1).

For peripheral pulse pressure monitoring, an adequate fast-flush test usually corresponds to a resonant frequency of 10 to 20 Hz coupled with a damping coefficient of 0.5 to 0.7 [19]. To ensure the continuing fidelity of a monitoring system, dynamic response validation by fast-flush test should be performed frequently: with every significant change in patient hemodynamic status, after each opening of the system (zeroing, blood sampling, tubing change), whenever the waveform appears dampened, and at least every 8 hours.

With consideration of the above concepts, components of the monitoring system are designed to optimize the frequency response of the entire system. The 18- and 20-gauge catheters used to gain vascular access are not a major source of distortion but can become kinked or occluded by thrombus, resulting in overdamping of the system. Connecting tubing with stopcocks is the major source of underdamped tracings. Standard, noncompliant tubing is provided with most disposable transducer kits and should be as short as possible to minimize signal amplification [17]. Air bubbles in the tubing and connecting stopcocks are a notorious source of overdamping of the tracing and can be cleared by flushing through a stopcock. Currently available disposable transducers incorporate microchip technology, are very reliable, and have relatively high resonant frequencies [8]. The transducer is attached to the electronic monitoring equipment by a cable. Modern monitors have internal calibration and filter artifacts and print the oscilloscope display on request. The digital readout display is an average of values over time and may not be an accurate representation of beat-to-beat variability. Most monitors can freeze a display and provide onscreen calibration with a cursor to measure beat-to-beat differences in amplitude precisely. This allows measurement of the effect of ectopic beats on blood pressure or assessment of the severity of pulsus paradoxus.

When one is presented with pressure data or readings that are believed to be inaccurate, or which are significantly different from indirect readings, a few quick checks can ensure sys-

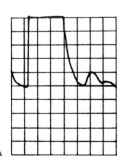 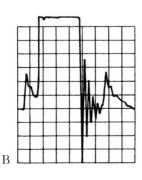 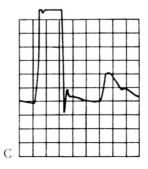

A   B   C

Fig. 3-1. Fast-flush test. **A:** Overdamped system. **B:** Underdamped system. **C:** Optimal damping.

tem accuracy. Improper zeroing of the system is the single most important source of error. Zeroing can be checked by opening the transducer stopcock to air and aligning with the midaxillary line, confirming that the monitor displays zero. Zeroing should be repeated with patient position changes, when significant changes in blood pressure occur, and routinely every 6 to 8 hours because of zero drift. Calibration of the system is usually not necessary due to standardization of current disposable transducers [8]. Transducers are faulty on occasion, however, and calibration can be checked by attaching a mercury manometer to the stopcock and applying 100, 150, and/or 200 mm Hg pressure. If the monitor does not display the pressure within an acceptable range (±5 mm Hg), the transducer should be replaced.

If zero referencing and calibration are correct, a fast-flush test can assess the system's dynamic response. Overdamped tracings are usually caused by air bubbles, kinks, clot formation, compliant tubing, loose connections, a deflated pressure bag, or anatomic factors that affect the catheter. All of these are usually correctable. An underdamped tracing results in systolic overshoot and can be secondary to excessive tubing length or patient factors such as increased inotropic or chronotropic state. Many monitors can be adjusted to filter out frequencies above a certain limit, which can eliminate frequencies in the input signal that cause ringing. However, this may also cause inaccurate readings if important frequencies are excluded.

Technique of Arterial Cannulation

SITE SELECTION. Several factors are important in selecting the site for arterial cannulation. The ideal artery has extensive collateral circulation that will maintain the viability of distal tissues if thrombosis occurs. The site should be comfortable for the patient, accessible for nursing care, and close to the monitoring equipment. Sites involved by infection or disruption in the epidermal barrier should be avoided. Certain procedures, such as coronary artery bypass grafting, may dictate preference for one site over another. Larger arteries and catheters provide more accurate (central aortic) pressure measurements. Physicians should also be cognizant of differences in pulse contour recorded at different sites. As the pressure pulse wave travels outward from the aorta, it encounters arteries that are smaller and less elastic, with multiple branch points, causing reflections of the pressure wave. This results in a peripheral pulse contour with increased slope and amplitude, causing recorded values to be artificially elevated. As a result, distal extremity artery recordings yield higher systolic values than central aortic or femoral artery recordings. Diastolic pressures tend to be less affected, and mean arterial pressures measured at the different sites are similar [21,22].

The most commonly used sites for arterial cannulation in adults are the radial, femoral, axillary, dorsalis pedis, and brachial arteries. Peripheral sites are cannulated percutaneously with a 2-in., 20-gauge, nontapered Teflon catheter-over-needle and larger arteries using the Seldinger technique with a prepackaged kit, typically containing a 6-in., 18-gauge Teflon catheter and appropriate introducer needles and guidewire.

Critical care physicians should be able to perform arterial cannulation easily at all sites, but the radial and femoral arteries are used for more than 90% of all arterial catheterizations. Although each site has unique complications, available data do not indicate a preference for any one site [23–27]. Radial artery cannulation is usually attempted initially unless the

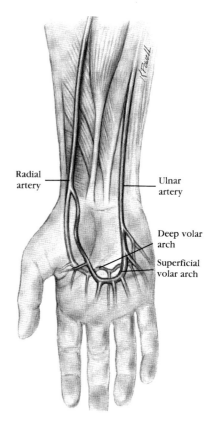

Fig. 3-2. Anatomy of the radial artery. Note the collateral circulation to the ulnar artery through the deep volar arterial arch and dorsal arch.

patient is in shock or pulses are not palpable, or both. If this fails, femoral artery cannulation should be performed.

RADIAL ARTERY CANNULATION. A thorough understanding of normal arterial anatomy and common anatomic variants greatly facilitates insertion of catheters and management of unexpected findings at all sites. The reader is referred elsewhere for a comprehensive review of arterial anatomy [28]; only relevant anatomic considerations are presented here. The radial artery is one of two final branches of the brachial artery. It courses over the flexor digitorum sublimis, flexor pollicis longus, and pronator quadratus muscles and lies just lateral to the flexor carpi radialis in the forearm (Fig. 3-2). As the artery enters the floor of the palm, it ends in the deep volar arterial arch at the level of the metacarpal bones and communicates with the ulnar artery. A second site of collateral flow for the radial artery occurs via the dorsal arch running in the dorsum of the hand.

The ulnar artery runs between the flexor carpi ulnaris and flexor digitorum sublimis in the forearm, with a short course over the ulnar nerve. In the hand the artery runs over the transverse carpal ligament and becomes the superficial volar arch, which forms an anastomosis with a small branch of the radial artery. These three anastomoses provide excellent collateral flow to the hand. Not all individuals, however, are born with three patent arches, and disease processes such as atherosclerosis and scleroderma may compromise previously existing channels. A competent superficial or deep palmar arch must be present to ensure adequate collateral flow. At least one of these arches may be absent in up to 20% of individuals.

Modified Allen's Test. Before placement of a radial or ulnar arterial line, it must be demonstrated that the blood supply to the hand would not be eliminated by a catheter-induced

thrombus. In 1929, Allen [29] described a technique of diagnosing occlusive arterial disease. His technique has been
modified and serves as the most common screening test
before radial artery cannulation. The examiner compresses
both radial and ulnar arteries and asks the patient to clinch
and unclinch the fist repeatedly until pallor of the palm is produced. Hyperextension of the hand is avoided, as it may
cause a false-negative result, suggesting inadequate collateral
flow [30]. One artery is then released and the time to blushing
of the palm noted. The procedure is repeated with the other
artery. Normal palmar blushing is complete before 7 seconds
(positive test); 8 to 14 seconds is considered equivocal, and 15
or more seconds abnormal (negative test).

The modified Allen's test is not an ideal screening procedure. In one study comparing the Allen's test to Doppler
examination, Allen's test had a sensitivity of 87% (i.e., it
detected ulnar collateral flow in 87% of cases in which Doppler study confirmed its presence) and a negative predictive
value of only 0.18 (i.e., only 18% of patients with no collateral
flow by Allen's test had this confirmed by Doppler study) [31].
Other studies have compared Allen's test to plethysmography,
with similar results [32]. Thus, the modified Allen's test does
not necessarily predict the presence of collateral circulation,
and many centers, including the author's, have abandoned its
use as a routine screening procedure. Each institution should
establish its own guidelines regarding routine Allen's testing
and the evaluation and management of negative results. If a
lack of collateral circulation is verified by confirmatory testing,
it is advisable to avoid arterial cannulation on that hand.

Percutaneous Insertion. Following evaluation for adequate
collateral circulation, the hand is placed in 30 to 60 degrees of
dorsiflexion with the aid of a roll of gauze and armband, avoiding hyperabduction of the thumb. The volar aspect of the wrist
is prepared and draped using sterile technique, and approximately 0.5 mL lidocaine is infiltrated on both sides of the artery
through a 25-gauge needle. Lidocaine serves to decrease
patient discomfort and the likelihood of arterial vasospasm [33].

A 20-gauge, nontapered, Teflon 1½- or 2-in. catheter-over-
needle apparatus is used for the puncture. Entry is made at a
30- to 60-degree angle to the skin approximately 3 to 5 cm
proximal to the distal wrist crease. The needle and cannula
are advanced until blood return is noted in the hub, signifying
intraarterial placement of the tip of the needle (Fig. 3-3). A
small amount of further advancement is necessary for the cannula to enter the artery as well. With this accomplished, needle and cannula are brought flat to the skin, and the cannula
is advanced to its hub with a firm, steady rotary action. Correct positioning is confirmed by pulsatile blood return on
removal of the needle. If the initial attempt is unsuccessful,
anatomic considerations indicate that subsequent attempts
should be more proximal rather than closer to the wrist crease
[28], although this may increase the incidence of catheters
becoming nonpatent [34].

If difficulty is encountered when attempting to pass the
catheter, carefully replacing the needle and slightly advancing
the whole apparatus may remedy the problem. Alternately, a
fixation technique can be attempted (Fig. 3-3). The artery is
purposely transfixed by advancing the needle and catheter
through the far wall of the vessel. The needle is then removed
and the cannula pulled back until vigorous arterial blood
return is noted. The catheter can then be advanced into the
arterial lumen, although occasionally the needle must be partially reinserted carefully (never forced, to avoid shearing the
catheter) to serve as a rigid stent.

Catheters with self-contained guidewires to facilitate passage of the cannula into the artery are available. Percutaneous
puncture is made in the same manner, but when blood return

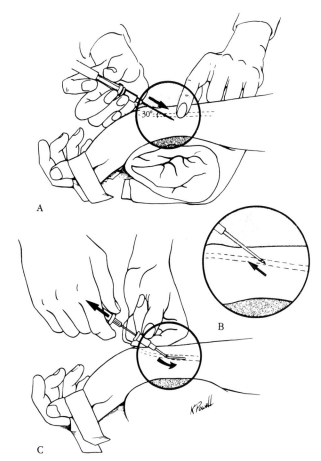

Fig. 3-3. Cannulation of the radial artery. **A:** A towel is placed
behind the wrist, and the hand is immobilized with tape. The radial
artery is fixated with a 20-gauge angiocath connected to a 5-mL
syringe (optional). **B:** The angiocath is withdrawn until pulsatile
blood return is noted. **C:** The trocar is withdrawn as the Teflon catheter is simultaneously advanced.

is noted in the catheter hub, the guidewire is passed through
the needle into the artery, serving as a stent for subsequent
catheter advancement. The guidewire and needle are then
removed and placement confirmed by pulsatile blood return.
The cannula is then secured firmly, attached to transducer
tubing, antiseptic ointment applied, and the site bandaged.

DORSALIS PEDIS ARTERY CANNULATION. Dorsalis pedis
artery catheterization is uncommon in most critical care units;
compared to the radial artery, the anatomy is less predictable
and the success rate lower [35,36]. The dorsalis pedis artery is
the main blood supply of the dorsum of the foot. The artery
runs from the level of the ankle to the great toe. It lies very
superficial and just lateral to the tendon of the extensor hallucis
longus (Fig. 3-4). The dorsalis pedis anastomoses with branches
from the posterior tibial (lateral plantar artery) and, to a lesser
extent, peroneal arteries, creating an arterial arch network analogous to that in the hand. Collateral circulation is assessed by
occluding the dorsalis pedis and posterior tibial pulses and
blanching the great toe by repeated flexion. Release of the posterior tibial artery should result in blushing of the toe within 10
seconds; longer blushing times may represent poor collateral
circulation. Tests using Doppler probes or pneumatic cuffs
around the great toe have also been proposed.

The foot is placed in plantar flexion and prepared in the
usual fashion. Vessel entry is obtained approximately halfway

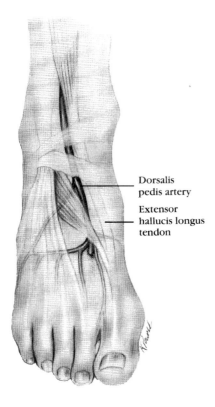

Fig. 3-4. Anatomy of dorsalis pedis artery and adjacent structures.

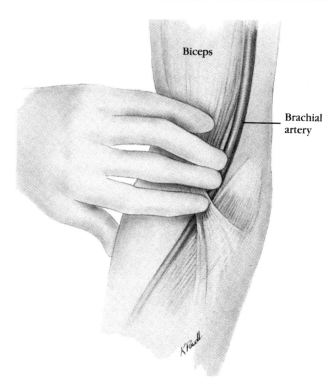

Fig. 3-5. Palpation of the brachial artery. The arm is fully extended at the elbow and the artery palpated in the antecubital fossa as indicated. The brachial artery is then cannulated at this site.

up the dorsum of the foot; advancement is the same as with cannulation of the radial artery. Patients usually find insertion here more painful but less physically limiting. Systolic pressure readings are usually 5 to 20 mm Hg higher with dorsalis pedis catheters than with radial artery catheters, but mean pressure values are generally unchanged.

BRACHIAL ARTERY CANNULATION. Cannulation of the brachial artery is infrequently performed because of concern regarding the lack of effective collateral circulation. Centers experienced in the use of brachial artery catheters, however, have reported complication rates that are no higher than with other routes [28,37,38]. Even when diminution of distal pulses occurs, either because of proximal obstruction or distal embolization, clinical ischemia is unlikely [37]. An additional anatomic consideration is the median nerve, which lies in close proximity to the brachial artery in the antecubital fossa and may be punctured in 1% to 2% of cases [38]. This usually causes only transient paresthesias, but median nerve palsy has been reported. Median nerve palsy is a particular risk in patients with coagulopathy because even minor bleeding into the fascial planes can produce compression of the median nerve [39]. Coagulopathy should be considered a relative contraindication to brachial artery cannulation.

It is good practice to perform a modified Allen's test or Doppler studies of the ulnar and radial arteries before brachial artery cannulation. An alternative site should be selected if one is missing or collateral circulation is inadequate. Cannulation of the brachial artery can be performed with a 2-in. catheter-over-needle as described for the radial artery, but most centers use the Seldinger technique (see Femoral Artery Cannulation). Inserting a 6-in. catheter into the brachial artery places the catheter tip in the axillary artery, and pressures obtained are more representative of aortic pressures. The brachial artery is punctured by extending the arm at the elbow

and locating the pulsation in or slightly proximal to the antecubital fossa, just medial to the bicipital tendon (Fig. 3-5). Once the catheter is established, the elbow must be kept in full extension to avoid kinking or breaking the catheter. Clinical examination of the hand, and Doppler studies if indicated, should be repeated daily while the brachial catheter is in place. The catheter should be promptly removed if diminution of any pulse occurs.

FEMORAL ARTERY CANNULATION. The femoral artery is usually the next alternative when radial artery cannulation fails or is inappropriate [23–27,40]. The femoral artery is large and often palpable when other sites are not, and the technique of cannulation is easy to learn. The most common reason for failure to cannulate is severe atherosclerosis or prior vascular procedures involving both femoral arteries, in which case axillary or brachial artery cannulation is appropriate. Complications unique to this site are rare but include retroperitoneal hemorrhage and intraabdominal viscus perforation. These complications occur because of poor technique or in the presence of anatomic variations (i.e., large inguinal hernia). Ischemic complications from femoral artery catheters are very rare.

The external iliac artery becomes the common femoral artery at the inguinal ligament (Fig. 3-6). The artery courses under the inguinal ligament near the junction of the medial and the middle third of a straight line drawn between the pubis and the anterior superior iliac spine. The artery is cannulated using the Seldinger technique and any one of several available prepackaged kits. Kits contain the equivalent of a 19-gauge thin-wall needle, appropriate guidewire, and 6-in., 18-gauge Teflon catheter. The patient lies supine with the leg extended and slightly abducted. Site preparation includes clipping of pubic hair if necessary. Skin puncture should be 3 to 5 cm caudal to the inguinal ligament to minimize the risk of retroperitoneal hematoma or bowel perforation, which can

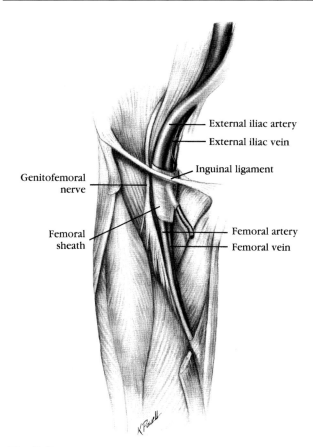

External iliac artery

External iliac vein

Inguinal ligament

Genitofemoral nerve

Femoral sheath

Femoral artery

Femoral vein

Fig. 3-6. Anatomy of the femoral artery and adjacent structures. The artery is cannulated below the inguinal ligament.

occur when needle puncture of the vessel is cephalad to the inguinal ligament. The thin-wall needle is directed, bevel up, cephalad at a 45-degree angle. When arterial blood return is confirmed, the needle and syringe are brought down against the skin to facilitate guidewire passage. The guidewire should advance smoothly, but minor manipulation and rotation are sometimes required if the wire meets resistance at the needle tip or after it has advanced into the vessel. Inability to pass the guidewire may be due to an intimal flap over the needle bevel or atherosclerotic plaques in the vessel. In the latter instance, cannulation of that femoral artery might not be possible. When the guidewire cannot pass beyond the needle tip, it should be withdrawn and blood return reestablished by advancing the needle or repeat vascular puncture. The guidewire is then inserted, the needle withdrawn, and a stab incision made with a scalpel at the skin puncture site. The catheter is next threaded over the guidewire to its hub and the guidewire withdrawn. The catheter is then sutured securely and connected to the transducer tubing.

AXILLARY ARTERY CANNULATION. Axillary artery catheterization in the ICU occurs infrequently, but centers that are experienced with its use report a low rate of complications [41,42]. The axillary artery is large and frequently palpable when all other sites are not and has a rich collateral circulation. The tip of a 6-in. catheter inserted through an axillary approach lies in the subclavian artery, and thus accurate central pressures are obtained. The central location of the tip makes cerebral air embolism a greater risk; therefore, left axillary catheters are preferred for the initial attempt, because air bubbles that pass into the right subclavian artery are more

likely to traverse the aortic arch [43]. Caution should be exercised in flushing axillary catheters, which is best accomplished manually using low pressures and small volumes.

The axillary artery begins at the lateral border of the first rib as a continuation of the subclavian artery and ends at the inferior margin of the teres major muscle, where it becomes the brachial artery. The optimal site for catheterization is the junction of the middle and lower third of the vessel, which usually corresponds to its highest palpable point in the axilla. At this point the artery is superficial and is located at the inferior border of the pectoralis major muscle. The artery is enclosed in a neurovascular bundle, the axillary sheath, with the medial, posterior, and lateral cords of the brachial plexus. Medial to the medial cord is the axillary vein. Not surprisingly, brachial plexus neuropathies have been reported from axillary artery cannulation [44]. Coagulopathy is a relative contraindication, as the axillary sheath can rapidly fill with blood from an uncontrolled arterial puncture, resulting in a compressive neuropathy.

The axillary artery is cannulated using the Seldinger technique and a prepackaged kit. The arm is abducted, externally rotated, and flexed at the elbow by having the patient place the hand under his or her head. Axillary hair should be clipped and the site prepared in standard fashion. The artery is palpated at the lower border of the pectoralis major muscle and fixed against the shaft of the humerus. After local infiltration with lidocaine, the thin-wall needle is introduced at a 30- to 45-degree angle to the vertical plane until return of arterial blood. The remainder of the catheterization proceeds as described for femoral artery cannulation.

Complications of Arterial Cannulation

Arterial cannulation is a relatively safe invasive procedure. Although estimates of the total complication rate range from 15% to 40%, clinically relevant complications occur in 5% or fewer (Table 3-2). Risk factors for infectious and noninfectious complications have been identified [45–53] (Table 3-3), but

Table 3-2. Complications Associated with Arterial Cannulation

Site	Complication
All sites	Pain and swelling
	Thrombosis
	Asymptomatic
	Symptomatic
	Embolization
	Hematoma
	Hemorrhage
	Limb ischemia
	Catheter-related infection
	Local
	Systemic
	Diagnostic blood loss
	Pseudoaneurysm
	Heparin-associated thrombocytopenia
Radial artery	Cerebral embolization
	Peripheral neuropathy
Femoral artery	Retroperitoneal hemorrhage
	Bowel perforation
	Arteriovenous fistula
Axillary artery	Cerebral embolization
	Brachial plexopathy
Brachial artery	Median nerve damage
	Cerebral embolization

Table 3-3. Factors Predisposing to Complications with Arterial Cannulation

Large tapered cannulas (>20 gauge except at the large artery sites)
Hypotension
Coagulopathy
Low cardiac output
Multiple puncture attempts
Use of vasopressors
Atherosclerosis
Hypercoagulable state
Placement by surgical cutdown
Site inflammation
Intermittent flushing system
Bacteremia

the clinical impact of most of these factors is minimal given the overall low incidence of complications.

THROMBOSIS. Thrombosis is the single most common complication of intraarterial catheters. The incidence of thrombosis varies with the site, method of detection, size of the cannula, and duration of cannulation. Thrombosis is common with radial and dorsalis pedis catheters but very rare with femoral or axillary catheters. The incidence of radial artery thrombosis after cannulation has progressively declined because of recognition of the importance of catheter size and composition and the use of continuous versus intermittent heparin flush systems [45,47,49–53]. The incidence probably increases significantly with duration of cannulation [53]. When a 20-gauge nontapered Teflon catheter with a continuous 3 mL per hour heparinized saline flush is used to cannulate the radial artery for 3 to 4 days, thrombosis of the vessel can be detected by Doppler study in 5% to 25% of cases [50,52]. Use of a flush solution containing heparin is standard and may reduce the incidence of thrombosis, but in patients with relative or absolute contraindications to heparin use, sodium citrate or saline alone can be substituted [54,55].

Thrombosis often occurs after decannulation. Women represent a preponderance of patients who experience flow abnormalities after radial artery cannulation, probably because of smaller arteries and a greater tendency to exhibit vasospasm [34]. Most patients eventually recanalize, generally by 3 weeks after removal of the catheter. Despite the high incidence of Doppler-detected thrombosis, clinical ischemia of the hand is rare and usually resolves after catheter removal. Symptomatic occlusion requiring surgical intervention occurs in fewer than 1% of cases. Most patients in whom clinical ischemia develops have an associated contributory cause, such as prolonged circulatory failure with high-dose vasopressor therapy [51].

Significant ischemic complications are minimized by regular inspection of the extremity for unexplained pain or signs of ischemia and immediate withdrawal of the catheter when they appear. If evidence of ischemia persists after catheter removal, thrombolytic therapy, radiologic or surgical embolectomy, or cervical sympathetic blockade is a treatment option [51].

CEREBRAL EMBOLIZATION. Continuous flush devices used with arterial catheters are designed to deliver 3 mL per hour heparinized saline (generally 1 to 5 U heparin per mL saline) from an infusion bag pressurized to 300 mm Hg. Lowenstein et al. [56] demonstrated that, with rapid flushing of radial artery lines with relatively small volumes of radiolabeled solution, traces of the solution could be detected in the central arterial circulation in a time frame representative of retrograde flow. Chang et al. [57] demonstrated that injection

of greater than 2 mL of air into the radial artery of small primates resulted in retrograde passage of air into the vertebral circulation. Factors that increase the risk for retrograde passage of air are patient size and position (air travels up in a sitting patient), injection site, and flush rate. Air embolism has been cited as a risk mainly for radial arterial catheters [57] but logically could occur with all arterial catheters, especially axillary and brachial artery catheters. The risk is minimized by clearing all air from tubing before flushing, opening the flush valve for no more than 2 to 3 seconds, and avoiding overaggressive manual flushing of the line.

DIAGNOSTIC BLOOD LOSS. DBL is patient blood loss that occurs as a result of frequent blood sampling obtained for laboratory testing. The significance of DBL is underappreciated. It is a particular problem in patients with standard arterial catheter setups that are used as the site for sampling, because 3 to 5 mL blood is typically wasted (to avoid heparin/saline contamination) every time a sample is obtained. In patients with frequent arterial blood gas determinations, DBL can be substantial and result in a transfusion requirement [58,59]. DBL can be minimized in several ways, including tubing systems that use a reservoir for blood sampling [60,61], continuous intraarterial blood gas monitoring [62], point of care microchemistry analysis, and the use of pediatric collection tubes. Given the expense and risks of blood component therapy, any or all of the above techniques should be routinely implemented in every ICU. Protocols that are designed to optimize laboratory use have resulted in significant cost savings and reduced transfusion requirements [63].

HEPARIN-ASSOCIATED THROMBOCYTOPENIA. Thrombocytopenia is very common in critically ill adults and usually not due to heparin [64]. However, when the platelet count falls below 80,000 to 100,000 per mL, it is advisable to discontinue all heparin, even the small amount contained in continuous flush devices, because of the possibility of heparin-associated thrombocytopenia [65]. Although the data are conflicting, heparin probably is beneficial in minimizing the risk of thrombosis with arterial catheters, and its routine use should be continued. In the presence of thrombocytopenia, however, sodium citrate, saline, and lactated Ringer's solution are suitable replacements.

OTHER MECHANICAL AND TECHNICAL COMPLICATIONS. Other noninfectious complications reported with arterial lines are pseudoaneurysm formation [66], hematoma, local tenderness, hemorrhage, neuropathies, and embolization.

INFECTION. Infectious sequelae are the most important clinical complications that occur because of arterial cannulation, and many of the concepts and definitions applied to central venous catheter–related infection (see Chapter 82) are also relevant to arterial catheters. Catheter-associated infection is usually initiated by skin flora that invade the intracutaneous tract, causing colonization of the catheters and, ultimately, bacteremia. An additional source of infection from pressure-monitoring systems is contaminated infusate or equipment, which generally causes epidemic nosocomial bacteremia [67]. Arterial pressure-monitoring systems have been the cause of a number of epidemics in the past [68] and are at greater risk for this type of infection than central venous catheters for several reasons: (a) The transducer can become colonized because of inadequate sterilization or stagnant flow, (b) the flush solution is infused at a slow rate (3 mL per hour) and may hang for several hours, and (c) multiple blood samples are obtained by several different personnel from stopcocks in the system, which can serve as entry sites for bacteria [69,70].

Appreciation of the mechanisms responsible for initiating arterial catheter–related infection is important in understanding how to minimize infection. Thorough operator and site preparation is paramount. Chlorhexidine has a broader antibacterial spectrum and longer duration of action than 10% povidone-iodine solution and has demonstrated an impressive reduction in catheter-related infection [71,72]. Operators must wash their hands and wear sterile gloves during insertion and care of the catheter. Breaks in sterile technique during insertion mandate termination of the procedure and replacement of the compromised equipment. Nursing personnel should follow strict guidelines when drawing blood samples or manipulating tubing. Ideally, stopcocks are covered with diaphragms instead of caps. Blood that is withdrawn to clear the tubing before drawing samples should not be reinjected unless a specially designed system is in use [73]. Daily inspection of the site is mandatory, and the catheter should be removed promptly if abnormalities are noted. Dressings are changed every 48 to 72 hours. Application of a polymicrobial ointment to the insertion site during dressing changes is standard but may not reduce the incidence of clinically important infection [74].

Finally, older recommendations to change the monitoring setup completely every 48 hours as a means of infection control are obsolete. Similar to recent experience with other medical equipment such as ventilator circuits, it appears that routine frequent changes of the pressure-monitoring system do not reduce infectious complications and may simply be another opportunity to introduce colonization. Studies have documented the safety of prolonging the interval of routine changes [75]; in our institution, the monitoring setup is changed every 96 hours.

These measures have contributed to an impressive decrease in arterial catheter–related infection. *Arterial catheter–related infection*, defined as 15 or more colonies on semiquantitative culture of a catheter segment [76], occurs in 4% to 20% of catheters but contributes to bacteremia or septicemia in 0% to 3% of cases [23–25,48,71,77,78]. The site of insertion does not appear to be an important factor impacting on the incidence of infection [24,25,36,79]; duration of catheterization continues to be important, but recommendations are changing. It is no longer necessary to change arterial catheters routinely, as studies of catheters remaining in place a week or longer have not demonstrated a higher rate of clinically important infection [41,78,79]. Each institution should determine its own catheter-associated infection rate so that rational policies can be formulated based on existing infection rates.

When arterial catheter infection does occur, *Staphylococcus* species, especially *S. epidermidis*, are commonly isolated. Gram-negative organisms are seen less frequently but predominate in contaminated infusate or equipment-related infection [67,80]. *Candida* species are a greater risk in prolonged catheterization of the glucose-intolerant patient on multiple systemic broad-spectrum antibiotics. Catheter-associated bacteremia should be treated with a 7- to 14-day course of appropriate antibiotics. In complicated cases, longer courses are sometimes necessary.

The optimal evaluation of febrile catheterized patients is a challenging problem. The decision to discontinue or change an arterial catheter differs from the approach with central venous catheters discussed in Chapter 2 in some fundamental ways. Arterial catheters are less likely to be the source of fever than central venous catheters, and changing of arterial lines is frequently not indicated. If the site appears abnormal or the patient is in septic shock with no other etiology, the catheter should be removed. More specific guidelines are difficult to recommend, and individual factors should always be consid-

ered. In general, arterial catheters that are in place for fewer than 4 days will not be the source of fever unless insertion was contaminated. Catheters that are in place for 7 days or longer should be changed to a different site because of the small but measurable chance of infection. Guidewire exchanges have limited utility in the management of arterial catheters unless alternative sites are not available.

Recommendations

Either the radial or femoral artery is an appropriate initial site for percutaneous arterial cannulation. Most centers have more experience with radial artery cannulation, but femoral artery catheters are reliable and have a comparable incidence of complication. In more than 95% of patients, one of these two sites is adequate to achieve arterial pressure monitoring. When these sites are not appropriate, the dorsalis pedis artery is a good alternative, but cannulation is frequently not possible, especially if radial artery cannulation failed because of poor perfusion. Under these circumstances, the axillary or brachial artery can be safely cannulated unless a coagulopathy is present. The site selected for any given patient may not be of prime importance, as centers experienced in the use of alternative sites report excellent results with low rates of complication. Recent experience indicates that arterial catheters can be left in place for longer than 4 days without significantly increasing infection, but each institution needs to conduct its own studies to standardize policies and document catheter-associated infection rates. Iatrogenic anemia and overuse of blood tests are real phenomena associated with arterial catheters, and they should be discontinued promptly when they are no longer required for patient management.

References

1. Gronbeck C, Miller EL: Nonphysician placement of arterial catheters: experience with 500 insertions. *Chest* 104:1716, 1993.
2. Farinas PL: A new technique for arteriographic examination of the abdominal aorta and its branches. *AJR Am J Roentgenol* 46:641, 1941.
3. Lambert E, Wood E: The use of a resistance wire strain gauge manometer to measure intra-arterial pressure. *Proc Soc Exp Biol Med* 64:186, 1947.
4. Peterson LH, Dripps RD, Risman GC: A method for recording the arterial pressure pulse and blood pressure in man. *Am Heart J* 37:771, 1949.
5. Massa DJ, Lundy JS, Faulconer A Jr, et al: A plastic needle. *Mayo Clin Proc* 25:413, 1950.
6. Barr PO: Percutaneous puncture of the radial artery with a multipurpose Teflon catheter for intravenous use. *Acta Physiol Scand* 51:353, 1961.
7. Seldinger SI: Catheter replacement of the needle in percutaneous arteriography. *Acta Radiol* 39:368, 1953.
8. Gardner RM: Accuracy and reliability of disposable pressure transducers coupled with modern pressure monitors. *Crit Care Med* 24:879, 1996.
9. Muakkassa FF, Rutledge R, Fakhry SM, et al: ABGs and arterial lines: the relationship to unnecessarily drawn arterial blood gas samples. *J Trauma* 30:1087, 1990.
10. Low LL, Harrington GR, Stoltzfus DP: The effect of arterial lines on blood-drawing practices and costs in intensive care units. *Chest* 108:216, 1995.
11. Zimmerman JE, Seneff MG, Sun X, et al: Evaluating laboratory utilization in the intensive care unit: patient and institutional characteristics that influence frequency of blood sampling. *Crit Care Med* 25:737, 1997.

12. Roberts D, Ostryzniuk P, Loewen E, et al: Control of blood gas measurements in intensive care units. *Lancet* 337:1580, 1991.
13. Clark JS, Votteri B, Ariagno RL, et al: Noninvasive assessment of blood gases. *Am Rev Respir Dis* 145:220, 1992.
14. Cohn JN: Blood pressure measurement in shock: mechanism of inaccuracy in auscultatory and palpatory methods. *JAMA* 199:972, 1967.
15. Bur A, Hirschl MM, Herkner H, et al: Accuracy of oscillometric blood pressure measurement according to the relation between cuff size and upper-arm circumference in critically ill patients. *Crit Care Med* 28:371, 2000.
16. Gardner RM: Direct arterial pressure monitoring. *Curr Anaesth Crit Care* 1:239, 1990.
17. Boutros A, Albert S: Effect of the dynamic response of transducer-tubing system on accuracy of direct-blood pressure measurement in patients. *Crit Care Med* 11:124, 1983.
18. Rothe CF, Kim KC: Measuring systolic arterial blood pressure. Possible errors from extension tubes or disposable transducer domes. *Crit Care Med* 8:683, 1980.
19. Gardner RM: Direct blood pressure measurement: dynamic response requirements. *Anesthesiology* 54:227, 1981.
20. Billiet E, Colardyn F: Pressure measurement evaluation and accuracy validation: the Gabarith test. *Intensive Care Med* 24:1323, 1998.
21. Pauca AL, Wallenhaupt SL, Kon ND, et al: Does radial artery pressure accurately reflect aorta pressure? *Chest* 102:1193, 1992.
22. O'Rourke MF, Yaginuma T: Wave reflections and the arterial pulse. *Arch Intern Med* 144:366, 1984.
23. Soderstrom CA, Wasserman DH, Dunham CM, et al: Superiority of the femoral artery for monitoring: a prospective study. *Am J Surg* 44:309, 1982.
24. Gurman GM, Kriemerman S: Cannulation of big arteries in critically ill patients. *Crit Care Med* 13:217, 1985.
25. Russell JA, Joel M, Hudson RJ, et al: Prospective evaluation of radial and femoral artery catheterization sites in critically ill adults. *Crit Care Med* 11:936, 1983.
26. Norwood SH, Cormier B, McMahon NG, et al: Prospective study of catheter-related infection during prolonged arterial catheterization. *Crit Care Med* 16:836, 1988.
27. Gordon LH, Brown M, Brown OW, et al: Alternative sites for continuous arterial monitoring. *South Med J* 77:1498, 1984.
28. Mathers LH Jr: Anatomical considerations in obtaining arterial access. *J Intensive Care Med* 5:110, 1990.
29. Allen EV: Thromboangiitis obliterans: method of diagnosis of chronic occlusive arterial lesions distal to the wrist with illustrative cases. *Am J Med Sci* 178:237, 1929.
30. Ejrup B, Fischer B, Wright IS: Clinical evaluation of blood flow to the hand: the false-positive Allen test. *Circulation* 33:778, 1966.
31. Glavin, RJ, Jones HM: Assessing collateral circulation in the hand: four methods compared. *Anaesthesia* 44:594, 1989.
32. Fuhrman TM, Reilley TE, Pippin WD: Comparison of digital blood pressure, plethysmography, and the modified Allen's test as means of evaluating the collateral circulation of the hand. *Anaesthesia* 47:959, 1992.
33. Giner J, Casan P, Belda J, et al: Pain during arterial puncture. *Chest* 110:1443, 1996.
34. Kaye J: Patency of radial artery catheters. *Am J Crit Care* 10:104, 2001.
35. Husum B, Palm T, Eriksen J: Percutaneous cannulation of the dorsalis pedis artery: a prospective study. *Br J Anaesth* 51:1055, 1979.
36. Martin C, Saux P, Papazian L, et al: Long-term arterial cannulation in ICU patients using the radial artery or dorsalis pedis artery. *Chest* 119:901, 2001.
37. Barnes RW, Foster EJ, Janssen GA, et al: Safety of brachial arterial catheters as monitors in the intensive care unit: a prospective evaluation with the Doppler ultrasonic velocity detector. *Anesthesiology* 44:260, 1976.
38. Mann S, Jones RI, Miller-Craig MW, et al: The safety of ambulatory intra-arterial pressure monitoring: A clinical audit of 1000 studies. *Int J Cardiol* 5:585, 1984.
39. Macon WL, Futrell JW: Median nerve neuropathy after percutaneous puncture of the brachial artery in patients receiving anticoagulants. *N Engl J Med* 288:1396, 1973.
40. Ersoz CJ, Hedden M, Lain L: Prolonged femoral arterial catheterization for intensive care. *Anesth Analg* 49:160, 1970.
41. DeAngelis J: Axillary artery monitoring. *Crit Care Med* 4:205, 1976.
42. Brown M, Gordon LH, Brown OW, et al: Intravascular monitoring via the axillary artery. *Anesth Intensive Care* 13:38, 1984.
43. Bryan-Brown CW, Kwun KB, Lumb PD, et al: The axillary artery catheter. *Heart Lung* 12:492, 1983.
44. Lipchik EO, Sugimoto H: Percutaneous brachial artery catheterization. *Radiology* 160:842, 1986.
45. Bedford RF, Wollman H: Complications of percutaneous radial artery monitoring. *Anesthesiology* 38:228, 1973.
46. Puri UK, Carlson RW, Bander JJ, et al: Complications of vascular catheterization in the critically ill. *Crit Care Med* 8:495, 1980.
47. Gardner RM, Schwartz R, Wong HC, et al: Percutaneous indwelling radial artery catheterization for monitoring cardiovascular function. *N Engl J Med* 290:1227, 1974.
48. Band JD, Maki DG: Infections caused by arterial catheters used for hemodynamic monitoring. *Am J Med* 67:735, 1979.
49. Davis FM: Radial artery cannulation: influence of catheter size and material on arterial occlusion. *Anesth Intensive Care* 6:49, 1978.
50. Bedford RF: Radial arterial function following percutaneous cannulation with 18- and 20-gauge catheters. *Anesthesiology* 47:37, 1977.
51. Wilkins RG: Radial artery cannulation and ischemic damage: a review. *Anaesthesia* 40:896, 1985.
52. Weiss BM, Galtiker RI: Complications during and following radial artery cannulation: a prospective study. *Intensive Care Med* 14:424, 1986.
53. Bedford RF: Long-term radial artery cannulation: effects on subsequent vessel function. *Crit Care Med* 6:64, 1978.
54. Clifton GD, Branson P, Kelly HJ, et al: Comparison of normal saline and heparin solutions for maintenance of arterial catheter patency. *Heart Lung* 20:115, 1990.
55. Hook ML, Reuling J, Luettgen ML, et al: Comparison of the patency of arterial lines maintained with heparinized and nonheparinized infusions. *Heart Lung* 16:693, 1987.
56. Lowenstein E, Little JW, Lo HH: Prevention of cerebral embolization from flushing radial artery cannulas. *N Engl J Med* 285:414, 1971.
57. Chang C, Dughi J, Shitabata P, et al: Air embolism and the radial arterial line. *Crit Care Med* 16:141, 1988.
58. Smoller BR, Kruskall MS: Phlebotomy for diagnostic laboratory tests in adults: patterns of use and effect on transfusion requirements. *N Engl J Med* 314:1233, 1986.
59. Henry ML, Garner WL, Fabri PJ: Iatrogenic anemia. *Am J Surg* 151:362, 1986.
60. Peruzzi WT, Parker MA, Lichtenthal PR, et al: A clinical evaluation of a blood conservation device in medical intensive care unit patients. *Crit Care Med* 21:501, 1993.
61. Silver MJ, Jubran H, Stein S, et al: Evaluation of a new blood-conserving arterial line system for patients in intensive care units. *Crit Care Med* 21:507, 1993.
62. Shapiro BA, Mahutte K, Cane RD, et al: Clinical performance of a blood gas monitor: a prospective, multicenter trial. *Crit Care Med* 21:487, 1993.
63. Roberts DE, Bell DD, Ostryzniuk T, et al: Eliminating needless testing in intensive care—an information-based team management approach. *Crit Care Med* 21:1452, 1993.
64. Wittels EG, Siegel RD, Mazur EM: Thrombocytopenia in the intensive care unit setting. *J Intensive Care Med* 5:224, 1990.
65. Warkintin TE, Levine MN, Hirsch J, et al: Heparin-induced thrombocytopenia in patients treated with low molecular weight heparin or unfractionated heparin. *N Engl J Med* 332:330, 1995.
66. Altin RS, Flicker S, Naidech HJ: Pseudoaneurysm and arteriovenous fistula after femoral artery catheterization: associated with low femoral punctures. *AJR Am J Roentgenol* 152:629, 1989.
67. Maki D: Nosocomial bacteremia: an epidemiologic overview. *Am J Med* 70:719, 1981.
68. Mermel LA, Maki DG: Epidemic bloodstream infections from hemodynamic pressure monitoring: Signs of the times. *Infect Control Hosp Epidemiol* 10:47, 1989.
69. Shinozaki T, Deane RS, Mazuzan JE, et al: Bacterial contamination of arterial lines: a prospective study. *JAMA* 249:223, 1983.
70. Stamm WE, Colella JJ, Anderson RL, et al: Indwelling arterial catheters as a source of nosocomial bacteremia. *N Engl J Med* 292:1099, 1975.
71. Maki DG, Ringer M, Alvarado CJ: Prospective, randomized trial of povidone-iodine, alcohol, and chlorhexidine for prevention of

infection associated with central venous and arterial catheters. *Lancet* 338:339, 1991.

72. Mimoz O, Pieroni L, Lawrence C, et al: Prospective, randomized trial of two antiseptic solutions for prevention of central venous or arterial catheter colonization and infection in intensive care unit patients. *Crit Care Med* 24:1818, 1996.

73. Peruzzi WT, Noskin GA, Moen SG, et al: Microbial contamination of blood conservation devices during routine use in the critical care setting: results of a prospective, randomized trial. *Crit Care Med* 24:1157, 1996.

74. Maki DG, Band JD: A comparative study of polyantibiotic and iodophor ointments in prevention of vascular catheter-related infection. *Am J Med* 70:739, 1981.

75. O'Malley MK, Rhame FS, Cerra FB, et al: Value of routine pressure monitoring system changes after 72 hours of continuous use. *Crit Care Med* 22:1424, 1994.

76. Maki DG, Weise CE, Sarafin HW: A semiquantitative culture method for identifying intravenous-catheter related infection. *N Engl J Med* 296:1305, 1977.

77. Leroy O, Billiau V, Beuscart C, et al: Nosocomial infections associated with long-term radial artery cannulation. *Intensive Care Med* 15:241, 1989.

78. Eyer S, Brummitt C, Crossley K, et al: Catheter-related sepsis: prospective randomized study of three methods of long-term catheter maintenance. *Crit Care Med* 18:1073, 1990.

79. Thomas F, Parker J, Burke J, et al: Prospective randomized evaluation of indwelling radial vs. femoral arterial catheters in high risk critically ill patients. *Crit Care Med* 10:226, 1982.

80. Ransjo V, Good Z: An outbreak of *Klebsiella oxytoca* septicemia associated with the use of invasive blood pressure monitoring. *Acta Anaesthesiol Scand* 36:289, 1992.

4. Pulmonary Artery Catheters

Stephen J. Voyce and
D. Robert McCaffree

Since their introduction into clinical practice in 1970 by Swan and associates [1], balloon-tipped, flow-directed pulmonary artery (PA) catheters have found widespread use in the clinical management of critically ill patients. However, in recent years, both the safety and efficacy of these catheters have been brought into question. In this chapter, we review the physiologic basis for their use, some history regarding their development and use, the concerns raised about their use, and suggestions for appropriate use of the catheters and the information obtained from them.

Physiologic Rationale for Use of the Pulmonary Artery Catheter

In unstable situations, during which hemodynamic changes often occur rapidly, clinical evaluation may be misleading [2–6]. PA catheters allow direct measurement of several major determinants and consequences of cardiac performance [preload, afterload, cardiac output (CO)], thereby supplying additional data to aid in clinical decision making [7–10].

Cardiac function depends on the relationship between muscle length (preload), the load on the muscle (afterload), and the intrinsic property of contractility. Until the development of the flow-directed PA catheter, there was no way to assess all of these using one instrument in a clinically useful way at bedside. The catheter allows the reflection of right ventricular (RV) preload (right atrial pressure), RV afterload (PA pressure), left ventricular preload [PA wedge pressure (PAWP)], and contractility (stroke volume or CO). Left ventricular afterload is reflected by the systemic artery pressure. This information allows the calculations of numerous parameters, including vascular resistances. No other tool allows the gathering of such a large amount of information.

Controversies Regarding Use of the Pulmonary Artery Catheter

Despite all its advantages, some clinicians elect to minimize the use of the PA catheter. The reason for this is that the benefit of using the catheter has been questioned. In fact, some studies even suggest increased mortality with catheter use.

The reasons that the increased physiologic information may not benefit many patients are not clear. However, this lack of benefit or even increased mortality is not easily explained by complications from catheter use. It has been hypothesized that these results could be due to erroneous or misused information obtained from the catheter or to the fact that use of the catheter reflects a more aggressive management style that could lead to greater mortality in critically ill patients.

Because the question of whether catheter use is beneficial—and if so, to which patients—is such a key issue, studies addressing both the benefits and the risks or lack of benefits of catheter use are reviewed first.

EVIDENCE OF BENEFIT. For the first several years after the introduction of the catheter, there were no studies discussing specific benefits, in large part because the increase in physiologic information seemed to confer an unquestionable benefit. In the 1980s, several reports appeared that seemed to support this benefit. Specifically, several studies found that the usual measures of trying to assess preload, afterload, and contractility were inaccurate and that the catheter affected clinical decisions in a significant way approximately one-half of the time [4,6,11,12]. The only one of these studies that looked at outcome as reflected by mortality found that in those patients in circulatory shock for whom the use of the catheter led to a significant change in therapy, mortality was significantly lower [12].

Many reports of the benefits of PA catheter use have been in surgical and anesthesia settings. The most compelling evidence of benefit in these populations is in the use of optimizing cardiovascular performance in the perioperative period or in the use of goal-directed therapy in high-risk surgical patients [i.e., attempting to drive the CO and oxygen delivery (DO_2) to supranormal levels] [13–19]. These strategies require the use of the PA catheter. The rationale is that patients with greater metabolic needs (e.g., postsurgery, trauma, burns, sepsis) require supranormal physiologic parameters to improve outcome. Using data derived from PA catheterization, investigators have retrospectively described the hemodynamic and oxygen transport variables of critically ill postoperative survivors versus nonsurvivors [16,17]. Subsequent application of these supranormal physiologic goals in some prospective studies [13,15] demonstrated favorable results. Although most of the success of this strategy has been demonstrated in surgical patients, there has been a study recently reported in patients with sepsis using goal-directed therapy instituted very early in the course of illness [20]. This was instituted in the emergency room (i.e., very early in the course of sepsis) and resulted in reduced mortality in this cohort of patients. It is important to recognize that these studies do not imply a causal relationship between improved patient outcome and increased DO_2. Indeed, others have suggested that the ability of the cardiovascular system to respond to fluid and pharmacologic manipulations is the ultimate determinant of the beneficial outcomes observed in these studies [205].

There has also been a recent metaanalysis of organ failure as an outcome end-point of catheter use [21]. This analysis of 1,610 patients in 12 randomized controlled trials using the PA catheter found that there was a significant reduction in morbidity in those patients in whom the catheter was used. However, the quality of the studies varied considerably, and eight of the 12 dealt with studies having supranormal values as their goals.

EVIDENCE OF HARM OR LACK OF BENEFIT. In contrast to the above evidence of benefit, there is growing evidence that the use of the catheter does not lead to improved outcomes [22,23]. In fact, in some groups of patients, it may be associated with an increased mortality. For example, in the discussion about supranormal goals, it has been argued that attempts to maintain supranormal physiologic parameters in the patients with left ventricular dysfunction or ischemic heart disease may, in fact, be detrimental [15,18]. More recent data have not convincingly demonstrated improved outcome or survival rates in patients randomized to augmentation of DO_2 to supranormal levels compared to those undergoing conventional therapy. Of clinical interest, an increased mortality recently has been reported in patients driven to supranormal hemodynamic levels [24,25]. The reason for the increased mortality cannot be attributed to the catheter itself, however, in these studies. Thus, for patients with systemic inflammatory response syndrome–related organ dysfunction, the Pulmonary Artery Catheter Consensus Statement [205] does not recommend PA catheter–guided hemodynamic intervention to achieve supranormal DO_2 levels.

Questions were first raised about the possibility of increased mortality associated with the use of the catheter as early as 1978 [26]. In 1980, in an editorial, Spodick [27] called for a randomized trial. Robin in 1985 [28] reviewed the reported complications of catheter use and noted no clear evidence of the risk to benefit ratio of using the catheter. He also called for randomized trials. In 1987, a retrospective study by Gore and colleagues [29] showed a higher mortality rate in patients with acute myocardial infarction complicated by heart failure, hypotension, or shock who underwent PA catheteriza-

tion than in patients with similar complications of myocardial infarction who were not catheterized. The difference in mortality rates persisted despite multivariate analysis of the data to adjust for infarct size. The authors acknowledged the difficulty in assessing whether the patients who received a PA catheter were actually sicker than those who did not, given the study's retrospective nature. No specific complication of PA catheterization could be related to the increased short-term mortality, and the authors were careful not to suggest that the increased mortality was due to the use of the PA catheter. This led to another call for controlled trials [30]. Subsequent reports also raised the question of the risk of catheter use in patients with acute myocardial infarction [31,32].

However, the most significant study raising questions about the usefulness of the catheter was that by Connors et al. [33]. This study has widely been quoted as showing evidence of increased risk of mortality associated with catheter use, but the authors actually interpret their findings more conservatively. They state simply that they found no benefit of catheter use. Because of the discussion generated by this study, it deserves a more detailed description.

The study by Connors et al. was a prospective cohort study of more than 5,700 patients with one of nine diagnoses and a life expectancy of less than 6 months, all of whom were enrolled in the Study to Understand Prognoses and Preferences for Outcomes and Risks of Treatment (SUPPORT). All were admitted to an intensive care unit (ICU) in one of the five participating centers. Approximately 40% received a PA catheter within the first 24 hours of ICU admission. All patients were evaluated according to a "propensity score" (i.e., the propensity to have a catheter placed), which was developed through the input of seven specialists in critical care. This score included more than 50 variables. Furthermore, the adequacy of adjustment by the propensity score was evaluated by sensitivity analysis, which ultimately assessed how substantial the effect of a missing variable would need to be to mask either a true relative hazard of death or a beneficial effect of the use of the catheter.

Connors et al. found that, in pairs of patients matched by their propensity scores, one of whom received the catheter and one of whom did not, catheter use increased the relative hazard of death in catheterized patients at 30, 60, and 180 days by approximately 25% overall. The in-hospital relative hazard of death increased by almost 40%. The 30-day relative hazard of death was greatest in patients with acute respiratory failure and multiple organ system failure (approximately 30%); these two categories accounted for almost 80% of the patients in the study and therefore heavily influenced the pooled data. The relative hazard of death was not significantly increased in those patients with congestive heart failure or the other six diagnoses. However, in no diagnostic category was there any demonstrated benefit from the use of the catheter. This is the major finding of the study, although they also found increased costs and longer hospital stays for catheterized patients (as have many others).

The sensitivity analysis confirmed the adequacy of the propensity score in identifying the most important variables associated with catheter use. This analysis revealed that any variable missing from consideration, which would also have to be independent from any other variable considered, would have to increase the relative hazard of death or the probability of catheter use sixfold to mask a benefit from the catheter. In the same vein, a missing variable would have to increase the relative hazard of death or the probability of catheter use more than threefold to make the reported increase in the relative hazard of death invalid.

Although this descriptive study could not evaluate the causes for the findings, the authors did speculate on possibilities. These included the possibility that complications from the catheter use itself could reduce any beneficial effect. This is unlikely, since the reported complication rates and types could not account for the level of risk found. Second, it may be that physicians using the catheter are not sufficiently knowledgeable in the interpretation and use of the information. There is some support for this possibility. Investigatiors [34–36] found in written questionnaires that experienced physicians and nurses misinterpreted pressure waveforms obtained from PA catheters. Third, it may be that use of the catheter marks a more aggressive approach that might be responsible for the greater mortality. This possibility is supported by the findings of Blumberg and Binns in patients with acute myocardial infarction [37]. They found that patients with PA catheters had higher Therapeutic Intervention Scoring System scores, even after removing the Therapeutic Intervention Scoring System points associated with the catheter itself, than those who did not receive the catheter. Moreover, Viellard-Baron et al. [38] reported that, in a small retrospective cohort study of patients with acute respiratory distress syndrome (ARDS) in two hospitals, one of which routinely used the PA catheter and one of which never used it, the use of epinephrine/norepinephrine and a nonpulmonary cause of ARDS were independently associated with mortality. They suggested that the use of vasopressors may be more important than the use of the PA catheter as a cause for mortality. A fourth possibility, which is related to the possibility proposed by Veillard-Baron et al., is that the information derived from the catheter leads to changes in therapy that may actually be harmful, such as more aggressive fluid therapy or use of inotropes. This could be reflected in those studies that have found that trying to achieve supranormal cardiovascular values in patients with medical illnesses is not beneficial and may be associated with increased mortality [23,24].

The results of the study conducted by Connors et al. generated even more calls either for a moratorium on the use of the catheter or for randomized controlled trials [39]. However, the importance of this study in increasing the perception of a need for randomized studies and a sense of clinical equipoise can be best illustrated by the experience of an earlier attempt at a randomized trial. Guyatt [40] reported the results of a randomized study in Ontario. Of 148 potentially eligible patients, only 33 were randomized. Of the 115 not randomized, 52 were not randomized because the attending physician believed that use of the catheter was ethically mandated, whereas 27 were not randomized because the attending physician felt it was unethical to use the catheter. After publication of the study by Connors et al., there seemed to be a greater consensus of the need for randomized controlled studies.

All the above studies dealt predominantly with patients with nonsurgical diseases. Recently, several studies have been reported in surgical patients addressing the use of the catheter and resultant outcomes and basically finding no benefit from the use of the catheter. Polanczyk et al. [41] reported the results of an observational study of the use of the PA catheter to prevent cardiac complications in patients undergoing noncardiac surgery. They found that patients undergoing catheterization had a threefold increase in major postoperative cardiac events. In a case-controlled analysis, those receiving a PA catheter also had a greater incidence of postoperative congestive heart failure. In a metaanalysis of routine perioperative PA catheterization in patients undergoing vascular surgery, Barone et al. [42] found no benefit of catheter use in preventing morbidity or mortality. Finally, in a study available only in abstract at the time of this writing, Sandham et al. [43] found in a large multicenter randomized controlled trial in 1,994 patients undergoing urgent or elective surgery that use of the catheter conferred no benefit in survival to hospital discharge.

CURRENT STATUS OF RECOMMENDATIONS FOR CATHETER USE. The studies detailed in this chapter have generated a great deal of discussion of the current role of the PA catheter. The only generally accepted conclusions are that randomized controlled trials are necessary and that education on the interpretation of information derived from the catheter and understanding of that information could be improved. At the present time, as per the recommendations of a workshop called by the National Heart, Lung, and Blood Institute (NHLBI) and the U.S. Food and Drug Administration (FDA) [44], two randomized control trials are under way, one in patients with ARDS and the other in patients with severe congestive heart failure (New York Heart Association classes III and IV). In addition, seven specialty organizations, along with the NHLBI and the FDA, have developed a Web-based educational program called the Pulmonary Artery Catheter Education Program (PACEP), which has recently been introduced. The URL is http://www.PACEP.org.

In the absence of definitive evidence of the relative risk to benefit ratios in specific groups of patients, and in light of the physiologic information available through the catheter, many critical care practitioners are continuing to use the catheter. The remainder of the chapter deals with the safe and rational use of the catheter.

Indications for Pulmonary Artery Catheter Use

The wide potential of the PA catheter should undergo a careful clinical assessment, since the use of the catheter entails a risk for the patient. Clinicians who use a PA catheter for monitoring should understand the fundamentals of the insertion technique, the equipment used, and the data that can be generated [9].

The use of the PA catheter for monitoring has four central objectives: (a) to assess left or right ventricular function, or both, (b) to monitor changes in hemodynamic status, (c) to guide treatment with pharmacologic and nonpharmacologic agents, and (d) to provide prognostic information. The conditions in which PA catheterization may be useful are characterized by a clinically unclear or rapidly changing hemodynamic status. Numerous sources review the indications for placement of PA catheters [9,45–47]. Table 4-1 is a partial listing of these indications. Use of PA catheters in specific disease entities is discussed in other chapters.

Other uses of PA catheters outside the ICU include applications in the anesthesia suite and cardiac catheterization laboratory [48–51]. These are not discussed further here.

Basic Catheter Features and Construction

The basic catheter is constructed from polyvinylchloride and has a pliable shaft that softens further at body temperature. Because polyvinylchloride has a high thrombogenicity, the catheters are generally coated with heparin. Heparin bonding of catheters, introduced in 1981, has been shown to be effective in reducing catheter thrombogenicity [53,57]. The standard catheter length is 110 cm, and the most commonly used external diameter is 5 or 7 French (Fr) (1 Fr = 0.0335 mm). A balloon is fastened 1 to 2 mm from the tip (Fig. 4-1); when inflated, it guides the catheter (by virtue of fluid dynamic

Table 4-1. General Indications for Pulmonary
Artery Catheterization

Management of complicated myocardial infarction
   Hypovolemia vs. cardiogenic shock
   Ventricular septal rupture vs. acute mitral regurgitation
   Severe left ventricular failure
   Right ventricular infarction
   Unstable angina
   Refractory ventricular tachycardia
Assessment of respiratory distress
   Cardiogenic vs. noncardiogenic (e.g., acute respiratory distress syndrome) pulmonary edema
   Primary vs. secondary pulmonary hypertension
Assessment of shock
   Cardiogenic
   Hypovolemic
   Septic
   Pulmonary embolism
Assessment of therapy in selected individuals
   Afterload reduction in patients with severe left ventricular function
   Inotropic agent
   Vasopressors
   Beta-blockers
   Temporary pacing (ventricular vs. atrioventricular)
   Intraaortic balloon counterpulsation
   Mechanical ventilation (e.g., with positive end-expiratory pressure)
Management of postoperative open heart surgical patients
Assessment of cardiac tamponade/constriction
Assessment of valvular heart disease
Perioperative monitoring of patients with unstable cardiac status during noncardiac surgery
Assessment of fluid requirements in critically ill patients
   Gastrointestinal hemorrhage
   Sepsis
   Acute renal failure
   Burns
   Decompensated cirrhosis
   Advanced peritonitis
Management of severe preeclampsia [198]

Adapted from JM Gore, JS Alpert, JR Benotti, et al: *Handbook of Hemodynamic Monitoring*. Boston, Little, Brown, 1984.

drag) from the greater intrathoracic veins through the right heart chambers into the PA. When fully inflated in a vessel of sufficiently large caliber, the balloon protrudes above the catheter tip, thus distributing tip forces over a large area and minimizing the chances for endocardial damage or arrhythmia induction during catheter insertion (Fig. 4-2). Progression of the catheter is stopped when it impacts in a PA slightly smaller in diameter than the fully inflated balloon. From this position, the PAWP is obtained. Balloon capacity varies according to catheter size, and the operator must be aware of the individual balloon's maximal inflation volume as recommended by the manufacturer. The balloon is usually inflated with air, but filtered carbon dioxide should be used in any situation in which balloon rupture might result in access of the inflation medium to the arterial system (e.g., if a right-to-left intracardiac shunt or a pulmonary arteriovenous fistula is suspected). If carbon dioxide is used, periodic deflation and reinflation may be necessary, since carbon dioxide diffuses through the latex balloon at a rate of approximately 0.5 cc per minute. Liquids should never be used as the inflation medium.

A variety of catheter constructions is available, each designed for particular clinical applications. Double-lumen catheters allow balloon inflation through one lumen, and a distal opening at the tip of the catheter is used to measure intravascular pressures and sample blood. Triple-lumen catheters have a proximal port terminating 30 cm from the tip of the catheter, allowing simultaneous measurement of right atrial

and PA or wedge pressures. The most commonly used PA catheter in the ICU setting is a quadruple-lumen catheter, which has a lumen containing electrical leads for a thermistor positioned at the catheter surface 4 cm proximal to its tip (Fig. 4-1) [54]. The thermistor measures PA blood temperature and allows thermodilution CO measurements. A five-lumen catheter is also available, with the fifth lumen opening 40 cm from the tip of the catheter. The fifth lumen provides additional central venous access for fluid or medication infusions when peripheral access is limited or when drugs requiring infusion into a large vein (e.g., dopamine, epinephrine) are used. Figure 4-2 shows the balloon on the tip inflated.

Several special-purpose PA catheter designs are available. Pacing PA catheters incorporate two groups of electrodes on the catheter surface, enabling intracardiac electrocardiographic (ECG) recording or temporary cardiac pacing [55]. These catheters are used for emergency cardiac pacing, although it is often difficult to position the catheter for reliable simultaneous cardiac pacing and PA pressure measurements. A five-lumen catheter (Paceport RV catheter; C.R. Bard, Billerica, MA) allows passage of a specially designed 2.4-Fr bipolar pacing electrode (probe) through the additional lumen, located 19 cm from the catheter tip. This allows emergency temporary intracardiac pacing without the need for a separate central venous puncture. The pacing probe is Teflon coated to allow easy introduction through the pacemaker port lumen; the intracavitary part of the probe is heparin impregnated to reduce the risk of thrombus formation. One report demonstrated satisfactory ventricular pacing in 19 of 23 patients using this catheter design (83% success rate) [56]. When a pacing probe is not in use, the fifth lumen may be used for additional central venous access or continuous RV pressure monitoring.

Continuous mixed venous oxygen saturation measurement is clinically available using a fiberoptic five-lumen PA catheter [57]. Segal and colleagues [58] described a catheter that incorporates Doppler technology for continuous CO determinations. Catheters equipped with a fast-response (95 milliseconds) thermistor and intracardiac ECG monitoring electrodes are also available. These catheters allow determination of the RV ejection fraction and RV systolic time intervals in critically ill patients [59–62]. The calculated RV ejection fraction has correlated well with simultaneous radionuclide first-pass studies [59]. The clinical utility of these and other catheter modifications is under investigation [58,63–66].

PRESSURE TRANSDUCERS. Hemodynamic monitoring requires a system able to convert changes in intravascular pressure into electrical signals suitable for interpretation. The most commonly used hemodynamic monitoring system is a catheter-tubing–transducer system. A fluid-filled intravascular catheter is connected to a transducer by a fluid-filled tubing system. (For more details, see the discussion in Chapter 3.)

Insertion Techniques

GENERAL CONSIDERATIONS. Techniques for insertion of Swan-Ganz catheters and handling of the monitoring equipment are described in many sources [67–71]. Manufacturers' recommendations should be carefully followed. All catheter manufacturers have detailed insertion and training materials. In addition, as already discussed, several specialty societies, the NHLBI, and the FDA have recently cooperated in producing a training program available on the Internet at http://www.PACEP.org. We only briefly describe the insertion technique.

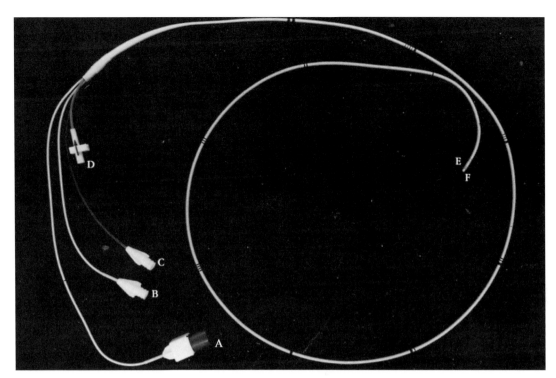

Fig. 4-1. Quadruple-lumen pulmonary artery catheter. Connection to thermodilution cardiac output computer (A). Connection to distal lumen (B). Connection to proximal lumen (C). Stopcock connected to balloon at the catheter tip for balloon inflation (D). Thermistor (E). Balloon (F). Note that the catheter is marked in 10-cm increments.

PA catheterization can be performed in any hospital location where continuous ECG and hemodynamic monitoring is possible and where equipment and supplies needed for cardiopulmonary resuscitation are readily available. Fluoroscopy is not essential, but it can facilitate difficult placements. Properly constructed beds and protective aprons are mandatory for safe use of fluoroscopic equipment. Meticulous attention to sterile technique is of obvious importance; all involved personnel must wear sterile caps, gowns, masks, and gloves, and the patient must be fully protected by sterile drapes.

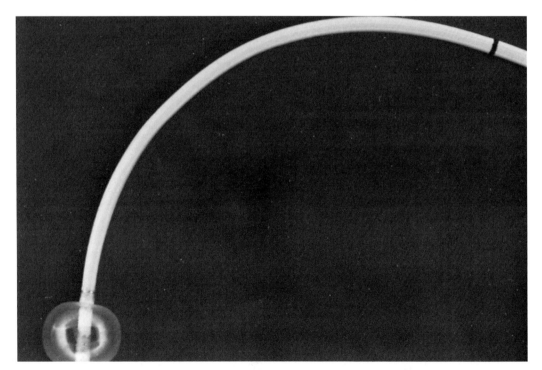

Fig. 4-2. Balloon properly inflated at the tip of a pulmonary artery catheter. Note that the balloon shields the catheter tip and prevents it from irritating cardiac chambers on its passage to the pulmonary artery.

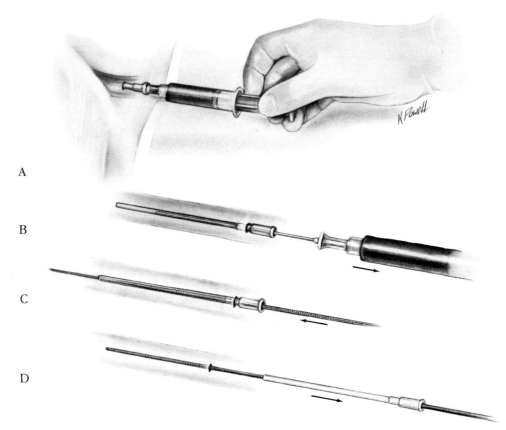

A

B

C

D

Fig. 4-3. A: Easy blood aspiration has been demonstrated using the guidewire introducer needle. **B:** The inner needle is removed. **C:** The spring guidewire is advanced, soft end first, through the cannula into the vessel. **D:** With the guidewire held in place, the cannula is withdrawn from the vessel by being pulled over and off the length of the guidewire.

The catheter may be inserted percutaneously or via cutdown into the basilic, brachial, femoral, subclavian, or internal jugular veins using techniques described in Chapter 2. For the following reasons, many clinicians prefer the percutaneous internal jugular approach: (a) patient arm movements are not encumbered and are unlikely to alter catheter tip position, (b) it can be used in patients undergoing intrathoracic surgery, and (c) fewer thrombotic and septic complications may occur. We often use a prepackaged catheter introducer kit (including a sheath vessel dilator, guidewire, sterile sleeve adapter, and related supplies).

TYPICAL CATHETER INSERTION PROCEDURE

1. Prepare and connect pressure tubing, manifolds, stopcocks, and transducers. Remove the sterile balloon-tipped catheter from its container and wipe the outside with gauze soaked in sterile water or saline. Test for balloon integrity by submerging it in a small amount of fluid and checking for air leaks as the balloon is inflated (using the amount of air recommended by the manufacturer). Deflate the balloon.
2. Insert a central venous cannula as described in Chapter 2. Using the Seldinger technique, remove the catheter and position the guidewire contained in the PA catheter kit in the vein (Figs. 4-3 and 4-4).
3. Make a small incision with a scalpel to enlarge the puncture site (Fig. 4-5) and thread a vessel dilator-sheath apparatus (the size should be 8 Fr if a 7-Fr catheter is to be used) over the guidewire and advance it into the vessel, using a twisting motion to get through the puncture site (Fig. 4-6).
4. Remove the guidewire and vessel dilator, leaving the introducer sheath in the vessel (Fig. 4-7).

5. Attach stopcocks to the right atrium and PA ports of the PA catheter and fill the proximal and distal catheter lumens with flush solution. Close the stopcocks to keep flush solution within the lumens and to avoid introduction of air into the circulation.
6. If a sterile sleeve adapter is to be used, insert the catheter through it and pull the adapter proximally over the catheter to keep it out of the way. Once the catheter is advanced to its desired intravascular location, attach the distal end of the sleeve adapter to the introducer sheath hub.

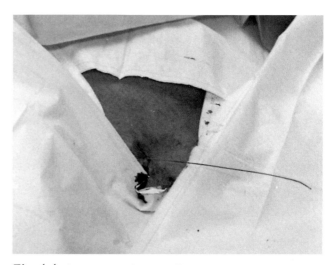

Fig. 4-4. The spring guidewire, stiff end protruding, is now located in the subclavian vein.

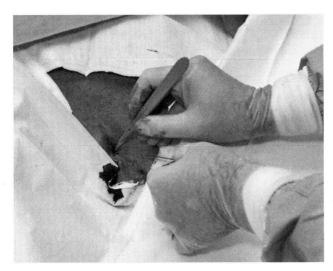

Fig. 4-5. A small incision is made with a scalpel to enlarge the puncture site.

7. Pass the catheter through the introducer sheath into the vein (Fig. 4-8). Advance it, using the marks on the catheter shaft indicating 10-cm distances from the tip, until the tip is in the right atrium. This requires advancement of approximately 35 to 40 cm from the left antecubital fossa, 10 to 15 cm from the internal jugular vein, 10 cm from the subclavian vein, and 35 to 40 cm from the femoral vein. A right atrial waveform on the monitor, with appropriate fluctuations accompanying respiratory changes or cough, confirms proper intrathoracic location (Fig. 4-9, center). Obtain right atrial blood for oxygen saturation from the distal port. Flush the distal lumen with heparinized saline and record the right atrial pressures. (Occasionally, it is necessary to inflate the balloon to keep the tip from adhering to the atrial wall during blood aspiration.)

8. With the catheter tip in the right atrium, inflate the balloon with the recommended amount of air or carbon dioxide (Fig. 4-9A). Inflation of the balloon should be associated with a slight feeling of resistance—if it is not, suspect balloon rupture and do not attempt further inflation or advancement of the catheter before properly reevaluating balloon integrity. If significant resistance to balloon inflation is encountered, suspect malposition of the catheter in a small vessel; withdraw the catheter and readvance it to a new position. Do not use liquids to inflate the balloon, as they might be irretrievable and could prevent balloon deflation.

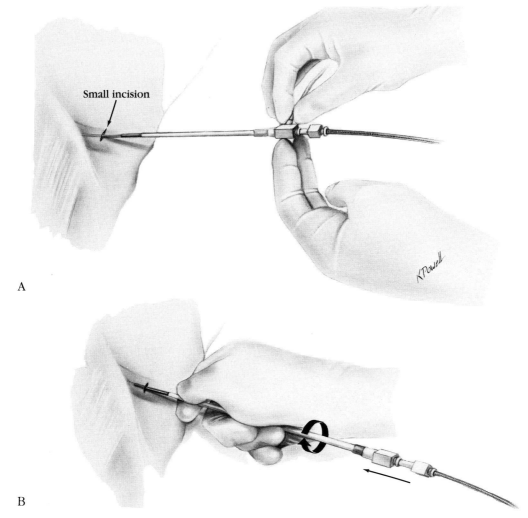

Fig. 4-6. **A:** The vessel dilator-sheath apparatus is threaded over the guidewire and advanced into the vessel. **B:** A twisting motion is used to thread the apparatus into the vessel.

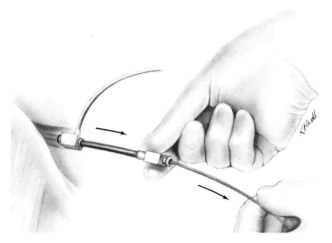

Fig. 4-7. The guidewire and vessel dilator are removed, leaving the introducer sheath in the vessel.

9. With the balloon inflated, advance the catheter until a RV pressure tracing is seen on the monitor (Fig. 4-9, center). Obtain and record RV pressures. Catheter passage into and through the RV is an especially risky time in terms of arrhythmias. Maintaining the balloon inflated in the RV minimizes ventricular irritation (Fig. 4-9B), but it is important to monitor vital signs and ECG throughout the entire insertion procedure.

10. Continue advancing the catheter until the diastolic pressure tracing rises above that in the RV (Fig. 4-9, center), indicating PA placement (Fig. 4-9C). If an RV trace still appears after the catheter has been advanced 15 cm beyond the original distance needed to reach the right atrium, suspect curling in the ventricle; deflate the balloon, withdraw it to the right atrium, then reinflate it and try again. Advancement beyond the PA position results in a fall on the pressure tracing from the levels of systolic pressure noted in the RV and PA. When this is noted, record the PAWP (Fig. 4-9, center, D) and deflate the balloon. Phasic PA pressure should reappear on the pressure tracing when the balloon is deflated. If it does not, pull back the catheter with the deflated balloon until the PA tracing appears. With the balloon deflated, blood may be aspirated for oxygen saturation measurement. Watch for intermittent RV tracings indicating slippage of the catheter backward into the ventricle.

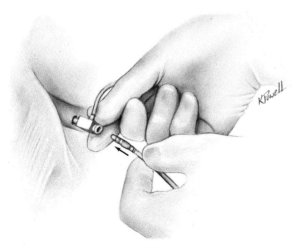

Fig. 4-8. The catheter is passed through the introducer sheath into the vein.

11. Carefully record the balloon inflation volume needed to change the PA pressure tracing to the PAWP tracing. If PAWP is recorded with an inflation volume significantly lower than the manufacturer's recommended volume, or if subsequent PAWP determinations require decreasing amounts of balloon inflation volume as compared to an initial appropriate amount, the catheter tip has migrated too far peripherally and should be pulled back immediately.

12. Secure the catheter in the correct PA position by suturing or taping it to the skin to prevent inadvertent advancement. Apply a germicidal agent and dress appropriately.

13. Order a chest radiograph to confirm catheter position; the catheter tip should appear no more than 3 to 5 cm from the midline. To assess whether peripheral catheter migration has occurred, daily chest radiographs are recommended to supplement pressure monitoring and checks on balloon inflation volumes. An initial cross-table lateral radiograph should be obtained in patients on positive end-expiratory pressure (PEEP) to rule out superior placements.

SPECIAL CONSIDERATIONS. In certain disease states (right atrial or RV dilatation, severe pulmonary hypertension, severe tricuspid insufficiency, low CO syndromes), it may be difficult to position a flow-directed catheter properly. These settings may require fluoroscopic guidance to aid in catheter positioning. Infusion of 5 to 10 mL of cold saline through the distal lumen may stiffen the catheter and aid in positioning. Alternatively, a 0.025-cm guidewire 145 cm long may be used to stiffen the catheter when placed through the distal lumen of a 7-Fr PA catheter. This manipulation should be performed only under fluoroscopic guidance by an experienced operator. Rarely, nonflow-directed PA catheters (e.g., Cournand catheters) may be required. Because of their rigidity, these catheters have the potential to perforate the right heart and must be placed only under fluoroscopy by a physician experienced in cardiac catheterization techniques.

Physiologic Data

Measurement of a variety of hemodynamic parameters and oxygen saturations is possible using the PA catheter. A summary of normal values for these parameters is found in Tables 4-2 and 4-3.

PRESSURES

Right Atrium. With the tip of the PA catheter in the right atrium (Fig. 4-9A), the balloon is deflated and a right atrial waveform recorded (Fig. 4-10). Normal resting right atrial pressure is 0 to 6 mm Hg. Two major positive atrial pressure waves, the *a* wave and *v* wave, can usually be recorded. On occasion, a third positive wave, the *c* wave, can also be seen. The *a* wave is due to atrial contraction and follows the simultaneously recorded ECG P wave [47,72]. The *a* wave peak generally follows the peak of the electrical P wave by approximately 80 milliseconds [73]. The *v* wave represents the pressure generated by venous filling of the right atrium while the tricuspid valve is closed. The peak of the *v* wave occurs at the end of ventricular systole when the atrium is maximally filled. This occurs near the end of the ECG T wave. The *c* wave is due to the sudden motion of the atrioventricular valve ring toward the right atrium at the onset of ventricular systole. The *c* wave follows the *a* wave by a time equal to the ECG P-R interval. The *c* wave is more readily visible in cases of P-R prolongation [73].

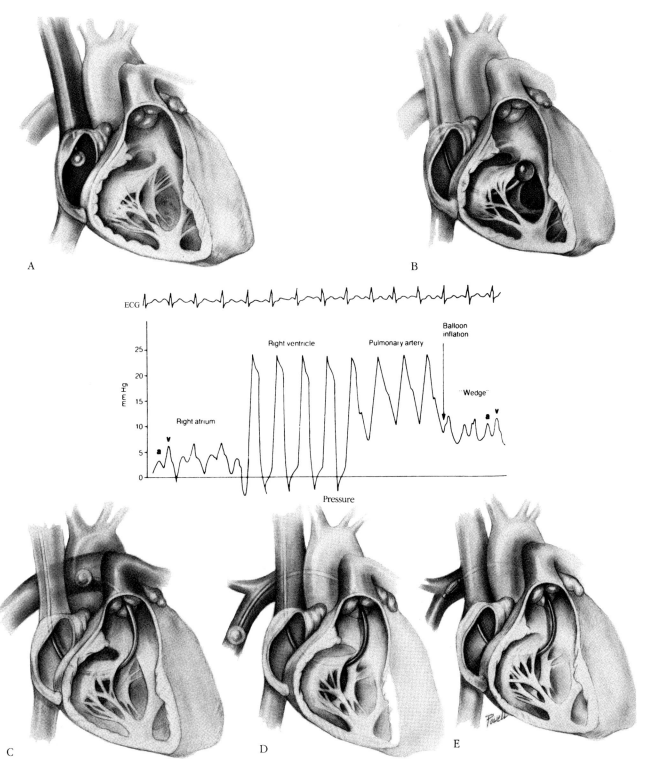

Fig. 4-9. **A:** With the catheter tip in the right atrium, the balloon is inflated. **B:** The catheter is advanced into the right ventricle with the balloon inflated, and right ventricle pressure tracings are obtained. **Center:** Waveform tracings are generated as the balloon-tipped catheter is advanced through the right heart chambers into the pulmonary artery. (Adapted from DK Cobb, KP High, RG Sawyer, et al: A controlled trial of scheduled replacement of central venous and pulmonary artery catheters. *N Engl J Med* 327:1062, 1992.) **C:** The catheter is advanced through the pulmonary valve into the pulmonary artery. A rise in diastolic pressure should be noted. **D:** The catheter is advanced to the pulmonary artery wedge pressure position. A typical pulmonary artery wedge pressure tracing should be noted with *a* and *v* waves. **E:** The balloon is deflated. Phasic pulmonary artery pressure should reappear on the monitor. (See text for details.)

Table 4-2. Normal Resting Pressures Obtained during Right Heart Catheterization

Cardiac chamber	Pressure (mm Hg)
Right atrium	
Range	0–6
Mean	3
Right ventricle	
Systolic	17–30
Diastolic	0–6
Pulmonary artery	
Systolic	15–30
Diastolic	5–13
Mean	10–18
Pulmonary artery wedge (mean)	2–12

Adapted from JM Gore, JS Alpert, JR Benotti, et al: *Handbook of Hemodynamic Monitoring.* Boston, Little, Brown, 1984.

The *x* descent follows the *a* wave and reflects atrial relaxation. The *y* descent is due to rapid emptying of the atrium after opening of the tricuspid valve. The mean right atrial pressure decreases during inspiration with spontaneous respiration (secondary to a decrease in intrathoracic pressure), whereas the *a* and *v* waves and the *x* and *y* descents become more prominent. Once a multilumen PA catheter is in position, right atrial blood can be sampled and pressure monitored using the proximal lumen. It should be noted that the pressures obtained via the proximal lumen may not accurately reflect right atrial pressure, due to positioning of the lumen against the atrial wall or within the introducer sheath. The latter problem is more frequently encountered in shorter patients [74].

Right Ventricle. The normal resting RV pressure is 17 to 30/0 to 6 mm Hg, recorded when the PA catheter crosses the tricuspid valve (Fig. 4-9B). The RV systolic pressure should equal the PA systolic pressure (except in cases of pulmonic stenosis or RV outflow tract obstruction). The RV diastolic pressure should equal the mean right atrial pressure during diastole when the tricuspid valve is open. Introduction of the RV Paceport catheter allows continuous monitoring of RV hemodynamics when the pacer probe is not in place. RV monitoring is increasingly used in the surgical critical care setting [75]. RV end-diastolic volume index and RV ejection fraction can now be accurately measured. A number of studies [76–78] have suggested that RV end-diastolic volume index may be a more accurate measure of ventricular preload and correlate better with cardiac index than does the PAWP. It is important to note that these studies did not include patients with underlying left ventricular dysfunction or arrhythmia; therefore, the conclusions may not apply to these

Table 4-3. Approximate Normal Oxygen Saturation and Content Values

Chamber sampled	Oxygen content (vol %)	Oxygen saturation (%)
Superior vena cava	14.0	70
Inferior vena cava	16.0	80
Right atrium	15.0	75
Right ventricle	15.0	75
Pulmonary artery	15.0	75
Pulmonary vein	20.0	98
Femoral artery	19.0	96
Atrioventricular oxygen content difference	3.5–5.5	—

Adapted from JM Gore, JS Alpert, JR Benotti, et al: *Handbook of Hemodynamic Monitoring.* Boston, Little, Brown, 1984.

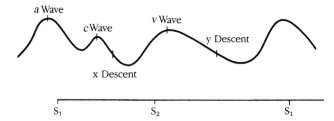

Fig. 4-10. Stylized representation of a right atrial waveform in relation to heart sounds. See text fort discussion of *a*, *c*, and *v* waves and *x* and *y* descents. S₁, first heart sound; S₂, second heart sound

latter groups. The role of RV monitoring in critically ill patients requires further investigation.

Pulmonary Artery. With the catheter in proper position and the balloon deflated, the distal lumen transmits PA pressure (Fig. 4-9E). Normal resting PA pressure is 15 to 30/5 to 13 mm Hg, with a normal mean pressure of 10 to 18 mm Hg. The PA waveform is characterized by a systolic peak and diastolic trough with a dicrotic notch due to closure of the pulmonic valve. The peak PA systolic pressure occurs in the T wave of a simultaneously recorded ECG.

Since the pulmonary vasculature is normally a low-resistance circuit, PA diastolic pressure (PADP) is closely related to mean PAWP (PADP is usually 1 to 3 mm Hg higher than mean PAWP) and thus can be used as an index of left ventricle filling pressure in patients in whom a wedge pressure is unobtainable or in whom PADP and PAWP have been shown to correlate closely. However, if pulmonary vascular resistance is increased, as in pulmonary embolic disease, pulmonary fibrosis, or reactive pulmonary hypertension (see Chapter 56), PADP may markedly exceed mean PAWP and thus become an unreliable index of left heart function [67–79]. Similar provisos apply when using PA mean pressure as an index of left ventricular function [2].

Pulmonary Artery Wedge Pressure. An important application of the balloon flotation catheter is the recording of PAWP. This measurement is obtained when the inflated balloon impacts into a slightly smaller branch of the PA (Fig. 4-9D). In this position, the balloon stops the flow, and the catheter tip senses pressure transmitted backward through the static column of blood from the next active circulatory bed—the pulmonary veins. Pulmonary venous pressure is a prime determinant of pulmonary congestion and thus of the tendency for fluid to shift from the pulmonary capillaries into the interstitial tissue and alveoli [68]. Also, pulmonary venous pressure and PAWP closely reflect left atrial pressure (except in rare instances, such as pulmonary venoocclusive disease, in which there is obstruction in the small pulmonary veins), and serve as indices of left ventricular filling pressure [79–81]. The PAWP is required to assess left ventricular filling pressure, since multiple studies have demonstrated that right atrial (e.g., central venous) pressure correlates poorly with PAWP [82–84].

The PAWP is a phase-delayed, amplitude-dampened version of the left atrial pressure. The normal resting PAWP is 2 to 12 mm Hg and averages 2 to 7 mm Hg below the mean PA pressure. The PAWP waveform is similar to that of the right atrium, with *a*, *c*, and *v* waves and *x* and *y* descents (Fig. 4-10). However, in contradistinction to the right atrial waveform, the PAWP waveform demonstrates a *v* wave that is slightly larger than the *a* wave [45]. Due to the time required for left atrial mechanical events to be transmitted through the pulmonary vasculature, PAWP waveforms are further delayed when recorded with a simultaneous ECG. The peak of the *a* wave follows the peak of the ECG P wave by approximately 240 milliseconds, and the

Table 4-4. Checklist for Verifying Position of Pulmonary Artery Catheter

	Zone 3	Zone 1 or 2
PAWP contour	Cardiac ripple (A + V waves)	Unnaturally smooth
PAD vs. PAWP	PAD > PAWP	PAD < PAWP
PEEP trial	ΔPAWP $<\frac{1}{2}$ ΔPEEP	ΔPAWP $>\frac{1}{2}$ ΔPEEP
Respiratory variation of PAWP	$<\frac{1}{2}$ ΔP_{ALV}	$\geq\frac{1}{2}$ ΔP_{ALV}
Catheter tip location	LA level or below	Above LA level

LA, left atrium; PAD, pulmonary artery diastolic pressure; P_{ALV}, alveolar pressure; PAWP, pulmonary artery wedge pressure; PEEP, positive end-expiratory pressure.
Adapted from RJ Schultz, GF Whitfield, JJ LaMura, et al: The role of physiologic monitoring in patients with fractures of the hip. *J Trauma* 25:309, 1985.

peak of the *v* wave occurs after the ECG T wave has been inscribed. Wedge position is confirmed by withdrawing a blood specimen from the distal lumen and measuring oxygen saturation. Measured oxygen saturation of 95% or more is satisfactory [81]. The lung segment from which the sample is obtained will be well ventilated if the patient breathes slowly and deeply.

A valid PAWP measurement requires a patent vascular channel between the left atrium and catheter tip. Thus, the PAWP approximates pulmonary venous pressure (and, therefore, left atrial pressure) only if the catheter tip lies in zone 3 of the lungs [47,85,86]. (The lung is divided into three physiologic zones, dependent on the relationship of PA, pulmonary venous, and alveolar pressures. In zone 3, the PA and pulmonary venous pressure exceed the alveolar pressure, ensuring an uninterrupted column of blood between the catheter tip and the pulmonary veins.) If, on portable lateral chest radiograph, the catheter tip is below the level of the left atrium (posterior position in supine patients), it can be assumed to be in zone 3. This assumption holds if applied PEEP is less than 15 cm H_2O and the patient is not markedly volume depleted. Whether the catheter is positioned in zone 3 may also be determined by certain physiologic characteristics (Table 4-4). A catheter wedged outside zone 3 shows marked respiratory variation, an unnaturally smooth vascular waveform, and misleading high pressures.

With a few exceptions [87], estimates of capillary hydrostatic filtration pressure from PAWP are acceptable [88]. It should be noted that measurement of PAWP does not take into account capillary permeability, serum colloid osmotic pressure, interstitial pressure, or actual pulmonary capillary resistance [88,89]. These factors all play roles in the formation of pulmonary edema, and the PAWP should be interpreted in the context of the specific clinical situation.

Mean PAWP correlates well with left ventricular end-diastolic pressure (LVEDP), provided the patient has a normal mitral valve and normal left ventricular function. In myocardial infarction, conditions with decreased left ventricular compliance (e.g., ischemia, left ventricular hypertrophy), and conditions with markedly increased left ventricular filling pressure (e.g., dilated cardiomyopathy), the contribution of atrial contraction to left ventricular filling is increased. Thus, the LVEDP may be significantly higher than the mean left atrial pressure or PAWP [47,86].

End expiration provides a readily identifiable reference point for PAWP interpretation because pleural pressure returns to baseline at the end of passive deflation (approximately equal to atmospheric pressure). Pleural pressure can exceed the normal resting value with active expiratory muscle contraction or use of PEEP. How much PEEP is transmitted to the pleural space cannot be estimated easily, since it varies depending on lung compliance and other factors. When normal lungs deflate passively, end-expiratory pleural pressure increases by approx-

imately one-half the applied PEEP. In patients with reduced lung compliance (e.g., patients with ARDS), the transmitted fraction may be one-fourth or less of the PEEP value. In the past, PEEP levels greater than 10 mm Hg were thought to interrupt the column of blood between the left atrium and PA catheter tip, causing the PAWP to reflect alveolar pressure more accurately than left atrial pressure. However, two studies suggest that this may not hold true in all cases. Hasan and colleagues [90] concluded that the PAWP–left atrial fluid column was protected by lung injury, and Teboul and co-workers [91] could find no significant discrepancy between PAWP and simultaneously measured LVEDP at PEEP levels of 0, 10, and 16 to 20 cm H_2O in patients with ARDS. They hypothesize that (a) a large intrapulmonary right-to-left shunt may provide a number of microvessels shielded from alveolar pressure, allowing free communication from PA to pulmonary veins, or (b) in ARDS, both vascular and lung compliance may decrease, reducing transmission of alveolar pressure to the pulmonary microvasculature and maintaining an uninterrupted blood column from the catheter tip to the left atrium.

Although it is difficult to estimate precisely the true transmural vascular pressure in a patient on PEEP, temporarily disconnecting PEEP to measure PAWP is not recommended. Because the hemodynamics have been destabilized, these measurements will be of questionable value. Venous return increases acutely after discontinuation of PEEP [91–94], and abrupt removal of PEEP will cause hypoxia, which may not reverse quickly on reinstitution of PEEP [94–96]. Additional discussion of measurement and interpretation of pulmonary vascular pressures on PEEP is found in Chapter 58.

CARDIAC OUTPUT

Thermodilution Technique. A catheter equipped with a thermistor 4 cm from its tip allows calculation of CO using the thermodilution principle [54,97]. Correlation with the Fick technique as applied in the cardiac catheterization laboratory is excellent [98]. The thermodilution principle holds that if a known quantity of cold solution is introduced into the circulation and adequately mixed (passage through two valves and a ventricle is adequate), the resultant cooling curve recorded at a downstream site allows calculation of net blood flow. CO is inversely proportional to the integral of the time-versus-temperature curve.

In practice, a known amount of cold solution (typically 10 mL of D_5W in adults and 5 mL of D_5W in children) is injected into the right atrium via the catheter's proximal port. The thermistor allows recording of the baseline PA blood temperature and subsequent temperature change. The resulting curve is usually analyzed by computer, although it can be analyzed manually by simple planimetric methods. Correction factors are added by catheter manufacturers to account for the mixture of cold indicator with warm residual fluid in the catheter injection lumen and the heat transfer from the catheter walls to the cold indicator.

Reported coefficients of variation using triplicate determinations, using 10 mL of cold injectate and a bedside computer, are approximately 4% or less [67,68]. Use of room-temperature injectate causes a slightly greater variability and is not recommended in states in which variations in PA blood temperature are expected (patients with severe shortness of breath, on mechanical ventilators, or in very-high-output states). Attempts to repeat the injection of cold solution during the same point in the respiratory cycle should be made in these patients [58]. Variations in the rate of injection can also introduce error into CO determinations, and it is thus important that the solution be injected as rapidly as possible. Careful attention must be paid to the details of this procedure; even then, changes of less than 10% to 15% above or below an initial value may not truly establish directional validity [69]. Thermodilution CO is inaccurate in low-output states, tricuspid regurgitation, and in cases of atrial or ventricular septal defects [99].

Fick Technique. When thermodilution technology is unavailable, CO can be estimated using the Fick principle. This principle states that the total release or uptake of a substance by an organ equals the product of blood flow through that organ multiplied by the difference of arteriovenous concentrations of the substance. Oxygen is the substance most conveniently used, and pulmonary blood flow is in practice assumed to be equal to CO. The formula used is as follows:

CO = oxygen consumption (mL/minute)/arterial O_2 content – venous O_2 content

Oxygen consumption ($\dot{V}O_2$) varies according to individual as well as by age and sex; accurate measurement in the cardiac catheterization laboratory involves collection of expired oxygen in a Douglas bag over a specified period. $\dot{V}O_2$ is estimated in the ICU setting, for practical reasons, as being 250 mL per minute for a 70-kg man. It can be more generally estimated as 130 mL times body surface area (BSA) if fat accounts for 15% or more of body weight, or 140 mL times BSA if fat content is estimated at 5% or less. BSA can be estimated using the patient's height and weight (Fig. 4-11).

Blood oxygen content refers to the total oxygen, both that bound to hemoglobin and that dissolved in plasma. However, the small amount of dissolved oxygen (0.003 mL of oxygen per 100 mL of blood per mm Hg partial pressure of oxygen) is usually ignored in clinical practice. Therefore, a simplified formula for oxygen content using the patient's hemoglobin content and the theoretic oxygen-carrying capacity of hemoglobin (and ignoring the small amount of dissolved oxygen) is as follows:

Oxygen content = % saturation × Hgb (g/dL) × 1.39 (mL O_2/g hemoglobin) × 10

This equation to determine mixed venous oxygen content in the PA cannot be used when any right-to-left, left-to-right, or bidirectional intracardiac shunt exists, since these situations violate the fundamental assumption that pulmonary blood flow equals CO. Also, since both $\dot{V}O_2$ and blood oxygen content are estimated in the ICU setting, absolute values for CO using this technique should be treated with caution. The utility of the Fick technique lies in its convenience and ability to provide an accurate sense of trends in CO changes. Normal values for arterial-venous oxygen content difference, mixed venous oxygen saturation, and CO can be found in Table 4-5.

A sample calculation of CO for a 70-kg man on room air with a hemoglobin of 14 g per dL, an arterial oxygen saturation of 95%, and a mixed venous oxygen saturation of 70% is as follows:

CO = 250 mL/minute/(0.95)(14)(1.39)(10) – (0.70)(14)(1.39)(10)

= 250 mL/minute/181–136 mL/L

= 5.55 L/minute

ANALYSIS OF MIXED VENOUS BLOOD. CO can be approximated merely by examining mixed venous (PA) oxygen saturation. If CO rises, then the mixed venous oxygen partial pressure will rise, since peripheral tissues need to exact less oxygen per unit of blood. Conversely, if CO falls, peripheral extraction from each unit will increase to meet the needs of metabolizing tissues. Thus, there is a direct proportionality, and serial determinations of mixed venous oxygen saturation can display trends in CO. Normal mixed venous oxygen saturation is 70% to 75%; values of less than 60% are associated with heart failure and values of less than 40% with shock

[100]. Potential sources of error in this determination include extreme low-flow states where poor mixing may occur and contamination of desaturated mixed venous blood by saturated pulmonary capillary blood when the sample is aspirated too quickly through the nonwedged catheter [48]. Fiberoptic reflectance oximetry PA catheters can continuously measure and record mixed venous oxygen saturations in appropriate clinical situations [57,64].

DERIVED PARAMETERS. Useful hemodynamic parameters that can be derived using data with PA catheters include the following:

1. Cardiac index = CO (L/minute)/BSA (m^2)
2. Stroke volume = CO (L/minute)/heart rate (beats/minute)
3. Stroke index = CO (L/minute)/heart rate (beats/minute) × BSA (m^2)
4. Mean arterial pressure (mm Hg) = (2 × diastolic) + systolic/3
5. Systemic vascular resistance (dyne/second/cm^{-5}) = mean arterial pressure – mean right atrial pressure (mm Hg)/CO (L/minute) × 80
6. Pulmonary arteriolar resistance (dyne/second/cm^{-5}) = mean PA pressure – PAWP (mm Hg)/CO (L/minute) × 80
7. Total pulmonary resistance (dyne/second/cm^{-5}) = mean PA pressure (mm Hg)/CO (L/minute) × 80
8. Left ventricular stroke work index = 1.36 (mean arterial pressure – PAWP) × stroke index/100
9. DO_2 (mL/minute/m^2) = cardiac index × arterial O_2 content

Normal values are listed in Table 4-5.

Clinical Applications of the Pulmonary Artery Catheter

Table 4-6 summarizes specific hemodynamic patterns for a variety of disease entities in which PA catheters are indicated. The examples given here illustrate the types of data generated and how they influence clinical decisions.

NORMAL RESTING HEMODYNAMIC PROFILE. The finding of normal CO associated with normal left and right heart filling pressures is useful in establishing a noncardiovascular basis to explain abnormal symptoms or signs and as a baseline to gauge a patient's disease progression or response to therapy. Right atrial pressures of 0 to 6 mm Hg, PA systolic pressures of 15 to 30 mm Hg, PADPs of 5 to 12 mm Hg, PA mean pressures of 9 to 18 mm Hg, PAWP of 5 to 12 mm Hg, and a cardiac index exceeding 2.5 L per minute per m^2 characterize a normal cardiovascular state at rest.

HYPOVOLEMIA. Decreases in cardiac index, right atrial pressure, and PAWP (with or without an accompanying fall in systemic blood pressure and the clinical picture of shock) are consistent with hypovolemia. Overvigorous diuretic therapy, hemorrhage, and third-space fluid losses are common etiologies. At a PAWP of less than 15 to 18 mm Hg, particularly in patients with acute myocardial infarction and decreased left ventricular compliance, small increases in PAWP/LVEDP resulting from volume replacement therapy may cause marked increases in stroke volume as ventricular function moves along the steep portion of the Starling curve. Attainment of slightly higher left heart filling pressures (18 to 24 mm Hg) may prove optimal for improving cardiac index in patients in whom relative hypovolemia complicates acute myocardial infarction. RV

BSA

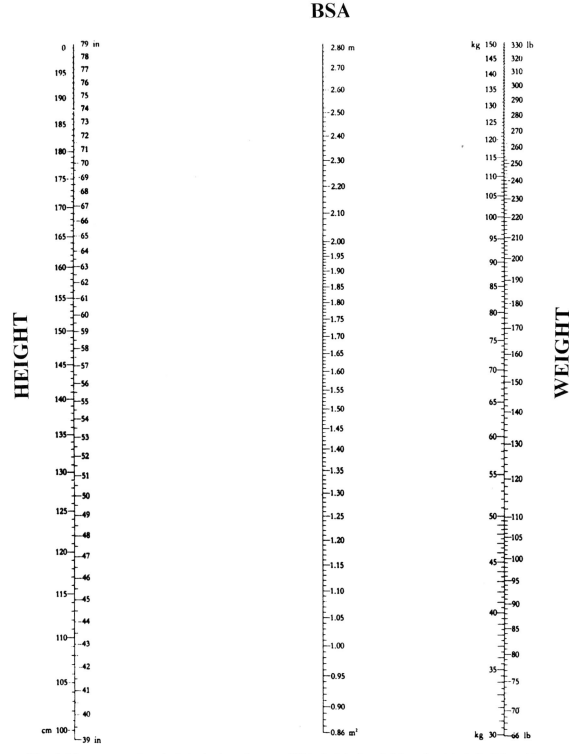

HEIGHT

WEIGHT

Fig. 4-11. Nomogram for calculating body surface area (BSA) of adults from height and weight (m²). (Adapted from JM Gore, JS Alpert, JR Benotti, et al: *Handbook of Hemodynamic Monitoring.* Boston, Little, Brown, 1984.)

failure (as manifested by elevated right atrial and RV end-diastolic pressures) may complicate hypovolemia and should not preclude volume loading in patients whose PAWP levels and other clinical signs indicate its requirement. Septic shock may cause the coexistence of a high cardiac index, a low PAWP, and a markedly low peripheral vascular resistance. Vasoconstricting agents and volume repletion may be helpful in such patients.

PULMONARY CONGESTION. Pulmonary congestion resulting from fluid overload or left ventricular failure is characterized by a PAWP in excess of 18 mm Hg or as high as 30 mm Hg or more in pulmonary edema. Diuretics in such circumstances tend to relieve congestion without alteration in CO, since changes occur on the flat portion of the Starling curve. Inotropic drugs, vasodilator agents, or both are added as indi-

Table 4-5. Selected Hemodynamic Variables Derived
from Right Heart Catheterization

Hemodynamic variable	Normal range
Arterial-venous content difference	3.5–5.5 mL/100 mL
Cardiac index	2.5–4.5 L/min/m^2
Cardiac output	3.0–7.0 L/min
Left ventricular stroke work index	45–60 g/beat/m^2
Mixed venous oxygen content	18.0 mL/100 mL
Mixed venous saturation	75% (approximately)
Oxygen consumption	200–250 mL/min
Pulmonary vascular resistance	120–250 dynes/sec/cm^{-5}
Stroke volume	70–130 mL/contraction
Stroke volume index	40–50 mL/contraction/m^2
Systemic vascular resistance	1,100–1,500 dynes/sec/cm^2

Adapted from JM Gore, JS Alpert, JR Benotti, et al: *Handbook of Hemodynamic Monitoring.* Boston, Little, Brown, 1984.

cated to attempt further preload or afterload reduction in cases of severe pump failure.

Pulmonary edema can occur at PAWP levels considerably lower than those listed above when the primary problem involves either a decrease in plasma colloid oncotic pressure or changes in the pulmonary capillary membranes. Examples include ARDS (with capillary leakage), severe hypoproteinemia, and overzealous administration of crystalloid solutions. Clinical evidence of respiratory distress and radiographic evidence of pulmonary edema with normal left heart filling pressures and function suggest the presence of noncardiac pulmonary edema.

HEART FAILURE. Cardiogenic shock is characterized by signs of peripheral hypoperfusion and shock in conjunction with hemodynamic data evidencing a markedly diminished cardiac index and markedly elevated PAWP. Milder degrees of left ventricular failure show correspondingly less depression in CO (diminished stroke volumes are often compensated by increases in heart rate) but are still characterized by elevated PAWP and varying degrees of pulmonary congestion.

RV failure is suggested by increases in RV end-diastolic and mean right atrial pressures. If it is caused by left ventricular failure, these increases are accompanied by an increased PAWP and a decreased CO. If caused by pulmonary vascular disease or occlusion, or in the setting of an isolated RV infarction, indices of left heart filling and function may be normal [101].

TRICUSPID INSUFFICIENCY. Tricuspid insufficiency generally occurs in the setting of pulmonary hypertension and RV dilatation, and usually presents as a chronic condition [102]. It causes accentuation of the right atrial *v* wave with a steep *y* descent and attendant elevation of the mean right atrial pressure. Tricuspid insufficiency interferes with measurement of thermodilution CO because of the back-and-forth flow of the indicator between the right atrium and RV.

ACUTE MITRAL REGURGITATION. Acute mitral regurgitation should be considered when a systolic murmur develops in the setting of acute ischemia or severe left ventricular failure of any origin. Left ventricular blood floods a normal-sized, noncompliant left atrium during ventricular systole, causing giant *v* waves in the wedge pressure tracing (Fig. 4-12). The giant *v* wave of acute mitral regurgitation may be transmitted to the PA tracing, yielding a bifid PA waveform composed of the PA systolic wave and the *v* wave. As the catheter is wedged, the PA systolic wave is lost, but the *v* wave remains. It is important to note that the PA systolic wave occurs earlier in relation to the QRS of a simultaneously recorded ECG (between the QRS and T waves) than does the *v* wave (after the T wave).

Although a large *v* wave is not diagnostic of acute mitral regurgitation and is not always present in this circumstance, acute mitral regurgitation remains the most common cause of giant *v* waves in the PAWP tracing. Prominent *v* waves may occur whenever the left atrium is distended and noncompliant due to left ventricular failure from any cause (e.g., ischemic heart disease, dilated cardiomyopathy) [103,104] or secondary to the increased pulmonary blood flow in acute ventricular septal defect [105]. Acute mitral regurgitation is the rare instance when the PA end-diastolic pressure may be lower than the computer-measured mean wedge pressure [73].

ACUTE VENTRICULAR SEPTAL RUPTURE. Acute ventricular septal perforation often occurs in the same clinical settings

Table 4-6. Hemodynamic Parameters in Commonly Encountered Clinical Situations (Idealized)

	RA	RV	PA	PAWP	AO	CI	SVR	PVR
Normal	0–6	25/0–6	25/6–12	6–12	130/80	≥2.5	1,500	≤250
Hypovolemic shock	0–2	15–20/0–2	15–20/2–6	2–6	≤90/60	<2.0	>1,500	≤250
Cardiogenic shock	8	50/8	50/35	35	≤90/60	<2.0	>1,500	≤250
Septic shock								
Early	0–2	20–25/0–2	20–25/0–6	0–6	≤90/60	≥2.5	<1,500	<250
Late[a]	0–4	25/4–10	25/4–10	4–10	≤90/60	<2.0	>1,500	>250
Acute massive pulmonary embolism	8–12	50/12	50/12–15	≤12	≤90/60	<2.0	>1,500	>450
Cardiac tamponade	12–18	25/12–18	25/12–18	12–18	≤90/60	<2.0	>1,500	≤250
AMI without LVF	0–6	25/0–6	25/12–18	≤18	140/90	≤2.5	1,500	≤250
AMI with LVF	0–6	30–40/0–6	30–40/18–25	>18	140/90	>2.0	>1,500	>250
Biventricular failure secondary to LVF	>6	50–60/>6	50–60/25	18–25	120/80	~2.0	>1,500	>250
RVF secondary to RVI	12–20	30/12–20	30/12	<12	≤90/60	<2.0	>1,500	>250
Cor pulmonale	>6	80/>6	80/35	<12	120/80	~2.0	>1,500	>400
Idiopathic pulmonary hypertension	0–6	80–100/0–6	80–100/40	<12	100/60	<2.0	>1,500	>500
Acute ventricular septal rupture[b]	6	60/6–8	60/35	30	≤90/60	<2.0	>1,500	>250

AMI, acute myocardial infarction; AO, aortic; CI, cardiac index; LVF, left ventricular failure; PA, pulmonary artery; PAWP, pulmonary artery wedge pressure; PVR, pulmonary vascular resistance; RA, right atrium; RV, right ventricle; RVF, right ventricular failure; RVI, right ventricular infarction; SVR, systemic vascular resistance.
[a]Hemodynamic profile seen in approximately one-third of patients in late septic shock.
[b]Confirmed by appropriate RA–PA oxygen saturation step-up. See text for discussion.
Adapted from JM Gore, JS Alpert, JR Benotti, et al: *Handbook of Hemodynamic Monitoring.* Boston, Little, Brown, 1984.

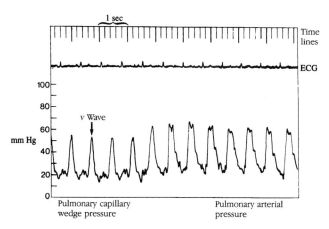

Fig. 4-12. Pulmonary artery and pulmonary artery wedge tracings with giant *v* waves distorting with pulmonary artery recording. ECG, electrocardiogram.

and produces physical findings similar to those of acute mitral regurgitation. Ventricular septal rupture can be rapidly demonstrated by documenting a marked oxygen saturation step-up in the PA or RV as compared to the right atrium [106]. An oxygen step-up greater than 1.0 volume percent (10% oxygen saturation step-up) between the right atrium and RV indicates a significant left-to-right shunt at the ventricular level.

Care must be taken when interpreting oxygen saturations obtained in acute ventricular septal rupture. Right atrial venous blood is from three sources: the inferior vena cava, the superior vena cava, and the coronary sinus. Right atrial oxygen saturation is misleadingly low if sampled adjacent to the coronary sinus. However, if significant tricuspid insufficiency is present in addition to acute ventricular septal rupture, the right atrial saturation will be misleadingly increased, since arterial blood will cross the ventricular septum and then regurgitate into the right atrium. In patients with an acute ventricular septal rupture, mixed venous blood should be sampled from the inferior and superior vena cavae [45]. As previously noted, a prominent *v* wave may be present in the PAWP tracing. Unusual causes of an oxygen step-up in the RV are coronary fistula to the RV, atrial septal defect primum, and patent ductus arteriosus with pulmonic regurgitation.

RIGHT VENTRICULAR INFARCTION. RV infarction typically occurs in the setting of inferior myocardial infarction. The hemodynamic findings are characteristic, although they may be confused with cardiac tamponade or constrictive pericarditis. The right atrial pressure is elevated (frequently greater than 10 mm Hg) and often disproportionately increased relative to the PAWP [107]. Right atrial waveform reveals prominent *x* and *y* descents, with the *y* descent occasionally exceeding the *x* descent due to a dilated noncompliant RV confined by a nondistensible pericardium [108,109]. These abnormalities may become exaggerated as right atrial pressure increases during volume expansion therapy. The right atrial pressure does not decline with inspiration and may actually increase (Kussmaul's sign). RV end-diastolic pressure and volume are elevated, and RV stroke volume is decreased, resulting in a narrowed PA pulse pressure. Tricuspid regurgitation may complicate RV infarction if RV dilatation or papillary muscle dysfunction occurs [110].

CARDIAC TAMPONADE. Cardiac tamponade constitutes a medical emergency, since rising intrapericardial pressure interferes with the diastolic filling of the heart. The hemody-

namic hallmarks of cardiac tamponade are elevation and equalization of the right atrial, RV diastolic, PA diastolic, and mean PAWPs. Examination of the right atrial pressure tracing reveals a dominant *x* descent due to the diminished cardiac volume during ventricular systole. The *y* descent is frequently absent, resulting in a unimodal right atrial pressure recording. Even in severe cardiac tamponade, the mean right atrial pressure declines with inspiration. This fact can be helpful for distinguishing cardiac tamponade from other conditions that result in elevated right-sided diastolic pressures, such as RV infarction and pericardial constriction. Hypovolemia and severe underlying left ventricular dysfunction may modify the hemodynamics of cardiac tamponade. The venous pressures are only modestly elevated in the former situation, while the PAWP may be significantly higher than the right atrial pressure in the latter [111,112].

PULMONARY HYPERTENSION. A mean PA pressure greater than 20 mm Hg defines pulmonary hypertension. Pulmonary hypertension can be classified as *passive* (when increases in left atrial or left ventricular end-diastolic pressure lead to increased pulmonary pressures), *active*, or *reactive*. For a comprehensive discussion of pulmonary hypertension and how to distinguish these three types, see Chapter 56.

PULMONARY EMBOLISM. Approximately 70% of patients with acute pulmonary embolism demonstrate some degree of pulmonary hypertension. Generally, 25% to 30% of a previously normal pulmonary vascular bed becomes obstructed [113]. The mean PA pressure is typically 20 to 40 mm Hg, with RV and PA systolic pressure rarely exceeding 50 mm Hg. Higher PA systolic pressures suggest a chronic component of pulmonary hypertension, since a previously normal RV lacks hypertrophy and cannot generate higher PA pressures acutely. The RV generally dilates and fails once RV systolic pressure reaches 50 to 60 mm Hg. Pulmonary vascular resistance is elevated in pulmonary embolism, with the PADP remaining significantly higher (greater than 5 mm Hg) than the mean PAWP. The PAWP is usually low or normal. The *a* and *v* waves of the PAWP tracing may disappear because the abnormal pulmonary vasculature may not allow retrograde transmission of these pressure waves from left atrium to catheter tip [73].

In patients with pulmonary emboli or respiratory distress of any cause, wide swings in intrathoracic pressure may be transmitted to the PAWP tracing and reduce the accuracy of the measurement. The true left ventricular filling pressure is usually overestimated in this setting. As previously mentioned, measurements should be made at end expiration [114].

Massive pulmonary embolism presenting as acute cor pulmonale with cardiogenic shock occurs when the pulmonary cross-sectional area is acutely obstructed by more than 60% [9]. In this setting, right atrial pressure is elevated (often greater than 10 mm Hg), RV and PA systolic pressures are increased, PAWP is usually low, pulmonary vascular resistance is significantly elevated (usually greater than two times normal), and CO is markedly decreased (Table 4-6).

ARRHYTHMIA DIAGNOSIS. The right atrial pressure tracing can be used both to diagnose arrhythmias and to aid in understanding their hemodynamic consequences. In atrial fibrillation, atrial systole is lost. This is reflected in the right atrial pressure tracing by disappearance of the *a* wave. Atrial flutter can be diagnosed by the presence of mechanical flutter waves in the right atrial pressure recording at a rate of approximately 300 waves per minute. During atrioventricular nodal reentrant tachycardia, the retrograde P wave is often hidden in the QRS complex on the ECG; however, atrial mechanical activity can be demonstrated by the presence of regular cannon *a* waves in the right atrial pressure tracing [73]. Cannon *a* waves are the result of atrial contraction at a time when the atrioventricular valves are closed during ventricular systole. The sequence of atrial and ventricular contraction is reversed, but the two events remain associated, causing the cannon *a* waves to be regular. Cannon *a* waves are also commonly encountered during ventricular arrhythmias. The presence of irregular cannon *a* waves during a wide-complex tachycardia suggests ventricular tachycardia.

PA catheters incorporating atrial and ventricular sensing electrodes on the catheter surface help in diagnosing complex cardiac arrhythmias by allowing the recording of the intracardiac electrogram. The pacing PA catheter and Paceport catheter also allow selective pacing and establishment of an optimal heart rate. The pacing PA catheter allows for atrioventricular synchronous pacing, whereas the Paceport allows only ventricular pacing. A Paceport catheter with separate atrial and ventricular probes is being designed [56].

Complications

Minor and major complications associated with bedside balloon flotation PA catheterization have been reported (Table 4-7). During the 1970s, in the first 10 years of clinical catheter use, a number of studies reported a relatively high incidence of certain complications. Consequent revision of guidelines for PA catheter use and improved insertion and maintenance techniques resulted in a decreased incidence of these complications in the 1980s [115]. The majority of complications are avoidable by scrupulous attention to detail in catheter placement and maintenance [116,117].

COMPLICATIONS ASSOCIATED WITH CENTRAL VENOUS ACCESS. The insertion techniques and complications of central venous cannulation are discussed in Chapter 2. Reported local vascular complications include local arterial or venous hematomas, inadvertent entry of the catheter into the carotid system, atrioventricular fistulas, and pseudoaneurysm formation [118–120]. Adjacent structures, such as the thoracic duct, can be damaged, with resultant chylothorax formation. Pneumothorax can be a serious complication of insertion, although the incidence is relatively low (1% to 2%) [73,121,122]. The incidence of pneumothorax is higher with the subclavian approach than with the internal jugular approach in some reports [123], but other studies demonstrate no difference between the two sites [124,125]. The incidence of complications associated with catheter insertion is generally considered to be inversely proportional to the operator's experience.

Table 4-7. Complications of Pulmonary Artery Catheterization

Associated with central venous access
Balloon rupture
Knotting
Pulmonary infarction
Pulmonary artery perforation
Thrombosis, embolism
Arrhythmias
Intracardiac damage
Infections
Miscellaneous complications

Some complications may be avoided by inserting the catheter from an arm vein under direct vision. Such placements, however, may be associated with a higher rate of thrombosis and make catheter manipulation more difficult; fluoroscopic guidance is generally required. To minimize the risk of mediastinal bleeding, peripheral placement should be considered in patients with abnormal hemostatic parameters and those with severe pulmonary hypertension.

BALLOON RUPTURE. This complication occurred more frequently in the early 1970s than it does now and was generally related to exceeding recommended inflation volumes. The main problems posed by balloon rupture are air emboli gaining access to the arterial circulation and balloon fragments embolizing to the distal pulmonary circulation. If rupture occurs during catheter insertion, the loss of the balloon's protective cushioning function can predispose to endocardial damage and attendant thrombotic and arrhythmic complications.

KNOTTING. Knotting of a catheter around itself is most likely to occur when loops form in the cardiac chambers and the catheter is repeatedly withdrawn and readvanced [126]. Knotting is avoided if care is taken not to advance the catheter significantly beyond the distances at which entrance to the ventricle or PA would ordinarily be anticipated. Knotted catheters usually can be extricated transvenously; guidewire placement [127], venotomy, or more extensive surgical procedures are occasionally necessary.

Knotting of PA catheters around intracardiac structures [128] or other intravascular catheters [129] has been reported. Rarely, entrapment of a PA catheter in cardiac sutures after open heart surgery has been reported, requiring varying approaches for removal [130].

PULMONARY INFARCTION. Peripheral migration of the catheter tip (caused by catheter softening and loop tightening over time) with persistent, undetected wedging in small branches of the PA is the most common mechanism underlying pulmonary ischemic lesions attributable to Swan-Ganz catheters [131]. These lesions are usually small and asymptomatic, often diagnosed solely on the basis of changes in the chest radiograph demonstrating a wedge-shaped pleural-based density with a convex proximal contour [132].

Severe infarctions are produced if the balloon is left inflated in the wedge position for an extended period, thus obstructing more central branches of the PA, or if solutions are injected at relatively high pressure through the catheter lumen in an attempt to restore an apparently damped pressure trace. Pulmonary embolic phenomena resulting from thrombus formation around the catheter or over areas of endothelial damage can also result in pulmonary infarction.

The reported incidence of pulmonary infarction secondary to PA catheters in 1974 was 7.2% [131], but recently reported rates of pulmonary infarction are much lower. Boyd and colleagues [133] found a 1.3% incidence of pulmonary infarction in a prospective study of 528 PA catheterizations. Sise and co-workers [134] reported no pulmonary infarctions in a prospective study of 319 PA catheter insertions. Use of continuous heparin flush solution and careful monitoring of PA waveforms are important reasons for the decreased incidence of this complication.

PULMONARY ARTERY PERFORATION. A serious and feared complication of PA catheterization is rupture of the PA leading to hemorrhage, which can be massive and sometimes fatal [135–143]. Rupture may occur during insertion or may be delayed a number of days [143]. PA rupture or perforation has been reported in approximately 0.1% to 0.2% of patients [133,144,145], although recent pathologic data suggest the true incidence of PA perforation is somewhat higher [146]. Proposed mechanisms by which PA rupture can occur include: (a) an increased pressure gradient between PAWP and PA pressure brought about by balloon inflation and favoring distal catheter migration, where perforation is more likely to occur; (b) a wedged catheter tip position favoring eccentric or distended balloon inflation with a spearing of the tip laterally and through the vessel; (c) cardiac pulsation causing shearing forces and damage as the catheter tip repeatedly contacts the vessel wall; (d) presence of the catheter tip near a distal arterial bifurcation where the integrity of the vessel wall against which the balloon is inflated may be compromised; and (e) simple lateral pressure on vessel walls caused by balloon inflation (this tends to be greater if the catheter tip was wedged before inflation began). Patient risk factors for PA perforation include pulmonary hypertension, mitral valve disease, advanced age, hypothermia, and anticoagulant therapy. In patients with these risk factors and in whom PADP reflects PAWP reasonably well, avoidance of subsequent balloon inflation altogether constitutes prudent prophylaxis.

Another infrequent but life-threatening complication is false aneurysm formation associated with rupture or dissection of the PA [147]. Technique factors related to PA hemorrhage are distal placement or migration of the catheter; failure to remove large catheter loops placed in the cardiac chambers during insertion; excessive catheter manipulation; use of stiffer catheter designs; and multiple overzealous or prolonged balloon inflations. Adherence to strict technique may decrease the incidence of this complication. In a prospective study reported in 1986, no cases of PA rupture occurred in 1,400 patients undergoing PA catheterization for cardiac surgery [123].

PA perforation typically presents with massive hemoptysis. Emergency management includes immediate wedge arteriogram and bronchoscopy, intubation of the unaffected lung, and consideration of emergency lobectomy or pneumonectomy. PA catheter balloon tamponade resulted in rapid control of bleeding in one case report [148]. Application of PEEP to intubated patients may also tamponade hemorrhage caused by a PA catheter [149,150].

THROMBOEMBOLIC COMPLICATIONS. Because PA catheters constitute foreign bodies in the cardiovascular system and can potentially damage the endocardium, they are associated with an increased incidence of thrombosis. Thrombi encasing the catheter tip and aseptic thrombotic vegetations forming at endocardial sites in contact with the catheter have been reported [131,151–153]. Extensive clotting around the catheter tip can occlude the pulmonary vasculature distal to the catheter, and thrombi anywhere in the venous system or right heart can serve as a source of pulmonary emboli. Subclavian venous thrombosis, presenting with unilateral neck vein distention and upper extremity edema, may occur in up to 2% of subclavian placements [154,155]. Venous thrombosis complicating percutaneous internal jugular vein catheterization is fairly commonly reported, although its clinical importance remains uncertain [156]. Consistently damped pressure tracings without evidence of peripheral catheter placement or pulmonary vascular occlusion should arouse suspicion of thrombi at the catheter tip. A changing relationship of PADP to PAWP over time should raise concern about possible pulmonary emboli.

If an underlying hypercoagulable state is known to exist, if catheter insertion was particularly traumatic, or if prolonged monitoring becomes necessary, one should consider cautiously anticoagulating the patient.

Heparin-bonded catheters reduce thrombogenicity [52] and have become the most commonly used PA catheters. An important complication of heparin-bonded catheters is heparin-induced thrombocytopenia [157,158]. Routine platelet counts are recommended for patients with heparin-bonded catheters in place.

RHYTHM DISTURBANCES. Atrial and ventricular arrhythmias occur commonly during insertion of PA catheters [159]. Premature ventricular contractions occurred during 11% of the catheter insertions originally reported by Swan and co-workers [1].

Recent studies have reported advanced ventricular arrhythmias (three or more consecutive ventricular premature beats) in approximately 30% to 60% of patients undergoing right heart catheterization [123,160–163]. Most arrhythmias are self-limited and do not require treatment, but sustained ventricular arrhythmias requiring treatment occur in 0% to 3% of patients [133,162,164]. Risk factors associated with increased incidence of advanced ventricular arrhythmias are acute myocardial ischemia or infarction, hypoxia, acidosis, hypocalcemia, and hypokalemia [162,163]. Prophylactic use of lidocaine in higher-risk patients may reduce the incidence of this complication [165]. A recent study [166] suggests that a right lateral tilt position (5-degree angle) during PA catheter insertion is associated with a lower incidence of malignant ventricular arrhythmias than is the Trendelenburg position.

Although the majority of arrhythmias occur during catheter insertion, arrhythmias may develop at any time after the catheter has been correctly positioned. These arrhythmias are due to mechanical irritation of the conducting system and may be persistent. Ventricular ectopy may also occur if the catheter tip falls back into the RV outflow tract. Evaluation of catheter-induced ectopy should include a portable chest radiograph to evaluate catheter position and assessment of the distal lumen pressure tracing to ensure that the catheter has not slipped into the RV. Lidocaine may be used but is unlikely to ablate the ectopy because the irritant is not removed [165]. If the arrhythmia persists after lidocaine therapy or is associated with hemodynamic compromise, the catheter should be removed. Catheter removal should be performed by physicians under continuous ECG monitoring, since the ectopy occurs almost as frequently during catheter removal as during insertion [167,168].

Right bundle-branch block (usually transient) can also complicate catheter insertion [169–172]. Patients undergoing anesthesia induction, those in the early stages of acute anteroseptal myocardial infarction, and those with acute pericarditis appear particularly susceptible to this complication. Patients with preexisting left bundle-branch block are at risk for developing complete heart block during catheter insertion [173,175].

The frequency of catheter-induced right bundle-branch block may be low, but the results may be disastrous. We suggest that these patients not be catheterized unless a temporary pacemaker can be inserted quickly or even prophylactically [173–175]. If a prophylactic temporary pacemaker is not selected, alternative considerations include use of an external transthoracic pacing device, a PA catheter with a specially designed Paceport, or a pacing PA catheter (electrodes mounted on the catheter surface). The operator should be familiar with the various limitations of these methods.

INTRACARDIAC DAMAGE. Damage to the right heart chambers, tricuspid valve, pulmonic valve, and their supporting structures as a consequence of PA catheterization has been reported [154,176–184]. The reported incidence of catheter-induced endocardial disruption detected by pathologic examination varies from 3.4% [184] to 75% [179], but most studies suggest a range of 20% to 30% [155,180,181]. These lesions consist of hemorrhage, sterile thrombus, intimal fibrin deposition, and nonbacterial thrombotic endocarditis. Their clinical significance is not clear, but there is concern that they may serve as a nidus for infectious endocarditis. Garrison and Freedman [185] demonstrated this theory in 1970. They produced infective endocarditis in rabbit hearts after induction of platelet-fibrin thrombi (created by intracardiac manipulation of polyethylene catheters) and subsequent catheter contamination with *Staphylococcus aureus.*

Direct damage to the cardiac valves and supporting chordae occurs primarily by withdrawal of the catheters while the balloon is inflated [1]. However, chordal rupture has been reported despite balloon deflation [149]. The incidence of intracardiac and valvular damage discovered on postmortem examination is considerably higher than that of clinically significant valvular dysfunction.

INFECTIONS. Catheter-related septicemia (the same pathogen growing from blood and the catheter tip) was reported in up to 2% of patients undergoing bedside catheterization in the 1970s [160,186]. However, the incidence of septicemia related to the catheter appears to have declined in recent years, with a number of studies suggesting a septicemia rate of 0% to 1% [123,187,188]. *In situ* time of more than 72 to 96 hours significantly increases the risk of catheter-related sepsis. Right-sided septic endocarditis has been reported [182,189], but the true incidence of this complication is unknown. Becker and colleagues [178] noted two cases of left ventricular abscess formation in patients with PA catheters and *S. aureus* septicemia. Incidence of catheter colonization or contamination varies from 5% to 20%, depending on the duration of catheter placement and the criteria used to define colonization [188,190]. Currently, it appears that there is no method to assess *in situ* bacterial colonization of PA catheters accurately and that there is no correlation between positive and negative blood cultures and catheter-related infection [149].

Pressure transducers have also been identified as an occasional source of infection [191]. The chance of introducing infection into a previously sterile system is increased during injections for CO determinations and during blood withdrawal. Approaches to reduce the risk of catheter-related infection include use of a sterile protective sleeve, antibiotic bonding to the catheter, and empiric changing of catheters over a guidewire [124,192–195].

OTHER COMPLICATIONS. Rare miscellaneous complications that have been reported include: (a) hemodynamically significant decreases in pulmonary blood flow caused by balloon inflation in the central PA in postpneumonectomy patients with pulmonary hypertension in the remaining lung [196], (b) disruption of the catheter's intraluminal septum as a result of injecting contrast medium under pressure [197], (c) artifactual production of a midsystolic click caused by a slapping motion of the catheter against the interventricular septum in a patient with RV strain and paradoxic septal motion [198], (d) thrombocytopenia secondary to heparin-bonded catheters [151,158], and (e) dislodgment of pacing electrodes [199]. Multiple unusual placements of PA catheters have also been reported, including in the left pericardiophrenic vein, via the left superior intercostal vein into the abdominal vasculature, and from the superior vena cava through the left atrium and left ventricle into the aorta after open heart surgery [200–202].

Guidelines for Safe Use of Pulmonary Artery Catheters

As experience with PA catheters and understanding of their potential complications increase, multiple revisions and changes in emphasis to the original recommended techniques and guidelines have emerged [68,70,86,115,116,121,136,139,151,175,203]. These precautions are summarized as follows:

1. Avoid complications associated with catheter insertion.
   a. Inexperienced personnel performing insertions must be supervised. Many hospitals require that PA catheters be inserted by a fully trained cardiologist.
   b. Keep the patient as still as possible. Restraints or sedation may be required.
   c. Strict sterile technique is mandatory.
   d. Avoid vein irritation by wetting the catheter and inserting it quickly, without undue manipulation.
   e. Examine the postprocedure chest radiograph for pneumothorax (especially after subclavian or internal jugular venipuncture) and for catheter tip position.
2. Avoid balloon rupture.
   a. Always inflate the balloon gradually. Stop inflation if no resistance is felt.
   b. Do not exceed recommended inflation volume. At the recommended volume, excess air will automatically be expelled from a syringe with holes bored in it that is constantly attached to the balloon port. Maintaining recommended volume also helps prevent the inadvertent injection of liquids.
   c. Keep the number of inflation-deflation cycles to a minimum.
   d. Do not reuse catheters designed for single usage, and do not leave catheters in place for prolonged periods.
   e. Use carbon dioxide as the inflation medium if communication between the right and left sides of the circulation is suspected.
3. Avoid knotting. Discontinue advancement of the catheter if entrance to right atrium, RV, or PA has not been achieved at distances normally anticipated from a given insertion site. If these distances have already been significantly exceeded, or if the catheter does not withdraw easily, use fluoroscopy before attempting catheter withdrawal. Never pull forcefully on a catheter that does not withdraw easily.
4. Avoid damage to pulmonary vasculature and parenchyma.
   a. Keep recording time of PAWP to a minimum, particularly in patients with pulmonary hypertension and other risk factors for PA rupture. Be sure the balloon is deflated after each PAWP recording. There is never an indication for continuous PAWP monitoring.
   b. Constant pressure monitoring is required each time the balloon is inflated. It should be inflated slowly, in small increments, and must be stopped as soon as the pressure tracing changes to PAWP or damped.
   c. If a wedge is recorded with balloon volumes significantly less than the inflation volume recommended on the catheter shaft, withdraw the catheter to a position where full (or nearly full) inflation volume produces the desired trace.
   d. Anticipate catheter tip migration. Softening of the catheter material with time, repeated manipulations, and cardiac motion make distal catheter migration almost inevitable.
      i. Continuous tip pressure monitoring is recommended, and the trace must be closely watched for changes from characteristic PA pressures to those indicating a PAWP or damped tip position.

ii. Decreases over time in the balloon inflation volumes necessary to attain wedge tracings should raise suspicion regarding catheter migration.

iii. Confirm satisfactory tip position with chest radiographs immediately after insertion, at the 6- to 12-hour mark, and then at least daily.

e. Do not use liquids to inflate the balloon. They may prevent deflation, and their relative incompressibility may increase lateral forces and stress on the walls of pulmonary vessels.

f. Hemoptysis is an ominous sign and should prompt an urgent diagnostic evaluation and rapid institution of appropriate therapy.

g. Avoid injecting solutions at high pressure through the catheter lumen on the assumption that clotting is the cause of the damped pressure trace. First, aspirate from the catheter. Then consider problems related to catheter position, stopcock position, transducer dome, transducers, pressure bag, flush system, or trapped air bubbles. Never flush the catheter in the wedge position.

5. Avoid thromboembolic complications.

a. Minimize trauma induced during insertion.

b. Use heparin-bonded catheters if there are no clinical contraindications.

c. Consider the judicious use of anticoagulants in patients with hypercoagulable states or other risk factors.

d. Avoid flushing the catheter under high pressure.

e. Watch for a changing PADP-PAWP relationship, as well as for other clinical indicators of pulmonary embolism.

6. Avoid arrhythmias.

a. Constant ECG monitoring during insertion and maintenance, as well as ready accessibility of all supplies for performing cardiopulmonary resuscitation, defibrillation, and temporary pacing, are mandatory.

b. Use caution when catheterizing patients with an acutely ischemic myocardium or preexisting left bundle-branch block. Use prophylactic antiarrhythmic drugs or a temporary pacemaker as indicated.

c. When the balloon is deflated, do not advance the catheter beyond the right atrium.

d. Avoid overmanipulation of the catheter.

e. Secure the catheter in place at the insertion site.

f. Watch for intermittent RV pressure tracings when the catheter is thought to be in the PA position. An unexplained ventricular arrhythmia in a patient with a PA catheter in place indicates the possibility of catheter-provoked ectopy.

7. Avoid valvular damage.

a. Avoid prolonged catheterization and excessive manipulation.

b. Do not withdraw the catheter when the balloon is inflated.

8. Avoid infections.

a. Use meticulously sterile technique on insertion.

b. Avoid excessive CO determinations and blood withdrawals.

c. Avoid prolonged catheterization.

Remove the catheter if signs of phlebitis develop. Culture the tip and use antibiotics as indicated.

Summary

Clinical use of the PA catheter has increased since its introduction in 1970. Approximately two million PA catheters were sold in 1996 [204]. Despite the popularity of the PA catheter, controversy regarding its appropriate use exists. Although it is generally agreed that hemodynamic monitoring enhances the understanding of cardiopulmonary pathophysiology in critically ill patients, the risk to benefit profile of PA catheterization in various clinical circumstances remains uncertain. Indeed, concrete evidence that information derived from PA catheterization improves patient outcome is scarce. There is increasing concern that PA catheterization may be overused and that the data obtained may not be optimally used.

Until the results of future studies are available, clinicians using hemodynamic monitoring should carefully assess the risk-to-benefit ratio on an individual patient basis. The operator should understand the indications, insertion techniques, equipment, and data that can be generated before undertaking PA catheter insertion. PA catheterization must not delay or replace bedside clinical evaluation and treatment.

References

1. Swan HJC, Ganz W, Forrester J, et al: Catheterization of the heart in man with use of a flow-directed balloon-tipped catheter. *N Engl J Med* 283:447, 1970.

2. Rutherford BD, McCann WD, O'Donovan TPB: The value of monitoring pulmonary artery pressure for early detection of left ventricular failure following myocardial infarction. *Circulation* 43:655, 1971.

3. Carabello B, Cohn PF, Alpert JS: Hemodynamic monitoring in patients with hypotension after myocardial infarction. *Chest* 74:5, 1978.

4. Connors AF, McCaffree DR, Gray BA: Evaluation of right heart catheterization in the critically ill patient without acute myocardial infarction. *N Engl J Med* 308:263, 1983.

5. Waller J, Johnson SP, Kaplan JA: Usefulness of pulmonary artery catheters during aortocoronary bypass surgery. *Anesth Analg* 61:221, 1982.

6. Iberti TJ, Fisher CJ: A prospective study on the use of the pulmonary artery catheter in a medical intensive care unit: its effects on diagnosis and therapy. *Crit Care Med* 11:238, 1983.

7. Gorlin R: Current concepts in cardiology: practical cardiac hemodynamics. *N Engl J Med* 296:203, 1977.

8. Dalen JE: Bedside hemodynamic monitoring. *N Engl J Med* 301:1176, 1979.

9. Gore JM, Alpert JS, Benotti JR, et al: *Handbook of Hemodynamic Monitoring*. Boston, Little, Brown, 1984.

10. Keefer FR, Barash PG: Pulmonary artery catheterization: a decade of clinical progress? *Chest* 84:241, 1984.

11. Eisenberg PR, Jaffe AS, Schuster DP: Clinical evaluation compared to pulmonary artery catheterization in the hemodynamic assessment of critically ill patients. *Crit Care Med* 12:549, 1984.

12. Mimoz O, Rauss A, Rekik N, et al: Pulmonary artery catheterization in critically ill patients: a prospective analysis of outcome changes associated with catheter-prompted changes in therapy. *Crit Care Med* 22:573, 1994.

13. Schultz RJ, Whitfield GF, LaMura JJ, et al: The role of physiologic monitoring in patients with fractures of the hip. *J Trauma* 25:309, 1985.

14. Del Guercia LRM: Does pulmonary artery catheter use change outcome? Yes. *Crit Care Clin* 12:553, 1996.

15. Shoemaker WC, Appel PL, Kram HB, et al: Prospective trial of supranormal values of survivors as therapeutic goals in high-risk surgical patients. *Chest* 94:1176, 1988.

16. Shoemaker WC, Appel PC, Kram HB: Oxygen transport measurements to evaluate tissue perfusion and titrate therapy: dobutamine and dopamine effects. *Crit Care Med* 19:672, 1991.

17. Shoemaker WC, Kram HB, Appel PL: Therapy of shock based on pathophysiology, monitoring, and outcome prediction. *Crit Care Med* 18:S19, 1990.

18. Bland RD, Shoemaker WC, Abraham E, et al: Hemodynamic and oxygen transport patterns in surviving and nonsurviving patients. *Crit Care Med* 13:85, 1985.

19. Bland R, Shoemaker WC, Shabot MM: Physiologic monitoring goals for the critically ill patient. *Surg Gynecol Obstet* 147:833, 1978.

20. Rivers E, Nguyen B, Haystad S, et al: Early goal-directed therapy in the treatment of severe sepsis and septic shock. *N Engl J Med* 345:1368, 2001.

21. Ivanov R, Allen J, Calvin J: The incidence of major morbidity in critically ill patients managed with pulmonary artery catheters: a meta-analysis. *Crit Care Med* 28:615, 2000.

22. Leibowitz A: Do pulmonary artery catheters improve patient outcome? No. *Crit Care Clinics* 3:559, 1996.

23. Valentine RJ, Duke ML, Inman MH, et al: Effectiveness of pulmonary artery catheters in aortic surgery: a randomized trial. *J Vasc Surg* 27:203, 1998.

24. Gattinoni L, Brazzi L, Pelosi P, et al: A trial of goal-oriented hemodynamic therapy in critically ill patients. *N Engl J Med* 333:1025, 1995.

25. Yu M, Levy M, Smith P: Effect of maximizing oxygen delivery on morbidity and mortality rates in critically ill patients. *Crit Care Med* 21:830, 1993.

26. Weber KT, Janicki JS, Russell RV, et al: Identification of high risk subsets of acute myocardial infarction. *Am J Cardiol* 41:197, 1978.

27. Spodick DH: Physiologic and prognostic complications of invasive monitoring: Undetermined risk/benefit ratios in patients with heart disease. *Am J Cardiol* 46:173, 1980.

28. Robin ED: The cult of the Swan-Ganz catheter: overuse and abuse of pulmonary flow catheters. *Ann Intern Med* 103:445, 1985.

29. Gore JM, Goldberg RJ, Spodick DH, et al: A community wide assessment of the use of pulmonary artery catheters in patients with acute myocardial infarction. *Chest* 92:721, 1987.

30. Robin ED: Death by pulmonary artery flow-directed catheter: time for a moratorium? *Chest* 92:727, 1987.

31. Zion MM, Balkin J, Rosenmann D, et al: Use of pulmonary artery catheters in patients with acute myocardial infarction: analysis of experience in 5841 patients in the SPRINT registry. *Chest* 98:1331, 1990.

32. Greenland P, Reicher-Reiss H, Goldbourt U, et al: In-hospital and 1-year mortality in 1524 women after myocardial infarction: comparison with 4315 men. *Circulation* 83:484, 1991.

33. Connors AF, Speroff T, Dawson NV, et al: The effectiveness of right heart catheterization in the initial care of critically ill patients. *JAMA* 276:889, 1996.

34. Iberti TJ, Fischer EP, Leibowitz AB, et al: A multicenter study of physicians' knowledge of the pulmonary artery catheter. *JAMA* 264:2928, 1990.

35. Trottier SJ, Taylor RW: Physicians' attitudes toward and knowledge of the pulmonary artery catheter: Society of Critical Care Medicine membership survey. *New Horiz* 5:201, 1997.

36. Burns D, Shively M: Critical care nurses' knowledge of the pulmonary artery catheter. *Am J Crit Care* 5:49, 1996.

37. Blumberg MS, Binns GS: Swans-Ganz catheter use and mortality of myocardial infarction patients. *Health Care Financ Rev* 15:91, 1994.

38. Viellard-Baron A, Girou E, Valente E, et al: Predictors of mortality in acute respiratory distress syndrome. *Am J Respir Crit Care Med* 161:1597, 2000.

39. Dalen JE, Bone RC: Is it time to pull the pulmonary artery catheter? *JAMA* 18:916, 1996.

40. Guyatt G: A randomized control trial of right heart catheterization in critically ill patients. Ontario Intensive Care Study Group. *J Intensive Care Med* 6:91, 1991.

41. Polanczyk CA, Rohde LE, Goldman L, et al: Right heart catheterization and cardiac complications in patients undergoing noncardiac surgery: an observational study. *JAMA* 286:348, 2001.

42. Barone JE, Tucker JB, Rassias D, et al: Routine perioperative pulmonary artery catheterization has no effect on rate of complications in vascular surgery: a meta-analysis. *Am Surg* 67:674, 2001.

43. Sandham JD, Hull RD, Brant R, et al: A randomized controlled trial of pulmonary artery catheter use in 1994 high-risk geriatric surgical patients. *Am J Respir Crit Care Med* 163:A16, 2001.

44. Bernard GR, Sopko G, Cerra F, et al: Pulmonary artery catheterization and clinical outcomes: National Heart, Lung and Blood Institute and Food and Drug Administration Workshop Report. Consensus statement. *JAMA* 283:2568, 2000.

45. Gore JM, Zwerner PL: Hemodynamic monitoring of acute myocardial infarction, in Alpert JS, Francis GS (eds): *Modern Coronary Care*. Boston, Little, Brown, 1990, p 139.

46. Wiedermann HP, Matthay MA, Matthay RA: Cardiovascular-pulmonary monitoring in the intensive care unit, 2. *Chest* 85:656, 1984.

47. Marini JJ: Hemodynamic monitoring with the pulmonary artery catheter. *Crit Care Clin* 2:551, 1986.

48. Pace NL: A critique of flow-directed pulmonary artery catheterization. *Anesthesiology* 47:455, 1977.

49. Steele P, Davies H: The Swan-Ganz catheter in the cardiac laboratory. *Br Heart J* 35:647, 1973.

50. Hesdorffer CS, Milne JF, Meyers AM, et al: The value of Swan-Ganz catheterization and volume loading in preventing renal failure in patients undergoing abdominal aneurysmectomy. *Clin Nephrol* 28:372, 1987.

51. Tuman KJ, McCarthy RJ, Spiess BD, et al: Effect of pulmonary artery catheterization on outcome in patients undergoing coronary artery surgery. *Anesthesiology* 70:199, 1989.

52. Hoar PF, Wilson RM, Mangano DT, et al: Heparin bonding reduces thrombogenicity of pulmonary-artery catheters. *N Engl J Med* 305:993, 1981.

53. Mangano DT: Heparin bonding long-term protection against thrombogenesis. *N Engl J Med* 307:894, 1982.

54. Forrester JS, Ganz W, Diamond G, et al: Thermodilution cardiac output determination with a single flow-directed catheter. *Am Heart J* 83:306, 1972.

55. Chatterjee K, Swan JHC, Ganz W, et al: Use of a balloon-tipped flotation electrode catheter for cardiac monitoring. *Am J Cardiol* 36:56, 1975.

56. Simoons ML, Demey HE, Bossaert LL, et al: The Paceport catheter: a new pacemaker system introduced through a Swan-Ganz catheter. *Cathet Cardiovasc Diagn* 15:66, 1988.

57. Baele PL, McMechan JC, Marsh HM, et al: Continuous monitoring of mixed venous oxygen saturation in critically ill patients. *Anesth Analg* 61:513, 1982.

58. Segal J, Pearl RG, Ford AJ, et al: Instantaneous and continuous cardiac output obtained with a Doppler pulmonary artery catheter. *J Am Coll Cardiol* 13:1382, 1989.

59. Vincent JL, Thirion M, Bumioulle S, et al: Thermodilution measurement of right ventricular ejection fraction with a modified pulmonary artery catheter. *Intensive Care Med* 12:33, 1986.

60. Guerrero JE, Munoz J, De Lacalle B, et al: Right ventricular systolic time intervals determined by means of a pulmonary artery catheter. *Crit Care Med* 20:1529, 1992.

61. Dhainaut JF, Brunet F, Monsallier JF, et al: Bedside evaluation of right ventricular performance using a rapid computerized thermodilution mode. *Crit Care Med* 15:148, 1987.

62. Vincent JL: Measurement of right ventricular ejection fraction. *Intensive Care World* 7:133, 1990.

63. Nishimura RA: Another measurement of cardiac output: is it truly needed? *J Am Coll Cardiol* 13:1393, 1989.

64. Rayput MA, Rickey HM, Bush BA, et al: A comparison between a conventional and a fiberoptic flow-directed thermal dilution pulmonary artery catheter in critically ill patients. *Arch Intern Med* 149:83, 1989.

65. Hankeln K, Michelsen H, Kubeak V, et al: Continuous, on-line, real-time measurement of cardiac output and derived cardiorespiratory variables in the critically ill. *Crit Care Med* 13:1071, 1985.

66. Normann RA, Johnson RW, Messinger JE, et al: A continuous cardiac output computer based on thermodilution principles. *Ann Biomed Eng* 17:61, 1989.

67. Buchbinder N, Ganz W: Hemodynamic monitoring: invasive techniques. *Anesthesiology* 45:146, 1976.

68. Swan HJC, Ganz W: Use of balloon flotation catheters in critically ill patients. *Surg Clin North Am* 55:501, 1975.

69. Hurst JW, Logue RB, Rackley CE, et al: *The Heart*. New York, McGraw-Hill, 1982.

70. Russel RO, Rackley CE: *Hemodynamic Monitoring in a Coronary Intensive Care Unit*. Mount Kisco, NY, Futura, 1981.

71. Ganz W, Swan HJC: Balloon-tipped flow-directed catheters, in Grossman W (ed): *Cardiac Catheterization and Angiography*. 2nd ed. Philadelphia, Lea & Febiger, 1980, p 78.

72. Barry WA, Grossman W: Cardiac catheterization, in Braunwald E (ed): *Heart Disease: A Textbook of Cardiovascular Medicine*. Philadelphia, WB Saunders, 1988, p 287 (vol 1).

73. Sharkey SW: Beyond the wedge: Clinical physiology and the Swan-Ganz catheter. *Am J Med* 83:111, 1987.
74. Bohrer H, Fleischer F: Errors in biochemical and haemodynamic data obtained using introducer lumen and proximal port of Swan-Ganz catheter. *Intensive Care Med* 15:330, 1989.
75. Huford WE, Zapol WM: The right ventricle and critical illness: a review of anatomy, physiology, and clinical evaluation of its function. *Intensive Care Med* 14:448, 1988.
76. Diebel LN, Wilson RF, Tagett MG, et al: End diastolic volume: a better indicator of preload in the critically ill. *Arch Surg* 127:817, 1992.
77. Martyn JA, Snider MT, Farago LF, et al: Thermodilution right ventricular volume: a novel and better predictor of volume replacement in acute thermal injury. *J Trauma* 21:619, 1981.
78. Reuse C, Vincent JL, Pinsky MR, et al: Measurements of right ventricular volumes during fluid challenge. *Chest* 98:1450, 1990.
79. Walston A, Kendall ME: Comparison of pulmonary wedge and left atrial pressure in man. *Am Heart J* 86:159, 1973.
80. Lange RA, Moore DM, Cigarroa RG, et al: Use of pulmonary capillary wedge pressure to assess severity of mitral stenosis: is true left atrial pressure needed in this condition? *J Am Coll Cardiol* 13:825, 1989.
81. Alpert JS: The lessons of history as reflected in the pulmonary capillary wedge pressure. *J Am Coll Cardiol* 13:830, 1989.
82. Mond HG, Hunt D, Sloman G: Hemodynamic monitoring in the coronary care unit using the Swan-Ganz right heart catheter. *Br Heart J* 35:635, 1973.
83. Scheinman MM, Aggott JA, Rapaport E: Clinical uses of a flow-directed right heart catheter. *Arch Intern Med* 124:19, 1969.
84. Forrester JS, Diamond G, McHugh TJ, et al: Filling pressures in the right and left sides of the heart in acute myocardial infarction. *N Engl J Med* 285:190, 1971.
85. O'Quin R, Marini JJ: Pulmonary artery occlusion pressure: clinical physiology, measurement, and interpretation. *Am Rev Respir Dis* 128:319, 1983.
86. Wiedermann HP, Matthay MA, Matthay RA: Cardiovascular-pulmonary monitoring in the intensive care unit, 1. *Chest* 85:537, 1984.
87. Timmis AD, Fowler MB, Burwood RJ, et al: Pulmonary edema without critical increase in left atrial pressure in acute myocardial infarction. *BMJ* 283:636, 1981.
88. Holloway H, Perry M, Downey J, et al: Estimation of effective pulmonary capillary pressure in intact lungs. *J Appl Physiol* 54:846, 1983.
89. Dawson CA, Linehan JH, Rickaby DA: Pulmonary microcirculatory hemodynamics. *Ann N Y Acad Sci* 384:90, 1982.
90. Hasan FM, Weiss WB, Braman SS, et al: Influence of lung injury on pulmonary wedge-left atrial pressure correlation during positive end-expiratory pressure ventilation. *Annu Rev Respir Dis* 131:246, 1985.
91. Teboul JL, Zapol WM, Brun-Buisson C, et al: A comparison of pulmonary artery occlusion pressure and left ventricular end diastolic pressure during mechanical ventilation with PEEP in patients with severe ARDS. *Anesthesiology* 70:261, 1989.
92. Quist J, Pontoppridan H, Wilson R, et al: Hemodynamic responses to mechanical ventilation with PEEP: The effect of hypervolemia. *Anesthesiology* 42:45, 1975.
93. Zarins CK, Virgilio RW, Smith DE, et al: The effect of vascular volume on positive end-expiratory pressure induced cardiac output depression and wedge-left atrial pressure discrepancy. *J Surg Res* 23:348, 1977.
94. Downs JB, Douglas ME: Assessment of cardiac filling pressure occurring in continuous positive-pressure ventilation. *Crit Care Med* 8:285, 1980.
95. DeCampo T, Civetta JM: The effect of short-term discontinuation of high-level PEEP in patients with acute respiratory failure. *Crit Care Med* 7:47, 1979.
96. Luterman A, Horovitz JH, Carrico CJ, et al: Withdrawal from positive end-expiratory pressure. *Surgery* 83:328, 1978.
97. Ganz W, Swan HJC: Measurement of blood flow by thermodilution. *Am J Cardiol* 29:241, 1972.
98. Branthwaite MA, Bradley RD: Measurement of cardiac output by thermal dilution in man. *J Appl Physiol* 24:434, 1968.
99. Grossman W: Blood flow measurement: the cardiac output, in Grossman W (ed): *Cardiac Catheterization and Angiography*. Philadelphia, Lea & Febiger, 1985, p 116.
100. Goldman RH, Klughaupt M, Metcalf T, et al: Measurement of central venous oxygen saturation in patients with myocardial infarction. *Circulation* 38:941, 1968.
101. Cohn JN, Guiha NH, Broder MI, et al: Right ventricular infarction: clinical and hemodynamic features. *Am J Cardiol* 33:209, 1974.
102. Ockene IS: Tricuspid valve disease, in Dalen JE, Alpert JS (eds): *Valvular Heart Disease*. Boston, Little, Brown, 1981, p 281.
103. Pichard AD, Kay R, Smith H, et al: Large V waves in the pulmonary wedge pressure tracing in the absence of mitral regurgitation. *Am J Cardiol* 50:1044, 1982.
104. Ruchs RM, Heuser RR, Yin FU, et al: Limitations of pulmonary wedge V waves in diagnosing mitral regurgitation. *Am J Cardiol* 49:849, 1982.
105. Bethen CF, Peter RH, Behar VS, et al: The hemodynamic simulation of mitral regurgitation in ventricular septal defect after myocardial infarction. *Cathet Cardiovasc Diagn* 2:97, 1976.
106. Meister SG, Helfant RH: Rapid bedside differentiation of ruptured interventricular septum from acute mitral insufficiency. *N Engl J Med* 287:1024, 1972.
107. Lopez-Senden J, Coma-Corella I, Gamallo C: Sensitivity and specificity of hemodynamic criteria in the diagnosis of acute right ventricular infarction. *Circulation* 64:515, 1981.
108. Arma-Canella I, Lopez-Sendon J: Ventricular compliance in ischemic right ventricular dysfunction. *Am J Cardiol* 45:555, 1980.
109. Lorell B, Leinback RC, Pohost GM, et al: Right ventricular infarction: clinical diagnosis and differentiation from cardiac tamponade and pericardial constriction. *Am J Cardiol* 43:465, 1979.
110. MacAllister RG, Friesinger GG, Sinclair-Smith BC: Tricuspid regurgitation following inferior myocardial infarction. *Arch Intern Med* 136:95, 1976.
111. Reddy PS, Antiss EL, O'Toole JD, et al: Cardiac tamponade: hemodynamic observations in man. *Circulation* 58:265, 1978.
112. Antman EM, Cargill V, Grossman W: Low pressure cardiac tamponade. *Ann Intern Med* 91:403, 1979.
113. McIntyre KM, Sasahara AA: The hemodynamic response to pulmonary embolism in patients without prior cardiopulmonary disease. *Am J Cardiol* 28:288, 1971.
114. Rice DL, Gaasch WH, Alexander JK, et al: Wedge pressure measurements in obstructive pulmonary disease. *Chest* 66:628, 1974.
115. Matthay MA, Chatterjee K: Bedside catheterization of the pulmonary artery: risks compared with benefits. *Ann Intern Med* 109:826, 1988.
116. Swan HJC, Ganz W: Complications with flow-directed balloon-tipped catheters. *Ann Intern Med* 91:494, 1979.
117. Swan HJC, Ganz W: Hemodynamic measurements in clinical practice: a decade in review. *J Am Cardiol* 1:103, 1983.
118. McNabb TG, Green CH, Parket FL: A potentially serious complication with Swan-Ganz catheter placement by the percutaneous internal jugular route. *Br J Anaesth* 47:895, 1975.
119. Hansbroyh JF, Narrod JA, Rutherford R: Arteriovenous fistulas following central venous catheterization. *Intensive Care Med* 9:287, 1983.
120. Shield CF, Richardson JD, Buckley CJ, et al: Pseudoaneurysm of the brachiocephalic arteries: a complication of percutaneous internal jugular vein catheterization. *Surgery* 78:190, 1975.
121. Patel C, LaBoy V, Venus B, et al: Acute complications of pulmonary artery catheter insertion in critically ill patients. *Crit Care Med* 14:195, 1986.
122. McNabb TG, Green LH, Parker FL: A potentially serious complication with Swan-Ganz catheter placement by the percutaneous internal jugular route. *Br J Anaesth* 47:895, 1975.
123. Damen J, Bolton D: A prospective analysis of 1,400 pulmonary artery catheterizations in patients undergoing cardiac surgery. *Acta Anaesthesiol Scand* 14:1957, 1986.
124. Senagere A, Waller JD, Bonnell BW, et al: Pulmonary artery catheterization: a prospective study of internal jugular and subclavian approaches. *Crit Care Med* 15:35, 1987.
125. Nembre AE: Swan-Ganz catheter. *Arch Surg* 115:1194, 1980.
126. Lipp H, O'Donoghue K, Resnekov L: Intracardiac knotting of a flow-directed balloon catheter. *N Engl J Med* 284:220, 1971.
127. Mond HG, Clark DW, Nesbitt SJ, et al: A technique for unknotting an intracardiac flow-directed balloon catheter. *Chest* 67:731, 1975.
128. Meister SG, Furr CM, Engel TR, et al: Knotting of a flow-directed catheter about a cardiac structure. *Cathet Cardiovasc Diagn* 3:171, 1977.

129. Swaroop S: Knotting of two central venous monitoring catheters. *Am J Med* 53:386, 1972.
130. Loggam C, Sanborn TA, Christian F: Ventricular entrapment of a Swan-Ganz catheter: a technique for nonsurgical removal. *J Am Coll Cardiol* 13:1422, 1989.
131. Foote GA, Schabel SI, Hodges M: Pulmonary complications of the flow-directed balloon-tipped catheter. *N Engl J Med* 290:927, 1974.
132. Wechsler RJ, Steiner RM, Kinori F: Monitoring the monitors: the radiology of thoracic catheters, wires and tubes. *Semin Roentgenol* 23:61, 1988.
133. Boyd KD, Thomas SJ, Gold J, et al: A prospective study of complications of pulmonary artery catheterizations in 500 consecutive patients. *Chest* 84:245, 1983.
134. Sise MJ, Hollingsworth P, Bumm JE, et al: Complications of the flow directed pulmonary artery catheter: a prospective analysis of 219 patients. *Crit Care Med* 9:315, 1981.
135. Barash PG, Nardi D, Hammond G, et al: Catheter-induced pulmonary artery perforation: mechanisms, management and modifications. *J Thorac Cardiovasc Surg* 82:5, 1981.
136. Pape LA, Haffajee CI, Markis JE, et al: Fatal pulmonary hemorrhage after use of the flow-directed balloon-tipped catheter. *Ann Intern Med* 90:344, 1979.
137. Lapin ES, Murray JA: Hemoptysis with flow-directed cardiac catheterization. *JAMA* 220:1246, 1972.
138. Haapaniemi J, Gadowski R, Naini M, et al: Massive hemoptysis secondary to flow-directed thermodilution catheters. *Cathet Cardiovasc Diagn* 5:151, 1979.
139. Golden MS, Pinder T, Anderson WT, et al: Fatal pulmonary hemorrhage complicating use of a flow-directed balloon-tipped catheter in a patient receiving anticoagulant therapy. *Am J Cardiol* 32:865, 1973.
140. Page DW, Teres D, Hartshorn JW: Fatal hemorrhage from Swan-Ganz catheter. *N Engl J Med* 291:260, 1974.
141. Chun GMH, Ellestad MH: Perforation of the pulmonary artery by a Swan-Ganz catheter. *N Engl J Med* 284:1041, 1971.
142. Fleischer AG, Tyers FO, Manning GT, et al: Management of massive hemoptysis secondary to catheter-induced perforation of the pulmonary artery during cardiopulmonary bypass. *Chest* 95:1340, 1989.
143. Carlson TA, Goldenberg IF, Murray PD, et al: Catheter-induced delayed recurrent pulmonary artery hemorrhage. *JAMA* 261:1943, 1989.
144. McDaniel DD, Stone JG, Faltas AN, et al: Catheter induced pulmonary artery hemorrhage: diagnosis and management in cardiac operations. *J Thorac Cardiovasc Surg* 82:1, 1981.
145. Shah KB, Rao TL, Laughlin S, et al: A review of pulmonary artery catheterization in 6245 patients. *Anesthesiology* 61:271, 1984.
146. Fraser RS: Catheter-induced pulmonary artery perforation: pathologic and pathogenic features. *Hum Pathol* 18:1246, 1987.
147. Declen JD, Friloux LA, Renner JW: Pulmonary artery false-aneurysms secondary to Swan-Ganz pulmonary artery catheters. *AJR Am J Roentgenol* 149:901, 1987.
148. Thoms R, Siproudhis L, Laurent JF, et al: Massive hemoptysis from iatrogenic balloon catheter rupture of pulmonary artery: successful early management by balloon tamponade. *Crit Care Med* 15:272, 1987.
149. Slacken A: Complications of invasive hemodynamic monitoring in the intensive care unit. *Curr Probl Surg* 25:69, 1988.
150. Scuderi PE, Prough DS, Price JD, et al: Cessation of pulmonary artery catheter-induced endobronchial hemorrhage associated with the use of PEEP. *Anesth Analg* 62:236, 1983.
151. Yorra FH, Oblath R, Jaffe H, et al: Massive thrombosis associated with use of a Swan-Ganz catheter. *Chest* 65:682, 1974.
152. Pace NL, Horton W: Indwelling pulmonary artery catheters: their relationship to aseptic thrombotic endocardial vegetations. *JAMA* 233:893, 1975.
153. Greene JF, Cummings KC: Aseptic thrombotic endocardial vegetations: a complication of indwelling pulmonary artery catheters. *JAMA* 225:1525, 1973.
154. Dye LE, Segall PH, Russell RO, et al: Deep venous thrombosis of the upper extremity associated with use of the Swan-Ganz catheter. *Chest* 73:673, 1978.
155. Elliot CG, Zimmerman GA, Clemmer TP: Complications of pulmonary artery catheterization in the care of critically ill patients: a prospective study. *Chest* 76:647, 1979.
156. Chastre J, Cornud F, Bouchama A, et al: Thrombosis as a complication of pulmonary artery catheterization via the internal jugular vein. *N Engl J Med* 306:278, 1982.
157. Laster JL, Nichols WK, Silver D: Thrombocytopenia associated with heparin-coated catheters in patients with heparin-associated antiplatelet antibodies. *Arch Intern Med* 149:2285, 1989.
158. Laster JL, Silver D: Heparin coated catheters and heparin-induced thrombocytopenia. *J Vasc Surg* 7:667, 1988.
159. Geha DG, Davis NJ, Lappas DG: Persistent atrial arrhythmias associated with placement of a Swan-Ganz catheter. *Anesthesiology* 39:651, 1973.
160. Elliot CG, Zimmerman GA, Clemmer TP: Complications of pulmonary artery catheterization in the care of critically ill patients. *Chest* 76:647, 1979.
161. Spring CL, Jacobs JL, Caralis PV, et al: Ventricular arrhythmias during Swan-Ganz catheterization of the critically ill. *Chest* 79:413, 1981.
162. Spring CL, Pozen PG, Rozanski JJ, et al: Advanced ventricular arrhythmias during bedside pulmonary artery catheterization. *Am J Med* 72:203, 1982.
163. Patel C, Laboy V, Venus B, et al: Acute complications of pulmonary artery catheter insertion in critically ill patients. *Crit Care Med* 14:195, 1986.
164. Iberti TJ, Benjamin E, Grupzi L, et al: Ventricular arrhythmias during pulmonary artery catheterization in the intensive care unit. *Am J Med* 78:451, 1985.
165. Spring CL, Marical EH, Garcia AA, et al: Prophylactic use of lidocaine to prevent advanced ventricular arrhythmias during pulmonary artery catheterization: Prospective, double blind study. *Am J Med* 75:906, 1983.
166. Keusch DJ, Winters S, Thys DM: The patient's position influences the incidence of dysrhythmias during pulmonary artery catheterization. *Anesthesiology* 70:582, 1989.
167. Johnston W, Royster R, Beamer W, et al: Arrhythmias during removal of pulmonary artery catheters. *Chest* 85:296, 1984.
168. Damen J: Ventricular arrhythmia during insertion and removal of pulmonary artery catheters. *Chest* 88:190, 1985.
169. Luck JC, Engel TR: Transient right bundle branch block with Swan-Ganz catheterization. *Am Heart J* 92:263, 1976.
170. Thomson IR, Dalton BC, Lappas DG, et al: Right bundle branch block and complete heart block caused by the Swan-Ganz catheter. *Anesthesiology* 51:359, 1979.
171. Abernathy WS: Complete heart block caused by the Swan-Ganz catheter. *Chest* 65:349, 1974.
172. Morris D, Mulvihill D, Lew WY: Risk of developing complete heart block during bedside pulmonary artery catheterization in patients with left bundle branch block. *Arch Intern Med* 147:2005, 1987.
173. Lavie CJ, Gersh BJ: Pacing in left bundle branch block during Swan-Ganz catheterization (letter). *Arch Intern Med* 148:981, 1988.
174. Kaye W: Invasive monitoring techniques, in McIntyre KM, Lewis AJ (eds): *Textbook of Advanced Cardiac Life Support*. Dallas, American Heart Association, 1983, p 165.
175. Moser KM, Spragg RG: Use of the balloon tipped pulmonary artery catheter in pulmonary disease. *Ann Intern Med* 98:53, 1983.
176. Smith WR, Glauser FL, Jenison P: Ruptured chordae of the tricuspid valve: the consequence of flow-directed Swan-Ganz catheterization. *Chest* 70:790, 1976.
177. O'Toole JD, Wurtzbacher JJ, Wearner NE, et al: Pulmonary valve injury and insufficiency during pulmonary artery catheterization. *N Engl J Med* 301:1167, 1979.
178. Becker RC, Martin RG, Underwood DA: Right-sided endocardial lesions and flow-directed pulmonary artery catheters. *Cleve Clin J Med* 54:384, 1987.
179. Ford SE, Manley PN: Indwelling cardiac catheters: an autopsy study of associated endocardial lesions. *Arch Pathol Lab Med* 106:314, 1982.
180. Lange HW, Galliani CA, Edwards JE: Local complications associated with indwelling Swan-Ganz catheters. *Am J Cardiol* 52:1108, 1983.
181. Sage MD, Koelmeyer TD, Smeeton WMI: Evolution of Swan-Ganz catheter related pulmonary valve nonbacterial endocarditis. *Am J Forensic Med Pathol* 9:112, 1988.
182. Rowley KM, Clubb KS, Smith GJW, et al: Right sided infective endocarditis as a consequence of flow directed pulmonary artery catheterization. *N Engl J Med* 311:1152, 1984.

183. Van der Belkahn J, Fowler NO, Doerger P: Right heart catheter lesions: any significance? *Am J Clin Pathol* 82:137, 1984.
184. Pace NL, Horton W: Indwelling pulmonary artery catheters: their relationship to aseptic thrombotic endocardial vegetations. *JAMA* 233:893, 1975.
185. Garrison PK, Freedman LR: Experimental endocarditis. I. Staphylococcal endocarditis in rabbit hearts resulting from placement of a polyethylene catheter in the right side of the heart. *Yale J Biol Med* 42:394, 1970.
186. Prochan H, Dittel M, Jobst C, et al: Bacterial contamination of pulmonary artery catheters. *Intensive Care Med* 4:79, 1978.
187. Pinella JC, Ross DF, Martin T, et al: Study of the incidence of intravascular catheter infection and associated septicemia in critically ill patients. *Crit Care Med* 11:21, 1983.
188. Michel L, Marsh HM, McMichan JC, et al: Infection of pulmonary artery catheters in critically ill patients. *JAMA* 245:1032, 1981.
189. Greene JF, Fitzwater JE, Clemmer TP: Septic endocarditis and indwelling pulmonary artery catheters. *JAMA* 233:891, 1975.
190. Myers ML, Austin TW, Sibbald WJ: Pulmonary artery catheter infections: a prospective study. *Ann Surg* 201:237, 1985.
191. Weinstein RA, Stamm WE, Kramer L: Pressure monitoring devices: overlooked source of nosocomial infection. *JAMA* 236:936, 1976.
192. Singh SJ, Puri VK: Prevention of bacterial colonization of pulmonary artery catheters. *Infect Surg* 853, 1984.
193. Kopman EA, Sandza JG Jr: Manipulation of the pulmonary artery catheter after placement: maintenance of sterility. *Anesthesiology* 48:373, 1978.
194. Heard SO, Davis RF, Skeretz RJ, et al: Influence of sterile protective sleeves on the sterility of pulmonary artery catheters. *Crit Care Med* 15:499, 1987.
195. Cobb DK, High KP, Sawyer RG, et al: A controlled trial of scheduled replacement of central venous and pulmonary artery catheters. *N Engl J Med* 327:1062, 1992.
196. Berry AJ, Geer RT, Marshall BE: Alteration of pulmonary blood flow by pulmonary artery occluded pressure measurement. *Anesthesiology* 51:164, 1979.
197. Schluger J, Green J, Giustra FX, et al: Complication with use of flow-directed catheter. *Am J Cardiol* 32:125, 1973.
198. Isner JM, Horton J, Ronan JAS: Systolic click from a Swan-Ganz catheter: phonoechocardiographic depiction of the underlying mechanism. *Am J Cardiol* 42:1046, 1979.
199. Lawson D, Kushkins LG: A complication of multipurpose pacing pulmonary artery catheterization via the external jugular vein approach (letter). *Anesthesiology* 62:377, 1985.
200. McLellan BA, Jerman MR, French WJ, et al: Inadvertent Swan-Ganz catheter placement in the left pericardiophrenic vein. *Cathet Cardiovasc Diagn* 16:173, 1989.
201. Allyn J, Lichtenstein A, Koski EG, et al: Inadvertent passage of a pulmonary artery catheter from the superior vena cava through the left atrium and left ventricle into the aorta. *Anesthesiology* 70:1019, 1989.
202. Lazzam C, Sanborn TA, Christian F: Ventricular entrapment of a Swan-Ganz catheter: a technique for nonsurgical removal. *J Am Coll Cardiol* 13:1422, 1989.
203. Swan HJC, Ganz W: Guidelines for use of balloon-tipped catheter. *Am J Cardiol* 34:119, 1974.
204. Ginosar Y, Sprung CL: The Swan-Ganz catheter: twenty-five years of monitoring. *Crit Care Clin* 12:771, 1996.
205. Pulmonary Artery Catheter Consensus Conference Participants: Pulmonary artery catheter consensus conference: consensus statement. *New Horiz* 5:175, 1997.

5. *Temporary Cardiac Pacing*

Seth T. Dahlberg and
Michael G. Mooradd

Because temporary cardiac pacing may be lifesaving in a number of disease states commonly treated in the intensive care unit (ICU), the indications and techniques for initiating and maintaining temporary cardiac pacing should be familiar to ICU personnel. Recommendations for training in the performance of transvenous pacing have been published by a Task Force of the American College of Physicians, the American Heart Association, and the American College of Cardiology [1].

Indications for Temporary Cardiac Pacing

As outlined in Table 5-1, temporary pacing is indicated in the diagnosis and management of a number of serious rhythm and conduction disturbances [2,3].

BRADYARRHYTHMIAS. Rate disturbances that respond to temporary cardiac pacing include sinus bradycardia and high-grade atrioventricular (AV) block, as well as ventricular tachycardia precipitated by episodic bradycardia [2].

Sinus bradycardia is commonly seen in patients with myocardial infarction, hyperkalemia, antiarrhythmic medication intoxication, myxedema, and increased intracranial pressure.

Bradyarrhythmias may also result from exaggerated vasovagal reactions to ICU procedures, such as suctioning of the tracheobronchial tree in the intubated patient. High-grade AV block may result from digitalis toxicity; hyperkalemia; or any other infectious, inflammatory, or metabolic process that impairs AV conduction. Bradycardia-dependent ventricular tachycardia may occur in association with ischemic heart disease and acute coronary insufficiency.

TACHYARRHYTHMIAS. Temporary cardiac pacing has been used in prevention and termination of supraventricular and ventricular tachyarrhythmias [4–8].

Atrial pacing is often effective in terminating atrial flutter and paroxysmal nodal supraventricular tachycardia [9]. A critical pacing rate (usually 125% to 135% of the flutter rate) and pacing duration (usually approximately 10 seconds) are important in the successful conversion of atrial flutter to sinus rhythm [10,11]. This method is often effective in patients with classic atrial flutter; however, it is typically ineffective for atypical or type II atrial flutter (rate 400 beats per minute, P waves upright in the inferior leads). Although pacing termination of atrial flutter may be more successful from sites in the low right atrium, this requires great care to avoid rapid ventricular stimulation, which may precipitate ventricular fibrillation with hemodynamic collapse.

In many clinical situations pacing termination of atrial flutter may be more attractive than synchronized cardioversion,

Table 5-1. Indications for Acute (Temporary) Cardiac Pacing

Conduction disturbances
  Symptomatic persistent third-degree AV block with inferior myocardial infarction
  Third-degree AV block, Mobitz type II AV block, new bifascicular block (e.g., right bundle branch block and left anterior hemiblock, left bundle branch block, first-degree AV block), or alternating left and right bundle branch block complicating acute anterior myocardial infarction
  Symptomatic idiopathic third-degree AV block, or high-degree AV block
Rate disturbances
  Hemodynamically significant or symptomatic sinus bradycardia
  Bradycardia-dependent ventricular tachycardia
  AV dissociation with inadequate cardiac output
  Polymorphic ventricular tachycardia with long QT interval (torsades de pointes)
  Recurrent ventricular tachycardia unresponsive to medical therapy
During electrophysiologic studies
  Evaluation of sinus node, AV node, and His bundle function
  Evaluation of wide QRS tachycardias
  Evaluation and treatment of supraventricular arrhythmias, including atrial flutter, AV nodal tachycardia, and Wolff-Parkinson-White syndrome
  Evaluation of therapeutic modalities for inducible ventricular and supraventricular tachycardia

AV, atrioventricular.

which requires anesthesia with its attendant risks. Pacing termination is the treatment of choice for atrial flutter in patients with epicardial atrial wires in place after cardiac surgery; it may also be preferred as the means to convert atrial flutter in patients on digoxin and those with sick sinus syndrome, as these groups often demonstrate prolonged sinus pauses after direct current cardioversion [12,13].

Rapid atrial pacing (at rates of 400 to 700 beats per minute) has also been used to prevent recurrent supraventricular tachycardias by inducing atrial fibrillation. This technique may be useful in situations in which the ventricular rate cannot be adequately controlled in response to an automatic or reentrant supraventricular tachycardia [14].

Temporary pacing has proved lifesaving in preventing paroxysmal ventricular tachycardia in patients with prolonged QT intervals (torsades de pointes), particularly when secondary to drugs. Temporary cardiac pacing is the treatment of choice to stabilize the patient while a type I antiarrhythmic agent exacerbating ventricular irritability is metabolized [15]. In this situation, the pacing rate is set to provide a mild tachycardia. The effectiveness of cardiac pacing probably relates to decreasing the dispersion of refractoriness of the ventricular myocardium (shortening the QT interval).

Temporary ventricular pacing is also frequently successful in terminating ventricular tachycardia [16–18]. If ventricular tachycardia must be terminated urgently, cardioversion is mandated (see Chapter 6). However, in less urgent situations, conversion of ventricular tachycardia via rapid ventricular pacing may be useful. The success of this technique depends on the setting in which ventricular tachycardia occurs as well as the type of pacing used (e.g., rapid overdrive pacing or programmed extrastimulation). Programmed stimulation techniques are usually effective in terminating ventricular tachycardia in a patient with remote myocardial infarction or in the absence of heart disease. This technique is less effective when ventricular tachycardia complicates acute myocardial infarction or cardiomyopathy. Rapid ventricular pacing is most successful in terminating ventricular tachycardia when the ventricle can be "captured" (asynchronous pacing for 5 to 10 beats at a rate of 50 beats per minute greater than that of the

underlying tachycardia). Extreme caution is advised, as it may be accompanied by acceleration of ventricular tachycardias in more than 40% of patients; a cardiac defibrillator should be available at the bedside.

DIAGNOSIS OF RAPID RHYTHMS. Temporary atrial pacing electrodes allow accurate diagnosis of tachyarrhythmias when the morphology of the P wave and its relation to the QRS complexes cannot be determined from the surface electrocardiogram (ECG) [19,20]. A recording of the intraatrial electrogram is particularly helpful in a rapid, regular, narrow-complex tachycardia in which the differential diagnosis includes atrial flutter with rapid ventricular response and in AV nodal reentrant or other supraventricular tachycardia. This technique is also useful to distinguish wide-complex tachycardias in which the differential diagnosis includes supraventricular tachycardia with aberrant conduction, sinus tachycardia with bundle-branch block, and ventricular tachycardia.

To record an intraatrial ECG, the limb leads are connected in the standard fashion and a precordial lead (usually V_1) is connected to the proximal electrode of the atrial pacing catheter. A rhythm strip is run at a rapid paper speed, simultaneously demonstrating two limb leads as well as the atrial electrogram obtained via lead V_1. This rhythm strip should reveal the conduction pattern between atria and ventricles as antegrade, simultaneous, retrograde, or dissociated.

ACUTE MYOCARDIAL INFARCTION. Temporary pacing may be used therapeutically or prophylactically in acute myocardial infarction. Recommendations for temporary cardiac pacing have been provided by a Task Force of the American College of Cardiology and the American Heart Association (Table 5-2) [21]. Bradyarrhythmias unresponsive to medical treatment that result in hemodynamic compromise require urgent treatment. Patients with anterior infarction and bifascicular block or Mobitz type II second-degree AV block, while hemodynamically stable, may require a temporary pacemaker, as they are at risk for sudden development of complete heart block with an unstable escape rhythm.

Because coordinated atrial transport may be essential for preservation and maintenance of effective stroke volume, AV sequential pacing is frequently the pacing modality of choice [22–24]. For example, when right ventricular involvement complicates inferoposterior infarction, transvenous AV sequential pacing may be necessary to ensure adequate cardiac output [25,26].

Prophylactic temporary cardiac pacing has aroused considerable debate for the role it may play in complicated anterior wall myocardial infarction [27,28]. Thrombolytic therapy, when indicated, should take precedence over placement of prophylactic cardiac pacing, as prophylactic pacing has not been shown to improve mortality. Transthoracic (transcutaneous) cardiac pacing is safe and usually effective [29–32] and would be a reasonable alternative to prophylactic transvenous cardiac pacing, particularly soon after thrombolytic therapy has been administered.

Equipment Available for Temporary Pacing

Several methods of temporary pacing are currently available for use in the ICU. Transvenous pacing of the right ventricle or right atrium with a pacing catheter or modified pulmonary

Table 5-2. American College of Cardiology/American Heart Association Guidelines for Temporary Pacing in Acute Myocardial Infarction

Guidelines for placement of transcutaneous patches[a] and active (demand) transcutaneous pacing[b]
  Class I (indicated)
    Sinus bradycardia (rate <50 beats/min) with symptoms of hypotension (systolic blood pressure <80 mm Hg) unresponsive to drug therapy[b]
    Mobitz type II second-degree AV block[b]
    Third-degree AV block[b]
    Bilateral BBB (alternating BBB, or RBBB and alternating LAFB, LPFB) (irrespective of time of onset)[a]
    Newly acquired or age-indeterminate LBBB, LBBB and LAFB, RBBB, and LPFB[a]
    RBBB or LBBB and first-degree AV block[a]
  Class IIa (probably indicated)
    Stable bradycardia (systolic blood pressure >90 mm Hg, no hemodynamic compromise, or compromise responsive to initial drug therapy)[a]
    Newly acquired or age-indeterminate RBBB[a]
  Class IIb (possibly indicated)
    Newly acquired or age-indeterminate first-degree AV block[a]
  Class III (not indicated)
    Uncomplicated AMI without evidence of conduction system disease
Guidelines for temporary transvenous pacing[c]
  Class I (indicated)
    Asystole
    Symptomatic bradycardia (includes sinus bradycardia with hypotension and type I second-degree AV block with hypotension not responsive to atropine)
    Bilateral BBB (alternating BBB or RBBB with alternating LAFB/LPFB) (any age)
    New or age-indeterminate bifascicular block (RBBB with LAFB or LPFB, or LBBB) with first-degree AV block
    Mobitz type II second-degree AV block
  Class IIa (probably indicated)
    RBBB and LAFB or LPFB (new or indeterminate)
    RBBB with first-degree AV block
    LBBB, new or indeterminate
    Incessant ventricular tachycardia, for atrial or ventricular overdrive pacing
    Recurrent sinus pauses (>3 sec) not responsive to atropine
  Class IIb (possibly indicated)
    Bifascicular block of indeterminate age
    New or age-indeterminate isolated RBBB
  Class III (not indicated)
    First-degree AV block
    Type I second-degree AV block with normal hemodynamics
    Accelerated idioventricular rhythm
    BBB or fascicular block known to exist before AMI

AMI, acute myocardial infarction; AV, atrioventricular; BBB, bundle-branch block; LAFB, left anterior fascicular block; LBBB, left bundle-branch block; LPFB, left posterior fascicular block; RBBB, right bundle-branch block.
[a]Transcutaneous patches applied; system may be attached and activated within brief time if needed. Transcutaneous pacing may be very helpful as an urgent expedient. Because it is associated with significant pain, high-risk patients likely to require pacing should receive a temporary pacemaker.
[b]Apply patches and attach system; system is in either active or standby mode to allow immediate use on demand as required. In facilities in which transvenous pacing or expertise are not available to place an intravenous system, consideration should be given to transporting the patient to one equipped for and competent in placing transvenous systems.
[c]It should be noted that in choosing an intravenous pacemaker system, patients with substantially depressed ventricular performance, including right ventricular infarction, may respond better to atrial/AV sequential pacing than ventricular pacing.
From Ryan TJ, Antman EM, Brooks NH, et al: 1999 update: ACC/AHA guidelines for the management of patients with acute myocardial infarction: executive summary and recommendations: a report of the American College of Cardiology/American Heart Association Task Force on Practice Guidelines (Committee on Management of Acute Myocardial Infarction). *Circulation* 100:1016–1030, 2001, with permission. Copyright 1999, American Heart Association.

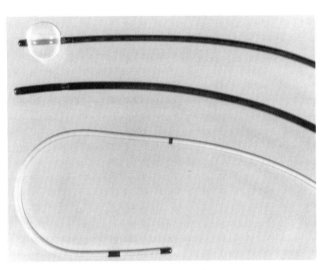

Fig. 5-1. Cardiac pacing catheters. Several designs are available for temporary pacing in the critical care unit. **Top:** Balloon-tipped, flow-directed pacing wire. **Middle:** Standard 5-French pacing wire. **Bottom:** Atrial J-shaped wire.

artery catheter is the most widely used technique; intraesophageal, transcutaneous, and epicardial pacing are also available.

TRANSVENOUS PACING CATHETERS. Some of the many transvenous pacing catheters available for use in the critical care setting are illustrated in Figure 5-1. Pacing catheters range in size from 4 French (Fr) (1.2 mm) to 7 Fr (2.1 mm). Stiff catheters (Fig. 5-1, middle) can be inserted under fluoroscopic guidance using standard central venous cannulation techniques. In more urgent situations, or where fluoroscopy is unavailable, a flow-directed flexible balloon-tipped catheter (Fig. 5-1, top) may be placed in the right ventricle using ECG guidance. The stiff catheter is easier to manipulate than the balloon-tipped catheter.

A flexible J-shaped catheter (Fig. 5-1, bottom) is available specifically for temporary atrial pacing [33]. This lead is positioned by "hooking" it in the right atrial appendage, providing stable contact with the atrial endocardium. Either the subclavian or internal jugular venous approach may be used. Fluoroscopic guidance is needed to achieve the proper pacing position.

A multilumen pulmonary artery catheter with a small (2.4 Fr) bipolar pacing lead through a right ventricular lumen allows intracardiac pressure monitoring and pacing through a single catheter [34]. Details on its use and insertion are described in Chapter 4.

ESOPHAGEAL ELECTRODE. An esophageal "pill" electrode allows atrial pacing and recording of atrial depolarizations without requiring central venous cannulation. As mentioned previously, detecting atrial depolarization aids in the diagnosis of tachyarrhythmias. Esophageal pacing has also been used to terminate supraventricular tachycardia and atrial flutter [35].

TRANSCUTANEOUS EXTERNAL PACEMAKERS. Transcutaneous external pacemakers have external patch electrodes that deliver a higher current (up to 200 mA) and longer pulse duration (20 to 40 milliseconds) than transvenous pacemakers. External pacing can be implemented immediately and the risks of central venous access avoided. Some patients may require sedation for the discomfort of skeletal muscle stimulation. Transcutaneous external pacemakers have been used to treat bradyasystolic cardiac arrest, symptomatic bradyarrhythmias, and overdrive pacing of tachyarrhythmias, and prophylactically for conduction abnormalities during myocardial infarction. They may be particularly useful when transvenous pacing is unavailable, as in the prehospital setting, or relatively contraindicated, as during thrombolytic therapy for acute myocardial infarction [29–31,36–38].

EPICARDIAL PACING. The placement of epicardial electrodes requires open thoracotomy. These electrodes are routinely placed electively during cardiac surgical procedures for use during the postoperative period [19,20].

PULSE GENERATORS FOR TEMPORARY PACING. Newer temporary pulse generators are now capable of ventricular, atrial, and dual-chamber sequential pacing with adjustable ventricular and atrial parameters that include pacing modes (synchronous or asynchronous), rates, current outputs (mA), sensing thresholds (mV), and AV pacing interval/delay (milliseconds). Because these generators have atrial sensing/inhibiting capability, they are also set with an upper rate limit (to avoid rapid ventricular pacing while "tracking" an atrial tachycardia); in addition, an atrial pacing refractory period may be programmed (to avoid pacemaker-mediated/endless loop tachyarrhythmias).

Earlier models may be limited to sensing only ventricular depolarization. Without atrial sensing, if the intrinsic atrial rate exceeds the atrial pacing rate, the atrial pacing stimulus fails to capture and AV sequential pacing is lost. Consequently, with these models, the pacing rate must be set continuously to exceed the intrinsic atrial rate to maintain AV sequential pacing.

Choice of Pacing Mode

A pacing mode must be selected when temporary cardiac pacing is initiated. Common modes for cardiac pacing are outlined in Table 5-3. The mode most likely to provide the greatest hemodynamic benefit should be selected. In patients with hemodynamic instability, establishing ventricular pacing is of paramount importance before attempts at AV sequential pacing.

Although ventricular pacing effectively counteracts bradycardia, it cannot restore normal cardiac hemodynamics because it disrupts the synchronous relationship between atrial and ventricular contraction [39–49]. In patients with diseases characterized by noncompliant ventricles (e.g., ischemic heart disease, hypertrophic or congestive cardiomyopathy, aortic stenosis, and right ventricular infarction), the atrial contribution to ven-

tricular stroke volume (the atrial "kick") may be quite substantial. In one study, loss of a properly timed atrial contraction in patients after inferior or anterior myocardial infarction was associated with a 25% decrease in systolic blood pressure and cardiac output [24].

Asynchronous contraction of the atria and ventricles (via random dissociation or retrograde ventriculoatrial conduction) results in increased left atrial pressure, reduced stroke volume and cardiac output, and intermittent mitral and tricuspid regurgitation.

In addition to the hemodynamic benefit of atrial or AV sequential pacing, the risk of atrial fibrillation or flutter may be reduced because of decreased atrial size, decreased atrial pressure, or both. This suggests that patients with intermittent atrial fibrillation may be better maintained in normal sinus rhythm with atrial or AV sequential pacing, rather than ventricular demand pacing.

Procedure to Establish Temporary Pacing

After achieving venous access (Chapter 2), the pacing catheter is advanced to the central venous circulation and then positioned in the right heart using fluoroscopic or ECG guidance [50,51]. To position the electrode using ECG guidance, the patient is connected to the limb leads of the ECG machine, and the distal (negative) electrode of the pacing catheter is connected to lead V_1 with an alligator clip or a special adaptor supplied with the lead. Lead V_1 is then used to continuously monitor a unipolar intracardiac electrogram. The morphology of the recorded electrogram indicates the position of the catheter tip (Fig. 5-2). The balloon is inflated in the superior vena cava,

Table 5-3. Common Pacemaker Modes for Temporary Cardiac Pacing

Mode	Definition
AOO	Atrial pacing: pacing is asynchronous.
AAI	Atrial pacing, atrial sensing: pacing is on demand to provide a minimum programmed rate.
VOO	Ventricular pacing: pacing is asynchronous.
VVI	Ventricular pacing, ventricular sensing: pacing is on demand to provide a minimum programmed rate.
DVI	Dual-chamber pacing, ventricular sensing: atrial pacing is asynchronous, ventricular pacing is on demand after a programmed atrioventricular delay.
DDD	Dual-chamber pacing and sensing: atrial and ventricular pacing is on demand to provide a minimum rate, ventricular pacing follows a programmed atrioventricular delay, and upper-rate pacing limit should be programmed.

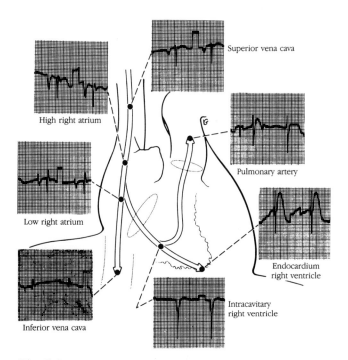

Fig. 5-2. Pattern of recorded electrogram at various locations in the venous circulation. [From Harthorne JW, McDermott J, Poulin FK: Cardiac pacing, in Johnson RA, Haber E, Austen WG (eds): *The Practice of Cardiology: The Medical and Surgical Cardiac Units at the Massachusetts General Hospital.* Boston, Little, Brown and Company, 1980, with permission.]

and the catheter is advanced while observing the recorded intra-cardiac electrogram. When the tip of the catheter is in the right ventricle, the balloon is deflated and the catheter advanced to the right ventricular apex. The ST segment of the intracardiac electrogram is elevated owing to a current of injury when the catheter tip contacts the ventricular endocardium.

After the tip of the pacing catheter is satisfactorily inserted in the right ventricular apex, the leads are connected to the ventricular output positions at the top of the pulse generator, with the pacemaker box in the off position. The pacemaker is then put on asynchronous mode and the ventricular rate set to exceed the patient's intrinsic ventricular rate by 10 to 20 beats per minute. The threshold current for ventricular pacing is set at 5 to 10 mA. Then, the pacemaker is switched on. Satisfactory ventricular pacing is evidenced by a wide QRS complex, with ST segment depression and T-wave inversion, immediately preceded by a pacemaker depolarization (spike). With pacing from the apex of the right ventricle, the paced rhythm usually demonstrates a pattern of left bundle-branch block on the surface ECG [52].

Ventricular pacing is maintained as the output current for ventricular pacing is slowly reduced. The pacing threshold is defined as the lowest current at which consistent ventricular capture occurs. With the ventricular electrode appropriately positioned at or near the apex of the right ventricle, a pacing threshold of less than 0.5 to 1.0 mA should be achieved. If the output current for continuous ventricular pacing is consistently greater than 1.0 to 1.5 mA, the pacing threshold is too high. Possible causes of a high pacing threshold include relatively refractory endomyocardial tissue (fibrosis) or, most commonly, unsatisfactory positioning of the pacing electrode. The tip of the pacing electrode should be repositioned in the region of the ventricular apex until satisfactory ventricular capture at a current of less than 1.0 mA is consistently maintained. After the threshold current for ventricular pacing has been established at a satisfactory level, the ventricular output is set to exceed the threshold current at least threefold. This guarantees uninterrupted ventricular capture despite any modest increase in the pacing threshold.

The pacemaker is now in VOO mode. However, the pacing generator generally should be set in the VVI ("demand") mode, as this prevents pacemaker discharge soon after an intrinsic or spontaneous premature depolarization, while the heart lies in the electrically vulnerable period for induction of sustained ventricular arrhythmias [53]. To set the pacemaker in VVI mode, the pacing rate is set at 10 beats per minute less than the intrinsic rate, and the sensitivity control is moved from asynchronous to the minimum sensitivity level. The sensitivity is gradually increased until pacing spikes appear. This level is the sensing threshold. The sensitivity is then set at a level slightly below the determined threshold and the pacing rate reset to the minimum desired ventricular rate.

If AV sequential pacing is desired, the atrial J-shaped pacing catheter should be advanced into the right atrium and rotated anteromedially to achieve a stable position in the right atrial appendage; positioning the atrial catheter usually requires fluoroscopy [51,54]. The leads are then connected to the atrial output of the pulse generator. The atrial current is set to 20 mA, and the atrial pacing rate adjusted to at least 10 beats per minute greater than the intrinsic atrial rate. The AV interval is adjusted at 100 to 200 milliseconds (shorter intervals usually provide better hemodynamics), and the surface ECG is inspected for evidence of atrial pacing (electrode depolarization and capture of the atrium at the pacing rate).

The manifestation of atrial capture on ECG is atrial depolarization immediately after the atrial pacing spike. In patients with intact AV conduction, satisfactory atrial capture can be verified by shutting off the ventricular portion of the pace-maker and demonstrating AV synchrony during atrial pacing. As long as the atrial pacing rate continually exceeds the intrinsic sinus rate, the atrial P wave activity should track with the atrial pacing spike.

The dual-chamber temporary pacemaker may not have atrial sensing capability. If not, the pacemaker will function in a DVI mode (Table 5-3). Should the intrinsic atrial rate equal or exceed the atrial pacing rate, the atrial stimulus fails to capture, and AV sequential pacing is lost. If the pacemaker has atrial sensing capability, the atrial sensing threshold should be determined and an appropriate level set. The pacer then functions in the DDD mode. The DDD mode is usually preferred, as it provides optimum cardiac hemodynamics through a range of intrinsic atrial rates. In this mode, an upper rate limit must be set to prevent rapid ventricular pacing in response to a paroxysmal supraventricular tachycardia.

Complications of Temporary Pacing

Although temporary endocardial pacing can be accomplished from several alternate venous access sites, rational selection of the optimal route requires understanding of the results and complications of each. A 43% incidence of pacemaker malfunction (i.e., failure to sense or capture the R wave properly) and a 16.9% incidence of pacemaker-related complications were reported in 142 episodes of temporary pacemaker insertion by the brachial (61 cases) or femoral (81 cases) approach [55]. Austin and associates reported pacemaker malfunction in 37 and complications in 20 of 100 patients requiring pacemaker insertion by the antecubital or femoral route [56]. The Mayo Clinic's early experience with temporary cardiac pacing in the coronary care unit revealed a 17.9% incidence of malfunction of the temporary pacemaker and a 13.7% incidence of complications [55]. Over the 4-year interval from 1976 to 1980, there was a decline in use of the basilic vein surgical approach (the initially preferred method for temporary pacemaker insertion) from 95.6% to 22.8%. As use of the antecubital route declined, so did the rate of complications (e.g., pacemaker malfunction, infection) when compared to the subclavian or internal jugular venous approaches. Using predominantly the subclavian or internal jugular approaches, Donovan and Lee reported a 7% rate of serious complications related to temporary cardiac pacing [57]. Complications of temporary pacing from any venous access route include pericardial friction rub, arrhythmia, right ventricular perforation, cardiac tamponade, infection, inadvertent arterial injury, diaphragmatic stimulation, phlebitis, and pneumothorax. The Mayo Clinic experience revealed that percutaneous cannulation of the right internal jugular vein provided the simplest, most direct route to the right-sided cardiac chambers. In addition, for selected patients, placement of the catheter in the coronary sinus provides the benefit of stable atrial stimulation. Temporary endocardial pacing via this route is convenient and may be associated with a lower rate of pacemaker complications [58].

Although insertion via direct cutdown of the brachial vein may be satisfactory for short-term pacing, percutaneous vascular access by the subclavian or internal jugular vein provides more stable long-term vascular access for temporary pacing (Chapter 2). Insertion from the brachial vein reduces the risk of arterial injury, hematoma formation, and pneumothorax, but the motion of the patient's arm relative to the torso increases the risk of dislodgement of the pacing electrode from a stable ventricular or atrial position [58]. The risk of infection may also be increased with this approach. The brachial approach is still preferred for the patient receiving thrombolytic therapy or full-dose anticoagulation.

Complications of internal jugular venous cannulation may include pneumothorax, carotid arterial injury, and pulmonary embolism (Chapter 2). These risks are minimized by knowledge of anatomic landmarks, adherence to proved techniques, and use of a small-caliber needle to localize the vein before insertion of the large-caliber needle (for full discussion, see Chapter 2). Full-dose systemic anticoagulation, thrombolytic therapy, and prior neck surgical procedures are relative contraindications to routine internal jugular vein cannulation [56,59]. The risk of venous thrombosis after temporary cardiac pacemaker insertion using the internal jugular or subclavian venous approach has not been prospectively studied [60].

Percutaneous subclavian venipuncture is also frequently used for insertion of temporary pacemakers [53,61,62]. When the operator has a good understanding of the subclavian anatomy, the latter procedure is relatively simple and safe (Chapter 2). This approach should be avoided in patients with severe obstructive lung disease or a bleeding diathesis (including thrombolytic therapy), in whom the risk of pneumothorax or bleeding is increased.

The femoral venous approach is used for electrophysiologic studies when the catheter is left in place for only a few hours. Although temporary cardiac pacing can be established through the percutaneous femoral approach, this approach is less desirable when long-term cardiac pacing is required, because there is a risk of deep venous thrombosis around the catheter. In one study, venographic or autopsy evidence of deep venous thrombosis was present in 34% and pulmonary embolism in 50% of patients in whom a temporary pacing catheter had been inserted by the femoral venous approach [63]. A more recent study showed that a 75% incidence of venous thrombosis, documented by Duplex ultrasound, was reduced to 12% by the use of intravenous heparin [64].

References

1. Francis GS, Williams SV, Achord JL, et al: Clinical competence in insertion of a temporary transvenous ventricular pacemaker: a statement for physicians from the ACP/ACC/AHA Task Force on Clinical Privileges in Cardiology. *Circulation* 89:1913, 1994.
2. Wiener I: Pacing techniques in the treatment of tachycardias. *Ann Intern Med* 93:326, 1980.
3. Silver MD, Goldschlager NG: Temporary transvenous cardiac pacing in the critical care setting. *Chest* 93:607, 1988.
4. Wellens HJJ, Bar F, Gorges AP, et al: Electrical management of arrhythmias with emphasis on the tachycardia. *Am J Cardiol* 41:1025, 1978.
5. Haft J: Treatment of arrhythmias by intracardiac electrical stimulation. *Prog Cardiovasc Dis* 16:539, 1974.
6. Batchelder JL, Zipes DP: Treatment of tachyarrhythmias by pacing. *Arch Intern Med* 135:1115, 1975.
7. Harold SS: Therapeutic uses of cardiac pacing in tachyarrhythmias, in Naruba O (ed): *His Bundle Electrocardiography and Clinical Electrophysiology.* Philadelphia, F.A. Davis, 1975.
8. Spurrell RAJ: Artificial cardiac pacemakers, in Kribler DC, Goodwin JF (eds): *Cardiac Arrhythmias.* London, WB Saunders, 1975, p 238.
9. Wellens HJJ: Value and limitations of programmed electrical stimulation of the heart in the study and treatment of tachycardias. *Circulation* 57:845, 1978.
10. Wills JI Jr, MacLean WAH, James TN, et al: Characterization of atrial flutter studies in man after open heart surgery using fixed atrial electrodes. *Circulation* 60:665, 1979.
11. Waldo AL, MacLean WAH, Karp RB, et al: Entrainment and interruption of atrial flutter with atrial pacing studies in man following open heart surgery. *Circulation* 56:737, 1977.
12. Das G, Anand K, Ankinfedu K, et al: Atrial pacing for cardioversion of atrial flutter in digitalized patients. *Am J Cardiol* 41:308, 1978.
13. Radford DJ, Julian DG: Sick sinus syndrome: experience of a cardiac pacemaker clinic. *BMJ* 3:504, 1974.
14. Waldo AL, MacLean WAH, Karp RB, et al: Continuous rapid atrial pacing to control recurrent or sustained supraventricular tachycardias following open heart surgery. *Circulation* 54:245, 1976.
15. Scarovsky S, Strasberg B, Lewin RF, et al: Polymorphous ventricular tachycardia—clinical features and treatment. *Am J Cardiol* 44:339, 1979.
16. Wellens HJJ, Schuilenburg RM, Durrer DL: Electrical stimulation of the heart in patients with ventricular tachycardia. *Circulation* 46:216, 1972.
17. Wellens HJJ, Duren DR, Lie KI: Observations on mechanisms of ventricular tachycardia in man. *Circulation* 54:237, 1976.
18. Josephson ME, Horowitz LN, Farshidi A, et al: Recurrent sustained ventricular tachycardia.1. Mechanisms. *Circulation* 57:431, 1978.
19. Waldo AL, MacLean WAH, Cooper TB, et al: Use of temporarily placed epicardial atrial wire electrodes for the diagnosis and treatment of cardiac arrhythmias following open-heart surgery. *J Thorac Cardiovasc Surg* 76:500, 1978.
20. Waldo AL: *Cardiac Arrhythmias: Their Mechanisms, Diagnosis, and Management.* Philadelphia, JB Lippincott Co, 1987.
21. Ryan TJ, Antman EM, Brooks NH, et al: 1999 update: ACC/AHA guidelines for the management of patients with acute myocardial infarction: executive summary and recommendations: a report of the American College of Cardiology/American Heart Association Task Force on Practice Guidelines (Committee on Management of Acute Myocardial Infarction). *Circulation* 100:1016, 2001.
22. Nimetz AA, Shubrooks SJ Jr, Hunter AM, et al: The significance of bundle branch block during acute myocardial infarction. *Am Heart J* 90:439, 1975.
23. Mullins CB, Atkins JM: Prognosis and management of ventricular conduction blocks in acute myocardial infarction. *Mod Concepts Cardiovasc Dis* 45:129, 1976.
24. Chamberlain DA, Leinbach RC, Vassau CE, et al: Sequential atrioventricular pacing in heart block complicating acute myocardial infarction. *N Engl J Med* 282:577, 1970.
25. Love JC, Haffajee CI, Gore JM, et al: Reversibility of hypotension and shock by atrial or atrioventricular sequential pacing in patients with right ventricular infarction. *Am Heart J* 108:5, 1984.
26. Topol EJ, Goldschlager N, Ports TA, et al: Hemodynamic benefit of atrial pacing in right ventricular myocardial infarction. *Ann Intern Med* 96:594, 1982.
27. Resnekov L, Lipp H: Pacemaking and acute myocardial infarction. *Prog Cardiovasc Dis* 14:475, 1972.
28. Lamas GA, Muller JE, Zoltan GT, et al: A simplified method to predict occurrence of complete heart block during acute myocardial infarction. *Am J Cardiol* 57:1213, 1986.
29. Falk RH, Ngai STA: External cardiac pacing: influence of electrode placement on pacing threshold. *Crit Care Med* 14:931, 1986.
30. Hedges JR, Syverud SA, Dalsey WC, et al: Prehospital trial of emergency transcutaneous cardiac pacing. *Circulation* 76:1337, 1987.
31. Madsen JK, Meibom J, Videbak R, et al: Transcutaneous pacing: experience with the Zoll noninvasive temporary pacemaker. *Am Heart J* 116:7, 1988.
32. Dunn DL, Gregory JJ: Noninvasive temporary pacing: experience in a community hospital. *Heart Lung* 1:23, 1989.
33. Littleford PO, Curry RC Jr, Schwartz KM, et al: Clinical evaluation of a new temporary atrial pacing catheter: results in 100 patients. *Am Heart J* 107:237, 1984.
34. Simoons ML, Demey HE, Bossaert LL, et al: The Paceport catheter: a new pacemaker system introduced through a Swan-Ganz catheter. *Cathet Cardiovasc Diagn* 15:66, 1988.
35. Benson DW: Transesophageal electrocardiography and cardiac pacing: the state of the art. *Circulation* 75:86, 1987.
36. Luck JC, Grubb BP, Artman SE, et al: Termination of sustained ventricular tachycardia by external noninvasive pacing. *Am J Cardiol* 61:574, 1988.
37. Kelly JS, Royster RL, Angert KC, et al: Efficacy of noninvasive transcutaneous cardiac pacing in patients undergoing cardiac surgery. *Anesthesiology* 70:747, 1989.
38. Blocka JJ: External transcutaneous pacemakers. *Ann Emerg Med* 18:1280, 1989.

39. Samet P, Bernstein W, Natha DA, et al: Atrial contribution to cardiac output in complete heart block. *Am J Cardiol* 16:1, 1965.
40. Romero LR, Haffajee CI, Doherty P, et al: Comparison of ventricular function and volume with A-V sequential and ventricular pacing. *Chest* 80:346, 1981.
41. Knuse I, Arnman K, Conradson TB, et al: A comparison of the acute and long-term hemodynamic effects of ventricular inhibited and atrial synchronous ventricular inhibited pacing. *Circulation* 65:846, 1982.
42. Judge RD, Wilson WJ, Siegel JH: Hemodynamic studies in patients with implanted cardiac pacemakers. *N Engl J Med* 270:1391, 1961.
43. Samet P, Bernstein WH, Levin S: Significance of atrial contribution to ventricular filling. *Am J Cardiol* 15:195, 1965.
44. Leinbach RC, Chamberlain DC, Kastor JA, et al: A comparison of the hemodynamic effects of ventricular and sequential A-V pacing in patients with heart block. *Am Heart J* 78:502, 1969.
45. DeSanctis RW: Diagnostic and therapeutic uses of atrial pacing. *Circulation* 43:748, 1971.
46. Haas JM, Strait GB: Pacemaker-induced cardiovascular failure. *Am J Cardiol* 33:295, 1974.
47. Patel AK, Yap VM, Thomsen JH: Adverse effects of right ventricular pacing in a patient with aortic stenosis. *Chest* 72:103, 1977.
48. Segel N, Samet P: Physiologic aspects of cardiac pacing, in Samet P (ed): *Cardiac Pacing*. New York, Grune & Stratton, 1980, p 111.
49. Murphy P, Morton P, Murtagh G, et al: Hemodynamic effects of different temporary pacing modes for the management of bradycardias complicating acute myocardial infarction. *Pacing Clin Electrophysiol* 15:391, 1992.
50. Bing OHL, McDowell JW, Hantman J, et al: Pacemaker placement by electrocardiographic monitoring. *N Engl J Med* 287:651, 1972.
51. Harthorne JW, McDermott J, Poulin FK: Cardiac pacing, in Johnson RA, Haber E, Austen WG (eds): *The Practice of Cardiology: The Medical and Surgical Cardiac Units at the Massachusetts General Hospital*. Boston, Little, Brown and Company, 1980.
52. Morelli RL, Goldschlager N: Temporary transvenous pacing: resolving postinsertion problems. *J Crit Illness* 2:73, 1987.
53. Donovan KD: Cardiac pacing in intensive care. *Anaesth Intensive Care* 13:41, 1984.
54. Holmes DR Jr: Temporary cardiac pacing, in Furman S, Hayes DL, Holmes DR Jr (eds): *A Practice of Cardiac Pacing*. Mount Kisco, NY, Futura Publishing, 1989.
55. Lumia FJ, Rios JC: Temporary transvenous pacemaker therapy: an analysis of complications. *Chest* 64:604, 1973.
56. Austin JL, Preis LK, Crampton RS, et al: Analysis of pacemaker malfunction and complications of temporary pacing in the coronary care unit. *Am J Cardiol* 49:301, 1982.
57. Donovan KD, Lee KY: Indications for and complications of temporary transvenous cardiac pacing. *Anaesth Intensive Care* 13:63, 1984.
58. Hynes JK, Holmes DR, Harrison CE: Five-year experience with temporary pacemaker therapy in the coronary care unit. *Mayo Clin Proc* 58:122, 1983.
59. Civetta JM, Gabel JC, Gemer M: Internal-jugular-vein puncture with a margin of safety. *Anesthesiology* 36:622, 1972.
60. Chastre J, Cornud F, Bouchama A, et al: Thrombosis as a complication of pulmonary-artery catheterization via the internal jugular vein: prospective evaluation by phlebography. *N Engl J Med* 306:278, 1982.
61. Davidson JT, Ben-Hur N, Nathen H: Subclavian venepuncture. *Lancet* 2:1139, 1963.
62. Linos DA, Mucha P Jr, van Heerden JA: Subclavian vein: a golden route. *Mayo Clin Proc* 55:315, 1980.
63. Nolewajka AJ, Goddard MD, Brown TC: Temporary transvenous pacing and femoral vein thrombosis. *Circulation* 62:646, 1980.
64. Sanders P: Effect of anticoagulation on the occurrence of deep venous thrombosis associated with temporary transvenous femoral pacemakers. *Am J Cardiol* 88:798, 2001.

6. Cardioversion and Defibrillation

Michael O. Sweeney

An interest in the use of electrical shocks to terminate cardiac arrhythmias dates back more than two centuries. However, the modern era of safe and routine use of direct current capacitive discharge electrical shocks for heart rhythm management began in the 1960s [1]. The term *cardioversion* refers to shocks synchronized to ventricular electrical systole. Synchronized shocks are used to terminate appropriately selected supraventricular (SVT) and ventricular (VT) tachycardias. The term *defibrillation* refers to the use of unsynchronized shocks to terminate ventricular fibrillation (VF). Direct current capacitive discharge electrical shocks are the preeminent therapy for appropriately selected persistent tachycardias due to their safety, efficacy, and immediacy of effect.

Understanding Cardioversion and Defibrillation

A rudimentary knowledge of capacitive discharge shocks and the application of basic electrical circuit theory to cardiac defibrillation is necessary to understand the effects of clinical variables and equipment on the outcome of electrical shocks for terminating cardiac arrhythmias.

UNITS OF ELECTRICITY. Electrical units are usually taught using fluid or hemodynamic analogies [2]. The fundamental electrical units necessary to understanding capacitive discharge electrical shocks are the ampere, volt, ohm, farad, and joule (J).

The *ampere* is the unit of current and is equal to a flow rate of 1 coulomb per second. This is analogous to a fluid flow rate of 1 L per minute.

The *volt* is the unit of voltage. This is the electrical "pressure" that forces current along its path. This is analogous to a fluid pressure such as mm Hg.

The *ohm* is the unit of electrical resistance. It is defined by "Ohm's Law," which expresses the ohm as the ratio of voltage to current (ohm = voltage/current). Thus, as pathway resistance increases, a higher voltage is necessary to force a given current through the pathway. The fluid analogy is peripheral resistance (mm Hg/L/minute).

The *farad* is the unit of capacitance, where capacitance measures the ability of a capacitor to store electrical charge. A simple capacitor is two electrical surfaces separated by an insulator. Capacitance is defined as the ratio of charge to voltage (charge = capacitance × voltage). Thus, to store greater charge on a capacitor, the surface area or voltage must be increased.

The *joule* is the unit of energy. The joule is the energy of 1 volt and 1 ampere lasting 1 second. This is expressed as energy = voltage × current × time.

When describing the effects of an electrical shock on myocardial tissue, it is useful to specify "space-normalized" units of electricity [2]. Thus, the electric field resulting from a shock delivered to a specific volume of tissue can be described as voltage difference per distance (volts per cm). Similarly, the current density can be described as the amperes per distance (amperes per cm²).

SHOCK WAVEFORMS. The initial use of electric shocks to terminate cardiac arrhythmias involved alternating current (AC shocks) derived from large transformers [3–5]. The pioneering work of Lown subsequently demonstrated that a damped sinusoidal waveform generated by a straight direct current (DC) capacitor discharge through a series inductor (paddle electrodes) and the resistor (the thorax) resulted in less myocardial damage, arrhythmias, and death versus AC shocks [6]. Variations on the damped sinusoidal waveform are used in most external defibrillators today.

Waveform shape influences defibrillation efficacy (Fig. 6-1). Monophasic waveforms deliver current in one direction. Damped sinusoidal waveforms allow the discharged current to fall gradually to zero. Such waveforms require large capacitors and are not practical for implantable cardioverter-defibrillators (ICDs), but are commonly used in external defibrillators. Truncated exponential waveforms cause the discharged current to fall to zero instantaneously. Monophasic truncated exponential waveforms are superior to untruncated monophasic waveforms for defibrillation. Truncation reduces the refibrillatory effects of the low voltage tail associated with untruncated (straight) capacitor discharges [7,8]. Biphasic waveforms deliver current in two directions. Current flows in the positive direction for a specified duration, then is instantaneously reversed to the negative direction for a specified duration. Biphasic waveforms are superior to monophasic waveforms for internal defibrillation using ICDs [9,10] and are superior to damped sinusoidal waveforms for external defibrillation [11,12]. The explanation for the superiority of biphasic waveforms is controversial. One hypothesis is the so-called charge-burping theory [13,14]: This states that the function of the first phase is to act as a monophasic shock (i.e., defibrillate), whereas the function of the second phase is to "burp" the residual charge on the cell membrane left behind by the first phase. This theory contends that the residual charge on the cell membrane after a monophasic shock may result in refibrillation. This effect can be minimized by large-amplitude monophasic shocks. Because the biphasic shock removes this residual charge (with its second phase), the amplitude requirement of the first phase is reduced relative to a monophasic shock.

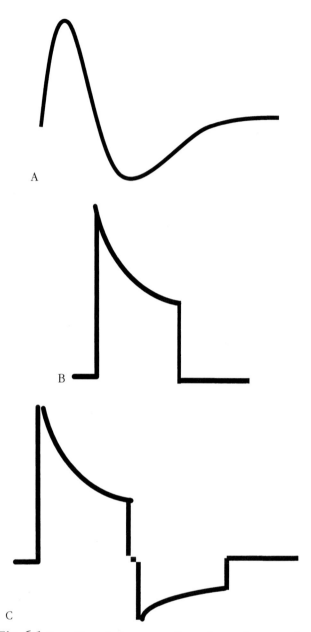

Fig. 6-1. Capacitive discharge waveform shapes (see text for details). **A:** Damped sinusoidal. **B:** Monophasic truncated exponential. **C:** Biphasic truncated exponential.

FACTORS THAT INFLUENCE DEFIBRILLATION EFFICACY. Many factors appear to influence defibrillation efficacy. Interpreting the mechanisms and relative contributions of the effects of these various factors requires a unifying theory of defibrillation. However, the mechanism of defibrillation by electrical shocks is unsettled. The two dominant theories of defibrillation are referred to as critical mass and upper limit of vulnerability (ULV). The critical mass theory states that a minimum mass of the fibrillating myocardium (at least 75%) must be exposed to current densities equal to or greater than the inexcitability threshold, which is the minimum current density (electric field) necessary to render a fibrillating myocyte inexcitable [15]. Thus, the critical mass hypothesis "guarantees" that the elimination of all fibrillating wavefronts would terminate fibrillation. ULV refers to the strongest shock capable of initiating fibrillation in a refibrillating ventricle, which has been shown to correlate with the defibrillation threshold [16].

The ULV hypothesis holds that the termination of fibrillation is "provisional" because the shock itself could simultaneously reinitiate fibrillation; a unifying theory referred to as "progressive defibrillation" has been proposed to reconcile these two theories [17].

From a practical perspective, the goal of transthoracic defibrillation is to achieve a sufficient current density in sufficient mass so as to render fibrillating myocytes inexcitable. Whether the fibrillating myocytes are ventricular or atrial is irrelevant. Current density delivered varies inversely with electrode surface area. Changing electrode positions may favorably alter the current path so that higher current densities are achieved in the target tissue (atrium or ventricle). Smaller electrodes result in higher current densities over a smaller area. Increasing electrode surface area disperses current over a larger area but the current density is reduced unless the voltage is increased. Higher transthoracic resistances reduce current delivery to the myocardium. Transthoracic resistance varies with size and composition of electrodes, contact medium between skin and electrodes, body size, phase of respiratory cycle, number of shocks delivered, and timing between shocks [18–21]. Electrolyte-impregnated electrode pads reduce the electrical resistance between the skin surface and the electrodes. Because air conducts current poorly, shock efficacy can be improved by delivery during expiration and with chest wall compression. Eliminating body hair beneath the electrodes reduces air trapping, which increases resistance and reduces efficacy.

Selection of Arrhythmias for Direct Current Cardioversion and Defibrillation

Electrical shocks are capable of terminating tachycardias that are due to reentry. Reentrant rhythms are characterized by three necessary conditions: (a) at least two functionally (or anatomically) distinct potential pathways that join proximally and distally to form a closed circuit of conduction, (b) unidirectional block in one of these potential pathways, and (c) slow conduction down the unblocked pathway, allowing the previously blocked pathway time to recover excitability. Reentry is maintained by a continuously circulating electrical wavefront along these pathways. The head of the electrical wavefront is followed sequentially by zones of tissue that are absolutely refractory (unresponsive to additional electrical stimuli) and relatively refractory (delayed response to electrical stimuli), and an excitable gap that is fully excitable. An electrical shock produces a second depolarizing wavefront that may interact with the conduction circuit supporting reentry. If properly timed and of sufficient strength, the shock wavefront enters the excitable gap anterogradely and retrogradely. Termination occurs because the shock wavefront collides retrogradely with the preceding tachycardia wavefront and blocks antegradely due to encroachment on the refractory period of the preceding wavefront. Arrhythmias that are due to reentry and capable of responding to electrical shocks are listed in Table 6-1.

Arrhythmias that are owing to focal automaticity or triggered activity are not terminated by electrical shocks or demonstrate only transient slowing. Such rhythms are shown in Table 6-2. It is often difficult to identify the mechanism of tachycardia using the surface electrocardiogram (ECG) unless examples of spontaneous initiation and termination are fortuitously observed. Initiation and termination by conduction block or delay (commonly associated with extrasystoles) are suggestive of reentry.

Table 6-1. Reentrant Rhythms That May Respond to Electrical Shocks

Supraventricular tachycardias
  Atrioventricular nodal reentry
  Atrioventricular reentry using accessory pathways
  Common atrial flutter
  Atrial fibrillation not owing to a focal source
Ventricular tachycardias
  Monomorphic ventricular tachycardia associated with chronic myocardial infarction
  Monomorphic ventricular tachycardia owing to bundle-branch reentry
  Monomorphic ventricular tachycardia owing to scar-related reentry in nonischemic cardiomyopathies
Polymorphic ventricular tachycardia and ventricular fibrillation

Table 6-2. Nonreentrant Rhythms That Do Not Respond to Electrical Shocks

Supraventricular tachycardias
  Sinus tachycardia
  Focal atrial tachycardias
  Atrial fibrillation due to a focal source
Ventricular tachycardias
  Idiopathic monomorphic ventricular tachycardia (right or left ventricular origin)
  Monomorphic ventricular tachycardia due to focal automaticity in nonischemic cardiomyopathies

Failure of SVT or VT to terminate with successive electrical shocks should raise suspicion of a nonreentrant mechanism. Further attempts at electrical termination should be withheld. This scenario is most commonly seen with sinus tachycardia that is misdiagnosed as some other SVT. True failure to terminate monomorphic VT owing to scar-related reentry must be distinguished from successful termination and immediate reinitiating: This can be very difficult to recognize on the surface ECG, but is often observed on retrieved intracardiac electrograms from ICDs.

Guidelines for Direct Current Cardioversion of Atrial Fibrillation and Other Supraventricular Tachycardias

COGNITIVE AND TECHNICAL SKILLS. Certain minimum cognitive and technical skills are mandatory for the safe application of direct current cardioversion (DCCV) techniques and are summarized in Tables 6-3 and 6-4 [22]. The overarching concern relates to patient safety and comfort. The physician should assume that the equipment will not work properly. The most important potentially life-threatening events after DCCV shock for SVT are the inadvertent initiation of ventricular tachycardia or ventricular fibrillation, asystole after tachycardia termination, myocardial depression after tachycardia termination (especially after multiple high-energy shocks), and acute respiratory failure related to sedation for the procedure. The physician must be sufficiently educated to minimize the likelihood of these adverse events, recognize them in a timely fashion when they occur, and take corrective measures

Table 6-3. Cognitive Skills Necessary to Perform External Direct Current Cardioversion (DCCV)

Electrophysiologic principles of DCCV
Indications for procedure
Anticoagulation management
Proper use and administration of antiarrhythmic therapy
Proper use and administration of sedation and management of overdose
DCCV equipment, including the selection of appropriate energy and synchronization
Knowledge to treat all possible complications, including the use of antibradycardia pacing, defibrillation, and advanced cardiovascular life support
Appropriate monitor display and recognition of adequate R-wave synchronization
Ability to interpret the baseline 12-lead electrocardiogram, recognition of acute changes, drug toxicity, and relative contraindications to DCCV

Table 6-4. Technical Skills Necessary to Perform
External Direct Current Cardioversion

Proper skin preparation and electrode placement
Recognition of artifact-free monitor strips and R-wave synchronization
  markers
Technically acceptable 12-lead electrocardiogram before and after
  direct current cardioversion
Temporary transcutaneous and/or transvenous antibradycardia pacing
  capabilities
Emergency defibrillation capabilities
Advanced cardiovascular life support training and certification

according to the nature of the adverse event. These sensibilities may be succinctly summarized by the remark, "If you don't know what you are doing, don't do it."

MINIMUM TRAINING REQUIREMENTS FOR COMPETENCY IN DIRECT CURRENT CARDIOVERSION. According to the American College of Cardiology, American Heart Association, and North American Society of Pacing and Electrophysiology, physicians performing DCCV must possess the cognitive and technical skills outlined above to meet requirements for minimum competence [22]. A minimum of eight supervised DCCVs is recommended, most often (but not necessarily) achieved in the context of formal training in cardiovascular disease. Further, a minimum of four external DCCVs annually is specified to maintain initial certification.

PREPARATION OF THE PATIENT FOR ELECTIVE DIRECT CURRENT CARDIOVERSION. Standards for preparation for DCCV have been published and are summarized in Table 6-5 [22,23]. This mandates a suitable period of fasting (typically 12 hours), reliable intravenous access for sedation, and strict attention to R-wave synchronization. The physician must be certain that the synchronization artifacts correspond to the peak of the QRS complex on the surface ECG. R-wave synchronization is necessary to ensure that electrical stimulation does not occur during the vulnerable phase of the cardiac cycle, from 60 to 80 milliseconds before to 20 to 30 milliseconds after the apex of the T wave [24]. It should be noted that during rapid ventricular rates (greater than 200 beats per minute) even perfectly synchronized R-wave shocks might fall within the T wave of the preceding R wave [25]. Thus, consideration should be given to slowing a rapid ventricular rate (using, for example, beta-blockers) before attempted cardioversion. Most external defibrillators nominally revert to unsynchronized shocks for safety reasons. Thus, if a charge is aborted or successive shocks are delivered, verification of synchronization is essential before continuing.

Sedation is usually achieved with intravenous fentanyl [26], midazolam [27], or propofol. The last agent has the virtues of

Table 6-5. Preparation for Elective External Direct
Current Cardioversion

Verify patient is in fasting, postabsorptive state.
Record baseline 12-lead ECG.
Establish reliable intravenous access.
Place electrodes (paddles) in anterior-posterior or base-apex location.
Confirm synchronization artifacts correspond to peak of the QRS
  complex.
Initiate sedation or general anesthesia.
Deliver synchronized shocks of increasing energy until arrhythmia is
  terminated or further attempts are deemed futile.
Record postcardioversion 12-lead ECG.

ECG, electrocardiogram.

producing rapid, deep sedation, amnesia, and a short half-life, but is generally administered by anesthesiologists, whereas nurses with special training in intravenous conscious sedation commonly administer the former two agents.

Most often an anterior-posterior (sternum–left scapula) electrode positioning is used initially, based on early reports of superior efficacy relative to alternative electrode positions [1,28]. The superiority of one electrode position over another has not been definitively established. Some reports suggest that an anterior-lateral (right infraclavicular–ventricular apex) position might be superior in some patients [18,19].

The starting DC shock energy is largely a matter of operator preference. The energy necessary to terminate a specific tachycardia in a specific patient is not predictable. Shock energies less than 100 to 200 J using a monophasic waveform are unlikely to be successful for atrial fibrillation (AF) [29] and may result in an increased number of shocks and delivered energy than if a higher energy been used initially [30]. Thus, DCCV is initially attempted at 200 J. Higher efficacy achieved with biphasic waveforms may allow the use of lower initial energies [29,31]. Failure to terminate tachycardia should result in iterative attempts at progressively higher energy settings until tachycardia is terminated or further attempts are deemed futile. At least 1 minute of rest should be allowed between successive high-energy attempts so as to minimize myocardial depression [32]. Organized tachycardias (e.g., atrial flutter or stable monomorphic VT) can often be terminated with very low energies (50 J) [29,33].

These guidelines apply for all supraventricular and ventricular tachycardias treated with DCCV. The special consideration of anticoagulation before and after DCCV for AF is discussed in the following sections.

ANTICOAGULATION FOR ELECTIVE DIRECT CURRENT CARDIOVERSION OF ATRIAL FIBRILLATION. Current recommendations for anticoagulation before elective DCCV for AF are shown in Table 6-6 [22,34–36]. Scrupulous attention to adequate anticoagulation minimizes, but does not eliminate, the risk of embolic stroke after restoration of organized atrial mechanical activity. If AF has been present for more than 48 hours and the patient has not been therapeutically anticoagulated with coumadin for a suitable period, anticoagulation with intravenous heparin and transesophageal echocardiography have been advocated [37]. Absence of visible clot in the left atrium and left atrial appendage, in particular, suggests a low risk of embolic complications. However, some patients with no demonstrable left atrial thrombus on transesophageal echocardiography before cardioversion have thromboembolic events [38]. This presumably relates to a period of mechanical "stunning" of the left atrium after cardioversion [39]. Thrombus may form during this period of mechanical inertia and embolize when organized mechanical function returns several days later. Presence of clot in the left atrial appendage is associated with a high risk of thromboembolism after cardioversion of AF. Such patients should be treated for at least 3 to 4 weeks before elec-

Table 6-6. Anticoagulation for Elective Direct
Current Cardioversion (DCCV) of Atrial Fibrillation (AF)

Patients with AF >48 h duration should receive warfarin for ≥3 wk
  before and 4 wk after DCCV.
Target INR of 2.5 (range, 2.0–3.0) is recommended for most patients.
For high-risk patients (e.g., those with mechanical heart valves,
  hypertrophic cardiomyopathy, prior embolic stroke) a target INR of
  3.0 (range, 2.5–3.5) is recommended.
Anticoagulation after DCCV for rhythms other than atrial fibrillation is
  controversial.

INR, international normalized ratio.

Table 6-7. Techniques for Direct Current Cardioversion of "Resistant" Atrial Fibrillation

Alternate pad location
Use of hand-held anterior paddle with downward pressure and large posterior paddle
Simultaneous high-energy shocks using two pathways
Biphasic shock waveform
Premedication with drugs to lower the atrial defibrillation threshold (ibutilide) or reduce vagal tone (atropine)
Internal direct current cardioversion using transvenous catheters

Table 6-8. Scenarios for Urgent Direct Current Cardioversion of Atrial Fibrillation (AF)

AF associated with ischemia due to acute myocardial infarction or unstable coronary syndrome
AF associated with hemodynamic instability due to rapid ventricular response over the atrioventricular node
AF associated with congestive heart failure due to rapid ventricular response over the atrioventricular node
AF causing hemodynamic instability due to a rapid ventricular response over an accessory pathway (Wolff-Parkinson-White)

trical cardioversion [29]. Whichever anticoagulation approach precedes DCCV for AF, all patients should receive routine anticoagulation for at least 3 to 4 weeks after cardioversion. Unresolved, however, is the risk of embolic complications when spontaneous contrast, rather than discrete thrombus, is seen.

MANAGEMENT OF ATRIAL FIBRILLATION "RESISTANT" TO DIRECT CURRENT CARDIOVERSION. DCCV using standard monophasic shocks fails to restore sinus rhythm in 5% to 30% of patients with AF. "Resistant" AF is defined as AF that cannot be terminated with at least two consecutive 360 J transthoracic monophasic shocks. The DCCV techniques for management of this condition are listed in Table 6-7. The simplest modification of the procedure that should be attempted first is to vary the current pathway by repositioning the skin electrodes. In some patients, a more superoanterior position of the left chest electrode facilitates atrial defibrillation. Applying direct pressure to the electrodes may reduce transthoracic resistance and increase current delivery to the heart, facilitating atrial defibrillation. Synchronization of high-energy shocks from two external defibrillators using electrical switches successfully restored sinus rhythm in 84% of patients with resistant AF [40]. "Nearly" simultaneous delivery of high-energy shocks from two electrode pairs using two operators has been advocated but should be avoided, however, because of an inability to guarantee shock synchronization using variations on the "ready, set, go" approach. There is clinical evidence that at least a one low-energy (120 J) rectilinear biphasic waveform improved cardioversion efficacy versus a standard escalating energy (greater than 200 J) damped sine-wave monophasic waveform (94% vs. 79%, respectively) [31]. Independent predictors of cardioversion success were rectilinear biphasic waveform, transthoracic resistance, and duration of AF. Pretreatment with ibutilide may facilitate DCCV, presumably due to favorable cell membrane effects [41,42]. Pretreatment with atropine may also facilitate DCCV, particularly amongst patients with structurally normal hearts in whom AF often occurs in the setting of high vagal tone [43]. Finally, internal DCCV, using two transvenous electrodes or a single transvenous electrode paired with a chest wall electrode, may terminate "resistant" AF when all other techniques fail [44–46]. This technique is generally reserved for trained clinical electrophysiologists in the electrophysiology laboratory.

APPROACH TO URGENT DIRECT CURRENT CARDIOVERSION FOR ATRIAL FIBRILLATION. The indications for urgent DCCV of AF are relatively rare and listed in Table 6-8. In many such instances, DCCV is used almost immediately after the onset of AF, and concerns about anticoagulation and embolic risk are minimal. When urgent DCCV is considered for AF of uncertain duration or exceeding 48 hours in the absence of suitable anticoagulation, the risk of systemic embolism must be carefully weighed against the immediate hemodynamic or electrical risk of AF.

Embolism Complications of Direct Current Cardioversion for Atrial Fibrillation and Other Supraventricular Tachycardias. The risk of thromboembolic events among patients who did not receive prophylactic anticoagulation before cardioversion of AF is between 1% and 7% [47,48]. This risk is probably reduced to 1% to 2% by anticoagulation pretreatment for 3 to 4 weeks as outlined previously [29].

Bradyarrhythmias. Benign, transient rhythm disturbances are common immediately after DCCV for AF. These include ventricular and atrial premature beats (probably owing to automaticity) and sinus arrest [49]. Sinus bradycardia and sinus arrest usually respond to pharmacologic support, such as atropine, isoproterenol, and dopamine. Rarely, temporary transcutaneous or transvenous pacing is necessary. A slow ventricular response during chronic AF may indicate significant underlying conduction system disease and should heighten alertness for postcardioversion bradycardia [50].

Ventricular Tachyarrhythmias. The induction of ventricular tachyarrhythmia during attempted DCCV of AF is almost always due to the delivery of an unsynchronized shock or inadequate synchronization, as outlined above. The risk of induction of ventricular arrhythmia is increased in the setting of hypokalemia and digitalis intoxication [51,52]. Hypokalemia should be corrected before DCCV. DCCV should be deferred in the presence of digitalis toxicity. However, it is not necessary to interrupt digoxin therapy before DCCV if there is no evidence of toxicity, as a serum digoxin level in the therapeutic range does not appear to increase the risk of ventricular arrhythmia [53].

Guidelines for Direct Current Cardioversion of Ventricular Tachycardia

APPROACH TO CARDIOVERSION OF MONOMORPHIC VENTRICULAR TACHYCARDIA. Cognitive skills, minimum training requirements, and patient preparation for DCCV of VT are similar to those listed for DCCV of AF. DCCV of VT is usually an urgent or semiurgent procedure, however, whereas DCCV of AF is usually elective. The urgency of the clinical scenario dictates modification in patient preparation and approach by necessity. From a practical perspective, considerations regarding patient monitoring, sedation, electrode position, synchronization, energy selection, and waveform type similarly apply. DCCV of monomorphic VT carries unique risks, however, which are reviewed in the following section.

COMPLICATIONS OF DIRECT CURRENT CARDIOVERSION FOR MONOMORPHIC VENTRICULAR TACHYCARDIA

Acceleration of Monomorphic Ventricular Tachycardia. Acceleration refers to an increase in rate of persistent ventricular tachyarrhythmia after failed cardioversion. Three types of acceleration are observed clinically: (a) monomorphic VT with similar morphology as the initial VT, (b) monomorphic VT with different morphology as the initial VT, and (c) polymorphic VT or VF. Acceleration caused by overdrive pacing is usually a fast monomorphic VT which can still be terminated by further pacing attempts. Acceleration by shock is usually rapid polymorphic VT or VF that requires a high-energy defibrillation shock. The risk of acceleration is directly related to the initial VT rate and is more common at rates exceeding 200 beats per minute [54,55].

Induction of Atrial Arrhythmias. AF is frequently initiated by synchronized shocks for VT. The incidence may be as high as 20% when transvenous shocks are used [56]. AF is also commonly initiated by low-energy T-wave shocks used to initiate VF during ICD testing. In either case, all that is required is that the "far-field" atrial shock strength resulting from the ventricular shock be less than the atrial ULV [57]. Such spuriously initiated AF may not terminate spontaneously and thus require DCCV.

Bradyarrhythmias. Transient bradyarrhythmias are common after DCCV for VT. Most often, these manifest as transient sinus bradycardia or sinus arrest for which no specific intervention is needed. Transient heart block is often seen after internal shocks for VT delivered by ICDs, and rarely, true electromechanical dissociation has been described in this situation [58]. This latter complication is probably a cause of sudden death despite termination of VT and VF in ICD patients [58].

Guidelines for Defibrillation Approach to Ventricular Defibrillation

Guidelines for defibrillation have been published [59] and are summarized in Table 6-9. The most important consideration in defibrillation is *time*. The probability of successful defibrillation and survival is inversely related to the time from onset of VF to the first shock [60–62]. All other considerations, including basic life support and advanced cardiac life support care, are secondary to the goal of rapid defibrillation [59].

Shock energies for defibrillation are delivered in an escalating fashion [59]. Historically, a first-shock energy of 200 J has been recommended for monophasic shocks [63]. If the first

Table 6-9. Guidelines for Ventricular Defibrillation

Attempt defibrillation using first-shock energy of 200 J.
If first attempt unsuccessful, reattempt defibrillation using 200 J.
If second attempt unsuccessful, reattempt defibrillation using 360 J.
If the first three shocks fail to achieve defibrillation, continue cardio-
  pulmonary resuscitation and follow advanced care life support
  guidelines for sudden ventricular fibrillation/ventricular tachycardia:
     Intravenous access.
     Tracheal intubation.
     Epinephrine.
     Repeat shocks if still in ventricular fibrillation.
     Consider intravenous amiodarone or lidocaine.

shock fails to defibrillate, the second-shock energy is a matter of debate but should be at least 200 J. A given shock energy may fail on the first attempt but succeed on the second attempt. This is possible because defibrillation is a probabilistic phenomenon [64]. This phenomenon refers to a definable probability that a particular energy delivered at a particular point in time results in successful defibrillation. Thus, the likelihood of successful defibrillation at a given shock energy increases with consecutive shocks. Additional shocks at the same energy may be increasingly efficacious due to a progressive fall in transthoracic resistance that increases transthoracic current densities [65,66]. If the first two shocks fail to defibrillate, a third shock of 360 J should be given immediately.

Biphasic truncated exponential waveforms are superior to monophasic waveforms for internal defibrillation [9,10] and have rendered monophasic waveforms obsolete in ICDs. External defibrillators using biphasic waveforms have recently become available and appear to be similarly superior to monophasic waveforms for transthoracic defibrillation [11,12]. Furthermore, repetitive lower-energy biphasic shocks (150 J) have equivalent or superior efficacy for defibrillation than escalating energy monophasic shocks (e.g., 200, 300, 360 J) [12]. Until further comparative clinical data are available, however, the use of lower energy biphasic shocks or escalating energy monophasic shocks cannot be preferentially recommended [59].

Special Considerations for Direct Current Cardioversion and Defibrillation in Patients with Pacemakers and Implantable Cardioverter-Defibrillators

The large electrical pulse during transthoracic cardioversion and defibrillation may adversely affect pacemaker and ICD operation. Such direct current pulses constitute a form of electromagnetic interference. Modern pacemaker and ICDs are remarkably resistant to all forms of electromagnetic interference owing to circuitry shielding and filtering techniques. The adverse manifestations of high-voltage electrical pulses on pacemakers and ICD systems include altered mode of operation; direct firmware and electronic component damage; and current shunting along the leads, causing cardiac tissue damage at the lead-endocardial interface.

Alteration of pacemaker operating mode may include inappropriate inhibition of pacing output, inappropriate triggering of pacing output, asynchronous pacing, and reprogramming to a backup mode [67]. Such resets of pacemaker operation are usually immediately evident during continuous electrocardiographic monitoring.

Firmware and circuitry damage owing to external cardioversion and defibrillation pulses is unusual in modern pacemakers and virtually never occurs in ICDs because of special designs (Zener diode) that regulate the voltage that enters the circuitry. Reports of catastrophic pacemaker failure after an external defibrillation pulse refer predominantly to older unipolar systems [67].

High current flow associated with cardioversion and defibrillation pulses may travel down the transvenous lead system, owing to capacitive coupling with the electrical pulse or shunting in the pacemaker circuit [67]. This can result in an effect similar to radiofrequency ablation at the endocardial-lead interface. Resistive heating of the endocardium may cause myocardial damage resulting in persistent pacing threshold elevation. Transient (a few seconds) pacing threshold elevations are common after cardioversion and defibrillation and generally not of clinical consequence.

Because this type of electromagnetic interference enters a pacemaker or ICD by conduction, it can be minimized by proper skin electrode position. The electrodes should not be placed in proximity to the device, which is usually in the left (or, less commonly, right) infraclavicular location. An anterior-posterior position is preferred. Pacemaker and ICD interrogation after transthoracic cardioversion or defibrillation is prudent, particularly if any abnormal behavior is noted during continuous electrocardiographic monitoring.

References

1. Lown B, Amarasingham R, Newman J: New method for terminating cardiac arrhythmias: use of synchronized capacitor discharge. *JAMA* 182:548–555, 1962.
2. Kroll MW, Lehmann MH, Tchou PJ: Defining the defibrillation dosage, in Kroll MW, Lehmann MH (eds): *Implantable Cardioverter Defibrillator Therapy: The Engineering-Clinical Interface.* Norwell, MA, Kluwer Academic Publishers, 1996, pp 63–89.
3. Hooker DR, Kouwenhoven WB, Langworthy OR: The effect of alternating currents on the heart. *Am J Physiol* 103:444–454, 1933.
4. Beck CS, Pritchard WH, Feil HS: Ventricular fibrillation of long duration abolished by electric shock. *JAMA* 135:985–986, 1947.
5. Zoll PM, Linenthal AJ, Gibson W, et al: Termination of ventricular fibrillation in man by externally applied electrical countershock. *N Engl J Med* 254:727–732, 1956.
6. Lown B, Newman J, Amarasingham R, et al: Comparison of alternating current with direct current electroshock across the closed chest. *Am J Cardiol* 1962:223–233, 1962.
7. Geddes LA, Tacker WA: Engineering and physiological considerations of direct capacitor-discharge ventricular defibrillation. *Med Biol Eng* 9:185–199, 1971.
8. Schuder JC, Stoeckle H, Keskar PY, et al: Transthoracic ventricular defibrillation in the dog with unidirectional rectangular double pulses. *Cardiovasc Res* 4:497–501, 1970.
9. Bardy GH, Ivey TD, Johnson G, et al: A prospective randomized evaluation of biphasic versus monophasic waveform pulses on defibrillation efficacy in humans. *J Am Coll Cardiol* 14:728–733, 1989.
10. Fain E, Sweeney M, Franz M: Improved internal defibrillation efficacy with a biphasic waveform. *Am Heart J* 117:358–364, 1989.
11. Bardy GH, Marchlinski FE, Sharma AD, et al: Transthoracic Investigators. Multicenter comparison of truncated biphasic shocks and standard damped sine wave monophasic shocks for transthoracic ventricular defibrillation. *Circulation* 94:2507–2514, 1996.
12. Poole JE, White RD, Kanz KG, et al: Low-energy impedance-compensating biphasic waveforms terminate ventricular fibrillation at high rates in victims of out-of-hospital cardiac arrest. *J Cardiovasc Electrophysiol* 8:1373–1385, 1997.
13. Kroll MW: A minimal model of the single capacitor biphasic waveform. *Pacing Clin Electrophysiol* 17:1782–1792, 1994.
14. Kroll MW: A minimal model of the monophasic defibrillation pulse. *Pacing Clin Electrophysiol* 16:769–777, 1993.
15. Zipes DP, Fischer J, King RM, et al: Termination of ventricular fibrillation in dogs by depolarizing a critical amount of myocardium. *Am J Cardiol* 36:37–44, 1975.
16. Chen PS, Shibata N, Dixon EG, et al: Comparison of the defibrillation threshold and the upper limit of ventricular vulnerability. *Circulation* 73:1022–1028, 1986.
17. Dillon SM, Kwaku KF: Progressive defibrillation: a unified hypothesis for defibrillation and fibrillation induction by shocks. *J Cardiovasc Electrophysiol* 9:529–552, 1998.
18. Kerber RE, Jensen SR, Grayzel J, et al: Elective cardioversion: influence of paddle-electrode position location and size on success rates and energy requirements. *N Engl J Med* 305:658–662, 1981.
19. Ewy GA: The optimal technique for electrical cardioversion of atrial fibrillation. *Clin Cardiol* 17:79–84, 1994.
20. Dalzell GW, Cunningham SR, Anderson J, et al: Electrode pad size, transthoracic impedance and success of external ventricular defibrillation. *Am J Cardiol* 64:741–744, 1989.
21. Connell PN, Ewy GA, Dahl CF, et al: Transthoracic impedance to defibrillator discharge: effect of electrode size and electrode chest wall interface. *J Electrocardiol* 6:313-M, 1973.
22. Tracy CM, Akhtar M, DiMarco JP, et al: American College of Cardiology/American Heart Association clinical competence statement on invasive electrophysiology studies, catheter ablation, and cardioversion. *J Am Coll Cardiol* 36:1725–1736, 2000.
23. Yurchak PM: Clinical competence in elective direct current (DC) cardioversion: a statement for physicians from the ACP/ACC/AHA Task Force on Clinical Privileges in Cardiology. *Circulation* 88:342–345, 1993.
24. Hou CJ, Chang-Sing P, Flynn E, et al: Determination of ventricular vulnerable period and ventricular fibrillation threshold by use of T-wave shocks in patients undergoing implantation of cardioverter/defibrillators. *Circulation* 92:2558–2564, 1995.
25. Ayers GM, Alferness CA, Ilina M, et al: Ventricular proarrhythmia effects of ventricular cycle length and shock strength in a sheep model of transvenous atrial defibrillation. *Circulation* 89:413–422, 1994.
26. Hagemeijer F, Van Mechelen R, Smalbraak DW: Fentanyl-etomidate anesthesia for cardioversion. *Eur Heart J* 3:155–158, 1982.
27. Khan AH, Malhotra R: Midazolam as intravenous sedative for electrocardioversion. *Chest* 95:1068–1071, 1989.
28. Lown B, Perlroth MG, Kaidbey S, et al: Cardioversion of atrial fibrillation: a report on the treatment of 65 episodes in 50 patients. *N Engl J Med* 269:325–331, 1963.
29. Fuster V, Ryden LE, Asinger RW, et al: ACC/AHA/ESC guidelines for the management of patients with atrial fibrillation: a report of the American College of Cardiology/American Heart Association Task Force on Practice Guidelines and the European Society of Cardiology Committee for Practice Guidelines and Policy Conferences (Committee to Develop Guidelines for the Management of Patients with Atrial Fibrillation). *J Am Coll Cardiol* 38:1–70, 2001.
30. Joglar JA, Hamdan MH, Ramaswamy K, et al: Initial energy for elective external cardioversion of persistent atrial fibrillation. *Am J Cardiol* 86:348–350, 2000.
31. Mittal S, Ayati S, Stein KM, et al: Transthoracic cardioversion of atrial fibrillation: comparison of rectilinear biphasic versus damped sine wave monophasic shocks. *Circulation* 101:1282–1287, 2000.
32. Dahl CF, Ewy GA, Warner ED, et al: Myocardial necrosis from direct current countershock: effect of paddle-electrode size and time interval between discharges. *Circulation* 50:956–961, 1974.
33. Pinski SL, Sgarbossa EN, Ching E, et al: A comparison of 50-J versus 100-J shock for direct current cardioversion of atrial flutter. *Am Heart J* 137:439–442, 1999.
34. Proceedings of the American College of Chest Physicians 5th Consensus on Antithrombotic Therapy. 1998. *Chest* 114:439S–769S, 1998.
35. Karlson BW, Herlitz J, Edvarsson N, et al: Prophylactic treatment after electroconversion of atrial fibrillation. *Clin Cardiol* 13(4):279–286, 1990.
36. Stein B, Halperin JL, Fuster V: Should patients with atrial fibrillation be anticoagulated prior to and chronically following cardioversion? *Cardiovasc Clin* 21:231–247, 1990.
37. Silverman DI, Manning WJ: Role of echocardiography in patients undergoing elective cardioversion of atrial fibrillation. *Circulation* 98[Suppl I]:479–486, 1998.
38. Black IW, Fatkin D, Sagar KB, et al: Exclusion of atrial thrombus by transesophageal echocardiography does not preclude embolism after cardioversion of atrial fibrillation: a multicenter study. *Circulation* 89:2509–2513, 1994.
39. Fatkin D, Kuchar DL, Thorburn CW, et al: Transesophageal echocardiography before and during direct current cardioversion of atrial fibrillation: evidence for "atrial stunning" as a mechanism of thromboembolic complications. *J Am Coll Cardiol* 23:307–316, 1994.
40. Saliba W, Juralti N, Chung MK, et al: Higher energy synchronized external direct current cardioversion for refractory atrial fibrillation. *J Am Coll Cardiol* 34:2031–2034, 1999.
41. Li H, Natale A, Tomassoni A, et al: Usefulness of ibutilide in facilitating external cardioversion of refractory atrial fibrillation. *Am J Cardiol* 84:1096–1098, 1999.

42. Oral H, Souza JJ, Michaud G, et al: Facilitating transthoracic cardioversion of atrial fibrillation with ibutilide pretreatment. *N Engl J Med* 340:1849–1854, 1999.
43. Sutton AGC, Khurana C, Hall JA, et al: The use of atropine for facilitation of direct current cardioversion from atrial fibrillation-results of a pilot study. *Clin Cardiol* 22:712–714, 1999.
44. Schmitt C, Alt E, Plewan A, et al: Low energy intracardiac cardioversion after failed external cardioversion of atrial fibrillation. *J Am Coll Cardiol* 28:994–999, 1996.
45. Levy S, Ricard P, Lau CP, et al: Multicenter low energy transvenous atrial defibrillation (XAD) trial results in different subsets of atrial fibrillation. *J Am Coll Cardiol* 29:750–755, 1997.
46. Levy S, Lauribe P, Dolla E, et al: A randomized comparison of external and internal cardioversion of chronic atrial fibrillation. *Circulation* 86:1415–1420, 1992.
47. Bjerkelund CJ, Orning OM: The efficacy of anticoagulant therapy in preventing embolism related to DC electrical conversion of atrial fibrillation. *Am J Cardiol* 23:208–216, 1969.
48. Arnold AZ, Mick MJ, Mazurek RP, et al: Role of prophylactic anticoagulation for direct current cardioversion in patients with atrial fibrillation or atrial flutter. *J Am Coll Cardiol* 19:851–855, 1992.
49. Rabbino MD, Likoff W, Dreifus LS: Complications and limitations of direct current countershock. *JAMA* 190:417–420, 1964.
50. Mancini GB, Goldberger AL: Cardioversion of atrial fibrillation: consideration of embolization, anticoagulation, prophylactic pacemaker, and long-term success. *Am Heart J* 104:617–621, 1982.
51. Lown B, Kleiger R, Williams J: Cardioversion and digitalis drugs: changed threshold to electric shock in digitized animals. *Circ Res* 17:519–531, 1965.
52. Aberg H, Cullhed I: Direct current countershock complications. *Acta Med Scand* 183:415–421, 1968.
53. Ditchey RV, Karliner JS: Safety of electrical cardioversion in patients without digitalis toxicity. *Ann Intern Med* 95:676–679, 1981.
54. Saksena S, Chandran P, Shah Y, et al: Comparative efficacy of transvenous cardioversion and pacing in patients with sustained ventricular tachycardia: a prospective, randomized crossover study. *Circulation* 72:153–160, 1985.
55. Saksena S, Calvo RA, Pantopoulos D: A prospective evaluation of single and dual current pathways for transvenous cardioversion in rapid ventricular tachycardia. *Pacing Clin Electrophysiol* 10:1130–1141, 1987.
56. Ciccone JM, Saksena S, Shah Y, et al: A prospective randomized study of the clinical efficacy and safety of transvenous cardioversion for termination of ventricular tachycardia. *Circulation* 71:571–578, 1985.
57. Florin TJ, Weiss DN, Peters RW, et al: The induction of atrial fibrillation with low-energy defibrillator shocks in patients with implantable cardioverter defibrillators. *Am J Cardiol* 80:960–962, 1997.
58. Sweeney MO, Ruskin JN, Garan H, et al: Influence of the implantable cardioverter-defibrillator on sudden death and total mortality in patients evaluated for cardiac transplantation. *Circulation* 92:3273–3281, 1995.
59. Advanced Life Support Working Group of the International Liaison Committee on Resuscitation. International guidelines 2000 for CPR and ECC. *Circulation* 102:I-90–I-94, 2000.
60. Eisenberg MS, Copass MK, Hallstrom AP, et al: Treatment of out-of-hospital cardiac arrest with rapid defibrillation by emergency medical technicians. *N Engl J Med* 302:1379–1383, 1980.
61. Stults KR, Brown DD, Schug VL, et al: Prehospital defibrillation performed by emergency medical technicians in rural communities. *N Engl J Med* 310:219–223, 1984.
62. Larsen MP, Eseinberg MS, Cummins RO, et al: Predicting survival from out-of-hospital cardiac arrest: a graphic model. *Ann Emerg Med* 22:1652–1658, 1993.
63. Weaver WD, Cobb LA, Copass ML, et al: Ventricular defibrillation: a comparative trial using 175-J and 360-J shocks. *N Engl J Med* 307:1101–1106, 1982.
64. McDaniel WC, Schuder JC: The cardiac ventricular DFT: inherent limitations in its application and interpretation. *Med Instrum* 21:170–176, 1987.
65. Kerber KE, Grayzel J, Hoyt R, et al: Transthoracic resistance in human defibrillation: influence of body weight, chest size, serial shocks, paddle size and paddle contact pressure. *Circulation* 63:676–682, 1981.
66. Sima SJ, Ferguson DW, Charbonnier F, et al: Factors affecting transthoracic impedance during electrical cardioversion. *Am J Cardiol* 62:1048–1052, 1988.
67. Levine PA, Barold SS, Fletcher RD, et al: Adverse acute and chronic effects of electrical defibrillation and cardioversion on implanted unipolar cardiac pacing systems. *J Am Coll Cardiol* 1:1413–1422, 1983.

7. Echocardiography in the Intensive Care Unit

Gerard P. Aurigemma and
Dennis A. Tighe

Echocardiography is commonly used to evaluate the critically ill patient in the intensive care unit (ICU) because of the wealth of information concerning cardiac structure and function that it can provide rapidly, and because studies can be performed at the patient's bedside. At the authors' institution, approximately 30% of all echocardiographic studies are performed emergently in the ICU or emergency room, principally to diagnose life-threatening conditions, such as aortic dissection, cardiac tamponade, and acute bacterial endocarditis, or to evaluate left ventricular function in patients with hypotension or congestive heart failure. In these and other clinical situations, echocardiography provides diagnostic information with excellent sensitivity and specificity and is frequently the only cardiac diagnostic test necessary.

Echocardiography may be performed either with the transducer placed directly on the patient's chest [transthoracic echocardiography (TTE)] or mounted on a gastroscope that is passed into the patient's esophagus and stomach [transesophageal echocardiography (TEE)]. TEE has extended the capabilities of echocardiography in the ICU by providing high-quality diagnostic images in situations in which TTE is technically limited. Thus at present, with few exceptions, echocardiography rapidly provides important clinical data, if not the answer to the major clinical question, in the ICU patient.

Ultrasonography Principles

Echocardiography uses ultrasonic energy to create real-time, two-dimensional (2-D) images of the beating heart. In this chapter, the term *echocardiography* is used to refer to ultrasonographic examination of the heart; a routine echocardiographic study consists of M-mode, 2-D, and Doppler echocardiographic examinations (discussed in the following paragraphs). Details about ultrasonographic physics may be found elsewhere [1,2]. The echocardiography machine consists of a device that transmits and receives ultrasonography (transducer), a central processor that converts the received ultrasonography into a 2-D image, and a video display. The echocardiographic examination is recorded by the operator on videotape and chart paper and reviewed off-line, on the machine or at a separate VCR/television viewing station. Increasingly, routine echocardiographic examinations are recorded and displayed using digital technology, which permits enhanced resolution and streamlined study storage, retrieval, and playback. Digital technology is already used extensively in stress echocardiography.

Transthoracic Echocardiographic Imaging

A 2-D echocardiogram depicts the beating heart on a video display from a series of viewpoints or "windows." The operator performs the examination using a standard routine and sequentially images the heart from each of these windows (see the following paragraphs and Figs. 7-1 and 7-2). The standard echocardiographic examination uses three separate ultrasonographic technologies: M-mode echo, 2-D echo, and Doppler flow analysis. The M-mode echocardiogram displays the motion of cardiac structures with respect to time, along a single ice-pick view (Fig. 7-3); this examination is recorded on strip-chart paper. At present, M-mode recordings are used principally for measurements of cardiac chamber sizes and to time events precisely in the cardiac cycle, because the temporal resolution of M-mode technique is superior to that of 2-D echo. This means, for example, that the M-mode recording may be used to detect diastolic collapse of the right ventricle in patients with cardiac tamponade or early closure of the mitral valve in patients with acute severe aortic regurgitation due to bacterial endocarditis. In most other respects, however, M-mode echo has been supplanted by 2-D echo, which images much more of the cardiac volume than M-mode echo and, therefore, permits a better spatial appreciation of cardiac structures (Fig. 7-2); however, the M-mode examination is still a vital part of the routine echocardiographic study in the laboratory for the analysis of dimensions and in situations that call for precise timing of cardiac events.

The third ultrasonographic technology used in routine echocardiographic studies is Doppler echocardiography. A detailed discussion of the physics of Doppler ultrasonography is provided elsewhere [3,4]. In brief, Doppler ultrasonography provides a measure of the velocity of flowing blood in the heart and great vessels. By use of the simplified Bernoulli equation, which relates the peak velocity of flow across valves or septal defects to the associated pressure drop, a pressure gradient may be estimated from the Doppler recording of peak velocity [3,4]. The Doppler technique is, therefore, used to estimate, from the velocity profile, the peak and mean pressure gradients associated with aortic and mitral stenosis [4,5]. The same principle is used to estimate the right ventricular (RV) sys-

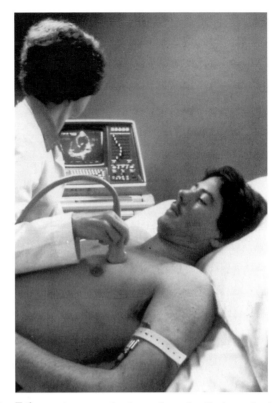

Fig. 7-1. Two-dimensional echo performed with the probe in the parasternal position. The patient is supine or in the left decubitus position, with electrocardiographic leads placed on the arms, shoulders, or chest. The ultrasonographer sits on the examination bed or stands at the bedside and continuously views the video display. The controls on the echocardiographic machine are set to optimize image quality. (Courtesy of Hewlett-Packard.)

tolic pressure from the peak velocity associated with tricuspid regurgitation (TR) [6]. The difference between RV and right atrial (RA) pressure can be derived from the TR velocity profile; this number is added to an estimate of RA pressure to derive the RV systolic pressure. In the absence of pulmonic stenosis, the RV pressure is equal to the pulmonary artery pressure.

Color-flow mapping [7,8] is another form of Doppler echocardiography that is used in virtually every echocardiographic examination. The principles underlying color-flow mapping are the same as those used in pulsed-wave Doppler. However, instead of a display of Doppler velocities with respect to time, color flow mapping provides a color-coded display of velocities superimposed on the 2-D echocardiographic image. In this manner, the spatial extent of disturbed flow may be appreciated in the context of the 2-D image. Color-flow Doppler therefore provides an immediate assessment of disturbed flow in valvular regurgitation, intracardiac shunts, and hypertrophic cardiomyopathy. Moreover, color-flow Doppler is the most widely used noninvasive technique to semiquantitate valvular regurgitation, providing results that are similar to semiquantitative angiographic grading of regurgitation [7,8].

TECHNIQUE. Echocardiographic imaging requires that the ultrasonographic transducer be placed in certain specific locations on the chest wall ("acoustic windows"); placement of the transducer in these locations permits the ultrasonographic beam to avoid interference by the lungs and ribs as it travels to and from the cardiac structures (Fig. 7-2). Routine echo is performed using several acoustic windows, as described in the following paragraphs. Transmission gel applied to the

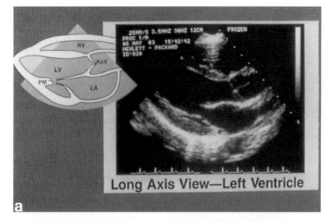

Long Axis View—Left Ventricle

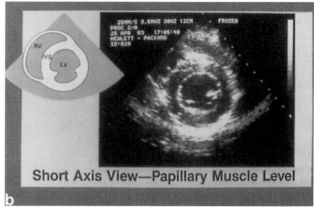

Short Axis View—Papillary Muscle Level

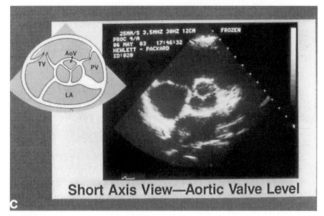

Short Axis View—Aortic Valve Level

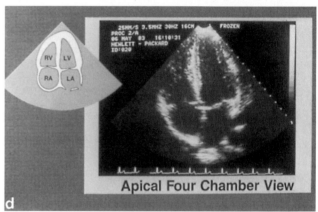

Apical Four Chamber View

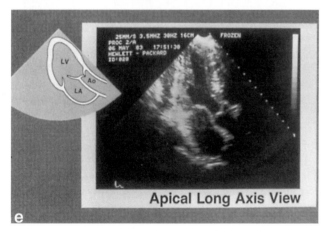

Apical Long Axis View

Fig. 7-2. Standard two-dimensional echo views with corresponding schematic diagrams to demonstrate cardiac anatomy. **A:** Parasternal long-axis view. **B:** Parasternal short-axis view at the level of the papillary muscle. **C:** Parasternal short-axis view at the level of the aortic valve (AoV). **D:** Apical four-chamber view. **E:** Apical long-axis view. The operator obtains sequential images from parasternal and apical windows. Thus, after a comprehensive examination, all four cardiac valves and all four cardiac chambers are completely examined. The combination of the parasternal short-axis view and the apical views permit a comprehensive examination of wall motion of the left ventricular myocardium in all three coronary perfusion beds. AO, aorta; LA, left atrium; LV, left ventricle; RA, right atrium; RV, right ventricle. (Courtesy of Hewlett-Packard.)

transducer serves as an interface between the transducer and the chest wall, because air transmits ultrasonography poorly.

An electrocardiogram (ECG) signal is recorded and displayed simultaneously with the echocardiographic examination; ECG timing is crucial for analysis of the motion of cardiac structures throughout the cardiac cycle. The ECG electrodes are usually placed on the patient's shoulders and lower part of the abdomen. Imaging is performed with the patient supine or in left lateral decubitus position, with the upper body lifted 30 to 40 degrees. This position is useful during imaging from the apical and parasternal windows (see the following sections).

In our laboratory, a routine examination comprises M-mode, 2-D, and Doppler echo; the examination is problem oriented, however, and is tailored to answer the major clinical questions. Routine examination includes imaging from four major acoustic windows to view the heart from different

angles. Additional images may be required to answer certain clinical questions; these images are obtained from any standard location by rotating and tilting the transducer. A complete examination generally takes 20 to 40 minutes but may be much longer in instances when precise Doppler quantitation of disturbed flow is required.

Parasternal Views. The transducer is first positioned at the second or third intercostal space just left of the sternum, with the patient in left lateral decubitus position; this positioning acts to shift the left lung to allow better visualization of the heart (Figs. 7-1 and 7-2). The reference point of the transducer is positioned toward the patient's right shoulder so that the plane of the image transects the heart along its long axis from apex to base. The resulting image, the parasternal long-axis view (Fig. 7-2A), displays the heart sagittally, with the left ven-

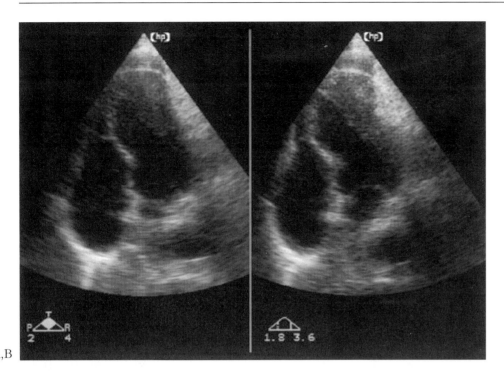

A,B

Fig. 7-3. Use of harmonic imaging. **A:** A suboptimal transthoracic echocardiography image, commonly obtained in intensive care unit patients. **B:** The same image, with the border between the left ventricular cavity and wall enhanced using harmonic imaging.

tricle (LV) at the center of the screen. The M-mode recording is made from this view.

A short-axis, or transverse, view of the heart is obtained by rotating the transducer 90 degrees from the long-axis view so the reference point is directed toward the patient's left shoulder (Fig. 7-2B,C). The resulting images depict the right side of the heart, including the tricuspid valve, on the left of the screen; the pulmonic valve on right side of the screen; and the three cusps of the aortic valve in the center of the screen. The transducer is tilted or rocked to a position that is more perpendicular to the chest wall so the ultrasonographic beam intersects the heart at the mitral valve level. Finally, the transducer is tilted inferiorly and toward the apex of the heart so the ultrasonographic beam bisects the midportion of the LV chamber and depicts the LV at the level of the papillary muscles. This view permits a comprehensive evaluation of LV function, because segmental wall motion abnormalities in all three coronary perfusion beds may be visualized at once.

Apical Views. The transducer is moved to the apical window, with the patient remaining in left lateral decubitus position, and placed at or near the cardiac apex and angled superiorly. The apical long-axis view is obtained by orienting the reference point on the transducer superiorly toward the patient's right shoulder. The resulting image displays the heart upside-down, with the apex of the heart displayed at the top of the monitor and the base displayed at the bottom. The apical four-chamber view is obtained by orienting the reference point on the transducer toward the patient's left shoulder. All four cardiac chambers (ventricles and atria) are seen simultaneously. This view is useful for evaluations of the LV lateral and septal walls, RV anterior wall, and mitral and tricuspid valves. The apical five-chamber view is obtained by tilting the transducer more anteriorly so the beam travels through the LV outflow tract and aortic valve.

Rotating the transducer so the reference point is directed toward the left side of the patient's neck causes the beam to bisect the chambers of the left side only. This positioning produces the apical two-chamber view, which displays the inferior and anterior walls of the LV.

Subcostal View. The transducer is positioned over the lower section of the chest just below the xiphoid. The ultrasonographic beam travels through the abdominal wall, liver, and diaphragm before reaching the heart. The reference point on the transducer is directed toward the right shoulder, with anterior and superior angulation of the transducer. The resulting image displays the base of the heart on the left and the apex on the right of the monitor. The anatomic relation of the plane of the interatrial septum to the path of the ultrasonographic beam is particularly important in evaluation of patients with suspected atrial septal defect. This view provides images that may supplement suboptimal images obtained from the parasternal or apical windows.

LIMITATIONS OF TRANSTHORACIC ECHOCARDIO-GRAPHY. Several important limitations of TTE should be noted. Imaging from the chest wall requires the use of relatively low-frequency transducers (usually 2.5 or 3.5 MHz for adults), which provides poor resolution of cardiac structures. Because air and the chest wall impede ultrasonographic transmission, high-quality TTE requires optimal acoustical windows. Consequently, patients who are obese, have obstructive lung disease, have suffered chest wall injury, or have undergone sternotomy may not be suitable ultrasonography subjects; similarly, patients who hyperventilate because of pain, anxiety, or poor gas exchange may be expected to have suboptimal studies. Prosthetic aortic and mitral valves present obstacles to the ultrasonographic beam transmission and result in acoustic shadowing. Such shadowing, for example, prevents the Doppler beam from reaching the left atrium on apical views and, therefore, prevents complete color-Doppler mapping of mitral regurgitation in most instances. Two new developments, however, permit improved diagnostic yield in the difficult-to-image patient. Harmonic imaging represents a major advance in diagnostic ultrasonography and greatly enhances signal to noise ratio, thereby improving the endocardial edge/blood pool interface [9,10] (Fig. 7-3). The second, related development is the advent of ultrasonographic contrast agents [11,12]. These compounds, several of which are now in clinical use in the United States and Europe, are often described as "microbubbles" which are administered intravenously and are small enough to traverse the pulmonary circulation and opacify the left atrium and LV. Contrast agents generally consist of an emulsion of an inert gas and an agent (e.g., polysaccharide), which helps to stabilize the bubbles and prevent destruction by ultrasonography.

Transesophageal Echocardiographic Imaging

Transesophageal echocardiographic imaging overcomes many of the technical limitations of TTE by imaging via the esophagus and avoiding the interference of the intervening chest wall structures and the lungs. In addition to providing a novel set of imaging windows, which permits examination of structures (e.g., the aorta and the left atrial appendage), the proximity of the esophagus to the heart and great vessels permits the use of higher-frequency transducers, providing better image resolution. For these reasons TEE images are, with few exceptions, of very high quality. Thus, the advantages of TEE (compared to TTE) include improved image quality and expanded diagnostic capabilities.

EQUIPMENT. The TEE probe consists of an ultrasonographic transducer mounted on the tip of a modified flexible gastroscope that is approximately 100 cm long (Fig. 7-4). The distal flexible tip of the scope houses the ultrasonographic transducer. The controls for manipulating the tip of the probe are located on the handle of the probe. Two lockable wheels on the handle control motion of the tip of the probe. A large outer wheel controls probe flexion (anteroposterior motion) while a smaller inner wheel controls lateral (right-left) motion. A cable connects the probe handle to an electrical transducer connector, which is inserted into the ultrasonographic imaging system. Controls for adjusting the echocardiographic image (e.g., sector size, depth, gain) and Doppler modalities are located on the echocardiographic machine.

The current generation of TEE transducers has multiplane imaging capabilities, often with multiple imaging frequencies, and full Doppler capabilities.

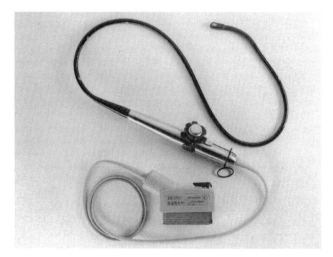

Fig. 7-4. Transesophageal echo probes. Shown here is the Hewlett-Packard OmniPlane probe, with a flexible probe, a handle with control wheels, a connecting cable, and an electrical transducer connector.

Table 7-1. Clinical Situations in which Transesophageal Echo Is Superior to Transthoracic Echo

Assessment of patients with suspected endocarditis, both native and prosthetic valve, and complications of endocarditis
Assessment of suspected prosthetic valve dysfunction, especially mitral prostheses
Evaluation of suspected thoracic aortic pathology, including aortic dissection
Evaluation of suspected intracardiac masses, especially in the atria (e.g., atrial myxoma, atrial thrombi)
Evaluation of patients with a suspected cardiac source of systemic emboli
Assessment of the interatrial septum (e.g., atrial septal defect, patent foramen ovale)
Diagnosis of central pulmonary emboli

INDICATIONS. TEE is indicated in the assessment of cardiac structure and function in patients in whom TTE images are inadequate to answer the clinical question. In addition, TEE has been shown to be superior to TTE for a variety of specific indications and is usually indicated as an adjunctive test to TTE. Table 7-1 lists indications for which TEE has been shown to be superior to TTE [13–21]. Transesophageal echo may also provide diagnostic information beyond that derived from a good-quality TTE in patients with native valve dysfunction, congenital heart disease, and complications of acute myocardial infarction. The precise role of TEE in many of these situations is rapidly evolving.

EXAMINATION. The TEE procedure has been described by several authors [22,23]. The authors' approach is described in the following paragraphs, with mention of special considerations when performing TEE in the critical care setting (Table 7-2).

Personnel. Whereas TTE is routinely performed by nonphysician sonographers, TEE is always performed by a physician who has extensive training in echocardiography and who has completed appropriate training in esophageal intubation and interpretation of TEE images [24].

For optimal patient safety, TEE requires the presence of one or two ancillary personnel to assist the physician operator and monitor the patient. A nurse or physician should be present to help position the patient, administer medications, monitor the patient's vital signs and respiratory status, and operate the suction device. It is helpful to have a second assistant (e.g., a sonographer or another physician) present to adjust the image settings on the echocardiography machine and to assist with videotaping.

Preparation. An appropriate patient history should be obtained to confirm the need for the study, screen for contraindications to the procedure, determine the need for endocarditis prophylaxis (see the section Endocarditis Prophylaxis), determine any

Table 7-2. Procedure for Transesophageal Echo

Patient preparation
  Screen for appropriate indications/contraindications
  Hemodynamic/respiratory status assessment
  Patient consent
  Non per os (nasogastric tube in selected patients)
  Intravenous access
Pharyngeal anesthesia
Sedation (midazolam and/or meperidine)
Monitor vital signs during and after procedure
Esophageal intubation
  Manual guidance or blind intubation
Image acquisition (goal-directed examination)
Equipment care

drug allergies, and assess the patient's respiratory and hemodynamic status. Patients with compromised respiratory status should be stabilized before TEE, because sedation, esophageal intubation, or both may result in further respiratory compromise. In such patients, the procedure should be delayed until the patient is stabilized; on occasion, intubation and controlled ventilation are required for airway protection and adequate oxygenation.

It is mandatory to review prior TTE studies; a careful review of the findings may sometimes obviate the need for TEE. In the authors' experience this is often the case when intracardiac masses are suspected: The TTE may demonstrate that the suspected mass is a Chiari network, prominent Eustachian valve, or imaging artifact.

The TEE probe should be inspected for damage to the probe and to ensure that the controls of the scope are operational, and it should be confirmed that the echocardiography machine is operating properly. An appropriate suction device, supplemental oxygen, resuscitation equipment, and appropriate medications must be readily available during the procedure.

Patient Preparation and Monitoring. The procedure should be explained to the patient and consent obtained from the patient or a surrogate. Dentures and other dental prostheses should be removed. To avoid the potential complication of aspiration of gastric contents, except in truly emergent situations, patients should fast a minimum of 4 hours before TEE and preferably take nothing orally (except medications) overnight before the study. Critically ill patients often develop a paralytic ileus and even with an adequate overnight fast may have retained gastric contents. If there is any question as to the presence of gastric contents, a nasogastric (NG) tube should be passed before TEE to decompress the stomach. The NG tube may remain in place during TEE if no difficulty is encountered in passing the probe; if there is difficulty in passing the TEE probe or if suboptimal images are obtained, the NG tube should be removed. For patients with an NG or feeding tube in place, the position of the tube should be confirmed after TEE, as it may be displaced during the procedure. Many patients in the ICU have central venous access present, which can be used to administer medications. If access is not present, a stable peripheral intravenous catheter (preferably located in an antecubital vein if a saline contrast study is to be performed) is needed to administer medications.

During the procedure, the patient's respiratory status, vital signs, and ECG should be continuously monitored. Continuous monitoring of the arterial oxygen saturation with pulse oximetry is routine in the authors' laboratory. After the procedure, patients must be observed to ensure that they have recovered from the effects of sedation and are stable. Food should be withheld until the effects of pharyngeal anesthesia have resolved, usually 1 to 2 hours.

Local Anesthesia. Local pharyngeal anesthesia is used to suppress the gag reflex, even in the intubated patient. For the paralyzed or unconscious patient, local anesthesia is not necessary. Patients who are able to swallow are asked to gargle and then swallow 15 to 30 mL of viscous lidocaine. After this, the pharynx is sprayed with a topical anesthetic, such as Cetacaine (Cetylite Industries, Pennsauken, NJ). The adequacy of the anesthesia is tested using a gloved finger to confirm that the gag reflex has been suppressed.

Sedation. Intravenous sedation is not mandatory [25], but we believe the procedure is much better tolerated with judicious use of conscious sedation [22,23]. The authors prefer a short-acting benzodiazepine, such as midazolam, given in 0.5- to 1.0-mg increments (to an average total dose of 4 mg). In addi-

tion, the authors frequently use meperidine in doses of 12.5 to 25.0 mg intravenously (average total dose 25 to 50 mg), or fentanyl (25 to 50 µg). In patients with renal failure, the authors prefer to use morphine sulfate in doses of 1 mg (to a total of 1 to 4 mg) in place of meperidine to avoid the accumulation of a major metabolite of meperidine that undergoes renal excretion. These drugs must be used with caution in critically ill patients who may have altered metabolism due to underlying disease (e.g., cardiac, renal, or hepatic failure), which may result in oversedation and respiratory depression. Hemodynamically unstable patients also may be more vulnerable to the potential hypotensive effects of these drugs. Adequate sedation is imperative in patients with suspected aortic dissection or acute myocardial infarction to avoid potentially deleterious increases in blood pressure and myocardial oxygen demand.

Endocarditis Prophylaxis. The need for endocarditis prophylaxis for TEE is controversial [26]. The incidence of bacteremia related to TEE and thus the risk of endocarditis should be similar to that of upper endoscopy without biopsy, a procedure thought to be low risk [27]. The patient population evaluated by TEE is at greater risk for endocarditis, however, because many patients have underlying valvular or congenital heart disease, or both. Although there have been reports of endocarditis apparently related to TEE [28], most prospective studies have found a low incidence of positive blood cultures related to TEE, most if not all of which were thought to represent contaminants [29]. Khandheria [26] summarized the results of several of these studies and concluded that the incidence of positive blood cultures related to TEE is no different than the rate of blood culture contamination; therefore, with the possible exception of patients with poor dentition and a history of endocarditis, antibiotic prophylaxis for TEE is not warranted. Patients at high risk (e.g., those with prosthetic heart valves, prior endocarditis, and surgically constructed systemic-pulmonary shunts) may be considered for prophylaxis. The authors' current practice is to administer prophylactic antibiotics only to patients with prosthetic valves, unless there is a clinical question of endocarditis, in which case such treatment could render diagnostic blood cultures negative.

Esophageal Intubation. The technique of inserting the probe (esophageal intubation) and performing the TEE procedure has been described in detail [22,23]. Here, the authors' approach is described. The nonintubated patient is asked to turn to the left lateral decubitus position; the intubated patient (see later) is usually studied in the supine position. The operator and assistant wear disposable gloves. In patients with teeth, a bite-guard is placed around the probe. The distal 10 to 15 cm of the probe is lubricated with a combination of a water-soluble lubricating gel and 2% lidocaine gel. The lock on the wheel controlling flexion/anteflexion is released while the medial/lateral control wheel is kept locked in the neutral position. Once the probe is inserted, this lock is released. After adequate conscious sedation and pharyngeal anesthesia, one or two fingers of one hand are placed in the posterior pharynx to guide the probe. Because fiberoptic guidance is not available for TEE, the probe is inserted with manual guidance, with care to keep the probe in the midline. Once the probe has been advanced to the posterior pharynx, the patient is asked to swallow to help advance the probe through the upper esophageal sphincter and into the distal esophagus (a depth of 25 to 35 cm as measured from the incisors), where the aortic valve and left atrium are visualized. The patient's neck may need to be flexed to facilitate probe placement. Gentle pressure may be used to pass the probe, but it should never be forcefully advanced. Once the probe is placed, the bite-guard is positioned and images obtained. An

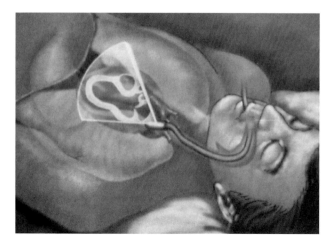

Fig. 7-5. Schematic drawing of a transesophageal echo probe in relationship to mediastinal structures. The probe is positioned in the esophageal imaging plane, providing a sagittal view of the heart. The probe may be further advanced into the stomach and retroflexed to image the heart in cross section. (Courtesy of Hewlett-Packard.)

alternative method of esophageal intubation is to place the bite-guard in the patient's mouth and insert the probe blindly through the opening in the bite-guard.

Intubated Patients. Probe insertion in the intubated patient is similar to that described previously. Because the airway is protected, patients are routinely studied in the supine position. As respiration is supported, sedatives and analgesics may be used somewhat more generously, though hypotension should be avoided. For patients who are awake, the posterior pharynx may be anesthetized with a topical anesthetic spray. If difficulty is encountered with esophageal intubation, the cuff of the endotracheal tube may be temporarily deflated to facilitate probe passage. The cuff is reinflated once the probe has been placed. A laryngoscope may be used to facilitate esophageal intubation in the intubated patient in whom there is extreme difficulty passing the probe blindly. We occasionally use vecuronium (Norcuron), a short-acting nondepolarizing neuromuscular-blocking agent, when the patient is extremely uncooperative despite maximal amounts of intravenous sedation; the usual dose of vecuronium is 0.05 to 0.10 mg per kg, given as an intravenous bolus.

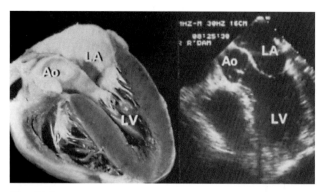

Fig. 7-6. Anatomic specimen and corresponding transesophageal echo image, illustrating the plane of the section when the probe is in the esophagus. Cardiac structures are labeled as follows: AO, aorta; LA, left atrium; LV, left ventricle. This view provides a coronal image of the LV with a view of the mitral apparatus, aortic valve, aortic outflow tract, and LA. (Courtesy of Hewlett-Packard.)

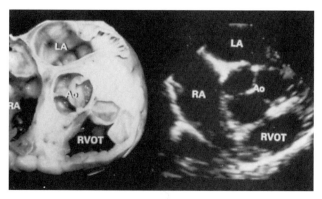

Fig. 7-7. Transesophageal view of the base of the heart, with the probe in the esophagus. Cardiac structures are labeled as follows: AO, aorta; LA, left atrium; RA, right atrium; RVOT, right ventricular outflow tract. Note the detail of the aortic valve leaflets. (Courtesy of Hewlett-Packard.)

Image Acquisition. Image acquisition commences with probe passage. Figures 7-5 to 7-8 show the standard TEE images recorded in a routine study. In the critical care setting, a brief, directed examination must sometimes suffice. On completion of the procedure, the probe is cleaned and disinfected with a 2% glutaraldehyde solution in accordance with the manufacturer's recommendations.

CONTRAINDICATIONS. The contraindications to TEE in the ICU patient are similar to those in the ambulatory patient [30]. A history of dysphagia should be elicited and if present evaluated to confirm that no significant esophageal disease is present. Esophageal pathology, such as strictures, varices, diverticula, scleroderma, prior surgery, or radiation is an absolute contraindication to TEE, as are gastric volvulus, perforation, and active upper gastrointestinal bleeding. If there are questions concerning the safety of TEE in a patient with known or suspected esophageal pathology, a gastroenterologist should be consulted.

Although the patient with a coagulopathy may be at increased risk of complications, therapeutic anticoagulation is not a contraindication to TEE. Relative contraindications to TEE include inability of the patient to cooperate, oropharyngeal distortion, and cervical spondylosis, which may make probe passing difficult. A hiatal hernia may interfere with image acquisition. Patients with head and neck trauma must be evaluated carefully to ensure that no oral/pharyngeal trauma exists that could interfere with safe passage of the probe. In patients with suspected cervical spine injury, cervical spine radiographs should be reviewed by a radiologist to exclude cervical spine fractures or dislocations before any attempt at probe passage or head positioning.

COMPLICATIONS. TEE has proven to be an extremely safe procedure, even in the critically ill patient [30–35]. The potential complications are similar to those encountered in the ambulatory patient and include pharyngeal and esophageal injury, aspiration, laryngospasm, tracheal intubation, respiratory depression, hypotension, and arrhythmias. Critically ill patients may be more susceptible to the untoward effects of intravenous sedation, and unconscious or heavily sedated patients may be at an increased risk of esophageal injury due to their inability to inform the operator of discomfort. In the largest series to date, Daniel et al. reported that the most common complication was failure to intubate the esophagus, which occurred in 201 (1.9%) of 10,419 procedures [36]. The procedure was prematurely aborted in 90 (0.86%), in most

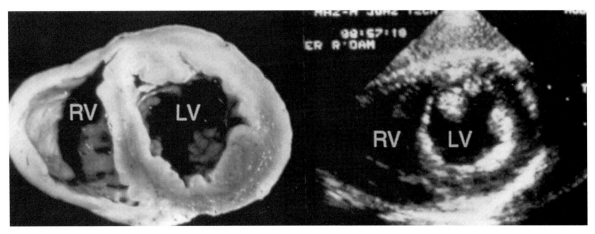

Fig. 7-8. The transesophageal echo probe has been advanced into the stomach and retroflexed to provide a short-axis image of the left ventricle (LV) similar to that obtained from transthoracic echo windows. From this transgastric window, wall motion of the myocardium in all three coronary perfusion beds may be visualized. The corresponding anatomy is labeled. RV, right ventricle. (Courtesy of Hewlett-Packard.)

cases due to patient intolerance (*n* = 65) or complications (*n* = 18). The complications included bronchospasm (*n* = 6), hypoxia (*n* = 2), arrhythmia (*n* = 7), severe angina (*n* = 1), pharyngeal bleeding (*n* = 1), and severe hematemesis resulting in death (*n* = 1). Thus the mortality rate in this series was 0.0098%. The patient who died had a lung tumor that eroded into the esophagus, resulting in uncontrollable bleeding. The Mayo Clinic reported their experience in 3,827 TEE studies performed over 4 years [32]. They reported complications in 2.9% of studies and death in one patient. The mortality rate was 0.026% (ventricular fibrillation in a patient with congestive heart failure). Several studies have shown that TEE is safe in the critical care setting [33–36].

Clinical Applications of Echocardiography in the Intensive Care Unit

This section reviews the application of echocardiography in ICU patients. The application of echocardiography in specific cardiovascular disorders is also discussed in Chapters 30 through 35, 37, and 39.

In the authors' experience, echocardiography is most commonly indicated in the ICU setting for the evaluation of LV function. Echocardiographic data are most helpful in guiding management in unexplained hypotension, congestive heart failure, and suspected mechanical complications after acute myocardial infarction. This experience is similar to that reported by other centers: In one study, hemodynamic instability was the indication for TEE in approximately one-half of ICU patients [35]. In these instances, a bedside echocardiogram (i.e., TTE, TEE, or both) rapidly furnishes information concerning LV size, systolic performance, and LV diastolic filling, and can depict disturbed flow resulting from valvular regurgitation or acquired ventricular septal defects.

UNEXPLAINED HYPOTENSION IN CRITICALLY ILL PATIENTS. TEE is a powerful diagnostic tool in the hemodynamically unstable ICU patient [34,35]. It has been suggested that TEE can predict mortality in critically ill patients with unexplained hypotension. In one study, 61 ICU patients

with unexplained hypotension were classified on the basis of their TEE findings: (a) nonventricular cardiac limitation to cardiac output (valvular, pericardial), (b) ventricular failure, and (c) noncardiac systemic disease (hypovolemia, low systemic vascular resistance, or both) [37]. The group with nonventricular limitation to cardiac output had improved survival compared to the other two groups (81% vs. 41% and 44%, respectively). In this same study, TTE was inadequate in 64% of the patients, compared to only 3% of inadequate TEEs. Therefore, it appears that TEE may play a pivotal role in the management of these patients, with both critical diagnostic information and prognostic risk stratification.

LEFT VENTRICULAR STRUCTURE AND FUNCTION

Hypotension. Comprehensive 2-D echo, using TEE where TTE is inadequate, rapidly provides an estimate of the ejection fraction (EF), the most widely used clinical index of LV systolic function. The EF may be estimated by visual inspection of the 2-D echo images or by computing LV end-diastolic and end-systolic volumes [38]. Most commercially available echocardiographic machines are equipped with software that allows for off-line computation of EF; these methods require that endocardial edges of the LV cavity be traced manually in systole and diastole. The EF is then calculated from the resulting cavity areas, using geometric assumptions about LV shape [38]. However, a study suggests that a visual estimate of EF by an experienced physician compares favorably with results of the more labor-intensive, off-line computer computation of EF from the same images [39]. There is much interest in the use of semiautomated border detection algorithms, which permit rapid determination of LV volumes and ejection fraction without the need for off-line, manual tracing of echocardiographic images. This technique appears to hold promise for the rapid quantitation of LV volumes and function in clinical practice (Fig. 7-9).

Because LV chamber dimensions and volumes may be estimated visually or by quantitative analysis, echocardiography can be used to diagnose hypovolemia. The echocardiogram demonstrates small end-diastolic and end-systolic LV volumes and normal or supranormal ejection fraction (Fig. 7-10). In the authors' experience, hypovolemia is an important cause of hypotension in the postoperative patient, particularly within the first 24 to 48 hours.

Echocardiography is an essential part of the evaluation and postoperative management of elderly patients after aortic

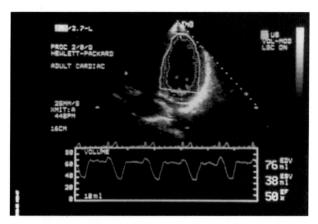

Fig. 7-9. The technique of automated boundary detection and its application to the study of cardiac volumes and ejection fraction. **Top:** Apical four-chamber view. **Bottom:** Corresponding beat-to-beat volume display. This technique may be used for on-line, rapid quantitation of end-diastolic and end-systolic volumes and ejection fraction. (Courtesy of Hewlett-Packard.)

valve replacement for aortic stenosis [40–43]. In a subset of these patients (generally older women) who had echocardiography to investigate hypotension, we have noted marked hypertrophy, hyperdynamic systolic function with an EF greater than 70%, small chamber volumes, and Doppler evidence consistent with outflow tract obstruction [40–43]. Often, these findings were completely unexpected and led to dramatic changes in postoperative management, such as discontinuation of positive inotropic agents and institution of fluid resuscitation; in some instances, institution of beta-blockers, calcium-channel blockers, or both was required. In the authors' experience, these changes are often associated with a restoration of adequate blood pressure, probably due to improved LV filling. Because proper management is predicated on correct diagnosis, there is a low threshold for performing an echocardiogram on postoperative aortic valve disease patients, as routine clinical, radiographic, and even Swan-Ganz catheter data may be misleading [40].

Congestive Heart Failure. Up to 40% of patients presenting with congestive heart failure have an EF of 45% or greater [44]. When the EF is normal, cardiac causes for congestive heart failure may include acute, severe mitral, or aortic regurgitation or impairment of LV filling (diastolic dysfunction) caused by myocardial ischemia, hypertensive heart disease, or both. Many patients with congestive heart failure and a normal EF have an antecedent history of hypertension [44]. In long-standing hypertension with or without myocardial ischemia, the LV loses its ability to fill completely at normal diastolic pressure [45]. Adequate filling of the LV is then associated with a rise in LV diastolic pressure, resulting in pulmonary congestion [45]. The Doppler mitral inflow velocity pattern has been used to identify abnormalities in diastolic function [46,47].

A pattern of abnormal relaxation (Fig. 7-11) generally accompanies patients with long-standing hypertension. However, a shift in the Doppler inflow pattern to a restrictive pattern generally indicates high LV filling pressures associated with abnormal LV compliance [46]. These diastolic filling profiles may be dynamic, as indicated by the fact that treatment with agents such as nitroglycerin or diuretics, which reduce filling pressures, results in a reversion of this restrictive pattern to the abnormal relaxation pattern [46]. The presence of an abnormal relaxation or restrictive filling pattern in the face of a normal LV ejection fraction signifies diastolic dysfunction as a possible etiology for congestive heart failure. Thus, 2-D echo coupled with Doppler mitral inflow analysis supports the diagnosis of diastolic dysfunction as a cause for congestive heart failure by demonstrating normal ejection fraction and an abnormal LV filling pattern.

Oh and coworkers demonstrated that the Doppler transmitral flow profile correlates with the presence of clinical heart failure in patients suffering an acute myocardial infarction [48]. This is presumably because the restrictive mitral inflow pattern is indicative of abnormally elevated LV diastolic pressures. Therefore, in patients with congestive heart failure, diastolic filling variables complement the assessment of systolic function and permit a comprehensive assessment of ventricular function.

Assessment of Pulmonary Venous Flow for Evaluation of Diastolic Function and Noninvasive Hemodynamics. In the ICU setting, mainly in mechanically ventilated patients, or in patients who have recently undergone open-heart surgery, it

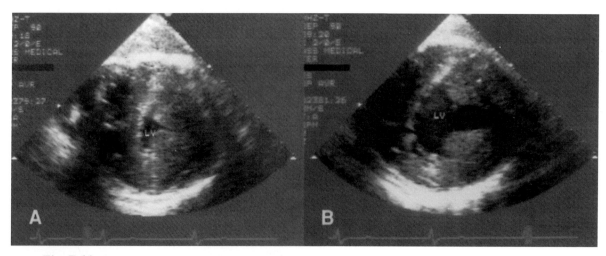

Fig. 7-10. A patient evaluated for hypotension after aortic valve replacement for aortic stenosis. Although systolic dysfunction was the suspected cause of hypotension, the study reveals that the ejection performance is supranormal, and there is very small end-systolic volume. **A:** End-systolic frame, demonstrating almost total cavity obliteration and small end-systolic volume. **B:** Diminished left ventricular cavity size on this diastolic frame. Posteromedial and anterolateral papillary muscles are shown at 1 and 5 o'clock, respectively. These findings led to discontinuation of intravenous pressor support and substitution of fluid resuscitation with subsequent hemodynamic improvement. LV, left ventricle.

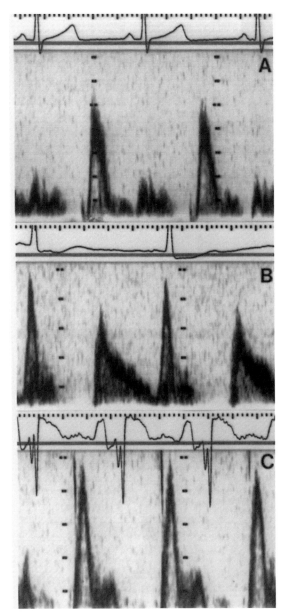

Fig. 7-11. Doppler mitral inflow patterns: strip chart recordings of mitral inflow velocities showing three commonly encountered patterns. Velocity is on the vertical axis and electrocardiogram (ECG) on the horizontal axis. **A:** A normal individual. In each cardiac cycle, denoted by the R wave, the first velocity profile is associated with passive filling of the left ventricle (LV) (E wave, occurring at the time of the T wave of the ECG), and the second profile is associated with atrial systole (A wave, occurring shortly after the P wave on the ECG). In normals, peak E exceeds peak A velocity. **B:** A patient with hypertensive left ventricular hypertrophy, showing reduced E velocity and enhanced A velocity. This pattern is consistent with abnormal LV relaxation. **C:** A patient with clinical congestive heart failure. This pattern (E velocity exceeding A velocity) is similar to normal, but the rapid deceleration of the E velocity profile reflects abnormal LV compliance and abnormal elevation in diastolic filling pressures.

is often difficult to obtain adequate mitral inflow velocity patterns for echocardiographic assessment of diastolic function and fluid status. This information can routinely be obtained with TEE. Although TEE can usually be used to evaluate most Doppler flows, it is especially useful for pulmonary venous flow in the determination of left ventricular filling pressures.

Measurement of the duration of the systolic fraction of pulmonary venous flow and the duration of the atrial systolic flow of the pulmonary vein flow relative to the duration of the mitral A wave can provide relevant bedside information. The change in systolic forward-flow velocity in the pulmonary vein correlates with changes in cardiac output, and the capillary wedge pressure correlates with the flow velocity reversal in the atrial contraction [49]. A prolonged duration of atrial flow reversal (relative to mitral A-wave duration) predicts an LV end-diastolic pressure of greater than 15 mm Hg, and the systolic fraction of pulmonary venous flow when markedly decreased (less than 0.4) indicates a pre-A pressure (left ventricular pressure before atrial systole) of greater than 18 mm Hg [50].

Myocardial Infarction. At the authors' institution, echocardiography is the principal method used to investigate suspected mechanical complications after myocardial infarction (see Chapter 40). Echocardiography can rapidly estimate LV ejection fraction and, therefore, determine whether hypotension in the patient after myocardial infarction is due to depressed pump function, RV infarction, hypovolemia, or a mechanical complication such as ventriculoseptal rupture.

The ability of echocardiography to detect wall motion abnormalities in myocardial infarction is well established [51–53]; in general, reduction in coronary flow of 20% or more is required to produce an abnormality in wall motion detectable by echocardiography [54]. The hallmark of such flow reduction is systolic thinning of the myocardium and an apparent outward motion of the endocardium. Coronary flow reductions of 50% or greater are reliably associated with a wall motion abnormality on the echocardiogram. An extensive literature has also documented that 2-D echo accurately diagnoses the site of acute myocardial infarction, with an excellent correlation between the location of the regional wall motion abnormality with coronary anatomy in patients with their first acute myocardial infarction [51].

Doppler color flow mapping enables the clinician rapidly to visualize flow disturbances complicating acute myocardial infarction. The echocardiographic examination can sensitively detect acute ventricular septal rupture as well as papillary muscle dysfunction or ruptured chordae tendineae complicating acute myocardial infarction [60]. Thus 2-D echo and color flow mapping are invaluable adjuncts to clinical examination in the postmyocardial infarction patient with a new holosystolic murmur. TEE supplements the transthoracic examination and in our experience has been particularly useful in diagnosing severe mitral regurgitation or ventricular septal rupture in patients with inadequate TTE studies. Echocardiography is also used to estimate the amount of myocardial damage by acute infarction. Although there has been an excellent correlation between echocardiographic and autopsy estimates of the extent of myocardial infarction in both experimental and human studies [54–56], echocardiography tends to overestimate the anatomic extent of infarction [57–58]. This phenomenon is most likely due to the fact that echocardiography depicts the abnormal function of anatomically normal myocardium that is tethered to the infarcted myocardium [59]. Despite this limitation, echocardiography is useful in estimating the extent of myocardial damage after infarction. In addition to diagnosing myocardial infarction and stratifying risk in patients presenting with chest pain syndromes, 2-D echo sensitively and accurately depicts mechanical complications of myocardial infarction [60] (Figs. 7-12 to 7-16).

CARDIAC VALVES

Stenosis and Regurgitation. Echocardiographic assessment of heart valve disease requires a combination of M-mode, 2-D, and Doppler techniques and a skilled ultrasonographer. For

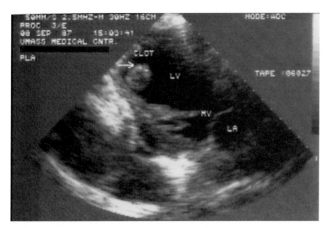

Fig. 7-12. A patient with a large apical myocardial infarction (apical long-axis orientation). The left ventricular cavity is enlarged and there is a pedunculated, large, freely mobile clot (*arrow*) attached to the inferoapical portion of the left ventricle (LV). LA, left atrium; MV, mitral valve.

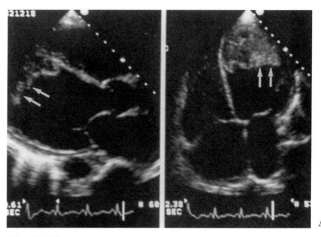

Fig. 7-13. A,B: A patient with an extensive apical myocardial infarction. Arrows demonstrate a large apical thrombus.

regurgitant lesions, the anatomical defect (e.g., flail mitral leaflet) is depicted by 2-D echo, and the location and spatial extent of the flow disturbance is semiquantitated by color-flow mapping [7,8].

Suspected Endocarditis. Echocardiography is commonly requested in the ICU to evaluate patients with suspected endocarditis. The reported sensitivity of TTE ranges from 44% to 80% in patients with clinically suspected endocarditis [61]; it has been shown to have excellent specificity and negative predictive value and can demonstrate abscess formation complicating endocarditis. However, false-positive results may be caused by nonspecific valve thickening, degenerative or rheumatic leaflet sclerosis, ruptured chordae tendineae, or severe myxomatous degeneration of valve leaflets. Pulsed and color-flow Doppler imaging supplement TTE in infective endocarditis by enabling the clinician to assess the site and severity of associated valvular regurgitation. Jaffe et al. demonstrated that when infective endocarditis is associated with minimal valvular regurgitation, the risk of in-hospital mortality is low and progression to valve replacement is unlikely [62].

Considering the high-quality images routinely obtained with TEE, it is not surprising that this procedure has an impressive incremental yield in sensitivity and specificity in patients with suspected endocarditis compared with TTE. Shively et al. showed that the sensitivity of TEE was much greater than that of TTE (94% vs. 44%, $p < .01$) when echocardiographic studies were considered "almost certainly" to demonstrate endocarditis [61]. At lesser levels of diagnostic certainty, TEE was still associated with a much higher sensitivity than TTE (94% vs. 69%), with no sacrifice in specificity. In the authors' experience, TEE is particularly helpful when TTE is suggestive but not diagnostic of vegetations (Fig. 7-17).

TEE may also demonstrate clinically unsuspected intracardiac abscesses (Fig. 7-18). Daniel and coworkers reported the findings of TEE examination in 118 consecutive patients with infective endocarditis of both native and prosthetic valves; 44 had one or more areas of intracardiac abscess, typically the result of *Staphylococcus aureus* infection of the aortic valve [20]. TEE successfully demonstrated 40 to 46 areas of abscess, compared with only 13 of 46 identified by TTE (sensitivity 87% for TEE vs. 28% for TTE).

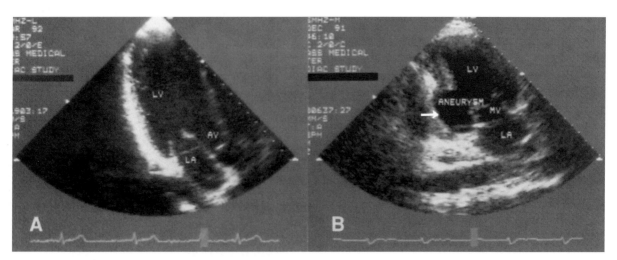

Fig. 7-14. Aneurysm of the inferoposterior wall of the left ventricle (LV). **A:** Normal LV inferoposterior wall. **B:** A patient with an inferior myocardial infarction. Large outpouching of the LV wall is seen in the vicinity of papillary muscle (*arrow*), which represents an aneurysm of the inferior wall. AV, aortic valve; LA, left atrium; MV, mitral valve.

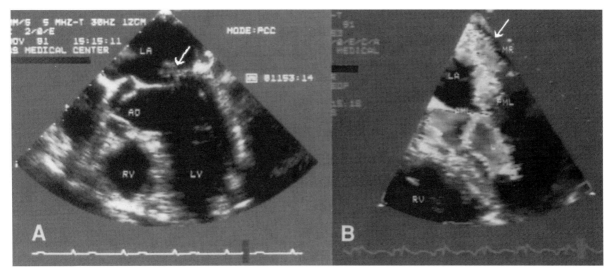

Fig. 7-15. Bacterial endocarditis. **A:** Large vegetation on the mitral valve (*arrow*). **B:** Turbulent flow indicative of mitral regurgitation (*arrow*). Cardiac structures are labeled as follows: AO, aorta; LA, left atrium; LV, left ventricle; PML, posterior mitral leaflet; MR, mitral regurgitation; RV, right ventricle.

Transthoracic echo also appears to identify endocarditis patients at increased risk of complications. Buda et al. [63] and Stafford et al. [64] observed more complicated clinical courses in endocarditis patients whose TTE studies demonstrated vegetations. In Buda's series, patients with maximal vegetation diameter exceeding 10 mm were at higher risk for the development of emboli, congestive heart failure, need for surgical intervention, and death than those with smaller vegetations [63]. Mugge and coworkers showed that 22 of 47 patients with a vegetation greater than 10 mm suffered embolic events, in comparison to 11 of 58 patients with a vegetation diameter of 10 mm or less [65]. Sanfilippo and coworkers retrospectively reviewed medical records and 2-D echo studies in 204 consecutive patients with a clinical diagnosis of endocarditis [66]. These investigators demonstrated that the probability of complications (e.g., antibiotic failure, congestive heart failure, embolization, need for surgery, in-hospital mortality) was related to vegetation size as a continuous variable. Moreover, echocardiographic descriptions of the vegetation (i.e., consistency, mobility, and extent) were predictors of complications. Jaffe and coworkers also demonstrated that in patients with vegetations greater than 10 mm as depicted by 2-D echo, the risk of subsequent embolism significantly exceeded that in patients with smaller vegetations [62].

Di Salvo and coworkers, using TEE, showed that the morphologic characteristics of vegetations by this technique are useful in predicting embolic risk [67]. Two factors—vegetation length and mobility—were found by these investigators to be significant predictors of embolic events. Specifically, vegetation length greater than 10 mm and moderately and severely mobile vegetations were associated with increased embolic potential. Large (greater than 15 mm) and severely mobile vegetations were associated with a very high risk (83%) of peripheral embolism. Other factors, including age, gender, vegetation location (aortic vs. mitral position), and valve type (native vs. prosthesis) were not associated with a significantly increased risk of embolism.

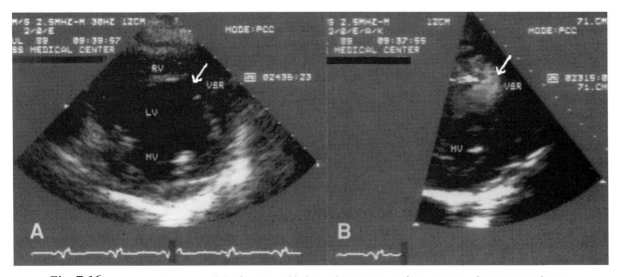

Fig. 7-16. A patient with a myocardial infarction and holosystolic murmur. **A:** Short-axis view, demonstrating discontinuity in the anteroseptal region (*arrow*). **B:** Turbulent flow, diagnostic of left ventricle–to–right ventricle septal rupture flow, is demonstrated (*arrow*). LV, left ventricle; MV, mitral valve; RV, right ventricle; VBR, ventricular-brain ratio.

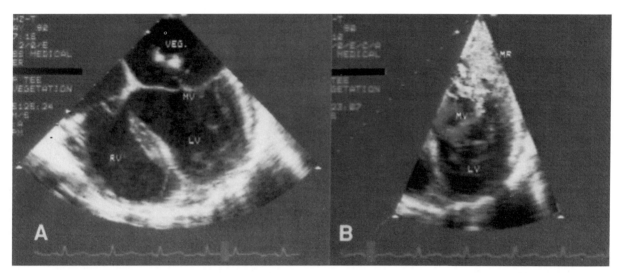

Fig. 7-17. Patient with clinical evidence of bacterial endocarditis. **A:** Transesophageal view, showing all four cardiac chambers. There is a large, freely mobile vegetation attached to the posterior mitral valve (MV) leaflet. **B:** Associated severe mitral regurgitation, denoted by mosaic color-flow pattern that completely fills the left atrium. This patient was taken to the operating room for MV replacement. LV, left ventricle; MR, mitral regurgitation; RV, right ventricle; VEG, vegetation.

In summary, TTE and TEE are complementary diagnostic techniques in infective endocarditis. A negative, high-quality TTE provides strong evidence against the diagnosis of bacterial endocarditis, particularly when valvular regurgitation is minimal. TEE offers an important increase in diagnostic sensitivity when the TTE is of poor quality or when the TTE is negative or equivocal in cases of high clinical suspicion for endocarditis. Certain TTE and TEE findings appear to identify infective endocarditis patients at high risk for embolic or other complications [66,67].

AORTA AND GREAT VESSELS

Thoracic Aortic Dissection. Thoracic aortic dissection is a catastrophic event in which a rapid, accurate diagnosis can be life saving. Until the 1990s, the evaluation of aortic dissection relied on aortography or contrast-enhanced computed tomog-

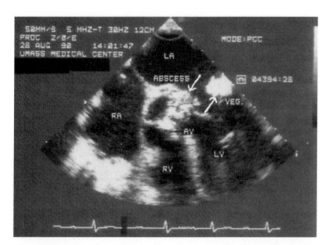

Fig. 7-18. Transesophageal image of a patient who had aortic valve surgery and subsequently developed bacterial endocarditis. The large mobile mass attached to the mitral valve represents a vegetation (VEG.) (*arrow*). There is also an aortic root abscess (*arrows*). The cardiac structures are labeled as follows: AV, aortic valve; LA, left atrium; LV, left ventricle; RA, right atrium; RV, right ventricle.

raphy. TEE and magnetic resonance imaging (MRI) have been introduced into use for diagnosis of aortic dissection. A complete discussion of aortic dissection is found in Chapter 34. TEE has greatly expanded the role of echocardiography in the evaluation of aortic dissection [68,69] and is also useful in detecting pulmonary embolism [70], conditions that often enter the differential diagnosis of the patient presenting with acute chest pain, dyspnea, or both.

Transthoracic echo has been used to evaluate patients with suspected aortic dissection [71,72], but its inadequate sensitivity, especially for descending aortic dissection, has until recently precluded the use of echocardiography as a definitive diagnostic test for aortic dissection. The diagnosis of aortic dissection by echocardiography depends on the identification of an intimal flap, an abnormal linear echo in the aortic lumen, which may be undulating or stationary [68,69]. If the false lumen is thrombosed, the presence of central displacement of intimal calcification may be used to diagnose aortic dissection.

Transthoracic echo is hampered by its inability to image the entire thoracic aorta, especially the descending aorta, as well as in obtaining adequate acoustic windows in critically ill patients. The reported sensitivity and specificity of TTE for diagnosing aortic dissection range from 59% to 100% and 63% to 96%, respectively [69]. TEE overcomes many of the limitations of TTE in assessment of the aorta. Due to the close proximity of the esophagus to the aorta, the entire thoracic aorta is well visualized by TEE, with the exception of a small blind spot in the distal ascending aorta that is obscured from view due to the interposition of the trachea between the esophagus and the aorta. Figure 7-19 demonstrates the appearance of aortic dissection on TEE.

Several studies comparing multiple imaging modalities have demonstrated that TEE is, with the possible exception of MRI, most accurate in the diagnosis of aortic dissection [69]. Two studies showed a lower specificity than originally reported, due to a significant number of false-positive findings in the ascending aorta [73]. False-positive studies are often due to the presence of imaging artifacts resulting from reverberations from vessel or aortic root calcification or atherosclerotic disease that mimics an intimal flap, as well as multiple path artifacts from ultrasound reflection in the left atrium [74]. The aorta-lung interface may cause mirror-image artifacts in the

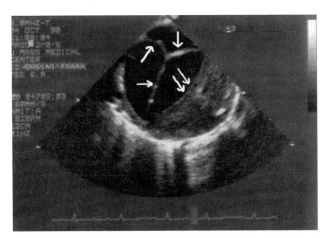

Fig. 7-19. Transesophageal study of a patient with Marfan syndrome. Transverse view of the descending aorta, demonstrating a complex intimal flap (*single arrows*) with thrombus in a false lumen (*double arrows*).

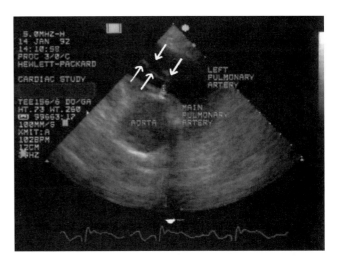

Fig. 7-20. Transverse view of the pulmonary artery bifurcation, demonstrating a large central pulmonary embolus (*arrows*). This patient presented with dyspnea and chest pain. Transesophageal echo was requested after inadequate transthoracic echo, to evaluate left ventricular function.

arch and descending aorta, giving the appearance of a double-lumen aorta [74]. Thus, accurate evaluation of the aorta while using TEE requires considerable operator experience and knowledge of the potential pitfalls.

TEE has several advantages over other imaging modalities: It is portable, thus allowing bedside diagnosis as well as ongoing treatment and monitoring of the patient's hemodynamic status; it is readily available; it allows rapid diagnosis (dissection can be excluded in minutes after the probe is placed); it is minimally invasive; it does not require the use of intravenous contrast material or ionizing radiation; and it is relatively inexpensive [69]. It can also assess LV function, the status of the aortic valve, degree of aortic regurgitation, and the presence of a pericardial effusion that may cause cardiac tamponade. With the possible exception of MRI, no other imaging modality shares all of these advantages, and MRI is hampered by the need for long scan times, which precludes its applicability to acutely ill patients. Thus, in many institutions, including that of the authors, TEE has become the imaging modality of choice in the initial evaluation of suspected aortic dissection, and in many circumstances has obviated the need for further diagnostic imaging, including aortography.

Acute Pulmonary Embolism. Transthoracic echo may demonstrate suggestive evidence of pulmonary embolus, such as right ventricular enlargement, abnormal right ventricular and interventricular septal wall motion, or evidence of pulmonary hypertension. Although it is not a primary imaging modality for the diagnosis of pulmonary embolus, TEE can detect central pulmonary embolus [70]. In patients undergoing TEE for chest pain syndromes and unexplained dyspnea or hypoxemia, careful scanning of the pulmonary arteries is warranted, especially if no other findings that may explain the patient's symptoms are detected (Fig. 7-20).

Trauma. Traumatic injury to the aorta commonly accompanies serious, nonpenetrating injury to the thorax. Several studies have demonstrated the use of TEE in the evaluation of patients with blunt thoracic trauma [75,76].

Traumatic valve injuries may result clinically in acute regurgitation. Most commonly, traumatic injury involves the aortic valve. The 2-D echo, either TTE or TEE, usually visualizes aortic valve rupture and aortic regurgitation. Echocardiography and color-flow Doppler mapping are also useful in penetrating chest injuries (Fig. 7-21).

PERICARDIAL DISEASE. Echocardiography is the principal method used in the ICU setting to evaluate the patient with suspected cardiac tamponade. M-mode and 2-D echo readily detect pericardial effusions and can help distinguish loculated from free-flowing collections (Figs. 7-22 and 7-23). Echocardiography may also be used at the bedside to guide pericardiocentesis and to help the clinician decide when an operative approach is advisable, in the case of localized collection of fluid.

In patients with sizable pericardial effusions, several echocardiographic signs indicate increased intrapericardial pressure, including early diastolic collapse of the RV free wall and diastolic collapse of the right atrial free wall. However, these are both sensitive signs of increases in intrapericardial pressure and do not necessarily diagnose cardiac tamponade, which is a clinical diagnosis made at the bedside. Additional signs of increased intrapericardial pressure include exaggerated respiratory variation in the Doppler mitral inflow and hepatic vein flow profiles.

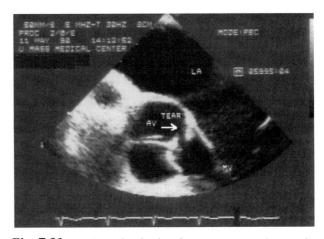

Fig. 7-21. A patient who developed acute, severe aortic regurgitation after blunt chest trauma during a motor vehicle accident. A tear in commissure between the noncoronary and left cusp is clearly demonstrated (*arrow*). Color-flow Doppler examination demonstrated severe aortic regurgitation. Based on this study, the patient was sent for urgent aortic valve replacement.

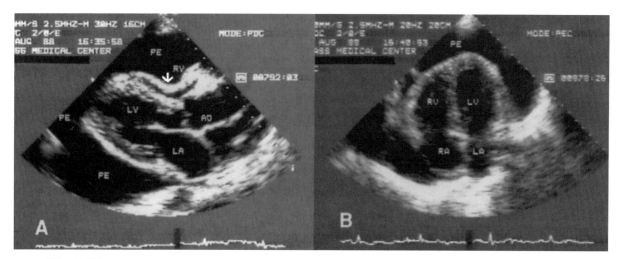

Fig. 7-22. A patient with hypotension. Panels **(A)** and **(B)** are parasternal and apical views, respectively. These images show a very large pericardial effusion (PE) and clear-cut compromise of right ventricular filling. Note the compression of the right ventricle (RV) in the diastolic frame shown in A (*arrow*). AO, aorta; LA, left atrium; LV, left ventricle; RA, right atrium.

Future Directions

Future directions in the use of echocardiography in the ICU setting include the potential development of miniaturized, indwelling TEE probes that make possible continuous assess-ment of LV function; expanded use of hand-held portable ultrasonographic devices by ICU staff with less extensive echo training to provide limited, but rapid point-of-care assessment of LV function; and the continued development of three-dimensional echocardiography technology that has the potential to provide real-time, on-line assessment of LV function and volumes.

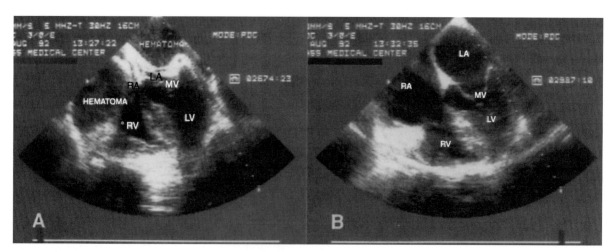

Fig. 7-23. A: Postoperative transesophageal study of a patient with profound hemodynamic compromise after cardiac surgery, demonstrating a large hematoma compressing the right atrium (RA) and left atrium (LA), limiting ventricular filling. **B:** Study obtained approximately 5 minutes later after drainage of large sanguineous pericardial effusion. Note the restoration of normal-sized RA and LA and increase in size of the right ventricle (RV). Pericardiocentesis was associated with dramatic increase in systolic pressure. LV, left ventricle; MV, mitral valve.

References

1. Feigenbaum H: *Echocardiography.* 4th ed. Philadelphia, Lea & Febiger, 1986.
2. Geiser EA: Echocardiography: physics and instrumentation, in Marcus M, et al (eds): *Cardiac Imaging.* Philadelphia, WB Saunders, 1991, p 348.
3. Hatle L, Angelsen B: *Doppler Ultrasound in Cardiology: Physical Principles and Clinical Applications.* 4th ed. Philadelphia, Lea & Febiger, 1984.
4. Cannon SR, Richards KL: Principles and physics of Doppler, in Marcus M, et al (eds): *Cardiac Imaging.* Philadelphia: WB Saunders, 1991, p 365.
5. Currie RJ, Seward JB, Reeder GS, et al: Continuous wave Doppler echocardiographic assessment of severity of calcific aortic stenosis. *Circulation* 79:1165, 1985.
6. Yock PG, Popp RL: Non-invasive estimation of right ventricular systolic pressure by Doppler ultrasound in patients with tricuspid regurgitation. *Circulation* 70:657, 1984.
7. Spain MG, Smith MD, Grayburn PA, et al: Quantitative assessment of mitral regurgitation by Doppler color flow imaging: angiographic and hemodynamic correlations. *J Am Coll Cardiol* 13:585, 1989.
8. Perry GJ, Helmcke F, Nanda NC, et al: Evaluation of aortic insufficiency by Doppler color flow mapping. *J Am Coll Cardiol* 9:952, 1987.
9. Aurigemma GP: Is harmonic imaging now fundamental? (Editorial). *Lancet* 352:1239–1240, 1998.
10. Caidahl K, Kazzam E, Lidberg J, et al: New concept in echocardiography: harmonic imaging of tissue without use of contrast agent. *Lancet* 352:1264–1270, 1998.
11. Grayburn PA, Weiss JL, Hack TC, et al: Multicenter trial comparing efficacy of 2% dodecafluoropentane emulsion (EchoGen) and 5% sonicated human albumin (Albunex) as ultrasound contrast agents in patients with suboptimal echocardiograms. *J Am Coll Cardiol* 32:230–236, 1998.
12. Kitzman DW, Goldman ME, Gillam LD, et al: Efficacy and safety of the novel ultrasound contrast agent perflutren (Definity) in patients with suboptimal baseline left ventricular echocardiographic images. *Am J Cardiol* 86:669–674, 2000.
13. Alton ME, Pasierski TJ, Orsinelli DA, et al: Comparison of transthoracic and transesophageal echocardiography in evaluation of 47 Starr-Edwards prosthetic valves. *J Am Coll Cardiol* 20:1503, 1992.
14. Nienaber C, Spielmann R, Kodolitsch Y, et al: Diagnosis of thoracic aortic dissection: magnetic resonance imaging versus transesophageal echocardiography. *Circulation* 85:434, 1992.
15. Pearson AC, Labovitz A, Tatineni S, et al: Superiority of transesophageal echocardiography in detecting cardiac source of embolism in patients with cerebral ischemia of uncertain etiology. *J Am Coll Cardiol* 17:66, 1991.
16. Khandheria BK, Takik AJ, Taylor CL, et al: Aortic dissection: review of value and limitations of two-dimensional echocardiography in a six-year experience. *J Am Soc Echocardiogr* 2:17, 1989.
17. van den Brink RBA, Visser CA, Basart DCG, et al: Comparison of transthoracic and transesophageal color Doppler flow imaging in patients with mechanical prostheses in the mitral valve position. *Am J Cardiol* 63:1471, 1989.
18. Wittlich N, Erbal R, Eichler A, et al: Detection of central pulmonary artery thromboemboli by transesophageal echocardiography in patients with severe pulmonary embolism. *J Am Soc Echocardiogr* 5:515, 1992.
19. Tunick PA, Kronzon I: Protruding atherosclerotic plaque in the aortic arch of patients with systemic embolization: a new finding seen by transesophageal echocardiography. *Am Heart J* 120:658, 1990.
20. Daniel WG, Mugge A, Martin RP, et al: Improvement in the diagnosis of abscesses associated with endocarditis by transesophageal echocardiography. *N Engl J Med* 324:795, 1991.
21. Reeder GS, Khandheria BK, Seward JB, et al: Transesophageal echocardiography and cardiac masses. *Mayo Clin Proc* 66:1101, 1991.
22. Seward JB, Khandheria BK, Oh JK, et al: Transesophageal echocardiography: technique, anatomic correlation, implementation, and clinical applications. *Mayo Clin Proc* 63:649, 1988.
23. Labovitz AJ, Pearson AC: *Transesophageal Echocardiography: Basic Principles and Clinical Applications.* Philadelphia, Lea & Febiger, 1992.
24. Pearlman AS, Gardin JM, Martin RP: Guidelines for physician training in transesophageal echocardiography: recommendations of the American Society of Echocardiography Committee for physician training in echocardiography. *J Am Soc Echocardiogr* 5:187, 1992.
25. Daniel WG, Erbel R, Kasper W, et al: Safety of transesophageal echocardiography. A multicenter survey of 10,419 examinations. *Circulation* 83:817, 1991.
26. Khandheria BK: Prophylaxis or no prophylaxis before transesophageal echocardiography? *J Am Soc Echocardiogr* 5:285, 1992.
27. Dajani AS, Bisno AL, Chung KJ, et al: Prevention of bacterial endocarditis. A statement for health professionals from the Committee on Rheumatic Fever, Endocarditis, and Kawasaki Disease of the Council of Cardiovascular Disease in the Young, the American Heart Association. *Circulation* 82:1170, 1991.
28. Foster E, Kusumoro FM, Sobol SM, et al: Streptococcal endocarditis temporally related to transesophageal echocardiography. *J Am Soc Echocardiogr* 3:424, 1990.
29. Nikutta P, Mantev-Stiers F, Becht I, et al: Risk of bacteremia induced by transesophageal echocardiography: analysis of 100 consecutive procedures. *J Am Soc Echocardiogr* 5:168, 1992.
30. Schiller NB, Maurer G, Ritter SB, et al: Transesophageal echocardiography. *J Am Soc Echocardiogr* 2:354, 1989.
31. Chan K, Cohen GI, Sochowski RA, et al: Complications of transesophageal echocardiography in ambulatory adult patients: analysis of 1500 consecutive examinations. *J Am Soc Echocardiogr* 4:577, 1991.
32. Seward JB, Khandheria BK, Oh JK, et al: Critical appraisal of transesophageal echocardiography: limitations, pitfalls, and complications. *J Am Soc Echocardiogr* 5:288, 1992.
33. Pearson AC, Castello R, Labovitz AJ: Safety and utility of transesophageal echocardiography in the critically ill patient. *Am Heart J* 119:1083, 1990.
34. Foster E, Schiller NB: The role of transesophageal echocardiography in critical care: UCSF experience. *J Am Soc Echocardiogr* 5:368, 1992.
35. Oh JK, Seward JB, Khandheria BK, et al: Transesophageal echocardiography in critically ill patients. *Am J Cardiol* 66:1492, 1990.
36. Daniel WG, Erbel R, Kasper W, et al: Safety of transesophageal echocardiography. A multicenter survey of 10,419 examinations. *Circulation* 83:817, 1991.
37. Heidenrich PA, Stainback RF, Redberg R, et al: Transesophageal echocardiography predicts mortality in critically ill patients with unexplained hypotension. *J Am Coll Cardiol* 26:152, 1995.
38. Schiller NB, Acquatella H, Ports TA, et al: Left ventricular volume from paired biplane two-dimensional echocardiography. *Circulation* 60:547, 1979.
39. Amico AF, Lichtenberg GS, Reisner SA, et al: Superiority of visual versus computerized echocardiographic estimation of radionuclide left ventricular ejection fraction. *Am Heart J* 118:1259, 1989.
40. Aurigemma G, Battista S, Orsinelli D, et al: Abnormal LV intracavity flow acceleration in patients undergoing aortic valve replacement for aortic stenosis: a marker for high post-operative morbidity and mortality. *Circulation* 86:926, 1992.
41. Vignon P, Boncoeur MP, Francois B, et al: Comparison of multiplane transesophageal echocardiography and contrast-enhanced

helical CT in the diagnosis of blunt traumatic cardiovascular injuries. *Anesthesiology* 94:615, 2001.

42. Laurent M, Leborgne O, Clement C, et al: Systolic intra-cavitary gradients following aortic valve replacement: an echo-Doppler study. *Eur Heart J* 12:1098, 1991.

43. Bartunek J, Vanderheyden M, De Bruyne B: Dynamic left ventricular outflow tract obstruction as a potential mechanism of myocardial rupture after acute myocardial infarction. *J Am Coll Cardiol* 34(7):2150, 1999.

44. Aurigemma GP, Gottdiener JS, Shemanski L, et al: Predictive value of systolic and diastolic function for incident congestive heart failure in the elderly: the cardiovascular health study. *J Am Coll Cardiol* 37(4):1042, 2001.

45. Zile MR, Gaasch WH, Carroll JD, et al: Heart failure with a normal ejection fraction: is measurement of diastolic function necessary to make the diagnosis of diastolic heart failure? *Circulation* 104(7):779, 2001.

46. Nishimura RA, Tajik AJ: Evaluation of diastolic filling of left ventricle in health and disease: Doppler echocardiography is the clinician's Rosetta Stone. *J Am Coll Cardiol* 30(1):8–18, 1997.

47. Stoddard MF, Pearson AC, Kern MJ, et al: Left ventricular diastolic function: comparison of pulsed Doppler echocardiographic and hemodynamic indexes in subjects with and without coronary artery disease. *J Am Coll Cardiol* 13:327, 1989.

48. Oh JK, Ding ZP, Gersh BJ, et al: Restrictive left ventricular diastolic filling identifies patients with heart failure after acute myocardial infarction. *J Am Soc Echocardiogr* 5:497, 1992.

49. Nishimura RA, Abel MA, Hatle LK, et al: Relation of pulmonary vein to mitral flow velocities by transesophageal Doppler echocardiography. *Circulation* 81:1488, 1990.

50. Rossvoll O, Hatle LK: Pulmonary venous flow velocities recorded by transthoracic Doppler ultrasound: relation to left ventricular diastolic pressures. *J Am Coll Cardiol* 21:1687, 1993.

51. Stamm RB, Gibson RS, Bishop HL, et al: Echocardiographic detection of infarct-localized asynergy and remote asynergy during acute myocardial infarction: correlation with the extent of angiographic coronary disease. *Circulation* 67:233, 1983.

52. Heger JJ, Weyman AE, Wann LS, et al: Cross-sectional echocardiography in acute myocardial infarction: detection and localization of regional left ventricular asynergy. *Circulation* 60:531, 1979.

53. Heger JJ, Weyman AE, Wann LS, et al: Cross-sectional echocardiographic analysis of the extent of left ventricular asynergy in acute myocardial infarction. *Circulation* 61:1113, 1980.

54. Pandian NG, Koyanagi S, Skorton DJ, et al: Relations between 2-dimensional echocardiographic wall thickening abnormalities, myocardial infarct size and coronary risk area in normal and hypertrophied myocardium in dogs. *Am J Cardiol* 52:1318, 1983.

55. Kerber RE, Marcus ML, Ehrhardt J, et al: Correlation between echocardiographically demonstrated segmental dyskinesis and regional myocardial perfusion. *Circulation* 52:1097, 1975.

56. Buda AL, Zotz RJ, LeMire MS, et al: Comparison of two-dimensional echocardiographic wall motion and wall thickening abnormalities in relation to the myocardium at risk. *Am Heart J* 111:587, 1986.

57. Guth BD, White FC, Gallagher KP, et al: Decreased systolic wall thickening in myocardium adjacent to ischemic zones in conscious swine during brief coronary artery occlusion. *Am Heart J* 107:458, 1984.

58. Force T, Kemper A, Perkins L, et al: Overestimation of infarct size by quantitative two-dimensional echocardiography: the role of tethering and of analytic procedures. *Circulation* 73:1360, 1986.

59. Armstrong WM, Francis GS (eds): *Modern Coronary Care.* Boston, Little, Brown, 1990, p 455.

60. Tighe DA, Paul J, Aurigemma GP: Echocardiography in the diagnosis and assessment of mechanical complications of myocardial infarction. *Cardiac Ultrasound Today* 7:107, 2001.

61. Shively BK, Gurule FT, Roldan CA, et al: Diagnostic value of transesophageal compared with transthoracic echocardiography in infective endocarditis. *J Am Coll Cardiol* 18:391, 1991.

62. Jaffe WM, Morgan ED, Pearlman AS, et al: Infective endocarditis, 1983–1988: echocardiographic findings and factors influencing morbidity and mortality. *J Am Coll Cardiol* 15:1227, 1990.

63. Buda AJ, Zotz RJ, LeMire MS, et al: Prognostic significance of vegetations detected by two-dimensional echocardiography in infective endocarditis. *Am Heart J* 112:1291, 1986.

64. Stafford WJ, Petch J, Radford DJ: Vegetations in infective endocarditis: clinical relevance and diagnosis by cross-sectional echocardiography. *Br Heart J* 53:301, 1985.

65. Mugge A, Daniel WG, Frank G, et al: Echocardiography in infective endocarditis: reassessment of prognostic implications of vegetation size determined by the transthoracic and the transesophageal approach. *J Am Coll Cardiol* 14:631, 1989.

66. Sanfilippo AJ, Picard MH, Newell JB, et al: Echocardiographic assessment of patients with infectious endocarditis: prediction of risk for complications. *J Am Coll Cardiol* 18:1191, 1991.

67. Di Salvo G, Habib G, Pergola V, et al: Echocardiography predicts embolic events in infective endocarditis. *J Am Coll Cardiol* 37:1069, 2001.

68. Nienaber CA, von Kodolitsch Y, Nicolas V, et al: The diagnosis of thoracic aortic dissection by noninvasive imaging procedures. *N Engl J Med* 328:1, 1993.

69. Cigarroa JE, Isselbacher EM, DeSanctis RW, et al: Diagnostic imaging in the evaluation of suspected aortic dissection. *N Engl J Med* 328:35, 1991.

70. Rittoo D, Sutherland GR, Flapan SL: Role of transesophageal echocardiography in diagnosis and management of central pulmonary artery thromboembolism. *Am J Cardiol* 71:1115, 1993.

71. Victor MF, Mintz GS, Kotler MN, et al: Two-dimensional echocardiographic diagnosis of aortic dissection. *Am J Cardiol* 48:1155, 1981.

72. Granato JE, Dee P, Gibson RS: Utility of two-dimensional echocardiography in suspected ascending aortic dissection. *Am J Cardiol* 56:123, 1985.

73. Nienaber C, Spielmann R, Kodolitsch Y, et al: Diagnosis of thoracic aortic dissection: magnetic resonance imaging versus transesophageal echocardiography. *Circulation* 85:434, 1992.

74. Appelbe AF, Walker PG, Yeoh JK, et al: Clinical significance and origin of artifacts in transesophageal echocardiography of the thoracic aorta. *J Am Coll Cardiol* 21:754, 1993.

75. Smith MD, Cassidy JM, Souther S, et al: Transesophageal echocardiography in the diagnosis of traumatic rupture of the aorta. *N Engl J Med* 332:356, 1995.

76. Vignon P, Gueret P, Verdinne JM, et al: Role of transesophageal echocardiography in the diagnosis and management of traumatic aortic disruption. *Circulation* 92:2959, 1995.

8. Pericardiocentesis

Glenn D. Focht and Richard C. Becker

Pericardiocentesis is an important and potentially life-saving procedure performed in the critical care setting. It is not carried out with enough frequency, however, to allow most physicians to master the procedure. This chapter reviews the indications for emergent and urgent pericardiocentesis, summarizes the pathobiology of pericardial effusions, and provides a step-by-step approach to pericardiocentesis, including management of patients after the procedure.

Indications for Pericardiocentesis

The initial management of a patient with known or suspected pericardial effusion is largely determined by overall clinical status. In the absence of hemodynamic instability or suspected purulent bacterial pericarditis, there is no need for emergent or urgent pericardiocentesis. It may, however, be performed for diagnostic purposes. A thorough noninvasive workup should be completed before consideration of an invasive diagnostic procedure [1]. Whenever possible, elective pericardiocentesis should be performed using ultrasonography or fluoroscopic guidance.

In contrast, the management of hemodynamically compromised patients requires *emergent* removal of pericardial fluid to restore adequate ventricular filling (pre-load) and hasten clinical stabilization. The exact method and timing of pericardiocentesis is ultimately dictated by the patient's overall degree of instability. Patients with hypotension unresponsive to fluid resuscitation and vasopressor support require immediate, often unguided (blind), pericardiocentesis. In this setting, there are no absolute contraindications to the procedure, and it should therefore be performed without delay at the patient's bedside.

Urgent pericardiocentesis is indicated for patients who are initially hypotensive but respond quickly to aggressive fluid resuscitation. The procedure should be performed within several hours of presentation while careful monitoring and hemodynamic support continue. As in elective circumstances, pericardiocentesis in these patients should be undertaken with appropriate visual guidance, the method of which depends on the physician's expertise and resources. The modalities used most commonly are ultrasonography, echocardiography, and fluoroscopy.

Three additional points must be stressed regarding patients undergoing expedited pericardiocentesis. First, coagulation parameters—prothrombin time activated, partial thromboplastin time, and platelet count—should be checked and, when possible, quickly normalized prior to the procedure. Second, some critical care authorities advocate performance of all pericardiocentesis procedures in the catheterization laboratory with concomitant right heart pressure monitoring to document efficacy of the procedure and to exclude a constrictive element of pericardial disease (see Chapter 33) [2]. The authors support this approach; however, excessive delays because of scheduling difficulties must be avoided. Finally, efforts to assure a cooperative and stationary patient during the procedure greatly facilitate the performance, safety, and success of pericardiocentesis.

The clinical presentation of hemodynamically significant pericardial effusions varies widely among patients. A compre-

hensive understanding requires knowledge of normal pericardial anatomy and physiology.

Anatomy

The pericardium is a membranous structure with two layers separated by a small potential space. The *visceral* pericardium is closely but loosely adherent to the epicardial surface. It is a monolayer of mesothelial cells and attaches to the epicardium by a loose collection of small blood vessels, lymphatics, and connective tissue. The *parietal* pericardium is a fibrous structure that defines the outer membrane: Its inner surface is also composed of a monolayer of mesothelial cells. The remainder of the parietal pericardium consists of a dense network of connective tissue that is relatively nondistendible; therefore, it defines the dimensions and shape of the pericardium [3].

Further anatomic definition of the pericardium is derived from multiple attachments of the parietal pericardium in the thorax. Superiorly, the fibrous parietal pericardium attaches to the ascending aorta just below the arch. The inferior portion adheres strongly to the fibrous center of the diaphragm on which it rests. Anteriorly, the outer membrane is anchored to the sternum and costal cartilages by ligaments, as well as by a less-organized collection of connective tissue. The posterior margin of the parietal pericardium abuts the esophagus and pleural sacs; here, the visceral pericardium is absent and the parietal pericardium attaches directly to the epicardium at the borders of the entrance of the inferior and superior vena cavae and pulmonary veins [4]. Beyond providing stability, these multiple attachments also limit the inherent elasticity and distensibility of the pericardium.

This complex anatomic arrangement provides an anchor for the contracting myocardium and results in a small space between the visceral and parietal layers (pericardial space). The pericardial space or sac usually contains a small volume (15 to 50 mL) of clear, serous fluid that is chemically similar to a plasma ultrafiltrate [5,6]. The mechanism responsible for the production of pericardial fluid is not well understood. A homeostasis usually exists between new production of pericardial fluid and its drainage into the venous circulation via lymphatics.

The major determinant of when and how pericardial effusions come to clinical attention is directly related to the speed at which they develop. Effusions that collect rapidly (over minutes to hours) may cause hemodynamic compromise with volumes of 250 mL or less. These effusions are usually located posteriorly and are often difficult to detect without echocardiography. In contrast, effusions developing slowly (over days to weeks) allow for hypertrophy and distention (stretch) of the fibrous parietal membrane. Volumes of 2,000 mL or greater may accumulate without significant hemodynamic compromise. These patients may present with symptoms owing to compression of adjacent thoracic structures, such as cough, dyspnea, dysphagia, or early satiety. Three other clinical conditions promote hemodynamic compromise, even in the absence of large pericardial effusions: intravascular hypovolemia, impaired ventricular systolic function, and ventricular hypertrophy with decreased elasticity of the myocardium (diastolic dysfunction).

Procedure

Since the first blind or closed pericardiocentesis in 1840 [7], several different approaches have been described [8]. These approaches have varied considerably, particularly in the needle apparatus entry site. Marfan described the subcostal approach in 1911 [9], which then became the standard approach for unguided pericardiocentesis.

The advent of clinically applicable ultrasonography has opened a new chapter in diagnostic and therapeutic approaches to pericardial disease, allowing clinicians to quantitate and localize pericardial effusions quickly and noninvasively [10,11]. Work by Callahan and colleagues at the Mayo Clinic established the efficacy and safety of two-dimensional echocardiography to guide pericardiocentesis [12,13]. This has resulted in two major trends in clinical practice: First, two-dimensional echocardiography is commonly used to guide pericardiocentesis. Second, approaches other than the subxiphoid method have been investigated owing to the ability to clearly define the anatomy (location and volume) of each patient's effusion [8,12,13]. Typically, a four-chamber view of the heart is obtained by positioning the transducer at the apex. After insertion of the pericardiocentesis needle (described later), appropriate positioning within the pericardial space can be confirmed by injecting 5 mL of agitated saline (contrast). Echocardiography can also be used to reposition the needle safely if fluid return is suboptimal. Standard fluoroscopy can be used to confirm needle and catheter positioning within the pericardial space.

Formulas for quantitating the amount of pericardial fluid by echocardiographic or fluoroscopic means have not been established. As a rule, however, an effusion of moderate size (at least 250 mL) is required for percutaneous pericardiocentesis.

Regardless of whether echocardiography or another guidance method is used, the subxiphoid approach remains the

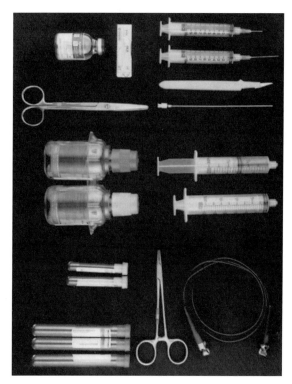

Fig. 8-1. Materials required for pericardiocentesis (clockwise from upper left): 1% lidocaine solution, suture material, 10-mL syringe with 25-gauge needle, 10-mL syringe with 22-gauge needle, No. 11 blade, 18-gauge 8-cm thin-walled needle, 20-mL syringe, 30-mL syringe, alligator clip, hemostat, three red-top tubes, two purple-top tubes, culture bottles, scissors.

standard of practice. The materials required for bedside pericardiocentesis are listed in Table 8-1 (Fig. 8-1). Table 8-2 (Fig. 8-2) lists the materials required for simultaneous placement of an intrapericardial drainage catheter. The materials are available in prepackaged kits or individually. The authors do not have a preference; the key to success is immediate availability of the necessary materials.

While the patient is being prepared for emergent or urgent pericardiocentesis, it is imperative that aggressive resuscitation measures are undertaken. Two large-bore peripheral intravenous lines should be placed for infusion of isotonic saline or colloid solutions. The use of inotropic agents and other vasoactive drugs (vasopressors) remains controversial [14–16], but when fluid resuscitation alone is inadequate, their use should be strongly considered.

Table 8-1. Materials for Pericardiocentesis

Site preparation
Antiseptic
Gauze
Sterile drapes and towels
Sterile gloves, masks, gowns, caps
5-mL or 10-mL syringe with 25-gauge needle
1% lidocaine (without epinephrine)
Code cart
Atropine (1-mg dose vial)
Procedure
No. 11 blade
20-mL syringe with 10 mL of 1% lidocaine (without epinephrine)
18-gauge, 8-cm, thin-walled needle with blunt tip
Multiple 20- and 40-mL syringes
Hemostat
Sterile alligator clip
Electrocardiogram machine
Three red-top tubes
Two purple-top (heparinized) tubes
Culture bottles
Postprocedure
Suture material
Scissors
Sterile gauze and bandage

Table 8-2. Materials for Intrapericardial Catheter

Catheter placement
Teflon-coated flexible J-curved guidewire
6-Fr dilator
8-Fr dilator
8-Fr, 35-cm flexible pigtail catheter with multiple fenestration (end and side holes)
Drainage system[a]
Three-way stopcock
Sterile IV tubing
500-mL sterile collecting bag (or bottle)
Sterile gauze and adhesive bag (or bottle)
Suture material

[a]System described allows continuous drainage.

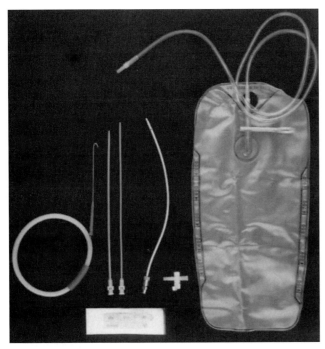

Fig. 8-2. Materials required for intrapericardial catheter placement and drainage (clockwise from lower left): Teflon-coated flexible 0.035-inch J-curved guidewire, 8-Fr dilator, 6.3-Fr dilator, 8-Fr catheter with end and side holes (35-cm flexible pigtail catheter not shown), three-way stopcock, 500-mL sterile collecting bag and tubing, suture material.

The subxiphoid approach for pericardiocentesis is as follows:

1. *Patient preparation.* Assist the patient in assuming a comfortable supine position with the head of the bed elevated to approximately 45 degrees from the horizontal plane. It is important for the patient to maintain this position during the procedure. Extremely dyspneic patients may need to be positioned fully upright, with a wedge if necessary. Elevation of the thorax allows free-flowing effusions to collect inferiorly and anteriorly, sites that are safest and easiest to access using the subxiphoid approach. The patient's bed should be placed at a comfortable height for the physician performing the procedure.

2. *Needle entry site selection.* Locate the patient's xiphoid process and the border of the left costal margin using inspection and careful palpation. The needle entry site should be 0.5 cm to the (patient's) left of the xiphoid process and 0.5 to 1.0 cm inferior to the costal margin (Fig. 8-3). It is essential that the surface anatomy be accurately defined before proceeding further. It is helpful to estimate (by palpation) the distance between the skin surface and the posterior margin of the bony thorax: This helps guide subsequent needle insertion. The usual distance is 1.0 to 2.5 cm, increasing with obesity or protuberance of the abdomen.

3. *Site preparation.* Strict sterile techniques must be maintained at all times in preparation of the needle entry site. Prepare a wide area in the subxiphoid region and lower thorax with a povidone-iodine solution and drape the field with sterile towels, leaving exposed the subxiphoid region. Raise a 1- to 2-cm subcutaneous wheal by infiltrating the needle entry site with 1% lidocaine solution (without epinephrine). Incise the skin with a No. 11 blade at the selected site after achieving adequate local anesthesia: This facilitates needle entry, which is at times difficult because of the absence of a bevel on the Teflon needle apparatus.

4. *Insertion of the needle apparatus.* Place the needle apparatus in the dominant hand (right-handed operators should

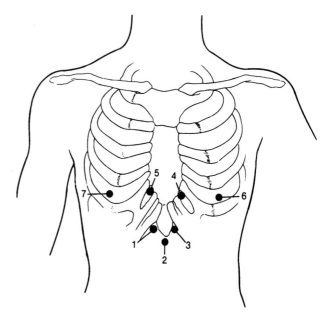

Fig. 8-3. Selected locations for pericardiocentesis. In most cases, the subxiphoid approach (1 to 3) is preferred. (From Spodick DH: *Acute Pericarditis.* New York, Grune & Stratton, 1959, with permission.)

stand to the patient's right and left-handed operators to the left) and insert it in the subxiphoid incision. The angle of entry (with the skin) should be approximately 45 degrees. Direct the needle tip superiorly, aiming for the patient's left shoulder. Continue to advance the needle posteriorly while alternating between aspiration and injection of lidocaine, until the tip has passed just beyond the posterior border of the bony thorax (Fig. 8-4). The posterior border usually lies within 2.5 cm of the skin surface. If the needle tip contacts the bony thorax, inject lidocaine after aspirating to clear the needle tip and anesthetize the periosteum. Then, walk the needle behind the posterior (costal) margin.

5. *Needle direction.* Reduce the angle of contact between the needle and skin to 15 degrees once the tip has passed the posterior margin of the bony thorax: This will be the angle of approach to the pericardium; the needle tip, however, should

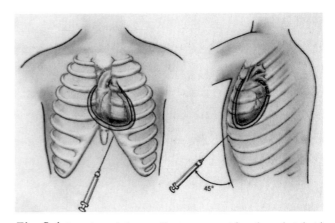

Fig. 8-4. Insertion of the needle apparatus. After the subxiphoid region and lower thorax are prepared and adequate local anesthesia is given, the pericardiocentesis needle is inserted in the subxiphoid incision. The angle of entry (with the skin) should be approximately 45 degrees. The needle tip should be directed superiorly, toward the patient's left shoulder.

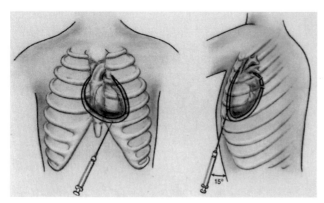

Fig. 8-5. Needle direction. The needle tip should be reduced to 15 degrees once the posterior margin of the bony thorax has been passed. Needle advancement: The needle is advanced toward the left shoulder slowly while alternating between aspiration and injection. A "give" is felt, and fluid is aspirated when the pericardial space is entered.

still be directed toward the patient's left shoulder. A 15-degree angle is used regardless of the height of the patient's thorax (whether at 45 degrees or sitting upright) (Fig. 8-5).

6. *Needle advancement.* Advance the needle slowly while alternating between aspiration of the syringe and injection of 1% lidocaine solution. If electrocardiographic guidance is used, apply the sterile alligator clip to the needle hub, being certain not to occlude the needle's lumen. Obtain a baseline lead V tracing and monitor a continuous tracing for the presence of ST-segment elevation or premature ventricular contractions (evidence of epicardial contact) as the needle is advanced. Advance the needle along this extrapleural path until either

a. A "give" is felt, and fluid is aspirated from the pericardial space (usually 6.0 to 7.5 cm from the skin) (Fig. 8-6). Some patients may experience a vasovagal response at this point and require atropine intravenously to increase their blood pressure and heart rate.

b. ST-segment elevation or premature ventricular contractions are observed on the electrocardiographic lead V tracing when the needle tip contacts the epicardium. If ST-segment elevation or premature ventricular complexes occur, immediately (and carefully) withdraw the needle toward the skin surface while aspirating. Avoid any lateral motion, which could damage the epicardial vessels. Completely withdraw the needle if no fluid is obtained during the initial repositioning.

The patient's hemodynamic status should improve promptly with removal of sufficient fluid. Successful relief of tamponade is supported by (a) a fall of intrapericardial pressure to levels between –3 and +3 mm Hg, (b) a fall in right atrial pressure and a separation between right and left ventricular diastolic pressures, (c) augmentation of cardiac output, (d) increased systemic blood pressure, and (e) reduced pulsus paradoxus to physiologic levels (10 mm Hg or less). An improvement may be observed after removal of the first 50 to 100 mL of fluid. If the right atrial pressure remains elevated after fluid removal, an effusive-constrictive process should be considered. The diagnostic studies performed on pericardial fluid are outlined in Table 8-3. Several options exist for continued drainage of the pericardial space. The simplest approach is to use large-volume syringes and aspirate the fluid by hand. This approach is not always practical (i.e., in large-volume effusions), however, and manipulation of the needle apparatus may cause myocardial trauma. Alternatively, some pericardiocentesis kits include materials and instructions for a catheter-over-

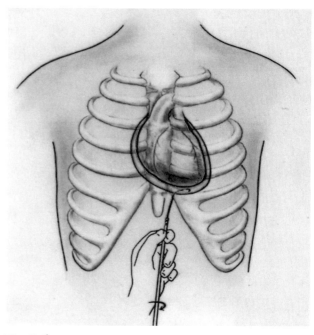

Fig. 8-6. Placement technique. Holding the needle in place, a Teflon-coated, 0.035-in. guidewire is advanced into the pericardial space. The needle is then removed. After a series of skin dilations, an 8-Fr, 35-cm flexible pigtail catheter is placed over the guidewire into the pericardial space. Passage of dilators and the pigtail catheter is facilitated by a gentle clockwise/counterclockwise motion.

needle technique for inserting a pericardial drain. Finally, the Seldinger technique may be used to place an indwelling pericardial drain.

7. *Placement technique.* Create a track for the catheter by passing a 6-Fr dilator over a firmly held guidewire. After removing the dilator, use the same technique to pass an 8-Fr dilator. Then advance an 8-Fr flexible pigtail catheter over the guidewire into the pericardial space. Remove the guidewire. Passage of the dilators is facilitated by use of a torquing (clockwise/counterclockwise) motion. A wider incision at the base of the guidewire may be required to pass the dilators. Proper positioning of the catheter using radiography, fluoroscopy, or bedside echocardiography can be used to facilitate fluid drainage.

8. *Drainage system* [17–20]. Attach a three-way stopcock to the intrapericardial catheter and close the system by attaching the stopcock to the sterile collecting bag with the connecting

Table 8-3. Diagnostic Studies Performed on Pericardial Fluid

Hematocrit
White blood cell count with differential
Glucose
Protein
Gram's stain
Routine aerobic and anaerobic cultures
Smear and culture for acid-fast bacilli
Cytology
Other studies as indicated
Cholesterol, triglyceride
Amylase
Lactate dehydrogenase
Special cultures (viral, parasite studies)
Antinuclear antibody
Rheumatoid factor
Total complement, C_3

Table 8-4. Complications of Pericardiocentesis

Cardiac puncture
Uncomplicated
Secondary hemopericardium, myocardial infarction
Pneumothorax
Arrhythmias
Bradycardia
Ventricular tachycardia
Trauma to abdominal organs (liver, gastrointestinal tract)
Cardiac arrest (predominantly electromechanical dissociation from myocardial perforation, but occasionally tachyarrhythmia or bradyarrhythmia)[a]
Rare
Coronary artery laceration (left anterior descending coronary artery, right coronary artery)
Infection
Fistula formation
Pulmonary edema

[a]Incidence has varied from 0% to 5% in studies and was less common in guided procedures, more common in "blind" procedures [1,21,22].

Table 8-6. Common Causes of Pericardial Effusion

Idiopathic
Malignancy
Uremia
Postpericardiotomy syndrome
Connective tissue disease
Trauma
Blunt
Penetrating
Infection
Viral
Bacterial
Fungal
Tuberculosis
Aortic dissection
Complication of cardiac catheterization or pacemaker insertion
Myxedema
Postirradiation

tubing. The catheter may also be connected to a transducer, allowing intrapericardial pressure monitoring. The system may be secured as follows:

a. Suture the pigtail catheter to the skin, making sure the lumen is not compressed. Cover the entry site with a sterile gauze and dressing.

b. Secure the drainage bag (or bottle) using tape at a level approximately 35 to 50 cm below the level of the heart. This system may be left in place for 48 to 72 hours. Echocardiography or fluoroscopic guidance may be used to reposition the pigtail catheter, facilitating complete drainage of existing pericardial fluid.

The catheter should be flushed every 4 to 6 hours using 10 to 15 cc of normal saline solution.

Short-Term and Long-Term Management

After pericardiocentesis, close monitoring is required to detect evidence of recurrent tamponade and procedure-related complications. Table 8-4 lists the most common serious complications associated with pericardiocentesis [1,21,22]. Factors associated with an increased risk of complications include (a) small effusion (less than 250 mL), (b) posterior effusion, (c) loculated effusion, (d) maximum anterior clear space (by echocardiography) less than 10 mm, and (e) unguided percutaneous

approach. All patients undergoing pericardiocentesis should have a portable chest radiograph performed immediately after the procedure to exclude the presence of pneumothorax. In addition, a transthoracic two-dimensional echocardiogram should be obtained within several hours to evaluate the adequacy of pericardial drainage. Echocardiography can also be used to confirm catheter placement.

Finally, careful technique is required to maintain the sterility of the pericardial catheter drainage system. With meticulous local care, the complication rate is exceptionally low, even when the catheter is left in place for 36 to 48 hours [12,18].

The long-term management of patients with significant pericardial fluid collections is beyond the scope of this chapter (see Chapter 33); however, the role of surgical intervention is reviewed briefly. The indications for surgical intervention are controversial and vary widely (Table 8-5) [2,23–28]. Several indications that have been established include (a) pericardial disease with concomitant constrictive physiology, (b) known loculated or posteriorly located effusions not amenable to pericardiocentesis, (c) suspected purulent pericarditis, (d) effusions not successfully drained by pericardiocentesis, and (e) rapidly recurring effusions [2,29]. The etiology of the pericardial effusion (Table 8-6) and the patient's functional status are of central importance for determining the preferred treatment. Aggressive attempts at nonsurgical management of chronically debilitated patients or those with metastatic disease involving the pericardium may be appropriate [25,30,31]. Pericardial sclerosis with tetracycline or other agents has benefited carefully selected patients with malignant pericardial disease [30,32,33]. Patients with a guarded prognosis who fail aggressive medical therapy should be offered the least invasive procedure.

Table 8-5. Major Surgical Options for the Management of Pericardial Effusions

Procedure	Approach	Resection Margins
Pericardial window		
Subxiphoid	Subxiphoid	<9 cm² block
Pleural	Thoracotomy	<9 cm² block
Partial pericardiectomy	Thoracotomy	Right phrenic nerve; great vessels to diaphragmatic reflection
Complete pericardiectomy	Thoracotomy or sternotomy	Right phrenic nerve to left pulmonary vein; great vessels to midportion of diaphragmatic pericardium

References

1. Permayer-Miulda G, Sagrista-Savleda J, Soler-Soler J: Primary acute pericardial disease: a prospective study of 231 consecutive patients. *Am J Cardiol* 56:623, 1985.
2. Lovell BH, Braunwald E: Pericardial disease, in Braunwald E (ed): *Heart Disease: A Textbook of Cardiovascular Medicine.* Philadelphia, WB Saunders, 1988, p 1484.
3. Tandler J: *Anatomie des Harsens.* Jeng, Fischer, 1913. Quoted by Elias H, Boyd LJ: Notes on the anatomy, embryology and histology of the pericardium. *J N Y Med Coll* 2:50, 1960.
4. Roberts WC, Spray TL: Pericardial heart disease: a study of its causes, consequences, and morphologic features, in Spodick D (ed): *Pericardial Diseases.* Philadelphia, FA Davis, 1976, p 17.

5. Shabatai R: Function of the pericardium, in Fowler NO (ed): *The Pericardium in Health and Disease*. Mount Kisco, NY, Futura, 1985, p 19.
6. Shabetai R: *The Pericardium*. New York, Grune & Stratton, 1981.
7. Schuh R: Erfahrungen uber de Paracentese der Brust und des Herz Beutels. *Med Jahrb Osterr Staates Wien* 33:388, 1841.
8. Tilkian AG, Daily EK: Pericardiocentesis and drainage, in Tilkian AG, Daily EK (eds): *Cardiovascular Procedures: Diagnostic Techniques and Therapeutic Approaches*. St. Louis, Mosby, 1986, p 231.
9. Marfan AB: Poncitian du pericarde par l espigahe. *Ann Med Chir Infarct* 15:529, 1911.
10. Pandian NG, Brockway B, Simonetti J, et al: Pericardiocentesis under 2-dimensional echocardiographic guidance in loculated pericardial effusion. *Ann Thorac Surg* 45:99, 1988.
11. Chandraratna PA, Reid CL, Nimalasuriya A, et al: Application of 2-dimensional contrast studies during pericardiocentesis. *Am J Cardiol* 52:1120, 1983.
12. Callahan JA, Seward JB, Nishimura RA: 2-dimensional echocardiography-guided pericardiocentesis: experience in 117 consecutive patients. *Am J Cardiol* 55:476, 1985.
13. Callahan JA, Seward JB, Tajik AJ: Pericardiocentesis assisted by 2-dimensional echocardiography. *J Thorac Cardiovasc Surg* 85:877, 1983.
14. Callahan M: Pericardiocentesis in traumatic and non-traumatic cardiac tamponade. *Ann Emerg Med* 13:924, 1984.
15. Fowler NO, Guberman BA, Gueron M: Cardiac tamponade, in Eliot RS (ed): *Cardiac Emergencies*. 2nd ed. Mount Kisco, NY, Futura, 1982, p 415.
16. Seldinger S: Catheter replacement of the needle in percutaneous angiography. *Acta Radiol Diagn (Stockh)* 39:368.
17. Kapoor AS: Technique of pericardiocentesis and intrapericardial drainage, in Kapoor AS (ed): *International Cardiology*. New York, Springer-Verlag, 1989, p 146.
18. Kopecky SL, Callahan JA, Tajik AJ, et al: Percutaneous pericardial catheter drainage: report of 42 consecutive cases. *Am J Cardiol* 58:633, 1986.
19. Massumi RA, Rios JC, Ewy GA: Technique for insertion of an indwelling pericardial catheter. *Br Heart J* 30:333, 1960.
20. Patel AK, Kogolcharoen PK, Nallasivan M, et al: Catheter drainage of the pericardium: practical method to maintain long-term patency. *Chest* 92:1018, 1987.
21. Wong B, Murphy J, Chang CJ, et al: The risk of pericardiocentesis. *Am J Cardiol* 44:1110, 1979.
22. Krikorian JG, Hancock EW: Pericardiocentesis. *Am J Med* 65:808, 1978.
23. Piehler JM, Pluth JR, Schaff HV, et al: Surgical management of effusive pericardial disease: Influence of extent of pericardial resection on clinical cause. *J Thorac Cardiovasc Surg* 90:506, 1985.
24. Little AG, Kremser PC, Wade JL, et al: Operation for diagnosis and treatment of pericardial effusions. *Surgery* 96:738, 1984.
25. Palatianos GM, Thuer RJ, Karser GA: Comparison of effectiveness and safety of operations on the pericardium. *Chest* 88:30, 1985.
26. Little AG, Fergusen MK: Pericardioscopy as adjunct to pericardial window. *Chest* 89:53, 1986.
27. Prager RL, Wilson CH, Border WH Jr: The subxiphoid approach to pericardial disease. *Ann Thorac Surg* 34:6, 1982.
28. Spodick DH: Pericardial windows are suboptimal. *Am J Cardiol* 51:607, 1983.
29. Rub RH, Moelleering RC: Clinical microbiologic and therapeutic aspects of purulent pericarditis. *Am J Med* 59:68, 1975.
30. Shepherd FA, Morgan C, Evans WK, et al: Medical management of malignant pericardial effusion by tetracycline sclerosis. *Am J Cardiol* 60:1161, 1987.
31. Morm JE, Hallonby D, Gonda A, et al: Management of uremia pericarditis: a report of 11 patients with cardiac tamponade and a review of the literature. *Ann Thorac Surg* 22:588, 1976.
32. Reitknecht F, Regal AM, Antkowiak JG, et al: Management of cardiac tamponade in patients with malignancy. *J Surg Oncol* 30:19, 1985.
33. Biran S, Brufman G, Klein E, et al: The management of pericardial effusion in cancer patients. *Chest* 71:182, 1977.

9. *The Intraaortic Balloon and Counterpulsation*

Bruce S. Cutler and Michael J. Singh

External left ventricular assist devices (LVADs) are of two types. The first type reduces left ventricular work by functioning as a pump in a parallel circuit with the heart. The second is the intraaortic balloon pump (IABP), which assists the ischemic left ventricle through improvement in coronary artery perfusion and reduction in systemic afterload by counterpulsation. The IABP is by far the most widely used LVAD because of its effectiveness, ease of application, and relative safety [1].

Equipment

The balloon is composed of a thin polyurethane or silicone membrane that provides strength and antithrombotic properties. Mechanical failures, including leaks, are rare. Intraaortic balloons are available in 25- to 50-cc volumes. The most commonly used size is 40 cc, which measures 15 mm × 263 mm (Table 9-1). The most common balloon catheter diameter is

6.5 French (Fr), which will pass through an 8-Fr introducer. This diameter is compatible with the insertion sheaths used for diagnostic and therapeutic cardiac catheterization, which facilitates intraaortic balloon (IAB) insertion in conjunction with other percutaneous cardiac procedures. Balloons are mounted on the end of a coaxial catheter. The smaller central lumen is used to pass a 0.020- or 0.025-in. guidewire during insertion and to monitor central aortic pressure. The outer lumen is the passageway for gas exchange and is connected to a console that synchronizes inflation and deflation with the cardiac cycle and makes automatic adjustments for changes in heart rate and rhythm. Circuitry in the console detects arrhythmias, gas leaks, and internal malfunctions. Helium is used as the driving gas because its low molecular weight allows the high gas velocities necessary at elevated heart rates without excessive generation of heat. Although the IAB can cycle as rapidly as 160 to 200 times per minute, the efficiency of counterpulsation is reduced at heart rates over 130 beats per minute. Pharmacologic control of tachycardia or other arrhythmia may be necessary for optimal IAB function.

Table 9-1. Fitting the Balloon to the Patient

Manufacturer	Patient height (cm)	Body surface area (m²)	IAB volume (cc)	IAB length (mm)
Datascope	<152	—	25	174
(Montvale, NJ)	153–162	—	34	219
	163–183	—	40	263
	>183	—	50	269
Arrow (Reading, PA)	—	<1.8	30	230
	—	>1.8	40	262

IAB, intraaortic balloon.

Physiology

Counterpulsation improves left ventricular performance through a favorable influence on the myocardial oxygen supply and demand ratio. Counterpulsation is timed so that the balloon inflates at the beginning of diastole and deflates during systole. Because the majority of coronary blood flow occurs during diastole, balloon inflation raises the diastolic pressure in the aortic root and enhances coronary perfusion. Improvement in coronary blood flow occurs without an increase in myocardial work and results in a 10% to 20% reduction in oxygen consumption. Counterpulsation also mechanically reduces impedance to ventricular ejection by deflating immediately before isovolumetric contraction, producing an intravascular volume deficit of approximately 40 cc in the aortic root. This allows the next ventricular contraction to occur against a reduced afterload, resulting in a further reduction in the myocardial oxygen requirement. Thus, the net effect of counterpulsation in a patient with cardiogenic shock is to increase coronary blood flow and myocardial oxygen supply while reducing myocardial work and oxygen consumption. Cardiac output may increase by as much as 50%.

In contrast to other types of circulatory assist devices, the IAB requires a minimum cardiac index of 1.2 to 1.4 L per minute per m² to be effective. Because of the requirement of minimum intrinsic left ventricular ejection, the IAB cannot assist the patient who is asystolic or in ventricular fibrillation. IAB counterpulsation has little effect on the perfusion of myocardium supplied by occluded coronary arteries [2].

Indications

CARDIOGENIC SHOCK. The IAB was developed in the hope of reversing cardiogenic shock after myocardial infarction. Clinical studies from a number of institutions have confirmed that counterpulsation is successful in reversing ventricular dysfunction, at least temporarily, in 80% to 85% of patients [3,4]. Postmortem studies of refractory patients show extensive infarction involving 50% or more of the left ventricle [5]. Although counterpulsation is initially effective in reversing shock after myocardial infarction, a disappointingly high percentage of such patients become dependent on the IAB, as demonstrated by a decrease in systemic arterial pressure and cardiac output and an increase in left atrial filling pressures when counterpulsation is temporarily discontinued. Under these circumstances, there is relatively little potential for spontaneous improvement in left ventricular function after myocardial infarction, and coun-

terpulsation by itself simply postpones the inevitable outcome. When the IAB is used alone in the treatment of cardiogenic shock after myocardial infarction, the 1-year survival rate is only 9% to 22% [6].

It is important that the anatomic and functional derangements responsible for cardiogenic shock be corrected if the high rate of IAB dependence is to be reduced. Animal and clinical studies indicate that infarcted myocardium is surrounded by a zone of ischemic tissue that may redevelop effective contractility if satisfactory coronary perfusion can be restored through thrombolytic therapy, angioplasty, or aortocoronary surgery. Counterpulsation should be initiated as soon as it is determined that the shock state is not responsive to volume expansion and drug therapy. Once stabilized, as indicated by improvement in the cardiac index, peripheral perfusion, and urinary output, the patient should undergo cardiac catheterization and, if feasible, revascularization. The IAB is usually removed a day or two later. Only approximately 40% of patients with cardiogenic shock after myocardial infarction are suitable candidates for revascularization. Although the overall mortality rate for early revascularization after myocardial infarction is 50%, this represents an improvement when compared with medical therapy alone.

REVERSIBLE MECHANICAL DEFECTS. Counterpulsation is very effective in the initial stabilization of patients with mechanical intracardiac defects complicating infarction, such as acute mitral regurgitation and ventricular septal perforation. Counterpulsation reduces pulmonary artery pressure and increases cardiac output for both of these lesions, and it also decreases the regurgitant V wave seen in mitral insufficiency. Mitral valve replacement with concomitant coronary revascularization is the usual treatment for rupture of a papillary muscle.

Acute ventricular septal defects are usually caused by infarction of the septum due to occlusion of the left anterior or posterior descending coronary artery, or both. The timing of surgical repair of an acute ventricular septal defect remains controversial. Some cardiologists have advocated early repair, before the development of multiple organ failure. Early operation poses the technical difficulty of suturing recently infarcted tissue and is associated with a surgical mortality of 36% [7]. With the delayed approach, mortality is reduced, but some patients die before operation. Both methods of treatment rely on counterpulsation to maintain pre- and postoperative hemodynamic stability [8].

UNSTABLE ANGINA. Counterpulsation is effective in the treatment of unstable angina. To be maximally effective, the IAB should be inserted before irreversible myocardial injury and cardiogenic shock occur. Some institutions use counterpulsation very liberally in the treatment of unstable angina and report surgical mortality rates approaching those for chronic stable angina—2% to 6% [9]. Such statistics are difficult to evaluate because the majority of patients with unstable angina also do well with aggressive medical therapy alone. Until more exact guidelines are developed from the results of randomized comparative trials, treatment of patients with unstable angina rests on clinical judgment. Counterpulsation should not be used as a substitute for vigorous pharmacologic therapy; however, counterpulsation is indicated when angina is persistent and when there is ongoing electrocardiographic evidence of ischemia, despite maximal medical therapy.

POSTCARDIOTOMY CARDIOGENIC SHOCK. One of the most useful and most common indications for counterpulsation is to aid in weaning patients from cardiopulmonary bypass who have sustained perioperative myocardial injury [10]. Postsurgical myocardial dysfunction is often reversible if the patient's circulation can be assisted for 24 to 48 hours. The best results are achieved when counterpulsation is used in conjunction with optimal preloading, reduction of afterload with vasodilators, and early institution of inotropic support to increase cardiac output. When used in this setting, approximately 75% of bypass-dependent patients can be successfully weaned, with a 50% 2-year survival rate. The best results are reported for patients with pure coronary artery disease, rather than for those requiring valve replacement or repair. Postcardiotomy patients who are refractory to counterpulsation usually require an LVAD to prevent further myocardial decompensation (see Chapter 10) [11].

PREOPERATIVE USE. Routine preoperative use of counterpulsation has been advocated by some centers for certain high-risk patients, including those with unstable angina requiring emergency procedures or left main coronary stenosis greater than 70%. It is also advocated for off-pump bypass to posterior coronary arteries [12], marked left ventricular dysfunction with an ejection fraction of less than 0.35, and redo coronary operations [13–15]. Patients who are placed on IAB support preoperatively are reported to have decreased cardiopulmonary bypass time, reduced mortality, and shorter intensive care unit stays. However, with improvements in anesthetic techniques and more sophisticated intraoperative monitoring, many institutions now report surgical mortality rates for left main coronary disease equivalent to those for other types of coronary surgery without preoperative support [16]. Because the incidence of peripheral vascular complications associated with the use of the IAB is significant, the risk of lower limb ischemia must be weighed against the potential benefits of routine counterpulsation. Most centers now use counterpulsation selectively for patients with diminished ejection fractions and complicated redo procedures [17].

BRIDGE TO TRANSPLANTATION. Counterpulsation has been used to provide mechanical support for patients in left ventricular failure while they await cardiac transplantation. The IAB may be used alone or in combination with other assist devices, such as an extracorporeal membrane oxygenator, LVAD, or implantable artificial heart. Not surprisingly, the incidence of bacteremia is higher and the survival rate reduced for bridged patients compared to those not requiring preoperative assistance [18].

PERCUTANEOUS CORONARY ANGIOPLASTY. The indications and experience with percutaneous coronary angioplasty have expanded to include patients with multiple coronary lesions and those with impaired left ventricular function [19]. Many centers now use counterpulsation to control unstable angina before and during coronary angioplasty and stenting [20,21]. The IAB has also been recommended for prophylactic use in patients with severe left ventricular dysfunction and during angioplasty and stenting of an unprotected left main coronary stenosis or a protected stenosis with reduced left ventricular function [22]. Some investigators have found that counterpulsation decreases the risk of acute coronary reocclusion after percutaneous transluminal coronary angioplasty, whereas others have found no benefit to the overall clinical outcome [23,24]. Nonetheless, counterpulsation may be lifesaving after a failed angioplasty to support the myocardium until emergency aortocoronary revascularization can be performed.

CHILDREN. Use of the extracorporeal membrane oxygenator has been the most widely used method to treat low cardiac output states in children because it provides biventricular and pulmonary support, whereas counterpulsation benefits only the left ventricle. At one time, there was concern that the greater elasticity of the aortic wall in children would prevent effective diastolic augmentation [25,26]. Recently, however, small-caliber balloons have been developed and consoles have been modified for the small volumes and high heart rates required for pediatric use. Counterpulsation has been effectively used in infants as young as 7 days [25]. Counterpulsation appears to be of value in treating perioperative left ventricular failure and appears to support low cardiac output states until the extracorporeal membrane oxygenator can be instituted.

LESS FREQUENT INDICATIONS. Counterpulsation is frequently used to stabilize patients in cardiogenic shock or with refractory angina during transit from a community hospital to a tertiary care facility, where more definitive treatment is available [27]. Successful use of IABs for treatment of heart failure after myocardial trauma has been reported [28]. Counterpulsation has also been used for perioperative support of high-risk noncardiac surgery, such as aortic aneurysm resection or general surgical procedures [29]. Under most circumstances, it is preferable to improve the cardiac status of such patients with preliminary percutaneous transluminal coronary angioplasty or aortocoronary surgery. In some instances, however, because of diffuse disease, limited ventricular function, or severe aortoiliac occlusive disease, coronary revascularization may not be feasible for patients in need of a major surgical procedure. Preliminary results from counterpulsation for noncardiac operations are encouraging, but experience is still too limited to recommend its widespread use in this setting [30,31].

Contraindications

Aortic valvular insufficiency, aortic dissection, and severe aortoiliac occlusive disease are absolute contraindications to counterpulsation. In the presence of aortic regurgitation, an IABP would cause transmission of the augmented diastolic pressure directly to the left ventricle, which could result in ventricular rupture in a patient with a recent myocardial infarction. The presence of prosthetic vascular grafts in the thoracic or abdominal aorta, thoracic or abdominal aortic aneurysms, and aortofemoral grafts are considered relative contraindications. The sheathless insertion technique should not be used in markedly obese patients or in the presence of severe scarring in the inguinal area. Because of the need for anticoagulation during counterpulsation, gastrointestinal bleeding, thrombocytopenia, and other bleeding diatheses are relative contraindications to counterpulsation.

Insertion Technique

The technique of IAB insertion described here, while generally applicable to all guidewire-directed IABs, is not intended to be a substitute for thorough familiarity with the manufacturer's instructions. New IAB devices are frequently introduced, each of which has its own variations in technique and list of precautions.

The following equipment is needed:

1. Manufacturer-supplied sterile insertion kit, including IAB, percutaneous insertion needle, guidewires, vessel dilators, introducer sheath, connector tubing, one-way valve, syringe, and three-way stopcock
2. Portable fluoroscope or transesophageal echocardiography (TEE)
3. Povidone-iodine prep solution, sterile drapes, gowns, gloves, and towel clips
4. 1% lidocaine with syringe and 22-gauge, 1.5-in. needle
5. Sterile gauze pads
6. No. 11 scalpel blade and handle
7. Dilute heparin solution (10,000 U in 500 mL of normal saline)
8. Two 0 silk sutures on curved cutting needles
9. Needle holder
10. 5,000 U heparin and a 10-mL syringe

Before insertion, the reasons for recommending counterpulsation therapy and potential complications should be fully explained to the patient and family and informed consent obtained. Because the IAB should be inserted on the side with the best circulation, any history suggesting vascular insufficiency, such as intermittent claudication or rest pain, should be ascertained. Femoral, popliteal, and pedal pulses in both lower extremities should be palpated. If pedal pulses are absent, the ankle arm index should be measured with a portable Doppler ultrasonic flow detector to determine the limb with the best circulation.

IABs are manufactured in several sizes to approximate the dimensions of the descending thoracic aorta. The appropriately sized balloon should be selected based on the patient's height or body surface area (Table 9-1). An indwelling cannula in the radial artery is very helpful to monitor arterial pressure and to time counterpulsation; it may be placed before insertion of the IAB (see Chapter 3). In an emergency, the IAB may be placed first and the central lumen of the balloon used to measure arterial pressure.

The procedure should be performed with the patient supine. Cannulation of the femoral artery is very difficult if the patient cannot lie perfectly flat. In the severely orthopneic patient, controlled respiration with a mechanical ventilator may be required. Insertion of the IAB should be carried out on a radiolucent bed, operating table, or cardiac catheterization table to permit the use of fluoroscopy. An assistant should be available to prepare a sterile field on which supplies can be arranged. Alternatively, TEE may be used instead of fluoroscopy to guide placement of the balloon. TEE is particularly useful when the IAB is inserted in conjunction with cardiac surgery.

Both inguinal areas are shaved and cleansed with povidone soap and water, followed by povidone-iodine solution. Sterile towels and sheets are used as drapes, leaving exposed a wide area over both femoral arteries. The contents of the insertion kit should be opened and arranged in order of use. The balloon should be handled very carefully to avoid damage to the delicate membrane and kinking of the catheter. The instructions for preparing the IAB should be followed closely, because the technique varies with the manufacturer. The most common method involves aspiration of a sterile one-way valve on the IAB Luer fitting with a 60-mL syringe. The syringe is removed from the valve when the IAB is fully collapsed. The balloon should be left in its protective sleeve until the femoral artery is cannulated. The central lumen of the balloon and the percutaneous angiographic needle should be flushed with dilute heparin saline.

Next, 10 mL of 1% lidocaine is infiltrated subdermally and subcutaneously over the femoral artery pulse. The puncture site should be 1 cm below the inguinal crease directly over the femoral pulsation. The femoral artery can be immobilized between

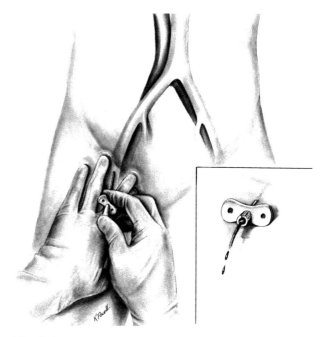

Fig. 9-1. The angiographic needle is inserted at a 45-degree angle into the common femoral artery. **Inset:** Pulsatile jet of blood indicates that the needle is properly located in the center of the arterial lumen.

the third and fourth fingers while the introducer needle is inserted at a 45-degree angle with the bevel pointing cephalad. The needle is passed through the anterior wall of the common femoral artery. Intraluminal placement is confirmed by a strong pulsatile jet of blood (Fig. 9-1). A weak jet of blood indicates that the needle is not properly located in the center of the arterial lumen; it should be withdrawn and replaced. When the needle is properly placed in the artery, a J guidewire, 145 cm long and 0.020 or 0.025 in. in diameter, is passed though the needle and advanced under fluoroscopic control until the tip is in the thoracic aorta (Fig. 9-2). The guidewire should easily pass through the cannula. Even minimal resistance may indicate that the guidewire is coiling. Under these circumstances, the guidewire should be removed, the needle repositioned for a brisk jet of blood, and another attempt made with a new wire. When the tip of the guidewire is satisfactorily positioned in the thoracic aorta, the patient should be intravenously anticoagulated with 5,000 U of heparin. The introducer needle is withdrawn, leaving the guidewire in place. To facilitate passage of the dilators and sheaths, a 4-mm incision is made at the puncture site using a no. 11 scalpel blade. A 6/8-Fr tapered dilator is passed over the guidewire and, with a rotating motion, passed through the skin and subcutaneous tissue into the femoral artery (Fig. 9-3). This dilator is removed and exchanged for a 8-Fr dilator with an overlying Teflon sheath. Pressure is maintained over the puncture site to control bleeding during the exchange. Approximately 2.5 cm of the sheath is left exposed caudal to the puncture site.

The IAB is removed from the protective sleeve with care not to touch the balloon surface with metal instruments, which can damage the polyurethane membrane. The dilator is removed, leaving the introducer sheath and guidewire in the artery. The sheath contains a valve to prevent back-bleeding during this maneuver. The free end of the guidewire is passed through the central lumen of the IAB. The IAB is advanced over the guidewire and through the sheath into the descending thoracic aorta, under fluoroscopic or TEE guidance (Fig. 9-4). As the IAB is advanced, a slight "give" or decrease in resistance is detected as the IAB exits from the distal end of the sheath. The tip of the balloon is radiopaque and readily visible by fluoros-

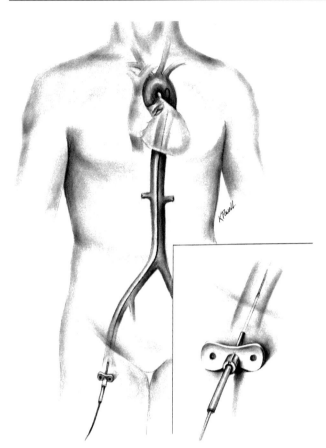

Fig. 9-2. When the angiographic needle is properly placed in the artery, the guidewire is advanced under fluoroscopic control until the tip is in the thoracic aorta (see **inset**).

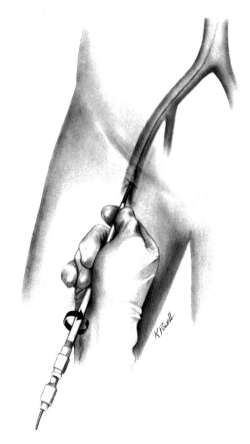

Fig. 9-3. A 8.0-French dilator with overlying Teflon introducer sheath is passed over the guidewire. A rotary motion and firm pressure are necessary to enter the lumen of the femoral artery.

copy or TEE. It should be positioned 2 cm distal to the origin of the left subclavian artery or at the caudal wall of the transverse aortic arch [31,32]. The IAB must be inserted to the level of the manufacturer's mark (usually a double line) on the IAB catheter to ensure that the entire membrane has emerged from the sheath to permit complete balloon opening. Failure of the balloon to completely exit the sheath will reduce diastolic augmentation, cause high balloon filling pressures, and lead to balloon fatigue and eventual rupture with gas embolization. When the IAB is properly positioned, the sheath seal is pushed over the hub of the sheath to control bleeding (Fig. 9-5). Return of blood though the central lumen of the IAB provides reassurance that the device has not caused a dissection. When in doubt, a small quantity of angiographic dye may be injected to confirm the final position of the IAB; thereafter, the central lumen should be carefully aspirated, flushed with heparinized saline, and used to monitor intraaortic pressure and to time counterpulsation. The one-way valve is removed and the female Luer fitting connected to the gas delivery line from the IAB console. The IAB and sheath should be secured to the inner thigh with heavy silk sutures. Antibiotic ointment should be applied to the puncture site, followed by a sterile occlusive dressing.

Alternatively, the IAB may be inserted without the use of the sheath, which reduces the intraluminal arterial obstruction and may decrease the risk of ischemic complications to the lower limb. Sheathless insertion of the IAB results in a 30% reduction in the cross-sectional area occupied by the catheter [33]. The sheathless technique is identical to that just described, except that insertion of the introducer, dilator, and sheath is omitted. The stepped dilator is advanced over the

wire to dilate the subcutaneous tunnel and arterial wall puncture. The dilator is then removed from the guidewire. Passage of the IAB without a sheath requires a more spacious subcutaneous tunnel, which can be produced by gently spreading a mosquito hemostat along the tract of the guidewire. The IAB should be moistened with sterile saline before insertion. The inner stylet is removed by rotating the Luer lock fitting one-half turn counterclockwise. The free end of the guidewire is inserted into the tip of the IAB until it exits from the female Luer fitting of the hub. The IAB is advanced over the guidewire through the skin and subcutaneous tissue, holding the IAB close to the insertion point to prevent kinking. As the IAB enters the artery, blood under arterial pressure runs back along the folds of the balloon but should stop once the IAB is completely inserted. The balloon is advanced to the proper position in the descending thoracic aorta. Sterility of the exposed catheter is maintained until its position has been confirmed by fluoroscopy or chest radiograph because it cannot be repositioned once it has been contaminated. The guidewire is removed, and the central lumen is aspirated and then flushed with dilute heparin. When the final position of the IAB has been verified, the hub is secured to the inner thigh with heavy silk sutures and covered with a sterile occlusive dressing. Counterpulsation is initiated as described earlier.

Insertion of the IAB is most safely performed with fluoroscopy. In emergency conditions, the IAB may be inserted without fluoroscopy. Under these circumstances, the length of the IAB to be inserted should be approximated by laying the device on the patient's chest so that the tip lies at the level of the third intercostal space and then marking the site on the catheter where it will exit the introducer with a silk tie. After

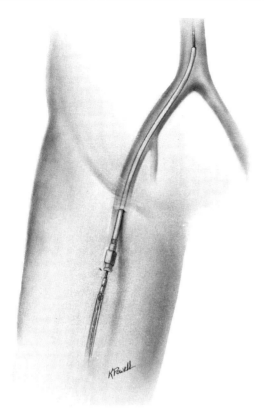

Fig. 9-4. The intraaortic balloon is advanced over the guidewire into the descending thoracic aorta under fluoroscopic guidance.

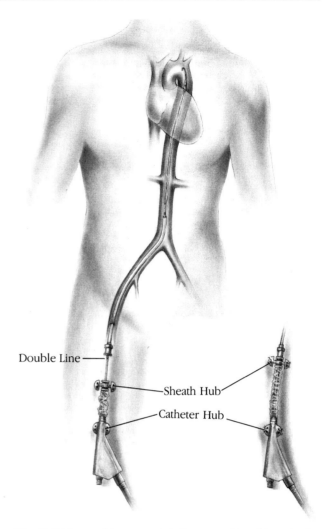

Fig. 9-5. The tip of the intraaortic balloon is positioned 2 cm distal to the origin of the left subclavian artery. The intraaortic balloon must be inserted to the level of the double line to be sure the entire membrane has emerged from the sheath. **Inset:** The sheath seal is pushed over the sheath hub to control bleeding. The sheath and catheter hubs are sutured in place.

insertion, the final position of the IAB must be verified with a portable chest radiograph and adjusted as necessary. TEE is frequently used to evaluate left ventricular function during cardiac operations [34,35]. Because of its ability to image the thoracic aorta in real time, it facilitates the insertion and positioning of the guidewire and balloon catheter. TEE can also confirm the presence of significant aortic valvular regurgitation, severe atherosclerotic aortic disease, acute aortic dissection, or misplacement of the IAB. It is a relatively noninvasive means to evaluate the position of the IAB in the thoracic aorta intraoperatively, and it can be used to monitor coronary blood flow velocity during counterpulsation [31,32].

The patient should be anticoagulated with a heparin infusion to maintain the partial thromboplastin time at twice the control value to reduce the risk of embolism from the surface of the balloon and to prevent thrombosis of the femoral artery at the puncture site. When anticoagulation is contraindicated because of thrombocytopenia, gastrointestinal bleeding, or recent surgery, an infusion of low-molecular-weight dextran at 20 mL per hour may be used. A prophylactic antibiotic effective against *Staphylococcus aureus*, such as cephalothin, is recommended to prevent bacterial seeding of the IAB.

As soon as the IAB is in position, the circulatory status of the limb should be checked. Due to partial obstruction of blood flow in the iliac and femoral arteries, it is not unusual for the IAB to cause previously palpable pedal pulses to decrease or even disappear. Usually, there is sufficient collateral flow to prevent severe ischemia. Adequacy of circulation is indicted by the preservation of sensation, motion, and normal color and by the absence of pain. Sedation or the residual effects of general anesthesia may make neurovascular assessment unreliable. Under these circumstances, measurement of the Doppler ankle arm index provides an objective evaluation of the circulation. The postinsertion ankle arm index should be compared with

the preinsertion value. A Doppler ankle pressure less than 40 mm Hg or an ankle arm index less than 0.25 indicates severe circulatory impairment. As long as the IAB is in position, it is imperative that the circulatory status be monitored every 1 to 2 hours. It is a common error to concentrate on the patient's cardiac problems and to overlook progressive limb ischemia.

Acute limb ischemia may occur at any time after initiation of counterpulsation but is most likely to occur immediately after IAB placement; after a decrease in cardiac output, especially if accompanied by an increase in inotropic support; or immediately after cardiac surgery. Some degree of ischemia occurs in many patients and is usually well tolerated and reversible when the IAB is removed. Consequently, initial management, particularly if the ischemia is mild, is conservative. Improvement in cardiac index, increase in systemic blood pressure and core temperature, and weaning from α-adrenergic agents often improve peripheral perfusion. Drawing the insertion sheath back until the distal end just emerges from the femoral artery may allow enough increased blood flow past the catheter to relieve limb ischemia.

Severe ischemia, indicated by the absence of an arterial Doppler signal over the dorsalis pedis or posterior tibial arteries at the ankle, requires prompt treatment. If the patient is not balloon dependent, the easiest solution is to wean rapidly and remove the IAB. If the patient is balloon dependent and the indication for counterpulsation is unstable or postinfarction angina, urgent cardiac catheterization and emergency coronary revascularization, followed by prompt removal of the IAB, should be considered. If coronary angiography and revascularization are not feasible, or if the ischemia is sufficiently severe that the circulation must be improved immediately to prevent tissue necrosis, transfer of the IAB to the opposite limb is the most expeditious treatment. Percutaneous or surgical removal of the IAB with thrombectomy should be considered for patients with acute leg ischemia. If the ischemia recurs on the contralateral side, the procedure may have allowed enough time to establish adequate pharmacologic support of the myocardium to proceed with cardiac catheterization and coronary revascularization. Return of a Doppler arterial signal in the distal vessels is an important indication that the acute leg ischemia has improved. Alternatively, a vascular bypass from the opposite common femoral artery to the superficial femoral artery distal to the IAB insertion site can restore nearly normal circulation. Although it may require transporting the patient to the operating room, the procedure is relatively minor and can be performed under local anesthesia. The procedure is highly successful in relieving limb ischemia, and the graft may be left in place when the IAB is removed. After establishing adequate arterial inflow, the limb must be closely observed for development of a compartment syndrome indicated by pain and tense swelling of the calf muscles. Surgical decompression of the swelling is necessary to prevent rhabdomyolysis, myoglobinuria, renal failure, and limb loss. The final option for the IAB-dependent patient is to accept the possibility of future amputation and to leave the device in place. Usually this choice is made only for the patient whose chances for survival are considered extremely poor.

Triggering and Timing of the Intraaortic Balloon Pump

The most important prerequisites for effective counterpulsation are a means to trigger deflation and proper timing of the inflation-deflation cycle. The R wave of the patient's electrocardiogram (ECG) is the most common means for timing balloon inflation. The IAB console is designed to detect the R wave of the ECG and is initially set so that inflation occurs at the peak of the T wave, which corresponds approximately with closure of the aortic valve. Deflation is then timed to occur just before the next QRS, which correlates with ventricular systole. It is important to select the ECG lead with the most pronounced R wave. Most triggering problems are due to an ECG with an R wave of low amplitude, dislodged electrodes, or electrical interference. If the patient has an implanted or external pacemaker, the pacing artifact may cause false triggering. In this setting, the lead in which the artifact has the minimum amplitude or is of a negative sign is selected. Most IAB consoles have circuitry designed to reject the pacing artifact. In addition, intermittent right bundle-branch block, in which the R wave is of varying amplitude, or atrial fibrillation, in which the R-R interval is variable, may interfere with effective ECG triggering. The arterial waveform may also be used to trigger the IAB. In this mode, the upstroke of the arterial wave is sensed by the console. A fairly sharp upstroke with a pulse pressure of at least 40 mm Hg is necessary for reliable arterial triggering. This mode is useful when ECG triggering is not feasible because of the lack of a consistently good R wave or when there is electrical interference, such as intraoperative use of electrocautery.

The IAB may be triggered by an external pacemaker. In this mode the pacing artifact, rather than the patient's R wave, is used to trigger inflation. This method is very useful when the ECG is of poor electrical quality or when pacing is necessary for bradycardia, complete heart block, or overdriving ventricular ectopy; however, it must be emphasized that this is a potentially lethal means of triggering. If pacing capture is lost, the timing of inflation and deflation will follow the pacemaker rather than the cardiac ejection pattern. Consequently, it is possible for the IAB to inflate during systole. Because of the potential hazards of pacemaker-triggering of the IAB, we recommend use of this mode only in an emergency, when triggering cannot be effected by ECG or arterial waveform, and then only with an IAB technician in constant attendance. Finally, counterpulsation can be triggered by an internally generated signal from the IAB console at a fixed rate. This triggering mode is used only to generate a pulse during cardiopulmonary bypass or cardiac arrest.

When initiating counterpulsation, the console should be set to a 1 to 2 assist ratio so that the effects of augmentation on every other beat can be analyzed. The IAB should be inflated to full volume right from the start so as to completely unfurl the IAB. Slide switches on the console permit adjustment of the timing of both inflation and deflation during the cardiac cycle (Fig. 9-6). If the IAB is inflated too early, when the aortic valve is still open, left ventricular workload is increased rather than reduced. If inflation occurs too late, diastolic aortic root pressure fails to rise significantly, and there is no improvement in coronary perfusion. Deflation should occur just before systole; consequently, it should be timed so that the intraaortic pressure is at a minimum when the aortic valve opens. If deflation occurs too early, the benefit of improved coronary filling in late diastole is lost. When deflation is too late, the left ventricle must contract against the residual pressure caused by a partially inflated IAB.

When the IAB technician and physician are satisfied with both triggering and timing, the IAB may be set to a 1 to 1 ratio to assist each cardiac cycle. The IAB inflation results in a diastolic pressure that exceeds the systolic pressure. Conversely, deflation of the balloon reduces end-diastolic pressure by 15 to 20 mm Hg and systolic pressure by 5 to 10 mm Hg. Timing should be rechecked every 1 to 2 hours and whenever there is a greater than 20% change in heart rate, change in cardiac output, development of arrhythmia, or change in triggering mode. When retiming, it is helpful to return the console to a 1 to 2 assist ratio.

Finally, the console should be switched from manual to automatic operation, which will activate internal monitoring circuits that will stop the IAB and sound an alarm when certain malfunctions are detected. The monitored functions include volume and pressure in the IAB, the presence of leaks causing loss of driving gas, loss of ECG or arterial trigger signal, detection of arrhythmias and changes in heart rate, and improper deflation of the IAB. Because many patients are adversely affected by even a brief loss of counterpulsation, it is important that physicians and intensive care nurses be completely familiar with the detection and prompt correction of common problems associated with the use of counterpulsation. An experienced IAB technician must be available on a 24-hour basis to manage the more complicated, but fortunately infrequent, equipment malfunctions.

Weaning from Counterpulsation

Cessation of counterpulsation involves two steps: weaning and IAB removal. The IAB console can provide counterpulsa-

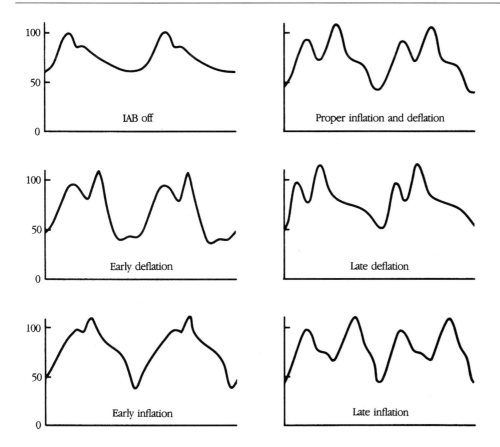

Fig. 9-6. Slide switches on the intraaortic balloon (IAB) console permit proper timing of inflation and deflation during the cardiac cycle.

tion ratios of 1 to 1, 1 to 2, 1 to 3, and 1 to 8. In addition, some consoles permit weaning by a gradual reduction in balloon volume. The patient may be progressively weaned by reducing the assist ratio or IAB volume and checking the cardiac index and filling pressures at each level. When the patient has been weaned to a 1 to 3 counterpulsation ratio and has been stable for a few hours, the IAB may be removed.

The heparin infusion should be stopped at least 2 hours before removing the percutaneous IAB. The prothrombin and partial thromboplastin times should be near normal and the platelet count greater than 60,000 per mm³ before removal of a percutaneous IAB. The IAB console should be turned to "standby" or "off." The dressing and securing sutures should be removed. The IAB catheter should be disconnected from the back of the console, and an assistant should use a 50-mL syringe to apply continuous negative pressure. The gasket is then removed from the sheath connector and the IAB is withdrawn until the balloon membrane abuts the sheath. The operator should not attempt to withdraw the balloon into the sheath. The IAB and sheath are then removed as a unit. Apply digital pressure *distal* to the arterial puncture site to allow free antegrade bleeding for 1 to 2 seconds to flush any residual thrombus. Firm pressure is then applied directly over the puncture site for 45 minutes to obliterate the femoral pulse before the operator checks for bleeding. If there is any evidence of bleeding, pressure should be reapplied for an additional 15 minutes. The use of sandbags or external compression clamps is not recommended because they do not apply sufficient localized pressure over the puncture site and can conceal a developing hematoma. Occasionally, particularly in obese or hypertensive patients, local pressure, even for 1 hour or more, will not control bleeding from the puncture site, and as a result a hematoma forms. This is best managed with early surgical exploration, evacuation of the hematoma, and direct surgical repair of the puncture site. As soon as the IAB is removed and

adequate hemostasis obtained, the circulatory status of the limb should be carefully checked.

Complications of Counterpulsation

Complications of counterpulsation may be grouped into three categories: (a) those that occur during the insertion procedure, (b) those that develop while the IAB is in place, and (c) those that are the consequence of IAB removal. The overall complication rate for percutaneous IAB placement is approximately 12%. The incidence of serious complications, such as amputation or death, related to the IAB has steadily decreased and is now less than 1% [36–38]. The most significant risk factors for limb ischemia are female gender and small body surface area, reflecting small-caliber vessels. Other risk factors are insulin-dependent diabetes, elevated end-diastolic pressure, history of smoking, postoperative insertion, and significant peripheral vascular occlusive disease as indicated by a preinsertion ankle arm index less than 0.6 [39]. Although the physician cannot select patients who are free of risk factors, earlier catheterization and revascularization can be considered for patients who are at increased risk of developing limb ischemia.

COMPLICATIONS DURING INSERTION. The most common complication related to insertion is failure of the IAB to pass the iliofemoral system because of atherosclerotic occlusive disease or marked tortuosity of the iliac artery. With the currently available 8.0-Fr percutaneous IAB, the reported failure rate is approximately 6% and may be slightly higher with the sheathless technique. If severe peripheral vascular disease precludes IAB placement, the balloon may be inserted from the ascending aorta at the time of cardiac surgery. The transthoracic route permits expeditious placement under direct vision and avoids potential ischemic complications to the lower extremities. The disadvantages of this approach are the risk of cerebral embolism during insertion, increased rate of balloon rupture, risk of mediastinal bleeding and infectious complications, and the need for a second operative procedure for its removal [40,41]. Although the complication rate of transthoracic placement is similar to that for the femoral route, the magnitude of the complications is potentially greater. Clearly, transthoracic placement of IAB is not available to nonsurgical patients [42].

There have been case reports of successful IAB insertion through the right subclavian and axillary artery. The usefulness of these approaches is limited by the fragility and relatively small caliber of the arteries [43]. Under emergency circumstances, an IAB may be inserted though the femoral limb of an aortobifemoral graft, with a reported infection rate of 12% [44]. Because of the potential for infection in a prosthetic graft, with its associated high morbidity and mortality, the duration of counterpulsation should be minimized when this method of access is used.

Other complications of IAB insertion include aortic or iliac dissection, arterial perforation, and bleeding. Perforation usually occurs in the common iliac artery because of difficulty in negotiating a tortuous vessel or angulation at the aortic bifurcation. Arterial perforation is an acute emergency requiring urgent surgical intervention. Retrograde dissection of the iliac artery can occur when the catheter elevates a large atherosclerotic plaque and is advanced in a subintimal plane [45]. Insertion of the IAB without fluoroscopic or TEE guidance has led to misplacement of the balloon in the left ventricle and subclavian, left common carotid, renal, and contralateral femoral arteries [46]. These types of arterial injuries and misplacements can be minimized by the use of wire-guided IAB and continuous fluoroscopy during the insertion procedure.

Complications while the Intraaortic Balloon Is in Place

Limb ischemia is the most common complication of counterpulsation and is sufficiently severe to require removal of the IAB in approximately 10% of patients. Early IABPs used a 12-Fr catheter placed though a surgical cutdown over the common femoral artery. Smaller catheters and the sheathless insertion technique have reduced the severity, but not the frequency, of complications [47]. It appears that the advantage of smaller-caliber balloons is offset by their use in higher-risk patients [48].

Because the IAB is a foreign body in continuous contact with the circulation, there is justifiable concern about infection. Surprisingly, septic complications are relatively unusual, even with prolonged periods of counterpulsation [49]. In one study of more than 700 patients, only 1.4% developed septicemia. However, when sepsis does occur in the presence of IAB, the mortality rate is high. Positive blood cultures in a patient on counterpulsation require prompt removal and culture of the IAB and treatment with appropriate intravenous antibiotics.

Some degrees of thrombocytopenia and hemolytic anemia are observed in most patients with an IAB, due to mechanical trauma from contact with the surface of the balloon. Platelet counts should be performed daily. Because heparin may also cause thrombocytopenia, low-molecular-weight dextran should be substituted for heparin if the platelet count falls below 100,000 per mm^3. There is usually no need to transfuse platelets unless the patient develops overt bleeding. The platelet count usually returns to normal soon after the IAB is removed.

There have been case reports of embolization of platelet aggregates from the surface of the balloon or dislodgment of atherosclerotic debris from the aortic wall to the mesenteric, renal, spinal, cerebral, and peripheral arteries. Such complications are unpredictable and are not preventable with the use of anticoagulation or antiplatelet drugs. Rupture of the IAB occurs in 2% to 4% of patients and may cause embolization of the helium driving gas, resulting in a cerebrovascular accident or death. Balloon rupture is probably not due to fatigue of the polyurethane membrane; one IAB was used for nearly a year (30 million cycles) in a single patient without leaking [50,51]. Balloon perforation seems to be most frequent in patients with a small-caliber aorta where there is intimate contact between the IAB and the wall of the aorta with each inflation. In this situation, a sharp plaque can abrade the balloon membrane, causing gas to escape into the circulation. An IAB rupture, therefore, may be heralded by console alarms detecting "gas loss." Blood in the connecting tubing is the hallmark of rupture and requires immediate cessation of counterpulsation, placement of the patient in the Trendelenburg position to prevent cerebral gas embolization, and IAB removal. Antibiotic coverage should be broadened, because the gas chamber of the IAB is not sterile. If the patient is dependent on counterpulsation, the IAB may be replaced over a guidewire.

A related, serious complication is IAB entrapment. A small perforation in the balloon membrane permits a slow leak of blood into the balloon lumen. The dry helium desiccates the collected blood, forming a rock-hard pellet that impinges against the orifice of the common iliac artery during attempted removal. The desiccated pellet can be rehydrated with a sterile saline solution instilled by syringe through the gas port of the IAB catheter [52]. Once the pellet is liquefied, the IAB may be withdrawn percutaneously. If resistance to removal is still present, the IAB should be removed by an open surgical procedure. Because entrapment can occur only if there is a balloon perforation, even a trace of blood in the tubing is an indication to remove or exchange the IAB.

COMPLICATIONS DURING OR AFTER REMOVAL. As noted earlier, the IAB may be removed percutaneously by withdrawing the balloon and sheath together, after which the puncture site is compressed for 45 to 60 minutes. A randomized prospective study showed that the incidence of vascular complications for IABs removed percutaneously was 4%, the same as with an open surgical procedure [53]. Although the majority of percutaneously placed IABs may be safely removed without an operation, surgical removal is still recommended for patients who are anticoagulated, who have a coagulopathy, or in whom the IAB was placed with an operative procedure. Arterial perfusion of the limb should be checked soon after removal of the IAB by palpation of pulses and measurement of the ankle arm index. The puncture site should be examined for hematoma, false aneurysm formation, and arteriovenous fistula. A characteristic continuous bruit heard over the puncture site indicates an arteriovenous fistula. Duplex ultrasound is a useful method to confirm the diagnosis.

Conclusions

The IAB is the most widely used external LVAD currently available. Its major value lies in its ability to buy time so that cardiac catheterization can be performed to look for remediable coronary artery disease or a surgically correctable mechanical defect.

In addition, it can often permit weaning from cardiopulmonary bypass of the cardiac surgical patient with depressed left ventricular function. Even in the most capable hands, there is probably an irreducible incidence of complications due to associated severe peripheral vascular disease and diminished cardiac output. The incidence of vascular complications from IAB placement has remained unchanged during the past 20 years despite advances in technology. However, the severity of the complications has significantly diminished. The incidence of complications can be minimized by limiting IAB use to well-accepted indications, maintaining meticulous insertion techniques, and carefully monitoring limb circulation after implantation.

Acknowledgment

Thanks to Kevin Cotter, C.C.P., for his assistance with the technical aspects of the manuscript.

References

1. Argenziano M, Mehmet CO, Rose EA: The continuing evolution of mechanical ventricular assistance. *Curr Probl Surg* 34:316, 1997.
2. Katz ES, Tunick PA, Kronzon I: Observations of coronary flow augmentation and balloon function during intraaortic balloon counterpulsation using transesophageal echocardiography. *Am J Cardiol* 69:1635, 1992.
3. Moulopoulos S, Stamatelopoulos S, Petrou P: Intraaortic balloon assistance in intractable cardiogenic shock. *Eur Heart J* 7:396, 1986.
4. Scheidt S, Wilner G, Mueller H, et al: Intra-aortic balloon counterpulsation in cardiogenic shock: report of a cooperative clinical trial. *N Engl J Med* 288:979, 1973.
5. O'Rourke MF, Norris RM, Campbell TJ, et al: Randomized controlled trial of intraaortic balloon counterpulsation in early myocardial infarction with acute heart failure. *Am J Cardiol* 47:815, 1981.
6. Sturm JT, Fuhrman TM, Igo SR, et al: Quantitative indices of intraaortic balloon pump (IABP) dependence during post-infarction cardiogenic shock. *Artif Organs* 4:8, 1980.
7. Lazar HL, Treanor P, Yang XM, et al: Enhanced recovery of ischemic myocardium by combining percutaneous bypass with intraaortic balloon pump support. *Ann Thorac Surg* 57:663, 1994.
8. Blanche C, Khan SS, Matloff JM, et al: Results of early repair of ventricular septal defect after an acute myocardial infarction. *J Thorac Cardiovasc Surg* 104:961, 1992.
9. Deja MA, Szostek J, Widenka K, et al: Post infarction ventricular septal defect—can we do better? *Eur J Cardiothorac Surg* 18:194, 2000.
10. Harris PL, Woollard K, Bartoli A, et al: The management of impending myocardial infarction using coronary artery bypass grafting and an intra-aortic balloon pump. *J Cardiovasc Surg* 21:405, 1980.
11. Mehta SM, Aufiero TX, Pae WE, et al: Results of mechanical ventricular assistance for the treatment of post cardiotomy cardiogenic shock. *ASAIO J* 42:211, 1996.
12. Goldstein DJ, Oz MC: Mechanical support for postcardiotomy cardiogenic shock. *Semin Thorac Cardiovasc Surg* 12:220, 2000.
13. Kim K, Lim C, Ahn H, et al: Intraaortic balloon pump therapy facilitates posterior vessel off pump coronary artery bypass grafting in high-risk patients. *Ann Thorac Surg* 71:1964, 2001.
14. Kang N, Edwards M, Larbalestier R: Preoperative intraaortic balloon pumps in high-risk patients undergoing open heart surgery. *Ann Thorac Surg* 72:54, 2001.
15. Dietl CA, Berkeimer MD, Woods EL, et al: Efficacy and cost-effectiveness of preoperative IABP in patients with ejection fraction of 0.25 or less. *Ann Thorac Surg* 62:401, 1996.
16. Spadoni S: Preoperative intraaortic balloon counterpulsation in high-risk coronary patients. *Canadiene Perfusion* 10:30, 2000.
17. Akins CW, discussion of Creswell LL, Rosenbloom M, Cox JL, et al: Intraaortic balloon counterpulsation: patterns of usage and outcome in cardiac surgery patients. *Ann Thorac Surg* 54:18, 1992.
18. Christenson JT, Badel P, Simonet F, et al: Preoperative intraaortic balloon pump enhances cardiac performance and improves the outcome of redo CABG. *Ann Thorac Surg* 64:1237, 1997.
19. Sapirstein JS, Pae WE, Aufiero TX, et al: Long-term left ventricular assist device use before transplantation. *ASAIO J* 41:530, 1995.
20. Aguirre FV, Kern MJ, Bach R, et al: Intraaortic balloon pump support during high-risk coronary angioplasty. *Cardiology* 84:175, 1994.
21. O'Murchu B, Foreman RD, Shaw RE, et al: Role of intraaortic balloon pump counterpulsation in high risk coronary rotational atherectomy. *J Am Coll Cardiol* 26:1270, 1995.
22. Kahn JK, Rutherford BD, McConahay DR, et al: Supported high risk coronary angioplasty using intraaortic balloon pump counterpulsation. *J Am Coll Cardiol* 15:1151, 1990.
23. Schreiber TL, Kodali UR, O'Neill WW, et al: Comparison of acute results of prophylactic intraaortic balloon pumping with cardiopulmonary support for percutaneous transluminal coronary angioplasty (PTCA). *Cathet Cardiovasc Diagn* 45:115, 1998.
24. Ishihara M, Sato H, Tateishi H, et al: Effects of intraaortic balloon pumping on coronary hemodynamics after coronary angioplasty in patients with acute myocardial infarction. *Am Heart J* 124:1133, 1992.
25. Stone GW, Marsalese D, Brodie B, et al: A prospective, randomized evaluation of prophylactic intraaortic counterpulsation in high risk patients with acute myocardial infarction treated with primary angioplasty. *J Am Coll Cardiol* 29:1459, 1997.
26. Akomea-Argyin C, Kejiriwal NK, Franks R, et al: Intraaortic balloon pumping in children. *Ann Thorac Surg* 67:1415, 1999.
27. del Nido PJ, Swan PR, Benson LN, et al: Successful use of intraaortic balloon pumping in a 2-kilogram infant. *Ann Thorac Surg* 45:574, 1998.
28. Reiss N, El-Banayosy A, Posival H, et al: Transport of hemodynamically unstable patients by a mobile mechanical circulatory team. *Artif Organs* 20:959, 1996.
29. Jacobs JP, Horowitz MD, Ladden DA, et al: Case report: intraaortic balloon counterpulsation in penetrating cardiac trauma. *J Cardiovasc Surg* 33:38, 1992.
30. Siu SC, Kowalchuk GJ, Welty FK, et al: Intra-aortic balloon counterpulsation support in the high-risk cardiac patient undergoing urgent noncardiac surgery. *Chest* 99:1342, 1991.
31. Masaki E, Takinami M, Kurata Y, et al: Anesthetic management of high-risk cardiac patients undergoing noncardiac surgery under the support of intraaortic balloon pump. *J Clin Anesth* 11:342, 1999.
32. Nishioka T, Freidman A, Cercek B, et al: Usefulness of transesophageal echocardiography for positioning the intraaortic balloon pump in the operating room. *Am J Cardiol* 77:105, 1996.
33. Shanewise JS, Sadel SM: Intraoperative transesophageal echocardiography to assist the insertion and positioning of the intraaortic balloon pump. *Anesth Analg* 79:577, 1994.
34. Nash IS, Larell BH, Fishman RF, et al: A new technique for sheathless intraaortic balloon catheter insertion. *Cathet Cardiovasc Diagn* 23:57, 1991.
35. Reichert CLA, Koolen JJ, Visser CA: Transesophageal echocardiographic evaluation of left ventricular function during intraaortic balloon pump counterpulsation. *J Am Soc Echocardiogr* 6:490, 1993.
36. Reference deleted.
37. Barnett MG, Swartz MT, Peterson GT, et al: Vascular complications from intraaortic balloons: risk Analysis. *J Vasc Surg* 19:81, 1994.
38. Eltchaninoff H, Dimas AP, Whitlow PL: Complications associated with percutaneous placement and use of intraaortic balloon counterpulsation. *Am J Cardiol* 71:328, 1993.
39. Minakata K, Konish Y, Matsumoto M, et al: Influence of peripheral vascular occlusive disease on the morbidity and mortality of coronary artery bypass grafting. *Jpn Circ J* 64:905, 2000.
40. Arafa OE, Pederson TH, Svennivig JL, et al: Vascular complications of the intraaortic balloon pump in patients undergoing open heart operations; a 15-year experience. *Ann Thorac Surg* 67:645, 1999.
41. Hazelrigg SR, Auer JE, Seifert PE: Experience in 100 transthoracic balloon pumps. *Ann Thorac Surg* 54:528, 1992.
42. Pinkard J, Utley JR, Leyland SA, et al: Relative risk of aortic and femoral insertion of intraaortic balloon pump after coronary artery bypass grafting procedures. *J Thorac Cardiovasc Surg* 105:721, 1993.

43. Burack JH, Uceda P, Cunningham JV, et al: Transthoracic intraaortic balloon pump: a simplified technique. *Ann Thorac Surg* 62:299, 1996.
44. McBride LR, Miller LW, Nauheim KS, et al: Axillary artery insertion of an intraaortic balloon pump. *Ann Thorac Surg* 48:874, 1989.
45. LaMuraglia GM, Vlahakes GJ, Moncure AC, et al: The safety of intraaortic balloon pump catheter insertion through suprainguinal prosthetic vascular bypass grafts. *J Vasc Surg* 13:830, 1991.
46. Isner JM, Cohen SR, Virmani R, et al: Complications of the intraaortic balloon counterpulsation device: clinical and morphologic observations in 54 necropsy patients. *Am J Cardiol* 45:260, 1980.
47. Coffin SA: The misplaced intraaortic balloon pump. *Anesth Analg* 78:1182, 1994.
48. Tatar H, Cicek S, Demirkilic U, et al: Vascular complications of intraaortic balloon pumping: unsheathed versus sheathed insertion. *Ann Thorac Surg* 55:1518, 1993.
49. Naunheim KS, Swartz MT, Pennington DG, et al: Intraaortic balloon pumping in patients requiring cardiac operations: risk analysis and long-term follow-up. *J Thorac Cardiovasc Surg* 104:1654, 1992.
50. Lazar JM, Ziady GM, Dummer SJ, et al: Outcome and complications of prolonged intraaortic balloon counterpulsation in cardiac patients. *Am J Cardiol* 69:955, 1992.
51. Freed PS, Wasfie T, Zado B, et al: Intraaortic balloon pumping for prolonged circulatory support. *Am J Cardiol* 61:554, 1988.
52. Horowitz MD, Otero M, de Marchena EJ, et al: Intraaortic balloon entrapment. *Ann Thorac Surg* 56:368, 1993.
53. Rohrer MJ, Sullivan CA, McLaughlin DJ, et al: A prospective randomized comparison of surgical and percutaneous intraaortic balloon pump removal. *J Thorac Cardiovasc Surg* 103:569, 1992.

10. Extracorporeal and Intracorporeal Support Technologies for Severe Cardiac and Respiratory Failure

Robert A. Lancey and
Harry L. Anderson III

A limited number of pharmacologic therapies are available for the treatment of respiratory and cardiac insufficiency in the intensive care unit. When cardiac or respiratory failure is sufficiently severe (end-organ failure) to require full support, the therapies available to the intensivist are actually mechanical. This chapter covers advanced extracorporeal, paracorporeal, and intracorporeal mechanical therapies for heart and lung failure. Although some of these techniques are considered "standard of care," we also cover other therapies that can be considered novel and extraordinary, and not simply experimental.

Cardiac Support

Cardiovascular disease continues to be the leading cause of death in the United States, with approximately two-thirds of these fatalities attributed to left ventricular failure. Cardiogenic shock occurs in 15% of patients who reach the hospital after an acute myocardial infarction. Despite maximum medical support and use of an intraaortic balloon pump (IABP), only 15% of these patients survive [1]. Likewise, of approximately 350,000 cardiac surgical procedures performed each year in the United States, 1% to 7% require placement of an IABP, with 65% surviving [2,3]. It is further estimated that 0.2% to 1.2% of patients undergoing cardiac surgery fail attempts at weaning from cardiopulmonary bypass (CPB), even with IABP support [4].

The patients identified above, as well as those with progressive cardiac failure awaiting transplantation, constitute a population in whom placement of a ventricular assist device (VAD) is potentially life-saving. These devices provide an improved means of support for a failing left ventricle and are often the only means of support to prevent progression to complete cardiac decompensation and death. This section focuses on the variety of mechanical assist devices used clinically for acute left ventricular failure (excluding IABPs, which are discussed in Chapter 9).

PATHOPHYSIOLOGY OF LEFT VENTRICULAR FAILURE. Cardiac function in both the normal and failing states is best described by Starling's law, which identifies cardiac performance as directly proportional to ventricular preload in a pressure-volume relationship. As ventricular volume is increased (producing a concomitant rise in end-diastolic filling pressure), the resultant stroke volume also increases within a normal physiologic range. The ability of the ventricle to respond with an increase in stroke volume (and thus an increase in cardiac output) depends on the ability of the myocardial fibril to respond to stretching with an increased force of contraction.

When the myocardial fibril stretches beyond twice its normal length, there is progressive loss of active tension and an increase in resting tension (a point marked by a shift to the descending limb of Starling's curve). Progressive cardiac failure and a decline in cardiac output ensue, as further volume loading simply produces a greater rise in left ventricular end-diastolic pressure and a decline in stroke volume. With profound myocardial ischemia or frank myocardial infarction, Starling's curve shifts downward and to the right, representing a progressive decline in myocardial contractility.

This model of progressive loss of ventricular power may begin with an imbalance between myocardial oxygen supply and demand. A reduction in high-energy phosphate stores in the myocardium results in a decline in velocity and extent of myocardial fibril shortening (depressed contractility), as well as an increase in ventricular wall tension. With rising wall tension, oxygen demand is increased while supply is decreased to the subendocardium. Progressive deterioration of left ventricular performance ultimately results in inadequate global tissue perfusion, accompanying acidosis, and eventual end-organ dysfunction. Left ventricular failure specifically results in pulmonary congestion and hypoxemia, compounding the insult to tissue perfusion.

Treatment is thus aimed at reducing myocardial oxygen demand, augmenting myocardial oxygen supply, and improving ventricular performance. Inotropic agents can increase cardiac contractile function, although at the expense of an increase in myocardial oxygen demand, potentially hastening the progression of ischemia. More effective treatment is provided by the IABP, which increases myocardial perfusion and reduces left ventricular wall tension and afterload [5]. For patients with postcardiotomy cardiogenic shock, a similar pattern may ensue. Aggressive pharmacologic support with inotropic agents and prompt use of an IABP can lead to successful weaning from CPB in the majority of these patients. For the remainder, either a VAD or extracorporeal membrane oxygenation (ECMO) may be indicated [6,7].

In experimental studies, left heart bypass has been shown to reduce infarct size [8–12] and decrease myocardial oxygen consumption and ventricular workload [11,12]. Left ventricular assist devices (LVADs) have also been found to be more effective than IABPs in reducing myocardial oxygen consumption [13] and more effective than a combination of IABP and pharmacologic inotropic support in preserving myocardial structure and function in an experimental model [14].

LVADs pump blood from the left atrium or left ventricle into the aorta. By reducing the workload of the heart (i.e., the wall tension), the LVAD allows a period of metabolic recovery for ischemic myocytes. High-energy phosphate stores are replenished, and ischemic myocardium on the border of an infarct zone may recover. Simultaneously, tissue perfusion is sustained.

HISTORICAL PERSPECTIVE.

The use of CPB is based on the pioneering work of Gibbon, who developed extracorporeal circulation and was the first to apply it clinically in 1953. Liotta was the first to use an LVAD clinically [15]. Although roller pumps were used initially [16,17], they were supplanted for use in adults in most centers by centrifugal pumps, which provided longer periods of support without the embolic and hemolytic consequences of roller pumps. Before 1985, most assist devices were used for postcardiotomy cardiogenic shock. Since then, they have also been used to support patients with acute myocardial infarctions complicated by cardiogenic shock and as bridges to cardiac transplantation [18].

Recent years have been characterized by tremendous growth in the research and technologic development of cardiac assist devices. Both nonpulsatile pumps (used in the operating room as components of CPB circuits) and pulsatile devices (containing prosthetic valves) are currently in use. As long-term support is becoming more widespread, fully implantable systems have gained popularity, both as bridges to transplantation and, in an experimental trial, as permanent replacements for the left ventricle. Their clinical and economic benefits are well documented [19].

FEATURES OF VENTRICULAR ASSIST DEVICES.

VADs may vary in location in relation to the patient, the pumping mechanism used, and the expected time course of support. They may be specifically used for short-term support (e.g., to provide perfusion during a time of ventricular recovery in the setting of an acute myocardial infarction or after failure to wean from CPB) or long-term support (e.g., as bridges to transplantation). Most recently, much research—as well as one clinical human trial—has focused on permanent implantation of total artificial hearts.

The pumps may be located extracorporeally (set apart from the body) or paracorporeally (in contact with the patient), or they may be implanted (usually in the abdominal wall), with

cannulae connecting them to the heart and great vessels. Pulsatile flow systems vary in their mode of function, with asynchronous systems pumping at a fixed, independent rate, and synchronous systems pumping in coordination with native ventricular contraction. Although synchronous pumping theoretically results in better decompression of the native ventricle, the intrinsic heart rate may be too fast and irregular for optimal filling [20]. Retrospective analyses comparing nonpulsatile and pulsatile modes have shown no significant statistical difference in terms of ability to wean from VADs and subsequent survival rates [21], likely due in part to the common use of an IABP with nonpulsatile VADs to provide a degree of pulsatile flow to the system.

TYPES OF VENTRICULAR ASSIST PUMPS.

Roller pumps were initially used and have shown acceptable patient survival rates when used for up to 48 hours [10]. Disadvantages include hemolysis and embolization during prolonged use and the ability to provide only a limited amount of flow (no greater than 3 L per minute) [22].

The Hemopump (Johnson & Johnson, Warren, NJ), developed in the late 1980s, was designed for short-term use. Using a rotary pump contained in a narrow 7-mm chamber on the end of a catheter, it provides for axial flow rates of up to 3.5 to 4.0 L per minute [23–25]. Inserted through a graft sewn onto the common femoral artery, the device tip is positioned in the left ventricle, from which blood is drawn and ejected into the aorta. This provides nonpulsatile flow over a short period and is perhaps most useful in a setting of acute hemodynamic deterioration from cardiogenic shock. Technical difficulties with this device include problems with insertion (lack of adequate vascular access) and kinking of the catheter at the insertion site [24].

Centrifugal pumps were commonly used as extracorporeal devices and result in less trauma to blood components than do roller pumps [26]. Although there was initial concern that centrifugal pumps would cause pump-induced trauma to blood components, studies on long-term use have not found this to be the case [27]. They provide nonpulsatile flow to one or both ventricles and are available in two types: vortex pumps (BioMedicus, Eden Prairie, MN) [28–32] and impeller pumps (Sarns/3M, Ann Arbor, MI) [33,34]. They are often used with standard CPB cannulation systems, and, although originally used for short-term support to recovery, their use in bridging to transplantation has been reported [28]. Use of centrifugal pumps with ECMO is becoming increasingly popular when support is required postcardiotomy, with survival rates as high as 72% in patients converted to an implantable system for bridging to transplantation [3].

The Abiomed B.V.S. System 5000 (Abiomed Cardiovascular, Danvers, MA) is an extracorporeal assist device that also supports one or both ventricles. Using a polyurethane pneumatically driven pump and bioprosthetic valves, the atrial chambers are gravity-filled from the patient's atrium, and blood is pumped back into either the pulmonary artery or aorta through a Dacron graft. Excellent clinical results have been obtained with this device in support-to-recovery after open heart surgery [35,36] and in bridging to transplantation [37].

The Thoratec VAD (Thoratec Laboratories, Berkeley, CA) [38,39] is a paracorporeal, pneumatically driven, pulsatile polyurethane pump that uses mechanical valves to provide single- or biventricular support. Cannulae penetrate the chest wall and connect to an atrium (or both atria) or the left ventricle and to the great vessels; connection to the great vessels is via a Dacron graft. In part due to the paracorporeal location of the pumps, which are secured to the skin on the abdominal wall, ambulation may be possible.

Fully implantable devices for left ventricular support only are used almost exclusively for bridging to transplantation, with the exceptions being rare patients who have been weaned unexpectedly from the devices, or those in whom they are placed permanently as part of an ongoing clinical trial (Randomized Evaluation of Mechanical Assistance for the Treatment of Congestive Heart Failure). The TCI Heartmate (Thermo Cardiosystems, Woburn, MA) is an implantable pulsatile pump placed within the abdomen or abdominal wall and connected to an external power source through a percutaneous lead [44,45]. It uses porcine valves and is connected to the left ventricular apex via a Dacron graft sewing ring. Minimal antithrombotic therapy is needed, as contact surfaces are impregnated with microspheres to promote formation of a biologic lining. Excellent clinical results have been reported [46,47], and investigations into its use over prolonged periods and as a permanent implant are ongoing [48]. The Novacor LVAS (Baxter Healthcare, Oakland, CA), an electrically driven pulsatile device for left ventricular support only, uses bioprosthetic valves, is placed in the abdominal cavity, and connects to the aorta and left ventricle with Dacron grafts [40]. Use of the device has also shown promising clinical results, with successful transplantation and discharge rates ranging from 56% to 83% [41–43].

INDICATIONS FOR USE. In an acute setting, VADs are often used in patients who do not wean from CPB after cardiac surgery or for those who develop left ventricular failure with cardiogenic shock secondary to myocardial ischemia or infarction [49–51]. Norman et al. defined cardiogenic shock by hemodynamic parameters that have since been modified and adapted for identifying patients requiring VAD support. When these conditions exist for more than a few hours, there is less than a 15% chance of survival [52].

Criteria have evolved for patient selection (Table 10-1) [18,30,53]. In addition to failing hemodynamics, surgically correctable lesions and metabolic abnormalities must first be corrected. Attention to adequate preload, maximal inotropic support, and use of an IABP should precede VAD placement.

Early institution of ventricular support has been identified as an important prognostic factor for success in eventual weaning from mechanical assistance [54]. Ideally, ventricular assistance should be instituted within 1 hour of the conclusion of the cardiac surgical procedure [1]. McGovern, in fact, noted no survivors if the device was placed after four or more attempts at weaning from CPB after unsuccessful cardiac surgery [55].

When a VAD is intended for short-term support, it is assumed that the heart will recover to a degree that will allow subsequent removal of the device. In the setting of cardiac failure after open heart surgery, it is often difficult to determine whether frank infarction or myocardial stunning is the cause of failure to wean from CPB. Although VADs will not resurrect infarcted myocardium, they may limit the amount of potentially infarcted tissue while also providing optimal conditions in which stunned myocardium may recover. A perioperative infarct is thus a poor prognostic factor for survival, as most patients with extensive myocardial necrosis do not survive even with VAD support [18].

Stunning is a state of reversible myocardial dysfunction secondary to ischemia [56]. During initial perfusion of ischemic myocardium, cellular and metabolic abnormalities may exist that produce impaired left ventricular function [57,58]. Such stunned myocardium often requires several days or weeks before baseline function is regained. Ellis and colleagues have shown that 15 minutes of acute coronary occlusion can produce detectable functional and metabolic derangements lasting up to a week [58]. However, no definitive method of

Table 10-1. Criteria for Left Ventricular Assist Device Insertion

Hemodynamic parameters
  Cardiac index <1.8 L/min/m^2
  Mean arterial pressure <60 mm Hg
  Left atrial pressure >20 mm Hg
  Urine output <20 mL/h
  Systemic vascular resistance >2,100 dyne • sec • cm^{-5}
No correctable surgical lesions
Metabolic abnormalities absent
Maximal inotropic support
Optimal preload
Use of intraaortic balloon pump

determining the presence and degree of myocardial infarction in the immediate postcardiotomy setting has been developed. Transesophageal echocardiography (TEE) may assist in identifying wall motion abnormalities, but these may also occur transiently as a result of ischemia. Myocardial biopsy is obviously more definitive but at present is neither feasible nor practical in the acute setting.

Patients with acute fulminant myocarditis may also be successfully supported to either recovery or transplant, often avoiding the latter with single- or biventricular assistance or ECMO. Survival in this setting may reach as high as 70% [59].

CONTRAINDICATIONS TO USE. Relative contraindications to VAD placement are well documented [18,53] (Table 10-2). Although massive myocardial infarction is obviously a contraindication, this condition may not be obvious in the immediate postoperative period. Sepsis may be an appropriate reason to avoid VAD placement, yet infections responding to antibiotic therapy should not absolutely preclude mechanical ventricular support. Because of the need to anticoagulate patients with VADs, those with bleeding disorders or active bleeding (such as from the gastrointestinal tract or the central nervous system) should be excluded as candidates for support.

Chronic debilitating diseases may also be contraindications to VAD placement. Metastatic cancer, severe pulmonary hypertension secondary to underlying pulmonary disease, severe peripheral vascular disease, and neurologic impairment are all relative contraindications, as are chronic renal or hepatic failure. Single-organ dysfunction, however, should not alone preclude placement of a VAD, because if organ dysfunction, rather than irreversible failure, is present, VAD support may in fact help to improve organ function [60].

Advanced age is a relative contraindication to VAD placement. Although a specific age above which VAD placement is absolutely contraindicated has not been defined (as a patient's general condition before left ventricular failure must also be considered), a retrospective analysis of prognostic factors revealed poor survival (13%) in patients older than 70 years [61]. Others have identified age older than 65 as a poor prog-

Table 10-2. Contraindications to Left Ventricular Assist Device Use

Massive myocardial infarction
Sepsis
Metastatic malignancy
Bleeding disorder
Active bleeding (gastrointestinal, central nervous system)
Severe pulmonary hypertension
Severe hepatic failure
Chronic renal failure
Severe peripheral vascular disease
Central neurologic impairment

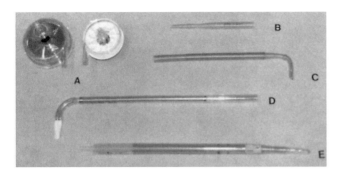

Fig. 10-1. Equipment for ventricular assist devices. **A:** Centrifugal pumps. **B:** Cannula for main pulmonary artery (right ventricular assist device inflow). **C:** Cannula for aorta (left ventricular assist device inflow). **D:** Cannula for left atrium (left ventricular assist device outflow). **E:** Cannula for right atrium (right ventricular assist device outflow).

nostic factor [53,54]. At the other end of the age spectrum, survival rates in children supported with VADs after cardiac surgery have exceeded those in adults [62].

TECHNIQUES OF PLACEMENT. Placement of a VAD is performed in the operating room, often after unsuccessful attempts to wean from CPB or in the setting of chronic end-stage heart failure (Figs. 10-1 and 10-2). A patent foramen ovale should be sought and closed, because unloading the left atrium with the VAD may result in significant right-to-left shunting. Centrifugal pumping systems generally use standard CPB cannulae for both inflow and outflow; purse-string sutures armed with Teflon pledgets passed through rubber tourniquets help secure cannulae in the left atrium and aorta [29]. Left atrial drainage is performed with a cannula placed through the right superior pulmonary vein, roof of the atrium, or left atrial appendage. Restriction of venous return at the time of cannulation helps raise the left atrial pressure (LAP) and evacuates air from the system. Meticulous care must be taken to protect against and identify bleeding from around the cannulae, as these sites are common sources of troublesome bleeding in the postoperative period.

Controversy exists as to the feasibility and efficacy of left ventricular unloading using left atrial cannulation versus left ventricular cannulation. The advantages of left atrial cannulation include relative technical simplicity and a notable reduc-

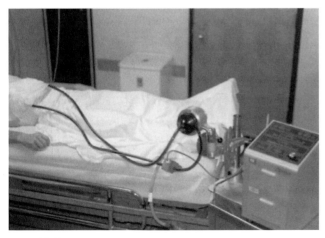

Fig. 10-2. Left ventricular assist device with console, centrifugal pumps, and tubing.

tion of inflow obstruction [1], as well as its association with improved survival rates when compared to left ventricular cannulation [18]. Left ventricular function is preserved by avoiding injury to the apex, whereas potential loss of future function may accompany left ventricular cannulation [1].

Left ventricular cannulation, however, provides greater flow rates than does left atrial cannulation (5.5 to 6.5 L per minute as opposed to 4.0 to 4.5 L per minute) [38], and animal studies have demonstrated better left ventricular decompression and greater reduction in myocardial infarct size with left ventricular cannulation [12,18,63]. Pulsatile pumps seem to fill better through the left ventricle than through the left atrium, probably due to the difference between active filling from left ventricular contraction and passive filling from the left atrium [18]. To avoid thrombosis, an LVAD with left ventricular cannulation is the preferred method of support in acute failure after mitral valve replacement and in cardiogenic shock after an acute myocardial infarction [7]. Although left atrial cannulation may be indicated in a support-to-recovery setting, left ventricular cannulation appears to be a more logical choice in the setting of bridging to transplantation, because the left ventricle will be sacrificed when a replacement heart becomes available.

POSTOPERATIVE MANAGEMENT. Cannulae must also be positioned with care in relation to the chest wall and bypass grafts, if present, to avoid compression of either the cannulae or grafts. To minimize infection, they should be placed through the chest wall rather than through the sternotomy wound, and every attempt should be made to approximate the skin edges over the mediastinum and to close the sternum itself.

Close monitoring of hemodynamic parameters, fluid and blood product intake, urine output, and blood loss is mandatory. Hemodynamic parameters are listed in Table 10-3 [18]. If biventricular assistance is required, left ventricular flow should exceed right ventricular flow by 500 to 1,000 mL to account for the return of bronchial flow to the left ventricle [18].

Pharmacologic inotropic support should be minimized as much as possible. In a setting of left ventricular assistance, its major purpose would be to support function of the right ventricle. Often only dopamine (1 to 3 µg per kg per minute) is necessary, to improve renal blood flow. Peripheral vasomotor tone may need support using vasodilators (e.g., sodium nitroprusside) or vasopressors (e.g., phenylephrine, norepinephrine). Drugs that vasodilate the pulmonary vasculature (isoproterenol, prostaglandin E, or inhaled nitric oxide) may be required either prophylactically or if signs of right ventricular failure develop.

Arrhythmias are commonly encountered due to electrolyte abnormalities, ischemia, infarction, and the use of inotropic agents. These are usually well tolerated when biventricular support is present; when only an LVAD is in use, their effects are often deleterious and require aggressive treatment because of the resulting loss of right ventricular output.

Because device contact surfaces are thrombogenic, anticoagulation is necessary in varying degrees, depending on the device and flow rates used. For centrifugal pumps, heparin or dextran may be used, with frequent monitoring of the activated clotting time (ACT) to achieve a goal of 180 to 200 seconds. The degree of anticoagulation must be strictly controlled, as

Table 10-3. Left Ventricular Assist Device Maintenance Parameters

Mean arterial pressure	65–80 mm Hg
Left and right arterial pressure	5–15 mm Hg
Cardiac index	2.2–3.0 L/min/m²
Mixed venous oxygen saturation	65–70%

bleeding remains one of the most common complications and worse prognostic factors for survival in VAD use. In the setting of long-term use (e.g., implantable left ventricular assist systems), aspirin or warfarin is indicated.

All cannulae and their connections must remain secured tightly to each other and to the patient without kinking. Dressings at the cannulation sites must be routinely changed under sterile conditions. Nutritional needs are addressed early in the postoperative course. Special attention must be paid to skin care, especially for patients who are limited in movement and have extracorporeal devices. Decubitus ulcers may develop rapidly; therefore, the use of specialized support beds is essential. In addition, the psychological needs of the patient and family involving anxiety about the device and fear of death must be addressed. Adequate care of a patient with a VAD requires a team of physicians, nurses, and perfusionists familiar with the device and the possible complications.

WEANING. The ultimate goal of ventricular assistance is removal of the device after ventricular recovery or replacement of it with a donor organ. Hemodynamic parameters, as well as TEE, are essential in the decision-making process.

Timing of VAD removal is critical. In the postcardiotomy setting, the device is placed to allow time for replenishment of high-energy phosphates and for resolution of myocardial edema that accompanies CPB [1]. Attempts to wean from mechanical ventricular support in less than 24 hours are usually unsuccessful [55], and retrospective analyses of large groups of patients requiring ventricular assistance postcardiotomy show that an average of 4 days of support is necessary [21]. In 90% of survivors, ventricular support is discontinued within 1 week [21]. In the setting of planned support-to-recovery, if no significant improvement in left ventricular function is identified by TEE within 72 hours, the chances of weaning are severely reduced [64]. Should failure to wean persist beyond 10 days, transplantation should be considered [18].

Initial assessment of suitability for VAD removal usually begins in the first 24 to 48 hours after insertion. Flow is decreased to no less than 1 L per minute until the LAP rises to 20 to 25 mm Hg while the arterial pressure waveform is continually monitored for evidence of left ventricular ejection. If none is present, full support is reinstituted. If there is evidence of recovery, TEE is performed to evaluate left ventricular function more precisely. Along with monitoring LAP as the flow is decreased, changes in right atrial pressure, pulmonary arterial pressures, mean arterial blood pressure, and cardiac index are observed. Removal of the device is frequently successful when, at low flow, right and left arterial pressures are less than 20 mm Hg, mean arterial blood pressure is maintained at greater than 70 mm Hg, and the cardiac index is greater than 2.2 L per minute per m². With reduction of flow during weaning efforts, the degree of anticoagulation should be increased. At 1 L per minute, the ACT should be greater than 180 seconds; this flow rate should not be maintained for more than 2 minutes [29].

An ejection fraction greater than 30% by TEE has been identified as a reliable indicator of successful weaning [18]. The use of TEE has also been extended to identification of intrapericardial clots compromising left ventricular function, intracavitary thrombi, and patent foramen ovale in hypoxic patients; it may also be used to evaluate the effects of epinephrine or dobutamine on severely hypokinetic segments to assess myocardial viability [64]. TEE also helps identify cannula position in the left atrium to maximize unloading of the left ventricle [65]. Radionuclide angiography has also been used to determine ejection fraction as an adjunct to hemodynamic parameters to assess ability to wean [18,66].

Table 10-4. Complications of Ventricular Assist Devices

Patient-related	Device-related
Bleeding	Thromboembolism
Infection	Hemolysis
Ventricular arrhythmias	Device failure
Stroke	Device infection
Respiratory failure	Right ventricular failure
Renal failure	

The most significant predictors of successful weaning are adequate mean arterial pressure and cardiac index, acceptable mixed venous oxygen saturation, improved ejection fraction, and normal LAP. Early signs of successful weaning include full recovery in less than 75 hours of ventricular support, some degree of left ventricular recovery within 24 hours, mild or absent right ventricular failure, and no evidence of postoperative myocardial infarction by electrocardiography and cardiac isoenzymes [47]. Patients who are weaned at the appropriate time and who attain adequate hemodynamic parameters have a 70% chance of survival [67].

COMPLICATIONS. Despite appropriate placement of VADs and meticulous management, numerous complications may occur. They are classified as patient-related or device-related (Table 10-4). Bleeding is the most common patient-related complication, occurring in up to 83% of patients requiring ventricular assistance [29,39], and is especially common after reoperative cardiac procedures [31]. Causes include thrombocytopenia, which occurs primarily in the first several days, platelet dysfunction, and hypofibrinogenemia. During VAD use, there is an increase in fibrin degradation products for the first 3 days [18]. Anticoagulation, both at the time of surgery and during ventricular assistance, contributes to excessive bleeding. Early institution of ventricular support has been found to carry fewer subsequent bleeding problems [18].

Heparin administered during CPB should be reversed with protamine and clotting allowed to normalize before institution of a heparin infusion in the intensive care unit. An adequate hemoglobin level must be maintained to optimize oxygen delivery, and transfusion of platelets is indicated if the platelet count is less than 100,000 [68]. If surgical bleeding is suspected, early exploration is mandatory. The application of fibrin glue at the site of cannulation at the time of insertion or during subsequent exploration may prove useful. Failure to control bleeding within the first 24 hours or the presence of bleeding at the time of weaning portends a poor chance of survival [53]. In addition to the hemodynamic compromise and potential deleterious effects on oxygen delivery that accompany massive bleeding, multiple transfusions in these patients are associated with acute respiratory distress syndrome (ARDS) and multiple organ dysfunction syndrome [18,69].

Infection is also a frequent complication and portends poor survival. The incidence is often related to the duration of support, occurring infrequently if support lasts less than 1 week [18] but occurring in as many as 70% of patients requiring support for up to 3 weeks [69]. Contributing causes include multiple blood transfusions, the presence of numerous invasive catheters (including pulmonary artery catheters and IABP), tissue edema, and reexploration for bleeding. Device-related infection must be aggressively treated but does not require immediate removal of the device. With appropriate antibiotic therapy, patients with infected devices have been successfully weaned or bridged to transplantation.

Prevention of infection entails control of bleeding and removal of invasive catheters as expeditiously as possible.

Frequent dressing changes at cannulation sites as well as routine surveillance cultures, including fungal titers, are helpful. Prophylactic antibiotics are administered, most commonly a cephalosporin for the first 3 days the device is in place, along with an aminoglycoside if the patient has been in the hospital more than 5 days before insertion [69].

Cerebrovascular accidents, from both inadequate cerebral blood flow and thromboemboli, are unfortunate consequences of VADs. Pulmonary insufficiency may occur in up to 60% of patients [70] and is usually related to volume overload, pulmonary edema secondary to multiple blood transfusions, prolonged periods of CPB, ARDS, or pneumonia. Renal failure, an important prognostic factor usually associated with a poor outcome, may occur in up to 60% of patients [69,70]. Contributing causes include low flow before and after insertion of the device, extended time on CPB, and multiple blood transfusions [18]. It may be progressive and unresponsive to therapy [18], although continuous arterial-venous hemofiltration, with or without dialysis, has been shown to be effective in treating hypervolemia and acute renal failure in this patient population [69,71].

Ventricular arrhythmias may complicate therapy in the VAD patient. Ventricular arrhythmias are often transient, and there is no significant difference in their occurrence before or during support with a VAD between survivors and nonsurvivors [72]. If severe and potentially lethal arrhythmias are present and persistent, bilateral ventricular assistance may be required [38].

Device-related complications are also numerous. Thromboembolism is inherent in the use of mechanical ventricular assistance, as the foreign surfaces all possess some degree of thrombogenicity [30,61,73–75]. Its incidence is related to the length of support and usually does not occur before day 4 [76]. Anticoagulation should be instituted when coagulation parameters have returned to normal after CPB and bleeding has been brought under control (less than 100 mL per minute) [68]. Textured surfaces have been developed (e.g., lining surfaces with microspheres) to enhance the formation of a neointimal lining [77]. The use of heparin-coated tubing has been studied, but results have been mixed [78,79]. Hemolysis occurs to a certain degree with most VADS but is rarely a major problem. Device failure is quite rare. Failure may be due to fractured valves, split tubing, or drive unit failures. Cannula obstruction may occur and present as low cardiac output.

Right ventricular failure may occur in up to 50% of those who receive an LVAD [18]. It is a common cause of mortality in LVAD patients, although its etiology is unclear [80,81]. Possible mechanisms include ventricular septal ischemia [82,83] and progressive elevation of pulmonary vascular resistance due to complement-mediated polymorphonuclear leukocyte activation and stasis in pulmonary capillaries [69,84,85]. However, not all investigators have found evidence for LVAD-induced right ventricular failure [86]. Although some surgeons routinely use biventricular assistance to avoid right heart failure, this practice is not universally adopted.

PROGNOSTIC FACTORS. Improved survival is associated with operator experience, use of biventricular assist devices, early institution of ventricular assistance, absence of perioperative myocardial infarction or right ventricular failure, and evidence of left ventricular recovery within 24 hours [29,73]. Conversely, factors associated with a poor outcome include arrival in the operating room in full cardiac arrest or cardiogenic shock, CPB of greater than 7 hours duration, biventricular failure, excessive bleeding during CPB, age older than 65 years, and an unsuccessful or incomplete operation [53,54].

OVERALL RESULTS. The American Society for Artificial and Internal Organs and the International Society for Heart Transplantation developed a database on the clinical application of VADs in 1985. The most recent report from this voluntary registry presents data from contributing centers up to January 1994 [87].

Data were collected on 1,279 patients who were supported with a VAD for postcardiotomy cardiogenic shock. In 70% of these cases, centrifugal pumps were used, with the remainder being supported by pneumatic pumps. Nearly 50% were supported with a left-sided device alone, and approximately 40% received biventricular assistance. The average length of support was 4 days. Those receiving centrifugal devices underwent significantly shorter periods of support compared to patients with pneumatic devices (3.0 days vs. 6.5 days, respectively). Patients who were weaned from ventricular assistance but died during hospitalization had a longer duration of circulatory support compared to those who were weaned and discharged from the hospital [87].

Differences were also noted between the complications seen with centrifugal and pneumatic devices. Bleeding or disseminated intravascular coagulation was associated most often with centrifugal devices, whereas renal failure, infection, hemolysis, and technical problems occurred significantly more frequently with pneumatic devices. Of those placed on mechanical support, 46% were ultimately weaned, and 25% were eventually discharged from the hospital. There was no significant difference in ultimate discharge rate between the modes of circulatory assistance (i.e., left, right, or biventricular). Both renal failure and advanced age correlated with lower early survival rates after institution of support and were also implicated as being the most predictive factors of failure to be discharged from the hospital alive [87].

Patients who survive to discharge can expect an acceptable lifestyle afterwards. A previous registry of patients who underwent mechanical support either postcardiotomy or as a bridge to transplantation demonstrated that, of those who were eventually discharged from the hospital, 86% were New York Heart Association functional class I or II [21]. Another study supports these findings: Two-thirds of survivors of VAD support felt they had returned to a normal lifestyle after discharge [88].

FUTURE DIRECTIONS. Clinical trials are presently under way to evaluate the utility of left ventricular assist systems as alternatives to cardiac transplantation in patients who are not candidates for the latter procedure [89]. These devices have already shown improved posttransplant survival when used for longer than 30 days, compared to a shorter time period, due to improved organ perfusion and function [90]. Interest has also been sparked by apparent ventricular recovery in patients who received LVADs for bridging to transplantation. There are as of yet, however, no reliable parameters that can predict success after weaning or the likelihood of explantation without transplantation in these patients [91,92]. The use of VADs is likely to continue and expand, given the successful clinical results that have been seen. In addition to being similar in cost to medical therapy for pretransplant patients, they offer an alternative to more conservative therapy with better clinical results [93].

Respiratory Support

ECMO, now more commonly referred to as *extracorporeal life support* (ECLS), is a modification of CPB for prolonged use at the bedside in the intensive care unit. ECLS became standard therapy for neonatal respiratory failure in 1986. Until recently, its successful use in pediatric and adult patients was anecdotal. In this section, the technique of ECLS is described, particularly as it applies to respiratory support of failing lungs. The indications, contraindications, and management of patients on ECLS are covered. Finally, future directions for extracorporeal and intracorporeal respiratory support are discussed.

BACKGROUND. As discussed earlier, it was Gibbon in 1937 [94] who described a system for cardiopulmonary support during operation on the heart. His machine, not unlike the ECLS circuit of today, consisted of a roller pump for perfusion of the blood through the system and a vertically mounted cylinder over which blood flowed, allowing exchange of carbon dioxide and oxygen between the thin film of blood and ambient air. Collected blood was then returned to the aorta. The technology of CPB quickly advanced, with a focus on refinement of the oxygenator. Various configurations have since evolved, including development of the bubble oxygenator, the disk oxygenator, the membrane oxygenator, and, more recently, the hollow-fiber oxygenator.

In 1972, Hill et al. [95] reported the first adult patient successfully treated with prolonged ECLS. Several other anecdotal reports of successes with ECMO followed. In 1979, Zapol et al. [96] reported the results of the National Institutes of Health (NIH)–sponsored multicenter comparison of ECMO to conventional mechanical ventilation in adult patients with respiratory failure due to ARDS. Patients from 11 medical centers were entered into the study based on having severe respiratory failure as predicted by strict entry criteria (mortality greater than 80%) and randomized to either continuing mechanical ventilation or ECMO. Although it was anticipated that 300 patients would be entered into the study, the study was terminated after 92 patients because of a meager 10% survival rate in each group. Based on these results, the use of ECMO for adult respiratory failure was essentially abandoned.

In 1976, Bartlett et al. [97] described the first newborn with neonatal respiratory distress syndrome successfully treated with ECMO. Several other centers reported the use of ECMO for treatment of persistent fetal circulation. Not until neonatal series from three centers were reported was ECMO considered standard therapy [98]. In one controversial randomized study of ECMO versus conventional management for treatment of neonatal respiratory failure, statistical significance was achieved with 13 patients treated with ECMO (who survived) and one patient in the control group (who died) [99,100].

When ECMO was recognized as standard therapy for neonatal respiratory failure, several encouraging reports describing its use for pediatric and adult respiratory failure began to appear [101–120]. In 1985, Gattinoni et al. [101] reported nearly 50% survival in 43 adult patients with respiratory failure treated by extracorporeal carbon dioxide removal ($ECCO_2R$). They used entry criteria similar to those used in the 1977 NIH-sponsored adult ECMO trial (i.e., entry threshold with predicted mortality of 80%). Their methodology incorporated percutaneous vascular access and a low-flow extracorporeal system that was particularly efficient at carbon dioxide removal. Several other European and U.S. centers reported similar successes with varying techniques of extracorporeal circulation. Because the technology of perfusion and the understanding of the pathophysiology and treatment of cardiac and pulmonary failure have improved in recent years (compared to the NIH-sponsored trial of the 1970s), the term

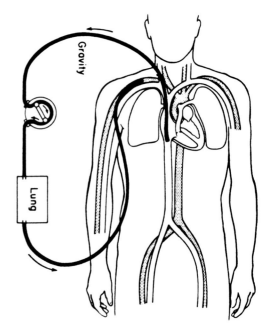

Fig. 10-3. Venoarterial extracorporeal life support perfusion. Blood is typically drained by a right internal jugular catheter with the tip in or near the right atrium and returned to the aorta by a catheter in the axillary, carotid, or femoral artery, or by direct cannulation of the aorta through the chest. (From RH Bartlett: Extracorporeal life support for cardiopulmonary failure. *Curr Probl Surg* 10:627, 1990, with permission.)

ECMO has been replaced by *ECLS* to acknowledge this modern approach to cardiopulmonary failure.

TECHNIQUE OF EXTRACORPOREAL LIFE SUPPORT PERFUSION. Because ECLS has its origin in open-heart surgery, the circuit is similar to the bypass perfusion equipment found in the operating room. The two modes of perfusion, venoarterial bypass and venovenous bypass, are depicted in Figures 10-3 and 10-4. Venoarterial perfusion is similar to CPB in that blood is drained from the right atrium, usually via a catheter placed via the right internal jugular vein, and pumped using a roller pump to the oxygenator, a device designed for gas exchange. Blood is returned to the aorta, usually via the common carotid artery or femoral artery, after warming by passage through a water-jacketed heat exchanger. This mode of perfusion is suitable for providing both cardiac and respiratory support. With venovenous bypass, blood is instead returned via a major vein (often the femoral vein), raising the oxygen content of venous blood before it enters the heart. Venovenous perfusion provides only respiratory support; cardiac function must be intact, because no cardiac support is provided. A comparison of venoarterial and venovenous perfusion can be found in Table 10-5.

Cannulation. Cannulation may be performed by surgical exposure and direct cannulation of vessels or by the percutaneous method described by Pesenti et al. [114,115]. With either cannulation technique for arterial access, repair of the artery is usually necessary at the time of decannulation.

Once a mode of perfusion has been selected, the patient is anticoagulated using 100 units of heparin per kilogram of body weight. Catheters are usually chosen on the basis of vessel size and the expected or required blood flow through the catheter. Montoya et al. [121] reported an indexing system describing the

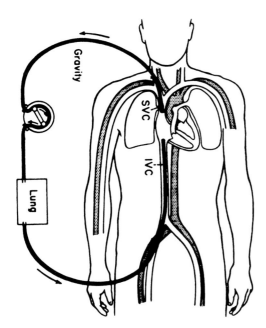

Fig. 10-4. Venovenous extracorporeal life support perfusion. Blood is typically drained by a right internal jugular catheter with the tip in or near the right atrium and returned to the vena cava by a catheter in the femoral vein. IVC, inferior vena cava; SVC, superior vena cava. (From RH Bartlett: Extracorporeal life support for cardiopulmonary failure. *Curr Probl Surg* 10:627, 1990, with permission.)

resistance to flow in various catheters based on a single number (the M number). Sinard et al. [122] tested and categorized various cannulae used today for extrathoracic cannulation. Thin-walled, wire-reinforced catheters manufactured by Bio-Medicus (Minneapolis, MN) typically provide low-resistance, high-flow access and are ideally suited for percutaneous access.

The limiting factor for bypass pump flow is the rate at which venous blood can be drained from the patient. Therefore, the largest possible catheter is selected for venous drainage. The internal jugular vein is typically used because it is the largest accessible extrathoracic vein leading to the right atrium. Additional catheters may be placed in the femoral vein or the right atrium by thoracotomy if additional venous drainage is necessary. Oxygenated warmed blood is typically returned to the femoral vein with venovenous perfusion. We recently incorporated a modification of the usual cannulation configuration, draining venous blood by cannulation of the

femoral veins and returning oxygenated blood to the right atrium by percutaneous cannulation of the right internal jugular vein. Recirculation of oxygenated blood delivered by the ECLS circuit appears to be reduced with this cannulation and perfusion method.

For venoarterial perfusion, oxygenated blood is returned to the carotid, femoral, or axillary arteries. Access is gained on the right side so that the internal jugular vein and common carotid artery each can be ligated distally and cannulae placed in each vessel proximally after a venotomy and arteriotomy, respectively, are created (Fig. 10-5). If the chest is open, direct cannulation of the aortic arch is performed, and this cannula is connected to the ECLS circuit. A separate operation is necessary for decannulation, at which time the sternum and chest wall are closed. The femoral and axillary arteries are considered end arteries, with minimal collateral supply to the distal limb. Therefore, distal perfusion of the limb must be provided when using these vessels for return of oxygenated blood. Usually, a small perfusion catheter can be taken off as a pigtail and placed adjacent to the perfusion cannula in the vessel (through the same arteriotomy) to perfuse the limb distally.

Unilateral ligation and cannulation of the common carotid artery is the usual method of cannulation in the neonate and is typically used for cannulation of pediatric and adult patients. Neurologic sequelae of occlusion of the common carotid artery are infrequent because of the generous collateral circulation from the external carotid artery and the circle of Willis to the ipsilateral hemisphere of the brain. Unilateral ligation of the common carotid artery is usually performed after removal of a carotid catheter; attempts at repair of the arteriotomy can be complicated by distal thromboembolization, carotid stenosis at the site of repair, and pseudoaneurysm formation. Several centers have attempted repair of the carotid artery in pediatric and neonatal patients with satisfactory results [123,124].

Pumping Systems. There are two types of pumps used for perfusion: the servo-controlled roller pump and the centrifugal pump. The roller pump has many years of laboratory and clinical use in the operating room. It is inexpensive and has no moving parts that contact the blood, but pump rotation speed must be regulated in response to changes in venous blood drainage from the patient. The centrifugal pump (of which type the Bio-Medicus Bio-Pump is the most commonly used) is a more expensive device that uses a spinning impeller that contacts and propels blood through the system. Although the centrifugal pump has no absolute requirement for servoregulation of the pump head rotational speed (based on venous drainage), periods of occlusion at the inlet can

Table 10-5. Comparison of Venoarterial and Venovenous Extracorporeal Life Support

	Venoarterial	Venovenous
Type of support provided	Cardiac and/or respiratory failure	Respiratory failure only
Vascular access	Vein to artery	Vein to vein
Decannulation	May require arterial ligation or repair	Typically catheter removal and pressure
Typical pump flow rates	80–100 mL/kg/min	100–120 mL/kg/min
Systemic oxygen delivery	Cardiac output + pump flow	Native cardiac output only
Inotrope requirements	None	Often required
Weaning of ventilator on initiation of bypass	Rapid	Gradual
Arterial waveform	Flattened pulse contour	Normal pulse contour
Central venous pressure	Inconsistent—dependent on pump flow	Accurate indicator of volume status
Pulmonary artery pressure	Low—dependent on pump flow	Accurate
Arterial oxygen saturation	95–100%—proportional to pump flow rates	80–95% common at maximum flow
Mixed venous oxygen saturation	Accurate	Artificially high due to recirculation

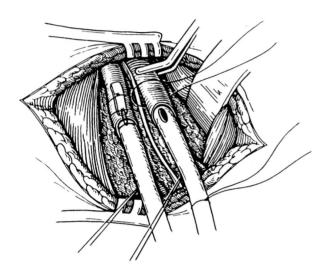

Fig. 10-5. Schematic drawing depicting cannulation of the right neck for venoarterial extracorporeal life support. After systemic anticoagulation, the distal common carotid artery and internal jugular vein are ligated, and then using proximal control, cannulae are inserted with tips in the aortic arch and right atrium, respectively (drawing orientation with the feet at the top of figure, head at the bottom). The vagus nerve is visualized between the neck vessels in the cannulation site. [From WP Dembitsky, DC Willms, BE Jaski: Peripheral vascular access for organ support, in JB Zwischenberger, RH Bartlett (eds): *ECMO: Extracorporeal Cardiopulmonary Support in Critical Care*. Ann Arbor, MI, Extracorporeal Life Support Organization, 1995, p 213, with permission.]

result in large variances in negative pressure (−200 to −700 mm Hg), resulting in cavitation of blood (gas bubble formation) in the pumping chamber. This results in hemolysis of blood and potential for air embolism [125,126]. The centrifugal pump head must also be replaced every few days because of wear of the impeller bearing, necessitating cessation of ECLS for a short period during the change. A pumping system incorporating the advantages of both systems is currently in use in Europe [127] and has been under development for use in ECLS in the United States [128].

Gas Exchange Devices (Oxygenators). The oxygenator is the key component of the ECLS system and the component of the circuit that continues to undergo continual modification and refinement. In contrast to the drum-type oxygenator used by Gibbon [94] and the disk or older plate-type oxygenators, modern oxygenators are of the spiral sandwich membrane (Kolobow membrane lung) or hollow-fiber type. Both oxygenator types are used in the operating room for cardiac perfusion. The spiral-wrapped membrane oxygenator consists of a single long envelope constructed of silicone, with gas ports at either end. This envelope is wound into a cylindrical shape, which is housed in a molded plastic container. Deoxygenated blood flows from one end of the device to the other and, thus, has intimate contact (blood phase) with the inner wound membrane gas envelope (gas phase). Oxygen gas is supplied to the inlet port of the oxygenator and passes through the envelope in countercurrent fashion, allowing oxygen and carbon dioxide gas exchange with blood. Gas exchange capability of oxygenators is rated in terms of square meters of surface area available for gas exchange. This design has had decades of satisfactory clinical use. For extended periods of use, however, the membrane lung is limited by the higher resistance to flow in the blood path and areas of stagnant flow, which lead to clot formation.

The hollow-fiber oxygenator is best typified by the Medtronic Maxima (Medtronic, Minneapolis, MN) oxygenator. This device has hollow microporous fibers through which the oxygen sweep gas flows and around which blood passes, an arrangement that again allows gas exchange between blood and gas phases. This design offers relatively small size and low resistance to blood flow, but the priming volume is much higher than with the membrane-type oxygenator. This oxygenator is available with a heparin-bonded coating that is U.S. Food and Drug Administration–approved for short-term perfusion in the operating room. It has been used extensively in Europe and in some U.S. centers for prolonged ECCO$_2$R or ECLS [107,115,129]. In theory, the level of anticoagulation can be reduced with heparin-bonded components, but in practice, wetting of the microporous membrane in these hollow-fiber oxygenators leads to leakage of plasma to the gas phase. This typically presents as a sudden, profuse outpouring of serum-containing foam approximately 1 to 7 days after initiating ECLS. The oxygenator must be quickly replaced when plasma leak degrades oxygenating efficiency. The mechanism of this plasma leakage appears to be related to elevated levels of plasma phospholipids, which alter the blood phase surface tension in contacting the microporous hollow-fiber material [130].

Heat Exchanger. The heat exchanger in the blood path warms the returned blood by using water supplied by a constant-temperature water bath. The heat exchanger is placed at the end (reinfusion side) of the circuit, warming the blood back to physiologic temperature before its return to the patient. Several available devices incorporate long, cylindrical chambers in which the blood enters the top and exits the bottom. Water warmed to just above physiologic temperature (38°C) is ported to the bottom of the same device, exiting the top and warming the blood in countercurrent fashion. There is a small visible reservoir of blood at the top of the heat exchanger, which doubles as a trap for bubbles that may make their way beyond the oxygenator, preventing passage to the patient.

PATIENT SELECTION. One of the more difficult aspects of using this technology is deciding which patients with early reversible cardiac or respiratory failure might benefit from ECLS support. The key terms here are *early* and *reversible*. It appears that early intervention, particularly after the initiation of mechanical ventilation in patients with respiratory failure, is important for a successful ECLS outcome [108,110]. For patients with primary cardiac dysfunction, ECLS intervention must begin early enough to avoid the inevitable deterioration of other organ systems (e.g., kidney, brain) when systemic perfusion is low.

Entry criteria for the neonate with persistent fetal circulation from primary pulmonary hypertension are well described. Entry is based on the patient attaining 50% to 80% or greater mortality with continued conventional management. Each neonatal ECLS center defines its mortality rate for any given patient with given physiologic parameters. For example, the alveolar-arterial oxygen gradient [P(A-a)O$_2$] can be used, although the more common method uses the oxygenation index (OI), defined as

$$OI = [FIO_2] \times [MAP \ (cm \ H_2O)]/[PaO_2 \ (mm \ Hg)] \times 100$$

where *F*IO$_2$ is the inspired oxygen fraction, *MAP* is the mean airway pressure, and *P*aO$_2$ is the arterial partial pressure of oxygen [131]. According to the University of Michigan's parameters, three successive calculations at 2-hour intervals resulting in OI values of 25 or greater predict at least 50% mortality, and OI

Table 10-6. Indications and Contraindications for the Institution of Extracorporeal Life Support for Pediatric and Adult Patients

Indications
  Total static lung compliance <0.5 mL/cm H_2O/kg
  Transpulmonary shunt >30% on inspired oxygen fraction of ≥0.6
  Reversible respiratory failure
  Time on mechanical ventilation ≤10 d (14 d relative maximum)
Contraindications
  Potential for severe bleeding
  Time on mechanical ventilation ≥15 d
  Necrotizing pneumonia
  Poor quality of life (those patients with metastatic malignancy,
    major central nervous system injury, or quadriplegia)
  Age >60 yr

values greater than 40 predict 80% mortality. A neonate consistently at the 50% mortality threshold for several hours, or one who reaches the 80% mortality threshold, may be placed on ECLS if no contraindication to anticoagulation exists.

Selection of the pediatric or adult patient for ECLS is less straightforward because the many disease processes that result in cardiac or respiratory failure in these older age groups do not result in a common pathophysiology of cardiorespiratory failure (such as the persistent fetal circulation of the newborn). During the NIH-sponsored ECMO trial of the 1970s, criteria were developed to predict mortality at the 80% level or greater. Most ECLS centers still use these physiologic criteria for the selection of pediatric and adult patients. We currently use a PaO_2 to FIO_2 ratio consistently less than 100, both in spite of and after optimal therapy. A more complete summary of indications and contraindications for pediatric and adult patients can be found in Table 10-6.

ECLS is designed to allow lung rest, and, when instituted for severe respiratory failure, ECLS has the primary purpose of providing sufficient oxygen transfer and carbon dioxide removal so that ventilator settings (inspired oxygen concentration, peak inflating pressures) may be decreased to less injurious levels. This is predicated on the expectation of lung recovery, which sometimes is based on an educated guess. ECLS is more likely to reverse sudden onset and deterioration in a patient with previously healthy lungs than in a patient with an acute process superimposed on some other chronic pulmonary condition (e.g., pulmonary fibrosis, pulmonary hypertension) if these two patients present with identical degrees of respiratory dysfunction. Pure capillary leak syndromes, bronchoreactive disease (e.g., asthma), sepsis (e.g., postpartum, meningococcemia), and nonnecrotizing pneumonia (e.g., some viral pneumonias, *Legionella* infection) can be treated with ECLS, and these diseases would be expected to reverse within 1 to 2 weeks of ECLS support.

For primary cardiac failure, ECLS has been used extensively by some centers, particularly in pediatric cardiac patients [102–106,109]. Venoarterial perfusion is the mainstay of cardiac support for patients with right or left ventricular failure, or both. Similar to patients with respiratory failure, reversibility of the cardiac insult is a prerequisite to instituting ECLS for cardiac failure, and near full recovery is expected after a few days of ECLS support.

Typical cardiac conditions treated by ECLS are myocarditis and cardiomyopathy when these disease processes result in a cardiac index less than 2 L per minute per m^2 and a mixed venous oxygen saturation of 50% or less for 2 hours or more, despite optimal pharmacologic and mechanical support. The ability to provide ECLS cardiac support has been a useful addition to medical centers with active pediatric cardiothoracic and cardiac transplantation programs [105,132,133]. In

such cases, ECLS provides short-term support before cardiac operation for congenital disease or transplantation (i.e., bridge to transplant). After cardiac operation, ECLS provides support until myocardial stunning resolves. Hill et al. [134] reported on the use of extracorporeal cardiopulmonary support (often abbreviated ECPS or ECPR) in 187 patients from 17 medical centers. In this report, 90% of which was composed of surgical and nonsurgical patients in cardiac arrest or cardiogenic shock, the long-term survival (greater than 30 days) was 21.4%. For any postoperative patient requiring extracorporeal support of heart or lung function, the potential for severe bleeding may be a contraindication. Special consideration and techniques are used in these circumstances.

MANAGEMENT OF PATIENTS UNDERGOING EXTRACORPOREAL LIFE SUPPORT. Once the patient has undergone cannulation and initiation of bypass, several considerations are necessary to minimize the likelihood of complications and to optimize the physiologic support provided by ECLS. This technology is expensive in terms of both hospital resources and the combined effort of medical personnel in hour-to-hour management. Attention to certain details with regard to management improves the likelihood and rapidity of a successful outcome.

Anticoagulation. After the initial loading dose of heparin at the time of cannulation, the patient is started on a continuous systemic heparin infusion. The ACT is checked hourly and the rate of heparin administration modified, if necessary, to maintain the ACT within desired limits. The ACT is a measure of heparin activity on whole blood (involving the combined effect of coagulation factors, platelets, etc.) and is preferred over assays of partial thromboplastin time or thrombin clotting time, which are isolated measurements of heparin activity in plasma. Usually, the target ACT is 160 to 180 seconds (normal ACT is 90 to 120 seconds). The desired ACT range is selected as a balance between too much anticoagulation (a higher ACT) and inadequate anticoagulation, which results in circuit component clotting, particularly in the oxygenator. For patients at risk for bleeding, a lower ACT range of 150 to 170 seconds is usually sought.

For patients actively bleeding while on ECLS, one may consider stopping the administration of heparin for several hours—or, sometimes, for 1 to 2 days—and using higher pump flow rates, with the expectation that a membrane oxygenator will eventually need to be changed because of thrombosis in the blood path and deterioration of gas transfer. In such cases, an additional circuit should be primed and kept ready nearby to swap if complete circuit failure by thrombosis occurs. Whittlesey et al. [135] described ECLS conducted without systemic heparin for several days. Heparinized circuits may also be used.

To ensure sufficient anticoagulation and prothrombosis when using systemic heparinization, antithrombin III activity and fibrinogen levels are monitored with some regularity and increased by transfusion with fresh-frozen plasma or cryoprecipitate. The antifibrinolytic agents aprotonin and tranexamic acid show some promise for use during ECLS because several investigators found a reduction in bleeding with their use during CPB [136,137].

Blood Product Management. The most common complication of ECLS is bleeding, which can occur in up to 20% of cases. Pediatric and adult patients are most prone to bleeding, given the propensity for other severe and unrelated illnesses (e.g., gastric ulcer) or even conditions specific to the disease being treated (e.g., fractures, chest tubes, recent operation, and bleeding from a surgical site). Blood loss during the NIH-sponsored ECMO trial in the 1970s routinely exceeded 2 L per day. Blood products (red blood cells, platelets, clotting factors) must be administered as part of the ECLS routine because of bulk loss (due to bleeding and laboratory sampling), consumption (due to platelet activation and aggregation in the membrane oxygenator), and sequestration (usually noted as an increase in liver and spleen size in patients undergoing ECLS).

Packed red blood cells are transfused to maintain a hematocrit of 40% to 45% to maximize the amount of oxygen delivered to the patient per liter of perfused blood. The small but possible risk of transfusion-associated disease must be understood by all parties involved, because by necessity blood products are required during some phase of the patient's ECLS course, beginning with the priming of the circuit. Concentrated platelets are administered to keep platelet counts greater than 100,000 per mm^3, and if ongoing bleeding is present, a higher target platelet level of 150,000 per mm^3 or greater is used. Although the absolute numbers may appear adequate during ECLS, platelet function is usually impaired because of platelet activation with the foreign surface of the ECLS circuit and the ongoing addition of older, more senescent platelets found in banked platelet transfusions.

Fluid Management. Most critically ill patients, particularly those requiring resuscitation to maintain adequate blood pressure in the presence of higher airway pressures or additional preload to compensate for diminished cardiac contractility, are usually several kilograms above dry weight. One goal early in ECLS is to augment net fluid loss with the intention of achieving near dry weight at the time of decannulation. Fluid balance is carefully monitored during ECLS, and fluids are usually administered in an amount approximately 80% of maintenance. In addition, diuretics (bumetanide, furosemide, ethacrynic acid, and mannitol) are added to the daily medication regimen to force diuresis. If rapid fluid removal is necessary, a dialyzer/hemofilter membrane can be placed in the ECLS circuit and filtration driven by the higher pressure of the preoxygenator side of the circuit. Slow continuous ultrafiltration or conventional continuous arteriovenous hemofiltration without or with dialysis, in the case of renal failure, can be performed [118,138]. Parenteral nutrition may be administered, but full enteral feeding using a nasoduodenal tube is preferred with a functioning gastrointestinal tract.

Ventilator Management. The primary goal of ECLS for respiratory failure is to allow lung rest by taking over most oxygenation and ventilation, so mechanical ventilator settings can be decreased to moderate levels. For cardiac and respiratory fail-

ure patients, a modification of the approach used by Gattinoni et al. [101] has been adopted: limited pressure (plateau airway pressures no higher than 30 cm H_2O), low FIO_2 (no more than 0.5), low respiratory rate (6 to 10 breaths per minute) ventilation, and modest levels of positive end-expiratory pressure (5 to 15 cm H_2O). Inspiratory time is prolonged by reversal of the inspiratory to expiratory ratio (a 2-to-1 to 4-to-1 relationship between inspiration and expiration) to augment alveolar recruitment and expansion. For longer ECLS runs, percutaneous tracheostomy using the method of Ciaglia and Graniero is usually performed [139]. Standard and routine tracheal suctioning is continued, and prone positioning is used, as are other standard respiratory care and nursing maneuvers [118].

Weaning from Extracorporeal Life Support. During ECLS, improvement in pulmonary or cardiac function is usually obvious, because blood gases improve and pump flow can be decreased over time. When extracorporeal support is weaned to approximately 10% to 20% of metabolic requirement or cardiac output, a "trial off" ECLS is performed, with the anticipation of eventual decannulation. For patients on venoarterial bypass, moderate ventilatory settings are chosen (e.g., FIO_2 of 0.5) and any inotropes adjusted to modest rates of infusion. The catheters connecting the patient to the ECLS circuit are clamped and the bridge opened to allow idling of the blood to prevent thrombosis in the circuit. A modest trial off bypass of 2 to 4 hours without deterioration usually indicates that the patient is ready to be decannulated. If the patient shows signs of deterioration (decreasing blood pressure, cardiac output, arterial or mixed venous saturation), the patient is simply placed back on ECLS support. Failure during a trial off means the patient is not yet "ready," and another trial off is planned for 1 to 2 days later. The trial off during venovenous bypass is much simpler, because only the oxygen supply needs to be removed from the oxygenator, while the bypass circuit is allowed to circulate mixed venous blood away from and back to the patient. The ECLS circuit, with blood oxygen saturation monitoring capability in the drainage limb of the circuit, acts to give the same information a fiberoptic oxygen saturation catheter would give if left in the central venous position. Such monitoring is invaluable when following the progress of a trial off.

RESULTS. To date, more than 24,000 patients have been treated with ECLS at more than 95 centers worldwide [140]. A current summary of the use of ECLS, compiled by the Extracorporeal Life Support Organization (ELSO) Registry, is listed in Table 10-7. ELSO, an organization of health care

Table 10-7. Neonatal, Pediatric, and Adult Extracorporeal Life Support (ECLS) Data Compiled by the Extracorporeal Life Support Organization Registry (Ann Arbor, Michigan) as of January 2002

Group	Patients reported	Survived ECLS (%)		Survived to D/C or transfer (%)	
Neonatal					
Respiratory	16,941	14,507	86	13,198	78
Cardiac	1,605	897	56	618	39
ECPR	71	43	61	30	42
Pediatric					
Respiratory	2,216	1,386	63	1,210	55
Cardiac	2,281	1,237	54	929	41
ECPR	118	51	43	43	36
Adult					
Respiratory	721	409	57	370	51
Cardiac	343	145	42	111	32
ECPR	69	32	46	22	32
Totals	24,365	18,707	77	16,531	68

D/C, discharge from hospital; ECPR, extracorporeal cardiopulmonary resuscitation.
From ECMO Registry of the Extracorporeal Life Support Organization. Ann Arbor, MI. ECMO Quarterly Report, January 2002, with permission.

professionals involved with ECLS from centers around the world, was founded in 1989. The registry is maintained for and is useful to member centers by offering data analysis of the accumulated ECLS patient database, and under the direction of ELSO, several multicenter trials have been conducted. The Registry allows investigators to study ECLS problems and hypotheses rather than just relying on anecdotal experience.

Experience with ECLS is greatest in neonates with respiratory failure, and this group of patients also has the highest survival rate. The survival rate for meconium aspiration syndrome is the highest (94%); that for congenital diaphragmatic hernias is much lower (54%) because of the complex surgical nature of this disease [140]. Survival is higher in the more experienced centers, and survival rates typically improve slightly over time at any new center beginning an ECLS program, lending support to the concept of a learning curve with this technology. A recent prospective, randomized trial of ECMO for neonatal respiratory failure conducted in the United Kingdom demonstrated greater survival in the group treated with ECMO compared to the group treated with conventional therapy [141]. Currently, the annual number of neonates with respiratory failure treated with ECLS is decreasing, due to the use of inhaled nitric oxide and the oscillator for mechanical ventilation.

For pediatric patients, experience with cardiac and respiratory failure has grown as the number of centers has grown, and there is a natural tendency for neonatal centers to move up to ECLS support of larger pediatric cardiorespiratory failure patients in the pediatric critical care unit. This growth has been most notable for the treatment of pediatric patients after cardiac operation for congenital anomaly and transplantation.

After the report by Gattinoni et al. [101] of improved survival with $ECCO_2R$ for adults with respiratory failure, several centers returned to this technology as a technique for respiratory support for failing lungs. For patients with primary lung failure and a predicted survival of only 10% to 20% (by entry criteria), the approximate 50% survival offered by ECLS, although not at the 80% to 90% survival level of newborns, is nonetheless an improvement. Several large series of adult patients with respiratory failure treated with ECLS have been reported [110,112,120]. A prospective, randomized trial comparing conventional ventilation and ECMO—Conventional Ventilation or ECMO for Severe Adult Respiratory Failure—is currently under way in the United Kingdom (G. Peek, *personal communication*, March 2002).

Morris et al. [116] reported a unique approach to the ventilatory treatment of ARDS using a computer-driven algorithm to attempt to standardize ventilatory manipulations and changes during the testing of any new technology or technique. They also used this methodology in a comparison of mechanical ventilation with $ECCO_2R$ for treatment of respiratory failure due to ARDS. Although the extracorporeal technique in this study is now considered inadequate, these investigators achieved a 40% survival in the mechanical ventilation arm of the study [117]. This study, nonetheless, has made a significant contribution. A definitive test of any advantage of ECLS over conventional therapy still needs to be performed in centers experienced with prolonged perfusion and aggressive surgical management of bleeding. We have yet to fully answer the question: Is ECLS better than conventional therapy?

TECHNOLOGIC ADVANCES IN EXTRACORPOREAL LIFE SUPPORT. The development and testing of several new technologies related to ECLS deserve special mention because these innovations will simplify ECLS and automate the process to the point where minute-by-minute attendance by an ECLS specialist should not be necessary. ECLS could be maintained and monitored by the critical care nurse already at the bedside.

First and foremost on the horizon is the development of a suitable thromboresistant surface coating for perfusion components. Although success has been achieved with heparin coating of short-term cardioperfusion components used in the operating room, two processes currently have been incorporated in surface coatings for the blood path of oxygenators for long-term use: Carmeda Bio-Active Surface (Medtronic/Carmeda, Stockholm, Sweden) and DuraFlo II (Baxter-Bentley Laboratories, Irvine, CA) [107,142,143]. Leakage of plasma from the blood phase to the gas phase (as previously described) is unpredictable in the timing of its appearance during ECLS, but this peculiar event has been reported in several centers where hollow-fiber oxygenators with the Carmeda coating are routinely used [130,144]. Further work toward refinement of the physical interaction of blood with the heparin-coated membrane may yield satisfactory results.

The roller pump and centrifugal pump have remained the two primary options for perfusion in the United States. A third system, previously marketed in Europe by Rhone-Poulenc (Collin-Cardio, Paris, France), has been used successfully by several European ECLS centers, particularly by Durandy et al. in Paris [127]. A similar device now available in the United States for cardiac surgery also incorporates several advantages of the roller pump and the centrifugal pump. This pump (Affinity Pump System, Avecor Cardiovascular, Inc., Minneapolis, MN) can be purchased at low cost and has the durability of the roller pump system. Also inherent in the design are safety features to prevent cavitation during periods of decreased venous return and overpressuring (resulting in tubing rupture during accidental occlusion of higher pressure outlet lines). Ovoid, distensible tubing is used as a "raceway" that collapses flat during inlet occlusion, preventing further blood flow and thus cavitation, and becomes round during outlet occlusion, overcoming the occlusion of the rollers and thus preventing high pressures [128].

Advances in catheter technology have been driven primarily by the needs of cardiothoracic perfusion. The thin-walled, low-resistance catheters for percutaneous insertion allow relatively high flow. A double-lumen catheter has been designed for single-site cannulation and venovenous perfusion in the newborn [145]. This design allows both drainage and return of blood through a single catheter barrel. A larger design for percutaneous placement in pediatric and adult patients is under development.

The existing ECLS perfusion system requires both a specialist at the bedside full-time for routine monitoring of the circuit, assessment of the level of anticoagulation, and modification of the rate of heparin administration and someone knowledgeable about the circuit to intervene effectively and quickly in circuit emergencies (e.g., raceway tubing rupture, oxygenator failure) or patient emergencies (e.g., bleeding, tension pneumothorax, hypotension). A team of ECLS specialists is comprised of nurses, respiratory care personnel, perfusionists, and physicians who are specially trained to assemble, prime, monitor, and troubleshoot the ECLS circuit. The ECLS specialist remains at the bedside along with the critical care nurse. One objective has been to add sufficient automation and servoregulation to the system such that, once cannulation and initial operation of the circuit have been completed and confirmed, the critical care nurse can both continue critical care duties and monitor the ECLS circuit.

This servoregulated ECLS circuit would automatically wean the system based on data input of mixed venous oxygen saturation, arterial oxygen saturation (by pulse oximetry), pulmonary mechanics (from the ventilator), and assay of blood gases. Pump flow and oxygenator sweep gas composition and flow would be modulated based on feedback from these physiologic parameters. Safety mechanisms would be built in to detect the presence of air bubbles in the arterial return side or high pressures within the system [146].

The IVOX (CardioPulmonics, Inc., Salt Lake City, UT) was introduced in 1987 as an implantable device [147] but, because of its application, it is more correctly referred to as an *intracorporeal* respiratory support device. It is inserted transvenously by way of the right femoral or jugular vein after surgical exposure of the vessel and resides in the vena cava. Before insertion, the IVOX is wound tightly (similar to an IABP catheter) to decrease the diameter of the device. Once the IVOX is placed and its position is confirmed fluoroscopically, it is unwound or "unfurled," the hollow fibers expanding to occupy the lumen of the vena cava. Gas exchange between blood in the vena cava and the oxygen within the fibers occurs through diffusion across the fiber wall.

Although several groups had reported safety and efficacy of the IVOX device [148–150], during clinical investigation it was cumbersome to insert and remove. Furthermore, the maximal CO_2 removal capability was approximately one-third that of metabolically produced CO_2, and the device was even less efficient at oxygen transfer to venous blood. Recently, Hattler and colleagues [151] have expanded on the design of the IVOX to produce a respiratory assist catheter that uses a centrally placed balloon around which hollow fibers with a more biocompatible gas exchange surface are placed. This device surpassed the IVOX in gas exchange transfer rates during both bench and animal testing. Clinical trials of the respiratory assist catheter in Europe will begin soon.

Finally, Conrad [152] and Zwischenberger [153] have described and tested a pumpless extracorporeal system that incorporates a low-resistance oxygenator to augment CO_2 removal in patients with respiratory failure. Access catheters are placed percutaneously in the femoral artery and vein, with perfusion of the oxygenator accomplished using arterial blood pressure as the driving force. Hence the acronym $AVCO_2R$ (*a*rterio*v*enous CO_2 *r*emoval), by which the system is known. A clinical study evaluating the utility and safety of this system in critically ill patients is currently under way.

ECLS has undergone significant technologic advances in recent years. It remains in the armamentarium of the intensivist for neonatal respiratory failure and is used in pediatric and adult cardiorespiratory failure. Critical to success with ECLS is early intervention in the disease process before irreversible lung and other organ damage takes place. Proper application of this technology requires an organized and experienced team of surgeons, intensivists, ECLS specialists, respiratory care practitioners, and nurses. Recent improved success with ECLS can be attributed to improved perfusion technology and better patient selection.

Conclusions

As perfusion technology and our understanding of the physiology of heart and lung failure continue to advance, support systems for these organ systems will improve with added reliability and safety. The aforementioned technologies are examples of research that began in the laboratory and moved to clinical use, saving tens or perhaps hundreds of thousands of lives in recent years. Nonetheless, these technologies are only temporizing for patients in the intensive care unit, because either organ function recovers or the patient must be considered for heart transplantation. As the science of the treatment of organ failure continues to develop (e.g., xenotransplantation, gene therapy, tissue culture and engineering), these mechanical technologies will continue to play a role in the support of patients with severe cardiac and respiratory failure in the intensive care unit.

References

1. Jorge E, Pae WE, Pierce WS: Left heart and biventricular bypass. *Crit Care Clin* 2:267, 1986.
2. Pennington DG, Swartz MT: Temporary circulatory support in patients with post-cardiotomy cardiogenic shock, in Spence PA, Chitwood WR (eds): *Cardiac Surgery: State of the Art Reviews.* Philadelphia, Hanley & Belfus, 1991, p 373.
3. Smedira NG, Blackstone EH: Postcardiotomy mechanical support: risk factors and outcomes. *Ann Thorac Surg* 71:S60, 2001.
4. Torchiana DF, Hirsch G, Buckley MJ, et al: Intraaortic balloon pumping for cardiac support: trends in practice and outcome, 1968 to 1995. *J Thorac Cardiovasc Surg* 113:758, 1997.
5. Mundth ED: Assisted circulation, in Sabiston DC, Spencer FC (eds): *Surgery of the Chest.* Philadelphia, WB Saunders, 1990, p 1777.
6. Pae WE, Miller CA, Matthews Y, et al: Ventricular assist devices for post-cardiotomy cardiogenic shock. *J Thorac Cardiovasc Surg* 104:541, 1992.
7. Pennington DG, Smedira NG, Samuels LE, et al: Mechanical circulatory support for acute heart failure. *Ann Thorac Surg* 71:S56, 2001.
8. Catinella FP, Cunningham JN, Glassman E, et al: Left atrium-to-femoral artery bypass: effectiveness in reduction of acute experimental myocardial infarction. *J Thorac Cardiovasc Surg* 86:887, 1983.
9. Laschinger JC, Cunningham JN, Catinella FP, et al: Pulsatile left atrial-femoral artery bypass. *Arch Surg* 118:965, 1983.
10. Rose DM, Grossi E, Laschinger JC, et al: Strategy for treatment of acute evolving myocardial infarction with pulsatile left heart assist device. *Crit Care Clin* 2:251, 1986.
11. Grossi EA, Laschinger JC, Cunningham IN, et al: Time course of myocardial salvage with left heart assist in evolving myocardial infarction. *Surg Forum* 35:322, 1984.
12. Pennock JL, Pae WE, Pierce WS, et al: Reduction of myocardial infarct size: comparison between left atrial and left ventricular bypass. *Circulation* 59:275, 1979.
13. McDonnell MA, Kralior AC, Tsagarir TJ, et al: Comparative effect of counterpulsation and bypass on left ventricular myocardial oxygen consumption and dynamics before and after coronary occlusion. *Am Heart J* 97:78, 1979.
14. Mickleborough LL, Rebeyka I, Wilson GJ, et al: Comparison of left ventricular assist and intra-aortic balloon counterpulsation during early reperfusion after ischemic arrest of the heart. *J Thorac Cardiovasc Surg* 93:597, 1987.
15. Champseur G, Ninet J, Vigneron M, et al: Use of the Abiomed BVS System 5000 as a bridge to cardiac transplantation. *J Thorac Cardiovasc Surg* 100:122, 1990.
16. Spencer FC, Eisenman NG, Trinkle JK, et al: Assisted circulation for cardiac failure following intracardiac support with CPB. *J Thorac Cardiovasc Surg* 49:56, 1965.
17. DeBakey ME: Left ventricular bypass for cardiac assistance: clinical experience. *Am J Cardiol* 27:3, 1971.
18. Pennington DG, Swartz MT: Current status of temporary circulatory support, in Karp RB, Kouchoukos N, Laks H, et al. (eds): *Advances in Cardiac Surgery.* Chicago, Year Book, 1990, p 177.
19. Poirier VL: Can our society afford mechanical hearts? *ASAIO Trans* 37:540, 1991.
20. Lick SL, Copeland JG, Smith RG, et al: Use of the Symbion biventricular assist device in bridging to transplantation. *Ann Thorac Surg* 55:283, 1993.

21. Pae WE: Ventricular assist devices and total artificial hearts: a combined registry experience. *Ann Thorac Surg* 55:295, 1993.
22. Rose DM, Connolly M, Cunningham JN, et al: Technique and results with a roller pump left and right heart assist device. *Ann Thorac Surg* 47:124, 1989.
23. Scholz KH, Tebbe U, Chemnitius M, et al: Transfemoral placement of the left ventricular assist device Hemopump during mechanical resuscitation. *J Thorac Cardiovasc Surg* 38:69, 1990.
24. Frazier OH, Wampler RK, Duncan JM, et al: First human use of the Hemopump, a catheter-mounted ventricular assist device. *Ann Thorac Surg* 49:299, 1990.
25. Frazier OH, Nakatani T, Duncan JM, et al: Clinical experience with the Hemopump. *ASAIO Trans* 35:604, 1989.
26. Hoerr HR, Kraemer MF, Williams JL, et al: In-vitro comparison on the blood handling by the constrained vortex and twin roller blood pumps. *J Extra Corpor Technol* 19:316, 1987.
27. Taenaka Y, Inoue K, Masuzawa T, et al: Influence of an impeller centrifugal pump on blood components in chronic animal experiments. *ASAIO J* 38:M577, 1992.
28. Bolman RM, Cox JL, Marshall W, et al: Circulatory support with centrifugal pump as a bridge to cardiac transplantation. *Ann Thorac Surg* 47:108, 1989.
29. McGovern GJ: The Biopump and postoperative circulatory support. *Ann Thorac Surg* 54:245, 1993.
30. Hoy FB, Stables C, Gomez RC, et al: Prolonged ventricular support using a centrifugal pump. *Can J Surg* 32:342, 1989.
31. Killen DA, Piehler JM, Borkon AM, et al: Bio-Medicus ventricular assist device for salvage of cardiac surgical patients. *Ann Thorac Surg* 52:230, 1991.
32. Joyce LD, Kiser JC, Eules F, et al: Experience with generally accepted centrifugal pumps: personal and collective experience. *Ann Thorac Surg* 61:287, 1996.
33. Curtis JJ, Walls JT, Schmaltz R, et al: Experience with the Sarns centrifugal pump in postcardiotomy ventricular failure. *J Thorac Cardiovasc Surg* 104:554, 1992.
34. Curtis JJ, Walls JT, Demmy TL, et al: Clinical experience with the Sarns centrifugal pump. *Artif Organs* 17:630, 1993.
35. Kaan GL, Noyez L, Vincent JG, et al: Management of postcardiotomy cardiogenic shock with a new pulsatile ventricular assist device. *ASAIO Trans* 37:559, 1991.
36. Samuels LE, Holmes EC, Thomas MP, et al: Management of acute cardiac failure with mechanical assist: experience with the ABIOMED BVS 5000. *Ann Thorac Surg* 71:S67, 2001.
37. Castells E, Calbet JM, Fontanillas C, et al: Ventricular circulatory assistance with the Abiomed system as a bridge to heart transplantation. *Transplant Proc* 27:2343, 1995.
38. Farrar DJ, Hill JD: Univentricular and biventricular Thoratec VAD support as a bridge to transplantation. *Ann Thorac Surg* 55:276, 1993.
39. Pennington DG, McBride LR, Swartz MT, et al: Use of the Pierce-Donachy ventricular assist device in patients with cardiogenic shock after cardiac operations. *Ann Thorac Surg* 47:130, 1989.
40. Portner PM, Oyer PE, Pennington DG, et al: Implantable electrical left ventricular assist system: bridge to transplantation and the future. *Ann Thorac Surg* 47:142, 1989.
41. Kormos RL, Murali S, Dew MA, et al: Chronic mechanical circulatory support: rehabilitation, low morbidity, and superior survival. *Ann Thorac Surg* 57:51, 1994.
42. Vetter HO, Kaulbach HG, Schmitz C, et al: Experience with the Novacor left ventricular assist system as a bridge to cardiac transplantation, including the new wearable system. *J Thorac Cardiovasc Surg* 109:74, 1995.
43. Korfer R, el-Banayosy A, Posival H, et al: Mechanical circulatory support: the bad Oeynhausen experience. *Ann Thorac Surg* 59:S56, 1995.
44. Frazier OH: Chronic left ventricular support with a vented electric assist device. *Ann Thorac Surg* 55:273, 1993.
45. McGee MG, Paynis SM, Nakatani T, et al: Extended clinical support with an implantable left ventricular assist device. *ASAIO Trans* 35:614, 1989.
46. Frazier OH, Rose EA, McCarthy P, et al: Improved mortality and rehabilitation of transplant candidates treated with a long-term implantable left ventricular assist system. *Ann Surg* 222:327, 1995.
47. McCarthy PM, Sabik JF: Implantable circulatory support devices as a bridge to heart transplantation. *Semin Thorac Cardiovasc Surg* 6:174, 1994.
48. Rose EA, Goldstein DJ: Wearable long-term mechanical support for patients with end-stage heart disease: a tenable goal. *Ann Thorac Surg* 61:399, 1996.
49. Phillips SJ: Percutaneous CPB and innovations in clinical counterpulsation. *Crit Care Clin* 2:297, 1986.
50. Dembitsky WP, Moreno-Cabral RJ, Adamson RM, et al: Emergency resuscitation using portable extracorporeal membrane oxygenation. *Ann Thorac Surg* 55:304, 1993.
51. Moritz A, Wolner E: Circulatory support with shock due to acute myocardial infarction. *Ann Thorac Surg* 55:238, 1993.
52. Norman JC, Cooley DA, Igo SR, et al: Prognostic indices for survival during postcardiotomy intra-aortic balloon pumping. *J Thorac Cardiovasc Surg* 74:709, 1977.
53. Pennington DG: Circulatory support symposium: patient selection. *Ann Thorac Surg* 47:77, 1989.
54. Emery RW, Joyce LD: Direction in cardiac assistance. *J Cardiovasc Surg* 6:400, 1991.
55. McGovern GJ: Circulatory support symposium: weaning and bridging. *Ann Thorac Surg* 47:102, 1989.
56. Braunwald E, Kloner RA: The stunned myocardium: prolonged, post-ischemic ventricular dysfunction. *Circulation* 66:1146, 1982.
57. Kloner RA, Ellis ST, Lange R, et al: Studies of experimental coronary artery reperfusion: effects on infarct size, myocardial function, biochemistry, ultrastructure and microvasculature damage. *Circulation* 68(suppl 1):8, 1983.
58. Ellis SB, Henschke CI, Sandor T, et al: Time course of functional and biochemical recovery of myocardium salvaged by reperfusion. *J Am Coll Cardiol* 11:1047, 1983.
59. Acker MA: Mechanical circulatory support for patients with acute-fulminant myocarditis. *Ann Thorac Surg* 71:S73, 2001.
60. Burnett CM, Duncan JM, Frazier OH, et al: Improved multiorgan function after prolonged univentricular support. *Ann Thorac Surg* 55:65, 1993.
61. Miller CA, Pae WE, Pierce WS: Combined registry for the clinical use of mechanical ventricular assist devices: postcardiotomy cardiogenic shock. *Trans Am Soc Artif Intern Organs* 36:43, 1990.
62. Pennington DG, Swartz MT: Circulatory support in infants and children. *Ann Thorac Surg* 55:233, 1993.
63. Laks H, Hahn IW, Blair O, et al: Cardiac assistance and infarct size: left atrial-to-aortic vs. left ventricular-to-aortic bypass. *Surg Forum* 27:226, 1976.
64. Barzilai B, Davila-Roman VG, Eaton MH, et al: Transesophageal echocardiography predicts successful withdrawal of ventricular assist devices. *J Thorac Cardiovasc Surg* 104:1410, 1992.
65. Nasu M, Okada Y, Fujiwara H, et al: Transesophageal echocardiography findings of intracardiac events during cardiac assist. *Artif Organs* 14:377, 1990.
66. Verani MS, Sekela ME, Mahmarian JJ, et al: Left ventricular function in patients with centrifugal left ventricular assist device. *ASAIO Trans* 35:544, 1989.
67. Termuhlen DF, Swartz MT, Ruzevich SA, et al: Hemodynamic predictors for weaning patients from ventricular assist devices (VADS). *J Biomater Appl* 4:374, 1990.
68. Copeland JG: Circulatory support symposium: bleeding and anticoagulation. *Ann Thorac Surg* 47:88, 1989.
69. Pierce WS: Circulatory support symposium: other postoperative complications. *Ann Thorac Surg* 47:96, 1989.
70. Zumbro GL, Kitchens WR, Shearer G, et al: Mechanical assistance for cardiogenic shock following cardiac surgery, myocardial infarction, and cardiac transplantation. *Ann Thorac Surg* 44:11, 1987.
71. Macris MP, Barcenas CG, Parnis SM, et al: Simplified method of hemofiltration in ventricular assist device patients. *ASAIO Trans* 34:708, 1988.
72. Moroney DA, Swartz MT, Reedy JE, et al: Importance of ventricular arrhythmias in recovery patients with ventricular assist devices. *ASAIO Trans* 37:M516, 1991.
73. Adamson RM, Dembitsky WP, Reichman RT, et al: Mechanical support: Assist or nemesis? *J Thorac Cardiovasc Surg* 98:915, 1989.
74. Kanter KR, Ruzevich SA, Pennington DG, et al: Follow-up of survivors of mechanical circulatory support. *J Thorac Cardiovasc Surg* 96:72, 1988.
75. Icenogle TB, Smith RG, Cleavinger M, et al: Thromboembolic complications of the Symbion AVAD system. *Artif Organs* 13:532, 1989.

76. Termuhlen DF, Swartz MT, Pennington DG, et al: Thromboembolic complications with the Pierce-Donachy ventricular assist device. *ASAIO Trans* 35:616, 1989.

77. Graham TR, Dasse K, Coumbe A, et al: Neo-intimal development on textured biomaterial surfaces during clinical use of an implantable left ventricular assist device. *Eur J Cardiothorac Surg* 4:182, 1990.

78. Von Segesser LK, Weiss BM, Bisang B, et al: Ventricular assist with heparin surface coated devices. *ASAIO Trans* 37:M278, 1991.

79. Bianchi JJ, Swartz MT, Raithel SC, et al: Initial clinical experience with centrifugal pumps coated with the carmeda process. *ASAIO Trans* 38:M143, 1992.

80. Pennington DG, Reedy JE, Swartz MT, et al: Univentricular versus biventricular assist device support. *J Heart Lung Transplant* 10:258, 1991.

81. Elbeery JR, Owen CH, Savitt MA, et al: Effects of left ventricular assist device on right ventricular function. *J Thorac Cardiovasc Surg* 99:809, 1990.

82. Nishigaki K, Matsuda H, Hirose H, et al: The effect of left ventricular bypass on the right ventricular function: experimental analysis of the effects of ischemic injuries to the right ventricular free wall and interventricular septum. *Artif Organs* 14:218, 1990.

83. Daly RC, Chandrasekaran K, Cavarocchi NC, et al: Ischemia of the interventricular septum: a mechanism of right ventricular failure during mechanical left ventricular assist. *J Thorac Cardiovasc Surg* 103:1186, 1992.

84. Pennington DG, Merjavy JP, Swartz MT, et al: The importance of biventricular failure in patients with postoperative cardiogenic shock. *Ann Thorac Surg* 39:16, 1985.

85. Hammerschmidt DE, Stroncek DF, Bowers TK, et al: Complement activation and neutropenia occurring during CPB. *J Thorac Cardiovasc Surg* 81:370, 1981.

86. Farrar DJ, Compton PG, Hershon JJ, et al: Right ventricular function in an operating room model of mechanical left ventricular assistance and its effects in patients with depressed left ventricular function. *Circulation* 72:1279, 1985.

87. Mehta SM, Aufiero TX, Pae WE, et al: Results of mechanical ventricular assistance for the treatment of postcardiotomy cardiogenic shock. *ASAIO J* 42:211, 1996.

88. Ruzevich SA, Swartz MT, Reedy JE, et al: Retrospective analysis of the psychologic effects of mechanical circulatory support. *J Heart Transplant* 9:209, 1990.

89. DeRose JJ, Argenziano M, Sun BC, et al: Implantable left ventricular assist devices: an evolving long-term cardiac replacement therapy. *Ann Surg* 226:461, 1997.

90. Ashton RC, Goldstein DJ, Rose EA, et al: Duration of left ventricular assist device support effects transplant survival. *J Heart Lung Transplant* 15:1151, 1996.

91. Hetzer R, Muller JH, Weng Y, et al: Bridging-to-recovery. *Ann Thorac Surg* 71:S109, 2001.

92. Kumpati GS, McCarthy PM, Hoercher KJ: Left ventricular assist device bridge to recovery: a review of the current status. *Ann Thorac Surg* 71:S103, 2001.

93. Mehta SM, Aufiero TX, Pae WE, et al: Mechanical ventricular assistance: an economical and effective means of treating end-stage heart disease. *Ann Thorac Surg* 60:284, 1995.

94. Gibbon JH Jr: Artificial maintenance circulation during experimental occlusion of the pulmonary artery. *Arch Surg* 34:1105, 1937.

95. Hill JD, O'Brien TG, Murray JJ, et al: Extracorporeal oxygenation for acute post-traumatic respiratory failure (shock-lung syndrome): use of the Bramson membrane lung. *N Engl J Med* 286:629, 1972.

96. Zapol WM, Snider MT, Hill JD, et al: Extracorporeal membrane oxygenation in severe acute respiratory failure: a randomized prospective study. *JAMA* 242:2193, 1979.

97. Bartlett RH, Gazzaniga AB, Jefferies R, et al: Extracorporeal membrane oxygenation (ECMO) cardiopulmonary support in infancy. *ASAIO Trans* 22:80, 1976.

98. Short BL, Pearson GD: Neonatal extracorporeal membrane oxygenation: a review. *J Intensive Care Med* 1:47, 1986.

99. Bartlett RH, Roloff DW, Cornell RG, et al: Extracorporeal circulation in neonatal respiratory failure: a prospective randomized study. *Pediatrics* 4:479, 1985.

100. Cornell RG, Landenberger BD, Bartlett RH: Randomized play-the-winner clinical trials. *Communicat Stat Theory Methods* 1:159, 1986.

101. Gattinoni L, Pesenti A, Mascheroni D, et al: Low-frequency positive-pressure ventilation with extracorporeal CO_2 removal in severe acute respiratory failure. *JAMA* 256:881, 1986.

102. Anderson HL III, Attorri RJ, Custer JR, et al: Extracorporeal membrane oxygenation (ECMO) for pediatric cardiopulmonary failure. *J Thorac Cardiovasc Surg* 99:1011, 1990.

103. Adolph V, Heaton J, Steiner R, et al: Extracorporeal membrane oxygenation for nonneonatal respiratory failure. *J Pediatr Surg* 26:326, 1991.

104. Redmond CR, Graves ED, Falterman KW, et al: Extracorporeal membrane oxygenation for respiratory and cardiac failure in infants and children. *J Thorac Cardiovasc Surg* 93:199, 1987.

105. Pennington GD, Swartz MT: Circulatory support in infants and children. *Ann Thorac Surg* 55:233, 1993.

106. O'Rourke PP, Stolar CJ, Zwischenberger JB, et al: Extracorporeal membrane oxygenation: support for overwhelming pulmonary pediatric population. Collective experience from the Extracorporeal Life Support Organization. *J Pediatr Surg* 28:523, 1993.

107. Bindslev L: Adult ECMO performed with surface-heparinized equipment. *ASAIO Trans* 34:1009, 1988.

108. Anderson HL III, Steimle CN, Shapiro MB, et al: Extracorporeal life support for adult cardiorespiratory failure. *Surgery* 114:161, 1993.

109. Green TP, Timmons OD, Fackler JC, et al: The impact of extracorporeal membrane oxygenation on survival in pediatric patients with acute respiratory failure. *Crit Care Med* 24:323, 1996.

110. Kolla S, Awad SA, Rich PB, et al: Extracorporeal life support for 100 adult patients with severe respiratory failure. *Ann Surg* 226:544, 1997.

111. Peek GJ, Firmin RK: Extracorporeal membrane oxygenation, a favourable outcome? *Br J Anaesth* 78:235, 1997.

112. Lewandowski K, Lewandowski M, Pappert D, et al: Outcome and follow-up of adults following extracorporeal life support, in Zwischenberger J, Bartlett RH (eds): *ECMO: Extracorporeal Cardiopulmonary Support in Critical Care.* Ann Arbor, MI, Extracorporeal Life Support Organization, 1995.

113. Anderson HL III, Shapiro MB, Delius RE, et al: Extracorporeal life support for respiratory failure due to trauma—a viable alternative. *J Trauma* 37:266, 1994.

114. Pesenti A, Gattinoni L, Kolobow T, et al: Extracorporeal circulation in adult respiratory failure. *ASAIO Trans* 34:43, 1988.

115. Pesenti A, Gattinoni L, Bombino M: Long term extracorporeal respiratory support: 20 years of progress. *Intensive Crit Care Dig* 12:15, 1993.

116. Morris AH, Menlove RL, Rollins RJ, et al: A controlled clinical trial of a new 3-step therapy that includes extracorporeal CO_2 removal for ARDS. *ASAIO Trans* 34:48, 1988.

117. Morris AH, Wallace CJ, Menlove RL, et al: Randomized clinical trial of pressure-controlled inverse ratio ventilation and extracorporeal CO_2 removal for adult respiratory distress syndrome. *Am J Respir Crit Care Med* 149:295, 1994.

118. Bartlett RH, Roloff DW, Custer JR, et al: Extracorporeal life support: the University of Michigan experience. *JAMA* 283:904, 2000.

119. Conrad SA, Rycus PT: Extracorporeal life support 1997. *ASAIO J* 44:848, 1998.

120. Macha M, Griffith B, Kennan R: ECMO support for adult patients with acute respiratory failure. *ASAIO J* 42:M841, 1996.

121. Montoya JP, Merz SI, Bartlett RH: A standardized system for describing flow/pressure relationships in vascular access devices. *ASAIO Trans* 37:4, 1991.

122. Sinard JM, Merz SI, Hatcher MD, et al: Evaluation of extracorporeal perfusion catheters using a standardized measurement technique: the M-number. *ASAIO Trans* 37:60, 1991.

123. Spector ML, Wiznitzer M, Walsh-Sukys MC, et al: Carotid reconstruction in the neonate following ECMO. *J Pediatr Surg* 26:357, 1991.

124. Taylor BJ, Seibert JJ, Glasier CM, et al: Evaluation of the reconstructed carotid artery following extracorporeal membrane oxygenation. *Pediatrics* 90:568, 1992.

125. Steinhorn RH, Isham-Schopf B, Smith C, et al: Hemolysis during long-term extracorporeal membrane oxygenation. *J Pediatr* 115:625, 1989.

126. Pedersen TH, Videm V, Svennevig JL, et al: Extracorporeal membrane oxygenation using a centrifugal pump and a servo regula-

tor to prevent negative inlet pressure. *Ann Thorac Surg* 63:1333, 1997.

127. Durandy Y, Chevalier JY, Lecompte Y: Single cannula venovenous bypass for respiratory membrane lung support. *J Thorac Cardiovasc Surg* 99:404, 1990.

128. Montoya JP, Merz SI, Bartlett RH: Laboratory experience with a novel, non-occlusive, pressure-regulated peristaltic pump. *ASAIO J* 38:M406, 1992.

129. Anderson HL III, Delius RE, Sinard JM, et al: Early experience with adult extracorporeal membrane oxygenation in the modern era. *Ann Thorac Surg* 53:553, 1992.

130. Montoya JP, Shanley CJ, Merz SI, et al: Plasma leakage through microporous membranes: role of phospholipids. *ASAIO J* 38:M399, 1992.

131. Bartlett RH: Extracorporeal life support for cardiopulmonary failure. *Curr Probl Surg* 10:627, 1990.

132. Delius RE, Bove EL, Meliones JN, et al: Use of extracorporeal life support in patients with congenital heart disease. *Crit Care Med* 20:1216, 1992.

133. Klein MD, Shaheen KW, Whittlesey GC, et al: Extracorporeal membrane oxygenation for the circulatory support of children after repair of congenital heart disease. *J Thorac Cardiovasc Surg* 100:498, 1990.

134. Hill JG, Bruhn PS, Cohen SE, et al: Emergent applications of cardiopulmonary support: a multiinstitutional experience. *Ann Thorac Surg* 54:699, 1992.

135. Whittlesey GC, Kundu SY, Salley SO, et al: Is heparin necessary for extracorporeal circulation? *ASAIO Trans* 34:823, 1988.

136. Nakashima A, Matsuzaki K, Hisahara M, et al: Tranexamic acid decreases blood loss after cardiopulmonary bypass (abstract). *ASAIO Trans* 22:64, 1993.

137. Lavee J, Raviv Z, Smolinsky A, et al: Platelet protection by low-dose aprotonin in cardiopulmonary bypass: electron microscopic study. *Ann Thorac Surg* 55:114, 1993.

138. Heiss KF, Petit B, Hirschl RB, et al: Renal insufficiency and volume overload in neonatal ECMO managed by continuous ultrafiltration. *ASAIO Trans* 10:557, 1987.

139. Ciaglia P, Graniero KD: Percutaneous dilatational tracheostomy: results and long-term follow-up. *Chest* 101:464, 1992.

140. ECMO Registry of the Extracorporeal Life Support Organization: ECMO Quarterly Report. Ann Arbor, MI, January 2002.

141. UK Collaborative ECMO Trial Group: UK collaborative randomised trial of neonatal extracorporeal membrane oxygenation. *Lancet* 348:75, 1996.

142. Shanley CJ, Hultquist KA, Rosenberg DM, et al: Prolonged extracorporeal circulation without heparin: evaluation of the Medtronic Minimax oxygenator. *ASAIO Trans* 38:M311, 1992.

143. Toomasian JM, Hsu L-C, Hirschl RB, et al: Evaluation of Duraflo II heparin coating in prolonged extracorporeal membrane oxygenation. *ASAIO Trans* 34:410, 1988.

144. Mottaghy K, Oedekoven B, Starmans H, et al: Technical aspects of plasma leakage prevention in microporous capillary membrane oxygenators. *ASAIO Trans* 35:640, 1989.

145. Anderson HL III, Snedecor SM, Otsu T, et al: Multicenter comparison of conventional venoarterial access versus venovenous double lumen catheter access in newborn infants undergoing extracorporeal membrane oxygenation. *J Pediatr Surg* 28:530, 1993.

146. Merz S, Montoya PJ, Shanley CJ, et al: Implementation of a controller for extracorporeal life support (abstract). *ASAIO Trans* 22:69, 1993.

147. Mortensen JD: An intravenacaval blood gas exchange (IVCBGE) device—preliminary report. *ASAIO Trans* 33:570, 1987.

148. Cox CS Jr, Zwischenberger JB, Grave DF, et al: Intracorporeal CO_2 removal and permissive hypercapnia to reduce airway pressure in acute respiratory failure: the theoretical basis for permissive hypercapnia with IVOX. *ASAIO Journal* 39:97, 1993.

149. Jurmann JM, Demertzis S, Schaefers H-J, et al: Intravascular oxygenation for advanced respiratory failure. *ASAIO Journal* 38:120, 1992.

150. Conrad SA, Eggerstedt JM, Morris VF, et al: Prolonged intracorporeal support of gas exchange with an intravenacaval oxygenator. *Chest* 103:158, 1993.

151. Hattler BG, Federspiel WJ: Gas exchange in the venous system: support for the failing lung, in Vaslef SN, Anderson RW (eds): *The Artificial Lung*. Austin, TX, Landes Bioscience, 2001.

152. Conrad SA, Zwischenberger JB, Grier LR, et al: Total extracorporeal arteriovenous carbon dioxide removal in acute respiratory failure: a phase I clinical study. *Int Care Med* 27:1340, 2001.

153. Zwischenberger JB, Conrad SA, Alpard SK, et al: Percutaneous extracorporeal arteriovenous CO_2 removal for severe respiratory failure. *Ann Thorac Surg* 68:181, 1999.

11. Chest Tube Insertion and Care

Robert A. Lancey

Chest tube insertion (tube thoracostomy) involves placement of a sterile tube into the pleural space to evacuate air or fluid into a closed collection system to restore negative intrathoracic pressure, promote lung expansion, and prevent potentially lethal levels of pressure from developing in the thorax. Although it is not as complex as many surgical procedures, serious and potentially life-threatening complications may result if chest tube insertion is performed without proper preparation or instruction. Insertion and care of chest tubes are common issues not only in the intensive care unit but throughout the hospital and have become a required component of the training for Advanced Trauma Life Support [1].

Pleural Anatomy and Physiology

Because the primary goal of chest tube placement is drainage of the pleural space, a basic knowledge of its anatomy and physiology is useful. The lung fills all but 10 cc of the pleural space in the normal physiologic state. This space is a closed, serous sac surrounded by two separate layers of mesothelial cells (the parietal and visceral pleurae), which are contiguous at the pulmonary hilum and the inferior pulmonary ligament. Normally, there is a negative intrapleural pressure of –2 to –5 cm water.

The parietal pleura is subdivided into four anatomic sections: the costal pleura (lining the ribs, costal cartilages, and intercostal spaces), the cervical pleura (on the most superior aspect of the pleural space), the mediastinal pleura (covering the medial aspect of the pleural space), and the diaphragmatic pleura. The visceral pleura completely covers and is adherent to the pulmonary parenchyma, extending into the interlobar fissures to varying degrees. The pleural layers are in close apposition and under normal physiologic conditions allow free expansion of the lung in a lubricated environment. In some areas, potential spaces exist where parietal pleural surfaces are in contact during expiration, most notably in the costodiaphragmatic and costomediastinal sinuses [2].

Drainage of the pleural space is necessary when the normal physiologic processes are disrupted. Violation of the visceral pleura allows accumulation of air (pneumothorax) and possibly blood (hemothorax) in the pleural space. Disruption of the parietal pleura may also result in a hemothorax if an underlying vascular structure is disrupted or a pneumothorax if the defect communicates to the environment.

Derangements of normal fluid dynamics in the pleural space may result in the accumulation of clinically significant effusions. Fluid is secreted into and reabsorbed from the pleural space by the parietal pleura, the latter process through stomas that drain into the lymphatic system and ultimately through the mediastinal, intercostal, phrenic, and substernal lymph nodes. Although up to 500 mL per day may enter the pleural space, normally less than 3 mL fluid is present at any given time [3]. This normal equilibrium may be disrupted by increased fluid entry into the space due to alterations in hydrostatic pressures (e.g., congestive heart failure) or oncotic pressures or by changes in the parietal pleura itself (e.g., inflammatory diseases). A derangement in lymphatic drainage, as with lymphatic obstruction by malignancy, may also result in excess fluid accumulation.

Chest Tube Placement

INDICATIONS. The indications for closed intercostal drainage encompass a variety of disease processes in the hospital setting (Table 11-1). The procedure may be performed to palliate a chronic disease process (e.g., drainage of malignant pleural effusions) or to relieve an acute, life-threatening process (e.g., decompression of a tension pneumothorax). Chest tubes also may provide a vehicle for pharmacologic interventions, as when used with antibiotic therapy for treatment of an empyema or to instill sclerosing agents to prevent recurrence of malignant effusions.

Pneumothorax. Accumulation of air in the pleural space is the most common indication for chest tube placement. Symptoms include tachypnea, dyspnea, and pleuritic pain, although some patients (in particular, those with a small spontaneous pneumothorax) may be asymptomatic. Physical findings include diminished breath sounds and hyperresonance to percussion on the affected side.

Diagnosis is often confirmed by chest radiography, demonstrating a thin opaque line beyond which exists a hyperlucent area without lung markings. Although the size of a pneumothorax may be estimated, this is at best a rough approximation of a three-dimensional space based on a two-dimensional view. Inspiratory and expiratory films may be helpful in equivocal situations, as may a lateral decubitus film with the suspected side up. Detection of an anterior pneumothorax in blunt trauma may be especially difficult and yet may be easily detected by chest computed tomographic (CT) scanning [4].

The decision to insert a chest tube for a pneumothorax is based on the patient's overall clinical status and may be aided by serial chest radiographs. Tube decompression is indicated in those who are symptomatic, who have a large or expanding pneumothorax, or who are being mechanically ventilated (the latter of whom may present acutely with deteriorating oxygenation and an increase in airway pressures, necessitating immediate decompression).

A spontaneous pneumothorax occurs most commonly in tall, slender, young males secondary to rupture of apical alveoli and subsequent formation of subpleural blebs, which then

Table 11-1. Indications for Chest Tube Insertion

Pneumothorax
  Spontaneous
  Traumatic
  Necrotizing pneumonia
  Interstitial fibrosis
  Malignancy
    Primary
    Metastatic
  Bullous emphysema
  Pulmonary infarction
  Iatrogenic
    Central line placement
    Positive-pressure ventilation
    Thoracentesis
Hemothorax
  Traumatic
    Blunt
    Penetrating
  Iatrogenic
  Malignancy
    Primary
    Metastatic
  Infectious
  Pulmonary arteriovenous malformation
  Spontaneous pneumothorax
  Blood dyscrasias
  Ruptured thoracic aortic aneurysm
Empyema
  Parapneumonic
  Posttraumatic
  Postoperative
  Septic emboli
  Intraabdominal infection
Chylothorax
  Traumatic
    Blunt
    Penetrating
    Surgical
  Congenital
  Malignancy
  Miscellaneous
    Filariasis
    Tuberculosis
    Subclavian vein obstruction
Pleural effusion
  Transudate
  Exudate
    Malignancy
    Postoperative
    Iatrogenic
    Immunologic
    Inflammatory

rupture into the pleural space. An associated hemothorax from torn adhesions may occur in up to 5% of cases [5]. The risk of a recurrent ipsilateral spontaneous pneumothorax is as high as 50%, and the risk of a third episode is 60% to 80% [6].

A small, stable, asymptomatic pneumothorax can be followed with serial chest radiographs. Reexpansion occurs at the rate of approximately 1.25% of lung volume per day [7]. Definitive operative intervention beyond tube thoracostomy may include resection of apical blebs, pleurodesis, and/or pleurectomy via open thoracotomy or thoracoscopy. These procedures are often reserved for those with a persistent air leak or with recurrent spontaneous pneumothoraces.

Pneumothorax in trauma patients is often accompanied by bleeding (hemopneumothorax) and almost invariably requires tube decompression, especially if mechanical ventilation is planned, to avoid a life-threatening tension pneumothorax.

Persistent leaking of air into the pleural space with no route of escape will ultimately collapse the affected lung, flatten the diaphragm, and eventually produce contralateral shift of the mediastinum. Compression of the contralateral lung and compromise of venous return result in progressive hypoxemia and hypotension. Emergency decompression with a 14- or 16-gauge catheter in the midclavicular line of the second intercostal space may be lifesaving while preparations for chest tube insertion are being made. In a hypotensive trauma patient, such pleural space decompression may be required before radiographic diagnosis of tension pneumothorax is confirmed.

Additional potential sources of pneumothorax are bullous disease, malignancies (particularly soft tissue sarcoma metastases), and necrotizing pneumonia. Iatrogenic causes include thoracentesis and central venous catheter insertion. The incidence of pneumothorax associated with attempts at subclavian vein access has been reported to be as high as 6%, and although the incidence is lower with an internal jugular approach, pneumothorax still may result (as the lung apices rise above the clavicles) [8]. Patients on mechanical ventilation, especially with elevated levels of positive end-expiratory pressure, are also at risk. In this setting, a tension pneumothorax may rapidly develop and require emergency measures as described above. Although prophylactic insertion of bilateral pleural tubes has been reported for patients on extremely high levels of positive end-expiratory pressure (greater than 40 cm H_2O), no controlled study has yet documented its benefit [9].

Hemothorax. Accumulation of blood in the pleural space can be classified as spontaneous, iatrogenic, or traumatic. Attempted thoracentesis or tube placement may result in injury to the intercostal or internal mammary arteries or to the pulmonary parenchyma. Up to a third of patients with traumatic rib fractures may have an accompanying pneumothorax or hemothorax [10]. Pulmonary parenchymal bleeding from chest trauma is often self-limited due to the low pressure of the pulmonary vascular system. However, systemic sources (intercostal, internal mammary or subclavian arteries, aorta, or heart) may persist and become life threatening.

Indications for open thoracotomy in the setting of traumatic hemothorax include initial blood loss greater than 1,500 mL or continued blood loss exceeding 500 mL over the first hour, 200 mL per hour after 2 to 4 hours, or 100 mL per hour after 6 to 8 hours, or in an unstable patient who does not respond to volume resuscitation [11–13]. Placement of large-bore [36 to 40 French (Fr)] drainage tubes encourages evacuation of blood and helps determine the need for immediate thoracotomy. Although some have advocated clamping the tube in the face of significant intrathoracic hemorrhage, this practice should be discouraged, as it fails to prevent hypotension and instead hinders ventilation [14].

Incomplete drainage of a traumatic hemothorax due to poor tube positioning or tube "thrombosis" may result in a chronic fibrothorax. Subsequent significant reduction of pulmonary reserve may occur as a result of restricted lung expansion. Early, aggressive evacuation of a retained hemothorax (via thoracoscopy or open thoracotomy) encourages full reexpansion and prevents empyema formation [15,16] in those who are able to tolerate the procedure. If the patient's condition mandates nonoperative management, a waiting period of several weeks allows an organized "peel" to form, facilitating its removal (decortication).

Spontaneous pneumothoraces may result from necrotizing pulmonary infections, pulmonary arteriovenous malformations, pulmonary infarctions, primary and metastatic malignancies of the lung and pleura, and tearing of adhesions between the visceral and parietal pleurae.

Empyema. Empyemas are pyogenic infections of the pleural space that may result from numerous clinical conditions, including necrotizing pneumonia, septic pulmonary emboli, spread of intraabdominal infections, or inadequate drainage of a traumatic hemothorax. Pyothorax as a complication of pneumonia is less common now than in the preantibiotic era, with the common organisms now being *Staphylococcus aureus* and anaerobic and Gram-negative microbes.

Definitive management includes evacuation of the collection and antibiotic therapy. Chest tube drainage is indicated for pleural collections with any of the following characteristics: pH less than 7.0, glucose less than 40 mg per dL, lactate dehydrogenase greater than 1,000 IU per L, frank purulence, or culture-positive specimens [17]. Large-bore drainage tubes (36 to 40 Fr) are used, and success is evidenced by resolving fever and leukocytosis, improving clinical status, and eventual resolution of drainage. The tube can then be removed slowly over several days, allowing a fibrous tract to form. If no improvement is seen, rib resection and open drainage may be indicated. Chronic empyema may require decortication or, in more debilitated patients, open flap drainage (Eloesser procedure). Fibrinolytic enzymes (urokinase or streptokinase) can also be instilled through the tube to facilitate drainage of persistent purulent collections or for hemothorax or malignant effusions [18–20].

Chylothorax. A collection of lymphatic fluid in the pleural space is termed *chylothorax*. Due to the immunologic properties of lymph, the collection is almost always sterile. As much as 1,500 mL per day may accumulate and may result in hemodynamic compromise or adverse metabolic sequelae as a result of loss of protein, fat, and fat-soluble vitamins. The diagnosis is confirmed by a fluid triglyceride level greater than 110 mg per dL or a cholesterol-triglyceride ratio of less than 1 [21,22].

Primary causes of chylothorax include trauma, surgery, malignancy, and congenital abnormalities. Surgical procedures most often implicated are those involving mobilization of the distal aortic arch and isthmus (e.g., repair of aortic coarctation, ligation of a patent ductus arteriosus, or repair of vascular rings) and esophageal resections [23]. Its appearance in the pleural space may be delayed for 7 to 10 days if there are postoperative dietary restrictions; the fluid may also collect in the posterior mediastinum before rupturing into the pleural space (often on the right side) [22]. Traumatic causes include crush or blast injuries, those that cause sudden hyperextension of the spine or neck, or even a bout of violent vomiting or coughing.

In the absence of trauma, malignancy must always be suspected. Leak occurs secondary to direct invasion of the thoracic duct or from obstruction by external compression or tumor emboli. Lymphosarcoma, lymphoma, and primary lung carcinomas are those most frequently implicated [22].

Treatment involves tube drainage along with aggressive maintenance of volume and nutrition. With hyperalimentation and intestinal rest (to limit flow through the thoracic duct), approximately 50% will resolve without surgery [24]. Although no consensus exists as to the optimal time to intervene surgically, a minimum of 2 weeks of observation is usually appropriate unless the patient is already malnourished [25,26]. Open thoracotomy may be necessary to ligate the duct and close the fistula.

Pleural Effusion. Management of a pleural effusion often begins with thoracentesis to identify the collection as either a transudative or exudative process. Treatment of *transudative* pleural effusions is aimed at controlling the underlying cause (e.g., congestive heart failure, nephrotic syndrome, cirrhosis). Tube thoracostomy is rarely indicated. *Exudative* effusions, however, often require tube drainage. Decubitus chest films before drainage are useful in determining whether the fluid is free flowing or loculated. If loculated, localization of the collection for proper tube placement may require use of ultrasound or CT scanning.

Malignancies (most commonly of the lung, breast, or lymph system) are a common cause of exudative effusions. Recurrence of effusion following thoracentesis may be as high as 97% in a month, with most recurring within 1 to 3 days [27]. Chest tube insertion serves not only to relieve symptoms and allow lung expansion but also to allow instillation of sclerosing agents to facilitate adherence of visceral to parietal surfaces to obliterate potential spaces and prevent future fluid accumulation. Tube drainage alone without sclerosis may result in a recurrence rate as high as 100% within a month [27]. Chemical pleurodesis should be undertaken once apposition of pleural surfaces is complete and can be performed using any of a number of agents, including bleomycin, doxycycline, and talc [28–30].

CONTRAINDICATIONS. The most obvious contraindication to chest tube insertion seems obvious—lack of a pneumothorax or of a fluid collection in the pleural space—yet this distinction is not always clear. What may appear at first to be a pneumothorax may instead be a rib edge or a skinfold, the medial border of the scapula, or even the tract of a recently removed chest tube. A large bulla may also be mistaken for a pneumothorax, a circumstance in which attempted pleural tube placement may result in significant morbidity. An expiratory chest film, which highlights the pulmonary parenchyma by increasing its density, or a decubitus view with the suspected side up may help confirm the diagnosis, as may CT scanning. Likewise, an apparent pleural effusion may be a lung abscess or consolidated pulmonary parenchyma (e.g., pneumonia, atelectasis, etc.). Again, CT scanning or ultrasonography may prove helpful in delineating the pathology before tube placement.

History of a process that would promote pleural symphysis (such as a sclerosing procedure, pleurodesis, pleurectomy, or previous thoracotomy on the affected side) should raise caution and prompt evaluation with CT scanning to help identify the exact area of pathology and to direct tube placement away from areas where the lung is adherent to the chest wall. In a postpneumonectomy patient, the pleural tube should be placed above the original incision, as the diaphragm frequently rises to this height.

The possibility of herniation of abdominal contents through the diaphragm in patients with severe blunt abdominal trauma or stab wounds in the vicinity of the diaphragm requires more extensive evaluation before tube placement. In addition, coagulopathies should be corrected before tube insertion in a nonemergency setting.

TECHNIQUE. Chest tube insertion requires knowledge not only of the anatomy of the chest wall and intrathoracic and intraabdominal structures but also of general aseptic technique. The procedure should be performed or supervised only by experienced personnel, because the complications of an improperly placed tube may have immediate life-threatening results. Before tube placement, the patient must be evaluated thoroughly by physical examination and chest films to avoid insertion of the tube into a bulla or lung abscess, into the abdomen, or even into the wrong side. Particular care must be taken before and during the procedure to avoid intubation of the pulmonary parenchyma.

The necessary equipment is listed in Table 11-2. Sterile technique is mandatory whether the procedure is performed in the operating room, intensive care unit, emergency room or

Table 11-2. Chest Tube Insertion Equipment

Povidone-iodine solution
Sterile towels and drapes
Sterile sponges
1% lidocaine without epinephrine (40 mL)
10-mL syringe
18-, 21-, and 25-gauge needles
2 Kelly clamps
Mayo scissors
Standard tissue forceps
Towel forceps
Needle holder
0-Silk suture with cutting needle
Scalpel handle and No. 10 blade
Chest tubes (24, 28, 32, and 36 French)
Chest tube drainage system (filled appropriately)
Petrolatum gauze
2-in. adhesive tape
Sterile gowns and gloves, masks, caps

on the ward. Detailed informed consent is obtained and contributes to reducing patient anxiety during the procedure. Careful titration of parenteral narcotics or benzodiazepines as well as careful and generous administration of local anesthetic agents provide for a relatively painless procedure.

Standard, large-bore drainage tubes are made from either Silastic or rubber. Right-angled rubber tubes elicit more pleural inflammation, have fewer drainage holes, and are not easily identified on chest radiograph. Silastic tubes are either right angled or straight, have multiple drainage holes, and contain a radiopaque stripe with a gap to mark the most proximal drainage hole. They are available in sizes ranging from 6 to 40 Fr, with size selection dependent on the patient population (6 to 24 Fr for infants and children) and the collection being drained (24 to 28 Fr for air, 32 to 36 Fr for pleural effusions, and 36 to 40 Fr for blood or pus).

Before performing the procedure, it is important to review the steps to be taken and to ensure that all necessary equipment is available. Patient comfort and safety are paramount.

1. With the patient supine and the head of the bed adjusted for comfort, the involved side is elevated slightly with the ipsilateral arm brought up over the head (Fig. 11-1). Supplemental oxygen is administered as needed.
2. The tube is usually inserted through the fourth or fifth intercostal space in the anterior axillary line. An alternative entry site (for decompression of a pneumothorax) is the second intercostal space in the midclavicular line, but for cosmetic reasons and to avoid the thick pectoral muscles, the former site is preferable in adults.
3. Under sterile conditions, the area is prepared with 10% povidone-iodine solution and draped to include the nipple, which serves as a landmark. A 2- to 3-cm area is infiltrated with 1% lidocaine to raise a wheal two finger breadths below the intercostal space to be penetrated. (This allows for a subcutaneous tunnel to develop, through which the tube will travel, and discourages air entry into the chest following removal of the tube.)
4. A 2-cm transverse incision is made at the wheal, and additional lidocaine is administered to infiltrate the tissues through which the tube will pass, including a generous area in the intercostal space (especially the periosteum of the ribs above and below the targeted interspace). Care should be taken to anesthetize the parietal pleura fully, as it (unlike the visceral pleura) contains pain fibers. Each injection of lidocaine should be preceded by aspiration of the syringe to prevent injection into the intercostal vessels. Up to 30 to 40 mL lidocaine may be needed to achieve adequate local anesthesia (Fig. 11-1).

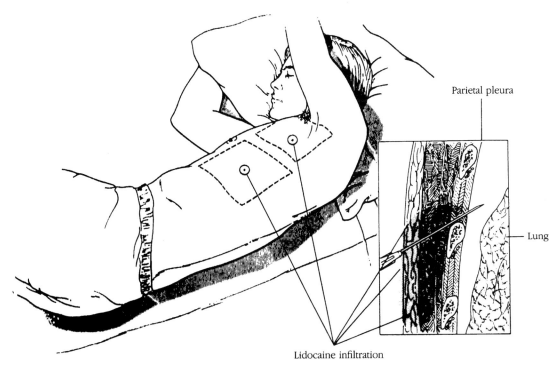

Fig. 11-1. Proper patient positioning for chest tube insertion. Note that the involved side is slightly elevated, and the arm is flexed over the head. Lidocaine infiltrates progressively through the tissue.

5. To confirm the location of air or fluid, a thoracentesis is then performed at the proposed site of tube insertion. If air or fluid is not aspirated, the anatomy should be reassessed and chest radiographs and CT scans reexamined before proceeding.

6. A short tunnel is created to the chosen intercostal space, using Kelly clamps. After the intercostal muscles are bluntly divided, the closed clamp is carefully inserted through the parietal pleura, hugging the superior portion of the lower rib to prevent injury to the intercostal bundle of the rib above. The clamp is placed to a depth of less than 1 cm to prevent injury to the intrathoracic structures and is spread open approximately 2 cm (Fig. 11-2).

7. A finger is inserted into the pleural space to explore the anatomy and confirm proper location and lack of pleural symphysis. Only easily disrupted adhesions should be broken. Bluntly dissecting strong adhesions may tear the lung and initiate potentially troublesome bleeding from the systemic circulation.

8. The chest tube is inserted into the pleural space and positioned apically for a pneumothorax and dependently for fluid removal. All holes must be confirmed to be within the pleural space. The use of undue pressure or force to insert the tube should be avoided (Fig. 11-3).

9. The location of the tube should be confirmed by observing flow of air (seen as condensation within the tube) or fluid from the tube. It is then sutured to the skin securely to prevent slippage (Fig. 11-4). A horizontal mattress suture can be used to allow the hole to be tied closed when the tube is removed. An occlusive petrolatum gauze dressing is applied, and the tube is connected to a drainage apparatus and securely taped to the dressing and to the patient. All connections between the patient and the drainage apparatus must be tight and securely taped also.

COMPLICATIONS. Chest tube insertion may be accompanied by significant complications. In one series, insertion and management of pleural tubes in patients with blunt chest trauma carried a 9% incidence of complications [31]. Insertion alone is usually accompanied by a 1% to 2% incidence of complications even when performed by experienced personnel [31,32] (Table 11-3).

Unintentional placement of the tube through intercostal vessels or into the lung, heart, liver, or spleen can result in considerable morbidity and possible mortality [32,33]. Malposition of tubes within the pleural space may potentially limit effectiveness. Baldt et al. [33] found that nearly one of four chest tubes placed in a trauma setting were not positioned correctly, with 75% of these not functioning properly. Adequate knowledge of the anatomy in general and of the pathologic process in particular should prevent such occurrences. Reexpansion pulmonary edema on the affected side in the setting of a large, chronic, pleural effusion may be avoided by incremental removal of the fluid, limiting initial removal to no more than 1 L over the first 30 minutes. Factors that contribute to this process include an inelastic lung and negative-pressure drainage [34,35].

A residual pneumothorax may follow removal of the tube as a result of a persistent air leak, entry of air through the tube site during or after removal, or restricted expansion of the lung. These conditions may be differentiated based on serial chest films, as a persistent leak results in an increasing pneumothorax and requires replacement of the tube. A small stable pneumothorax can be treated by sealing the wound securely and continued observation. If the pneumothorax is large or symptomatic, tube decompression is indicated.

Rarely, secondary infection of the pleural space may occur after chest tube insertion, resulting in an empyema. This is most common following treatment for a traumatic hemothorax. Numerous studies have examined the utility of prophylactic antibiotics for tube thoracostomy. Although it is generally accepted that antibiotics are of no benefit for decompression of a spontaneous pneumothorax [36], several investigations, including a metaanalysis of six randomized studies, suggested benefit of prophylactic antibiotic regimens directed against *Staphylococcus aureus* in patients undergoing tube thoracostomy in a trauma setting [37–39].

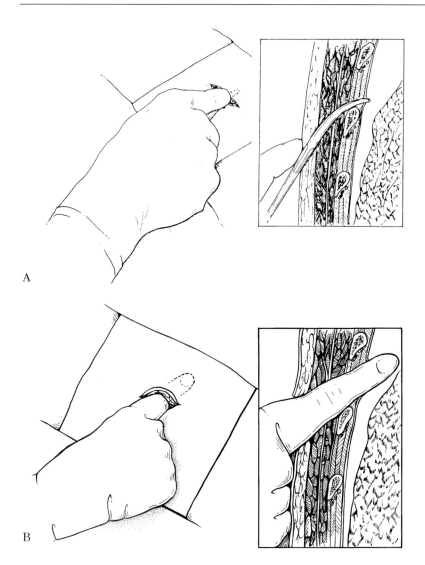

Fig. 11-2. A: The clamp penetrates the intercostal muscle. **B:** The index finger is gently inserted to explore the immediate area around the incision. No instruments are inserted into the pleural space at this time.

Because of their size and rigidity, chest tubes may limit ambulation and deep breathing. Pain associated with their presence as well as with their removal has come under scrutiny with efforts to encourage early ambulation and discharge [40,41], particularly following cardiac surgery [42]. They have also been found to impair pulmonary function, especially when placed through an intercostal space [43].

Chest Tube Management and Care

While a chest tube is in place, the tube and drainage system must be checked daily for adequate functioning. Most institutions use a three-chambered system that contains a calibrated collection trap for fluid, an underwater seal unit to allow escape of air while maintaining negative pleural pressure, and a suction regulator. Suction is routinely established at 15 to 20 cm water, controlled by the height of the column in the suction regulator unit, and maintained as long as an air leak is present. The drainage system is examined daily to ensure that appropriate levels are maintained in the underwater seal and suction regulator chambers. If suction is desired, bubbling should be noted in the suction regulator unit. Connections between the chest tube and the drainage system should be tightly fitted and securely taped. For continuous drainage, the chest tube and the tubing to the drainage system should remain free of kinks, should not be left in a dependent position, and should never be clamped. The tube can be milked and gently stripped, although with caution, as this may generate negative pressures of up to 1,500 mm Hg and can injure adjacent tissues [44]. Irrigation of the tube is discouraged. Dressing changes should be performed every 2 or 3 days and as needed. Adequate pain control is mandatory to encourage coughing and ambulation, to facilitate lung reexpansion.

Serial chest films are obtained routinely to evaluate the progress of drainage and to ensure that the most proximal drainage hole has not migrated from the pleural space (a situation that may result in pneumothorax or subcutaneous emphysema). If this occurs and the pathologic process is not corrected, replacement of the tube is usually indicated, especially if subcutaneous emphysema is developing. A tube should never be readvanced into the pleural space, and if a tube is to be replaced it should always be at a different site rather than through the same hole. If a pneumothorax persists, increasing the suction level may be beneficial, but an additional tube may be required if no improvement results. Proper positioning may also be confirmed by chest CT scanning [45].

Chest Tube Removal

Indications for removal of chest tubes include resolution of the pneumothorax or fluid accumulation in the pleural space, or

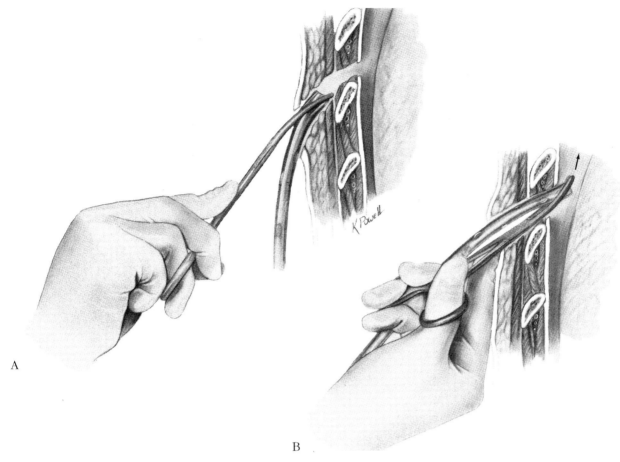

Fig. 11-3. A: The end of the chest tube is grasped with a Kelly clamp and guided with a finger through the chest incision. **B:** The clamp is rotated 180 degrees to direct the tube toward the apex.

both. For a pneumothorax, the drainage system is left on suction until the air leak stops. If an air leak persists, brief clamping of the chest tube can be performed to confirm that the leak is from the patient and not the system. If, after several days, an air leak persists, placement of an additional tube may be indicated. When the leak has ceased for more than 24 to 48 hours (or if no fluctuation is seen in the underwater seal chamber), the drainage system is placed on water seal by disconnecting the wall suction, followed by a chest film several hours later. If no pneumothorax is present and no air leak appears in the system with coughing, deep breathing, and reestablishment of suction, the tube can be removed. For fluid collections, the tube can be removed when drainage is minimal, unless sclerotherapy is planned.

Tube removal is often preceded by oral or parenteral analgesia at an appropriate time interval [46]. The suture holding the tube to the skin is cut. As the patient takes deep breaths, the tube is removed and the hole simultaneously covered with an occlusive petrolatum gauze dressing at peak inspiration (at which point only positive pressure can be generated in the pleural space, minimizing the possibility of drawing air in). A chest radiograph is performed immediately to check for a pneumothorax and is repeated 24 hours later to rule out reaccumulation of air or fluid.

Related Systems

Percutaneous aspiration of the pleural space to relieve a pneumothorax with no active air leak has been reported.

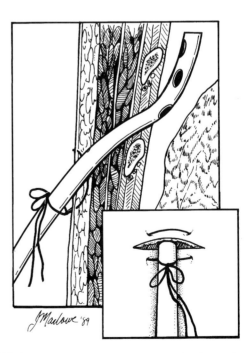

Fig. 11-4. The tube is securely sutured to the skin with a 1-0 or 2-0 silk suture. This suture is left long, wrapped around the tube, and secured with tape. To seal the tunnel, the suture is tied when the tube is pulled out.

Table 11-3. Complications of Chest Tube Insertion

Unintentional tube placement into vital structures (lung, liver, spleen, etc.)
Bleeding
Reexpansion pulmonary edema
Residual pneumothorax
Residual hemothorax
Empyema

Although successful in up to 75% of cases of needle-induced or traumatic pneumothoraces, the success rate is less for those with a spontaneous pneumothorax [47,48]. Small-bore catheters placed via Seldinger technique or using a trocar have been successful for treatment of spontaneous and iatrogenic pneumothoraces [49–51].

Heimlich valves (one-way flutter valves that allow egress of air from pleural tubes or catheters) have also gained more use by facilitating ambulation and outpatient care for those with persistent air leaks [52,53]. Small-caliber, soft, fluted drains have been used successfully to drain pleural and pericardial spaces after open heart surgery [54].

References

1. *Advanced Trauma Life Support Instructor Manual.* Chicago, American College of Surgeons, 1989, p 105.
2. DeMeester TR, Lafontaine E: The pleura, in Sabiston DC, Spencer FC (eds): *Surgery of the Chest.* Philadelphia, WB Saunders, 1990, p 444.
3. Sahn SA: Benign and malignant pleural effusions, in Shields TW (ed): *General Thoracic Surgery.* Philadelphia, Lea & Febiger, 1989, p 613.
4. Collins JA, Samra GS: Failure of chest x-rays to diagnose pneumothoraces after blunt trauma. *Anaesthesia* 53:69, 1998.
5. Deslauriers J, LeBlanc P, McClish A: Bullous and bleb diseases of the lung, in Shields TW (ed): *General Thoracic Surgery.* Philadelphia, Lea & Febiger, 1989, p 727.
6. Gobbel WG, Rhea WG, Nelson IA, et al: Spontaneous pneumothorax. *J Thorac Cardiovasc Surg* 46:331, 1963.
7. Kircher LT Jr, Swartzel RL: Spontaneous pneumothorax and its treatment. *JAMA* 155:24, 1954.
8. Bernard RW, Stahl WM: Subclavian vein catheterization: a prospective study, I. Non-infectious complications. *Ann Surg* 173:184, 1971.
9. Hayes DF, Lucas CE: Bilateral tube thoracostomy to preclude tension pneumothorax in patients with acute respiratory insufficiency. *Am Surg* 42:330, 1976.
10. Ziegler DW, Agarwal NN: The morbidity and mortality of rib fractures. *J Trauma* 37:975, 1994.
11. Sandrasagra FA: Management of penetrating stab wounds of the chest: assessment of the indications for early operation. *Thorax* 33:474, 1978.
12. McNamara JJ, Messersmith JK, Dunn RA, et al: Thoracic injuries in combat casualties in Vietnam. *Ann Thorac Surg* 10:389, 1970.
13. Boyd AD: Pneumothorax and hemothorax, in Hood RM, Boyd AD, Culliford AT (eds): *Thoracic Trauma.* Philadelphia, WB Saunders, 1989, p 133.
14. Ali J, Qi W: Effectiveness of chest tube clamping in massive hemothorax. *J Trauma* 38:59, 1995.
15. Collins MP, Shuck JM, Wachtel TL, et al: Early decortication after thoracic trauma. *Arch Surg* 113:440, 1978.
16. Meyer DM, Jessen ME, Wait MA, et al: Early evaluation of traumatic retained hemothoraces using thoracoscopy: a prospective, randomized trial. *Ann Thorac Surg* 64:1396, 1997.
17. Miller JI Jr: Infections of the pleura, in Shields TW (ed): *General Thoracic Surgery.* Philadelphia, Lea & Febiger, 1989, p 633.
18. Bouros D, Schiza S, Patsourakis G, et al: Intrapleural streptokinase versus urokinase in the treatment of complicated parapneu-monic effusions: a prospective double-blind study. *Am J Respir Crit Care Med* 155:291, 1997.
19. Roupie E, Bouabdallah K, Delclaux C, et al: Intrapleural administration of streptokinase in complicated purulent pleural effusion: a CT-guided strategy. *Intensive Care Med* 22:1351, 1996.
20. Robinson LA, Moulton AL, Fleming WH, et al: Intrapleural fibrinolytic treatment of multiloculated thoracic empyemas. *Ann Thorac Surg* 57:803, 1994.
21. Staats RA, Ellefson RD, Budahn LL, et al: The lipoprotein profile of chylous and unchylous pleural effusions. *Mayo Clin Proc* 55:700, 1980.
22. Miller JI Jr: Chylothorax and anatomy of the thoracic duct, in Shields TW (ed): *General Thoracic Surgery.* Philadelphia, Lea & Febiger, 1989, p 625.
23. Bessone LN, Ferguson TB, Burford TH: Chylothorax. *Ann Thorac Surg* 12:527, 1971.
24. Ross JK: A review of the surgery of the thoracic duct. *Thorax* 16:12, 1961.
25. Williams KR, Burford TH: The management of chylothorax. *Ann Surg* 160:131, 1964.
26. Selle JG, Snyder WA, Schreiber JT: Chylothorax. *Ann Surg* 177:245, 1977.
27. Anderson CB, Philpott GW, Ferguson TB: The treatment of malignant pleural effusions. *Cancer* 33:916, 1974.
28. Hausheer FH, Yarbro JW: Diagnosis and treatment of malignant pleural effusions. *Semin Oncol* 12:54, 1985.
29. Milanez RC, Vargas FS, Filomeno LB, et al: Intrapleural talc for the treatment of malignant pleural effusions secondary to breast cancer. *Cancer* 75:2688, 1995.
30. Heffner JE, Standerfer RJ, Torstveit J, et al: Clinical efficacy of doxycycline for pleurodesis. *Chest* 105:1743, 1994.
31. Daly RC, Mucha P, Pairolero PC, et al: The risk of percutaneous chest tube thoracostomy for blunt thoracic trauma. *Ann Emerg Med* 14:865, 1985.
32. Millikan JS, Moore EE, Steiner E, et al: Complications of tube thoracostomy for acute trauma. *Am J Surg* 140:738, 1980.
33. Baldt MM, Bankier AA, Germann PS, et al: Complications after emergency tube thoracostomy: assessment with CT. *Radiology* 195:539, 1995.
34. Trapneel DH, Thurston JGB: Unilateral pulmonary edema after pleural aspiration. *Lancet* 1:1367, 1970.
35. Janocik SE, Roy TM, Killeen TR: Re-expansion pulmonary edema: a preventable complication. *J Ky Med Assoc* 91:143, 1993.
36. Neugebauer MK, Fosburg RG, Trummer MJ: Routine antibiotic therapy following pleural space intubation: a reappraisal. *J Thorac Cardiovasc Surg* 61:882, 1971.
37. Evans JT, Green JD, Carlin PE, et al: Meta-analysis of antibiotics in tube thoracostomy. *Am Surg* 61:215, 1995.
38. Stone HH, Symbas PN, Hooper CA: Cefamandole for prophylaxis against infection in closed tube thoracostomy. *J Trauma* 21:975, 1981.
39. Nichols RL, Smith JW, Muzik AC, et al: Preventive antibiotic usage in traumatic thoracic injuries requiring closed tube thoracostomy. *Chest* 106:1493, 1994.
40. Gift AG, Bolgiano CS, Cunningham J: Sensations during chest tube removal. *Heart Lung* 20:131, 1991.
41. Carson MM, Barton DM, Morrison CC, et al: Managing pain during mediastinal chest tube removal. *Heart Lung* 23:500, 1994.
42. Kinney MR, Kirchhoff KT, Puntillo KA: Chest tube removal practices in critical care units in the United States. *Am J Crit Care* 4:419, 1995.
43. Hagl C, Harringer W, Gohrbandt B, et al: Site of pleural drain insertion and early postoperative pulmonary function following coronary artery bypass grafting with internal mammary artery. *Chest* 115:757, 1999.
44. Landolfo K, Smith P: Postoperative care in cardiac surgery, in Sabiston DC, Spencer FC (eds): *Surgery of the Chest.* 6th ed. Philadelphia, WB Saunders, 1996, p 230.
45. Cameron EW, Mirvis SE, Shanmuganathan K, et al: Computed tomography of malpositioned thoracostomy drains: a pictorial essay. *Clin Radiol* 52:187, 1997.
46. Puntillo KA: Effects of intrapleural bupivacaine on pleural chest tube removal pain: a randomized controlled trial. *Am J Crit Care* 5:102, 1996.

47. Delius RE, Obeid FN, Horst HM, et al: Catheter aspiration for simple pneumothorax. *Arch Surg* 124:883, 1989.
48. Andrevit P, Djedaini K, Teboul JL, et al: Spontaneous pneumothorax: comparison of thoracic drainage vs. immediate or delayed needle aspiration. *Chest* 108:335, 1995.
49. Conces DJ, Tarver RD, Gray WC, et al: Treatment of pneumothoraces utilizing small caliber chest tubes. *Chest* 94:55, 1988.
50. Peters J, Kubitschek KR: Clinical evaluation of a percutaneous pneumothorax catheter. *Chest* 86:714, 1984.
51. Minami H, Saka H, Senda K, et al: Small caliber catheter drainage for spontaneous pneumothorax. *Am J Med Sci* 304, 345: 1992.
52. McKenna RJ Jr, Fischel RJ, Brenner M, et al: Use of the Heimlich valve to shorten hospital stay after lung reduction surgery for emphysema. *Ann Thorac Surg* 61:1115, 1996.
53. Ponn RB, Silverman HJ, Federico JA: Outpatient chest tube management. *Ann Thorac Surg* 64:1437, 1997.
54. Lancey RA, Gaca C, Vander Salm TJ: The use of smaller, more flexible chest drains following open heart surgery. *Chest* 119:19, 2001.

12. Bronchoscopy

Stephen J. Krinzman and Richard S. Irwin

Bronchoscopy is the endoscopic examination of the tracheobronchial tree. Whether performed with a flexible or rigid instrument, it is a procedure of the trained specialist who is familiar with all of its potential indications, complications, and contraindications. Unless otherwise stated, this chapter focuses on the flexible instrument.

Since its commercial introduction for clinical use in 1968, flexible bronchoscopy has had a dramatic impact on the approach and management of patients with a wide variety of respiratory problems [1]. The procedure revolutionized the practice of clinical chest medicine. It offers a variety of features and capabilities that have fostered its widespread use: (a) It is easily performed; (b) it is associated with few complications [2]; (c) it is much more comfortable [3] and safer [4] for the patient than rigid bronchoscopy; (d) it exposes a far greater proportion of the tracheobronchial tree (especially the upper lobes) to direct visualization than does rigid bronchoscopy [5]; (e) it does not require general anesthesia or the use of an operating room [3]; and (f) it can be performed at the bedside [3]. For all of these reasons, flexible bronchoscopy has largely replaced rigid bronchoscopy as the procedure of choice for most endoscopic evaluations of the airway. On the other hand, rigid bronchoscopy may be the procedure of choice [1,6] for (a) brisk hemoptysis (200 mL per 24 hours); (b) extraction of foreign bodies; (c) endobronchial resection of granulation tissue that might occur after traumatic or prolonged intubation, or both; (d) biopsy of vascular tumors (e.g., bronchial carcinoid) in which brisk and excessive bleeding can be controlled by packing; (e) endoscopic laser surgery; and (f) dilation of tracheobronchial strictures and placement of airway stents.

Diagnostic Indications

GENERAL CONSIDERATIONS. Because flexible bronchoscopy can be performed easily even in intubated patients, the same general indications apply to critically ill patients on ventilators and to noncritically ill patients. However, only the indications most commonly encountered in critically ill patients are discussed here.

COMMON INDICATIONS

Hemoptysis. Hemoptysis is one of the commonest clinical problems for which bronchoscopy is indicated [7,8] (see Chapter 53 for a detailed discussion). Whether the patient complains of blood streaking or massive hemoptysis (expectoration of more than 600 mL in 48 hours) [9], bronchoscopy should be considered to localize the site of bleeding and to diagnose the cause. Localization of the site of bleeding is crucial if definitive therapy such as surgery becomes necessary. Bronchoscopy performed within 48 hours of the time that bleeding stops is more likely to localize the site of bleeding (34% to 91%) compared with delayed bronchoscopy (11% to 52%) [10]. Bronchoscopy is more likely to identify a bleeding source in patients with moderate or severe hemoptysis [11]. Clinical judgment must dictate whether and when bronchoscopy is indicated. For instance, it is not indicated in patients with obvious pulmonary embolism with infarction. Whenever patients have an endotracheal or tracheostomy tube in place, hemoptysis should always be evaluated, because it may indicate potentially life-threatening tracheal damage. Unless the bleeding is massive, a flexible bronchoscope, rather than a rigid bronchoscope, is the instrument of choice for evaluating hemoptysis.

Atelectasis. Although atelectasis may be due to mucous plugging, bronchoscopy should be performed in patents who do not improve after chest physiotherapy to rule out endobronchial obstruction by carcinoma, foreign body, mucoid impaction, or clot. When atelectasis occurs in critically ill patients who had a normal chest film on admission, mucous plugging is the most likely cause [12]. In intubated patients, the position of the endotracheal tube, which may have slipped down the right mainstem bronchus and obstructed the right upper lobe, should be determined on a chest radiograph [13].

Diffuse Parenchymal Disease. In patients with diffuse pulmonary disease, the clinical setting influences the choice of procedure. When diffuse pulmonary infiltrates suggest sarcoidosis, carcinomatosis, or eosinophilic pneumonia, transbronchoscopic lung forceps biopsy should be considered initially because it has an extremely high yield in these situations (see Chapter 69). Transbronchial lung biopsy has a low yield for the definitive diagnosis of inorganic pneumoconiosis and pulmonary vasculitides [14]; when these disorders are suspected, surgical lung biopsy is the procedure of choice. In the case of pulmonary fibrosis and acute interstitial pneumonitis, transbronchial biopsy does not provide adequate tissue for a specific histologic diagnosis, although by excluding infection the procedure may provide sufficient information to guide therapy.

When an infectious process is suspected, the diagnostic yield depends on the organism and the immune status of the patient. In immunocompetent patients, bronchoalveolar lavage (BAL) has a sensitivity of 87% for detecting respiratory pathogens [15], and a negative BAL quantitative culture has a specificity of 96% in predicting sterile lung parenchyma. For these reasons, bronchoscopic or surgical biopsy is not usually indicated to diagnose infections in this setting unless there is a suspicion for viral or fungal pathogens, where isolation of the organism within the airways does not always indicate clinically significant infection. In bone marrow transplant recipients with pulmonary complications, BAL is diagnostic in 31% to 66% of patients [16]. The addition of transbronchial biopsy has not been shown to increase the diagnostic yield significantly in this population [17]. In patients with acquired immunodeficiency syndrome, the sensitivity of lavage or transbronchial lung biopsy for identifying all opportunistic organisms can be as high as 87% [18,19]. Transbronchial biopsy adds significantly to the diagnostic yield in patients with acquired immunodeficiency syndrome and may be the sole means of making a diagnosis in up to 24% of patients, including diagnoses of *Pneumocystis carinii*, *Cryptococcus neoformans*, *Mycobacterium tuberculosis*, and nonspecific interstitial pneumonitis [20]. Lavage alone may have a sensitivity of up to 97% for the diagnosis of *P. carinii* pneumonia [21]. However, because induced sputum samples can also be positive for *P. carinii* in up to 79% of cases [21], induced sputum, when available, should be evaluated first for this organism before resorting to bronchoscopy.

Acute Inhalation Injury. In patients who are exposed to smoke inhalation, flexible nasopharyngoscopy, laryngoscopy, and bronchoscopy are indicated to identify the anatomic level and severity of injury [22,23]. Prophylactic intubation should be considered if considerable upper airway mucosal injury is noted early; acute respiratory failure is more likely in patients with mucosal changes seen at segmental or lower levels [24]. Upper airway obstruction is a life-threatening problem that usually develops during the initial 24 hours after inhalation injury. It correlates significantly with increased size of cutaneous burns, burns of the face and neck, and rapid intravenous fluid administration [25].

Blunt Chest Trauma. Flexible bronchoscopy has a high yield in the evaluation of patients after major chest trauma. Patients may present with atelectasis, pulmonary contusion, hemothorax, pneumothorax, pneumomediastinum, or hemoptysis. Prompt bronchoscopic evaluation of such patients has a diagnostic yield of 53%; findings may include tracheal or bronchial laceration or transection (14%), aspirated material (6%), supraglottic tear with glottic obstruction (2%), mucous plugging (15%), and distal hemorrhage (13%) [26]. Many of these diagnoses may not be clinically evident, and require surgical intervention.

Postresectional Surgery. Flexible bronchoscopy can identify a disrupted suture line that is causing bleeding and pneumothorax [27] following surgery and an exposed endobronchial suture that is causing cough [28].

Assessment of Intubation Damage. When a nasotracheal or orotracheal tube of the proper size is in place, the balloon can be routinely deflated and the tube withdrawn over the bronchoscope to look for subglottic damage. The tube is withdrawn up through the vocal cords and over the flexible bronchoscope, and glottic and supraglottic damage is sought. This technique may be useful after reintubation for stridor or when deflation of the endotracheal tube cuff does not produce a significant air leak, suggesting the potential for life-threatening upper airway obstruction when extubation takes place. In patients on long-term ventilatory assistance with cuffed tracheostomy tubes, flexible bronchoscopy can help differentiate aspiration from tracheoesophageal fistula. With the bronchoscope in the distal trachea, the patient is asked to swallow a dilute solution of methylene blue. The absence of methylene blue in the trachea and its presence leaking around and out of the tracheostomy stoma provide accurate evidence of a swallowing abnormality and the absence of a tracheoesophageal fistula.

Diagnosing Ventilator-Associated Pneumonia. The clinical diagnosis of ventilator-associated pneumonia continues to be problematic. Direct visualization of the bronchial tree in immunocompetent patients may be useful. A multivariate analysis showed that the presence of at least two of three factors [a decrease in partial arterial pressure of oxygen/inspired oxygen concentration (PaO_2/FIO_2) greater than or equal to 50 mm Hg, distal purulent secretions, and persistence of distal secretions surging from distal bronchi during exhalation in paralyzed patients] predicted pneumonia that was subsequently diagnosed by distal bacteriologic results, follow-up, and lung biopsy with a sensitivity of 78% and specificity of 89% [29].

With respect to cultures, transnasal or transoral flexible bronchoscopy aspirates from a nonintubated patient [30] are no more reliable than the inaccurate nasotracheal suction aspirates or expectorated sputum specimens for culture of routine aerobic and anaerobic organisms [31]. Bronchoscopy aspirates, however, may be extremely useful in identifying *M. tuberculosis* [32], *Nocardia* species [33], pathogenic fungi [33], and *Legionella* species [34] when patients are unable to expectorate adequate quantities of sputum. Although quantitative cultures of BAL fluid or a protected specimen brush improves specificity, the accuracy of these tests for the diagnosis of ventilator-associated pneumonia has varied greatly in published series. For protected specimen brush, the sensitivity ranges from 33% to 100%, with a median of 67%, and the specificity is between 50% and 100%, with a median of 95% [35]. The determination of the performance characteristics of these diagnostic studies has been hindered by lack of consensus on the "gold standard" for the diagnosis of ventilator-associated pneumonia. In one investigation comparing airway cultures with lung biopsy histology and culture, suctioned specimens from the lower trachea obtained via an endotracheal tube detected 87% of bacterial species that are simultaneously present in the lung parenchyma, and a negative BAL quantitative culture had a 63% sensitivity and 96% specificity in predicting sterile lung parenchyma [36].

Therapeutic Indications

EXCESSIVE SECRETIONS AND ATELECTASIS. When chest physiotherapy, incentive spirometry, and sustained maximum inspiration with cough fail to clear the airways of excessive secretions and reexpand lobar atelectasis [37], flexible bronchoscopy may be successful. Variable results have been reported, with improvements in radiographs or oxygenation in 19% to 44% of patients [38]. Occasionally, the direct instillation of acetylcysteine (Mucomyst) through the bronchoscope may be necessary to liquefy the thick, tenacious inspissated mucus [39]. Because acetylcysteine may induce bronchospasm in asthmatics, these patients must be pretreated with a bronchodilator.

FOREIGN BODIES. Although the rigid bronchoscope is considered by many to be the instrument of choice for removing foreign bodies, devices with which to grasp objects are available for use with the flexible bronchoscope [40].

ENDOTRACHEAL INTUBATION. In patients with ankylosing spondylitis and other mechanical problems of the neck, the flexible bronchoscope can be used as an obturator for endotracheal intubation [27]. The bronchoscope with an endotracheal tube passed over it can be passed transnasally (after proper local anesthesia) through the vocal cords into the trachea. Then the tube can be passed over the scope. This same technique can be used in patients with tetanus complicated by trismus and in patients with acute supraglottitis [41]. In the latter two instances, the procedure should preferably be done in the operating room with an anesthesiologist and otolaryngologist present.

HEMOPTYSIS. On the rare occasions on which brisk bleeding threatens asphyxiation, endobronchial tamponade may stabilize the patient's condition before definitive therapy is performed [42] (see Chapter 53). With the use of the flexible bronchoscope, usually passed through a rigid bronchoscope or endotracheal tube, a Fogarty catheter with balloon is passed into the bleeding lobar orifice. When the balloon is inflated and wedged tightly, the patient can be transferred to surgery or angiography for bronchial arteriography and bronchial artery embolization [43–45].

CENTRAL OBSTRUCTING AIRWAY LESIONS. Some patients with cancer and others with benign lesions that obstruct the larynx, trachea, and major bronchi can be treated by using bronchoscopy to deliver laser photoresection, cryotherapy, or phototherapy [46]. Flexible bronchoscopy can also be used to place catheters that facilitate endobronchial delivery of radiation (brachytherapy). Metal or silicone endobronchial stents can be placed bronchoscopically to relieve stenosis of large airways [47].

CLOSURE OF BRONCHOPLEURAL FISTULA. Bronchopleural fistula (BPF) is an acquired pathway between the bronchial tree and pleural space. After placement of a chest tube, drainage of the pleural space, and stabilization of the patient (e.g., infection, cardiovascular and respiratory systems), bronchoscopy can be used to visualize a proximal BPF or localize a distal BPF; it can also be used in attempts to close the BPF [48,49]. Although the published experience on bronchoscopically sealing BPFs is limited, a number of case reports have suggested that a variety of materials, injected through the bronchoscope, may successfully seal BPFs [48–51]. These materials have included doxycycline and tetracycline followed by autologous blood instillation to form an obstructive blood clot, lead fishing weights or shot, tissue adhesive, fibrin glue, absorbable gelatin sponge, angiographic occlusion coils, silver nitrate, and balloon occlusion. For an in-depth discussion of BPF and its management, see Chapter 57.

Complications

When performed by a trained specialist, routine flexible bronchoscopy is extremely safe. Mortality should not exceed 0.1% [2], and overall complications should not exceed 8.1% [2]. The rare deaths have been due to excessive premedication or topical anesthesia, respiratory arrest from hemorrhage, laryngospasm or bronchospasm, and cardiac arrest from acute myocardial infarction [52,53]. Nonfatal complications occurring within 24 hours of the procedure include fever (1.2% to 24.0%) [2,54,55], pneumonia (0.6% to 6.0%) [2,54], vasovagal reactions (2.4%) [2], laryngospasm and bronchospasm (0.1% to 0.4%) [2,52], cardiac arrhythmias (0.9 to 4.0%) [2,56], pneumothorax (4% after transbronchial biopsy) [56], anesthesia-related problems (0.1%) [2,52], and aphonia (0.1%) [2]. Fever may occur in up to 24% of patients after bronchoscopy and appears to be cytokine mediated and uncommonly indicative of a true infection or bacteremia [55]. Transient bacteremias often occur (15.4% to 33.0%) after rigid bronchoscopy [57,58], probably due to trauma to the teeth and airways. Most investigations have found that the incidence of bacteremia after transoral flexible bronchoscopy is much lower (0.7%) [59]. However, one larger prospective study that excluded patients with evidence of infection or receiving recent antibiotics found an incidence of 6.5% [59]. The most recent guidelines of the American Heart Association [60] recommend endocarditis prophylaxis for rigid but not for flexible bronchoscopy, except in high-risk cardiac patients such as those with prosthetic valves, in which case prophylaxis should be considered.

Although routine bronchoscopy is extremely safe, critically ill patients appear to be at higher risk of complications. Asthmatics are prone to development of laryngospasm and bronchospasm. Major bleeding is more likely to develop in bone marrow transplant recipients during bronchoscopy (0 to 6%) [17,61], particularly if protected specimen brush or transbronchial lung biopsy is performed (7.7% vs. 1.5% for BAL alone) [61]. Patients with uremia are at increased risk of bleeding [62]. In critically ill, mechanically ventilated patents, bronchoscopy causes a transient decrease in PaO_2 of approximately 25% [63], and transbronchial lung biopsy is more likely to result in pneumothorax (7% to 23%) [64,65]. Patients with the acute respiratory distress syndrome have more pronounced declines in oxygenation, with a mean decrease of more than 50% in the PaO_2 [63].

Contraindications

Bronchoscopy should not be performed (a) when an experienced bronchoscopist is not available; (b) when the patient will not or cannot cooperate; (c) when adequate oxygenation cannot be maintained during the procedure; (d) when coagulation studies cannot be normalized in patients in whom biopsies, brush or forceps, are to be taken; (e) in unstable cardiac patients [66–68]; and (f) in untreated symptomatic asthmatics [69]. In patients with recent cardiac ischemia, the major complication rate is low (3% to 5%) and is similar to that of other critically ill populations [70,71]. Although patients with stable carbon dioxide retention can safely undergo bronchoscopy with a flexible instrument [72], premedication, sedation during the procedure, and supplemental oxygen must be used with caution.

Consideration of bronchoscopy in neurologic and neurosurgical patients requires attention to the effects of bronchoscopy on intracranial pressure (ICP) and cerebral perfusion pressure (CPP). In patients with head trauma, bronchoscopy causes the ICP to increase by at least 50% in 88% of patients, and by at least 100% in 69% of patients, despite the use of deep sedation and paralysis [73]. Because mean arterial pressure tends to rise in parallel with ICP, there is often no change in CPP. No significant neurologic complications have been noted in patients with severe head trauma [73,74] or with space-occupying intracranial lesions with computed tomographic evidence of elevated ICP [75]. Bronchoscopy in such patients should be accompanied by deep sedation, paralysis, and medications for cerebral protection (thiopental, lidocaine). Cerebral hemodynamics should be continuously monitored to ensure that ICP and CPP are within acceptable levels. Caution is warranted in patients with markedly elevated baseline ICP or with borderline CPP.

Procedure

PREPROCEDURAL CONSIDERATIONS. The following is a checklist for use before performing the procedure:

1. Has a procedure consent form been signed?
2. Does the patient have asthma or cardiovascular disease?
3. Coagulation status: If brushings or biopsy are anticipated, have platelet counts and coagulation times been checked; is the patient taking anticoagulants; is there a history of bleeding disorders; is the patient uremic?
4. Does the patient have drug allergies?
5. Is proper monitoring in place: continuous pulse oximetry, electrocardiogram, and blood pressure monitoring at least every 5 minutes?
6. Is there stable intravenous access? Has the patient fasted for 3 to 4 hours before the procedure?
7. If the patient is mechanically ventilated, is the size of the endotracheal tube adequate, has the FIO_2 been increased to 100%, and has the ventilator been adjusted to assure adequate tidal volume?

PROCEDURAL CONSIDERATIONS

Airway and Intubation. In nonintubated patients, flexible bronchoscopy can be performed by the transnasal route or transoral route with a bite block [1]. In intubated and mechanically ventilated patients, the flexible bronchoscope can be passed through a swivel adapter with a rubber diaphragm that prevents loss of the delivered respiratory gases [76]. To prevent dramatic increases in airway resistance and an unacceptable loss of tidal volumes, the lumen of the endotracheal tube should be at least 2 mm larger than the outer diameter of the bronchoscope [77,78]. Thus, flexible bronchoscopy with an average adult-sized instrument (outside diameter of scope, 4.8 to 5.9 mm) can be performed in a ventilated patient if there is an endotracheal tube in place that is 8 mm or larger in internal diameter. If the endotracheal tube is smaller, a pediatric bronchoscope (outside diameter, 3.5 mm) or intubation endoscope (outside diameter, 3.8 mm) must be used.

Premedication. Topical anesthesia can be achieved by hand-nebulized lidocaine and lidocaine jelly as a lubricant [1] and by instilling approximately 3 mL 1% or 2% lidocaine at the main carina and, if needed, into the lower airways. Lidocaine is absorbed through the mucous membranes, producing peak serum concentrations that are nearly as high as when the equivalent dose is administered intravenously, although toxicity is rare if the total dose does not exceed 6 to 7 mg per kg. In patients with hepatic or cardiac insufficiency, lidocaine clearance is reduced, and the dose should be decreased to a maximum of 4 to 5 mg per kg [79]. Conscious sedation with incremental doses of midazolam, titrated to produce light sleep, produces amnesia in greater than 95% of patients, but adequate sedation may require a total of greater than 20 mg in some subjects [80]. Premedication with intravenous atropine has not been found to reduce secretions, decrease coughing, or prevent bradycardia [81,82].

Mechanical Ventilation. Maintaining adequate oxygenation and ventilation while preventing breath-stacking and positive

end-expiratory pressure (PEEP) may be challenging when insertion of the bronchoscope reduces the effective lumen of the endotracheal tube by more than 50%. PEEP caused by standard scopes and tubes approaches 20 cm H_2O with the potential for barotrauma [77]. PEEP, if already being delivered, must be discontinued before the scope is inserted [77]. The inspired oxygen concentration must be temporarily increased to 100% [77]. With the help of a respiratory care practitioner, expired volumes should be constantly measured to ensure that they are adequate (tidal volumes usually have to be increased 40% to 50%) [77]. Meeting these ventilatory goals may require increasing the high-pressure limit in volume-cycled ventilation to near its maximal value, allowing the ventilator to generate the force needed to overcome the added resistance caused by the bronchoscope. Although this increases the measured peak airway pressure, the alveolar pressure is not likely to change significantly because the lung is protected by the resistance of the bronchoscope [78]. Alternatively, decreasing the inspiratory flow rate in an attempt to decrease measured peak pressures may paradoxically increase alveolar pressures by decreasing expiratory time and thus increasing auto-PEEP. Suctioning should be kept to a minimum and for short periods of time, because suctioning decreases the tidal volumes being delivered [77].

References

1. Sackner MA: Bronchofiberoscopy. *Am Rev Respir Dis* 111:62, 1975.
2. Pereira W Jr, Kovnat DM, Snider GL: A prospective cooperative study of complications following flexible fiberoptic bronchoscopy. *Chest* 73:813, 1978.
3. Rath GS, Schaff JT, Snider GL: Flexible fiberoptic bronchoscopy: techniques and review of 100 bronchoscopies. *Chest* 63:689, 1973.
4. Lukomsky GI, Ovchinnikov AA, Bilal A: Complications of bronchoscopy: comparison of rigid bronchoscopy under general anesthesia and flexible fiberoptic bronchoscopy under topical anesthesia. *Chest* 79:316, 1981.
5. Kovnat DM, Rath GS, Anderson WM, et al: Maximal extent of visualization of bronchial tree by flexible fiberoptic bronchoscopy. *Am Rev Respir Dis* 110:88, 1974.
6. Prakash UBS, Stuffs SE: The bronchoscopy survey: some reflections. *Chest* 100:1660, 1991.
7. Khan MA, Whitcomb ME, Snider GL: Flexible fiberoptic bronchoscopy. *Am J Med* 61:151, 1976.
8. Selecky PA: Evaluation of hemoptysis through the bronchoscope. *Chest* 73[Suppl]:741, 1978.
9. Crocco JA, Rooney JJ, Fankushen DS, et al: Massive hemoptysis. *Arch Intern Med* 121:495, 1968.
10. Dweik RA, Stoller JK: Role of bronchoscopy in massive hemoptysis. *Clin Chest Med* 20:89, 1999.
11. Hirshberg B, Biran I, Glazer M, et al: Hemoptysis: etiology, evaluation, and outcome in a tertiary referral hospital. *Chest* 112:440, 1997.
12. Mahajan VK, Catron PW, Huber GL: The value of fiberoptic bronchoscopy in the management of pulmonary collapse. *Chest* 73:817, 1978.
13. Goodman LR, Putnam CE: Radiological evaluation of patients receiving assisted ventilation. *JAMA* 245:858, 1981.
14. Schnabel A, Holl-Ulrich K, Dahloff K, et al: Efficacy of transbronchial biopsy in pulmonary vasculitides. *Eur Respir J* 10:2738, 1997.
15. Kirtland SH, Corley DE, Winterbauer RH, et al: The diagnosis of ventilator-associated pneumonia: a comparison of histologic, microbiologic, and clinical criteria. *Chest* 112:445, 1997.
16. Gruson D, Hilbert H, Valentino R, et al: Utility of fiberoptic bronchoscopy in neutropenic patients admitted to the intensive care unit with pulmonary infiltrates. *Crit Care Med* 28:2224, 2000.
17. White P, Bonacum JT, Miller CB: Utility of fiberoptic bronchoscopy in bone marrow transplant patients. *Bone Marrow Transplant* 20:681, 1997.
18. Emanuel D, Peppard J, Stover D, et al: Rapid immunodiagnosis

of cytomegalovirus pneumonia by bronchoalveolar lavage using human and murine monoclonal antibodies. *Ann Intern Med* 104: 476, 1986.

19. Broaddus C, Dake MD, Stulbarg MS, et al: Bronchoalveolar lavage and transbronchial biopsy for the diagnosis of pulmonary infections in the acquired immunodeficiency syndrome. *Ann Intern Med* 102:747, 1985.

20. Raoof S, Rosen MJ, Khan FA: Role of bronchoscopy in AIDS. *Clin Chest Med* 20:63, 1999.

21. Hopewell PC: *Pneumocystis carinii* pneumonia: diagnosis. *J Infect Dis* 157:1115, 1988.

22. Wanner A, Cutchavaree A: Early recognition of upper airway obstruction following smoke inhalation. *Am Rev Respir Dis* 108:1421, 1973.

23. Hunt JL, Agree RN, Pruitt BA Jr: Fiberoptic bronchoscopy in acute inhalation injury. *J Trauma* 15:641, 1975.

24. Brandstetter RD: Flexible fiberoptic bronchoscopy in the intensive care unit. *Intensive Care Med* 4:248, 1989.

25. Haponik EF, Meyers DA, Munster AM, et al: Acute upper airway injury in burn patients: serial changes of flow-volume curves and nasopharyngoscopy. *Am Rev Respir Dis* 135:360, 1987.

26. Hara KS, Prakash UBS: Fiberoptic bronchoscopy in the evaluation of acute chest and upper airway trauma. *Chest* 96:627, 1989.

27. Landa JF: Indications for bronchoscopy. *Chest* 73[Suppl]:686, 1978.

28. Albertini RE: Cough caused by exposed endobronchial sutures. *Ann Intern Med* 94:205, 1981.

29. Timsit J-F, Misset B, Azoulay E, et al: Usefulness of airway visualization in the diagnosis of nosocomial pneumonia in ventilated patients. *Chest* 110:172, 1996.

30. Fossieck BE Jr, Parker RH, Cohen MH, et al: Fiberoptic bronchoscopy and culture of bacteria from the lower respiratory tract. *Chest* 72:5, 1977.

31. Irwin RS, Corrao WM: A perspective on sputum analyses in pneumonia. *Respir Care* 24:328, 1979.

32. Jett Jr, Cortese DA, Dines DE: The value of bronchoscopy in the diagnosis of mycobacterial disease: a five-year experience. *Chest* 80:575, 1981.

33. George RB, Jenkinson SG, Light RW: Fiberoptic bronchoscopy in the diagnosis of pulmonary fungal and nocardial infections. *Chest* 73:33, 1978.

34. Saravolatz LD, Russell G, Cvitkovich D: Direct immunofluorescence in the diagnosis of Legionnaire's disease. *Chest* 79:566, 1981.

35. Grossman RF, Fein A: Evidence-based assessment of diagnostic tests for ventilator associated pneumonia. *Chest* 117:177S, 2000.

36. Kirtland SH, Corley DE, Winterbauer RH, et al: The diagnosis of ventilator associated pneumonia: a comparison of histologic, microbiologic, and clinical criteria. *Chest* 112:445, 1997.

37. Marini JJ, Pierson DJ, Hudson LD: Acute lobar atelectasis: a prospective comparison of fiberoptic bronchoscopy and respiratory therapy. *Am Rev Respir Dis* 119:971, 1979.

38. Olapade CO, Prakash UBS: Bronchoscopy in the critical-care unit. *Mayo Clin Proc* 64:1225, 1989.

39. Lieberman J: The appropriate use of mucolytic agents. *Am J Med* 49:1, 1970.

40. Cunanan OS: The flexible fiberoptic bronchoscope in foreign body removal: experience in 300 cases. *Chest* 73:725, 1978.

41. Giudice JC, Komansky HJ: Acute epiglottitis: the use of a fiberoptic bronchoscope in diagnosis and therapy. *Chest* 75:211, 1979.

42. Saw EC, Gottlieb LS, Yokoyama T, et al: Flexible fiberoptic bronchoscopy and endobronchial tamponade in the management of massive hemoptysis. *Chest* 70:589, 1976.

43. Bredin CP, Richardson PR, King TKC: Treatment of massive hemoptysis by combined occlusion of pulmonary and bronchial arteries. *Am Rev Respir Dis* 117:969, 1978.

44. Remy J, Arnaud A, Fardou H, et al: Treatment of hemoptysis by embolization of bronchial arteries. *Radiology* 122:33, 1977.

45. White RI, Kaufman SL, Barth KH: Therapeutic embolization with detachable silicone balloons: early clinical experience. *JAMA* 241:1257, 1979.

46. Seijo LM, Sterman DH: Interventional pulmonology. *N Engl J Med* 344:740, 2001.

47. Prakash UBS: Advances in bronchoscopic procedures. *Chest* 116: 1404, 1999.

48. Powner DJ, Bierman MI: Thoracic and extrathoracic bronchial fistulas. *Chest* 100:480, 1991.

49. Baumann MH, Sahn SA: Medical management and therapy of bronchopleural fistulas in the mechanically ventilated patient. *Chest* 97:721, 1990.

50. Salmon CJ, Ponn RB, Westcott JL: Endobronchial vascular occlusion coils for control of a large parenchymal bronchopleural fistula. *Chest* 98:233, 1990.

51. Martin WR, Siefkin AD, Allen R: Closure of a bronchopleural fistula with bronchoscopic instillation of tetracycline. *Chest* 99:1040, 1991.

52. Credle WF, Smiddy JF, Elliott RC: Complications of fiberoptic bronchoscopy. *Am Rev Respir Dis* 109:67, 1974.

53. Suratt PM, Smiddy JF, Gruber B: Deaths and complications associated with fiberoptic bronchoscopy. *Chest* 69:747, 1976.

54. Pereira W, Kovnat DM, Khan MA, et al: Fever and pneumonia after flexible fiberoptic bronchoscopy. *Am Rev Respir Dis* 112:59, 1975.

55. Krause A, Hohberg B, Heine F, et al: Cytokines derived from alveolar macrophages induce fever after bronchoscopy and bronchoalveolar lavage. *Am J Respir Crit Care Med* 155:1793, 1997.

56. Stubbs SE, Brutinel WM: Complications of bronchoscopy, in Prakash UBS (ed): *Bronchoscopy*. New York, Raven Press, 1994, p 357.

57. Burman SO: Bronchoscopy and bacteremia. *J Thorac Cardiovasc Surg* 40:635, 1960.

58. Everett ED, Hirschmann JV: Transient bacteremia and endocarditis prophylaxis: a review. *Medicine* 56:61, 1977.

59. Yigla M, Oren I, Solomonov A, et al: Incidence of bacteraemia following fiberoptic bronchoscopy. *Eur Respir J* 14:789, 1999.

60. Dajani AS, Taubert KA, Wilson W, et al: Prevention of bacterial endocarditis: recommendations of the American Heart Association. *JAMA* 277:1794, 1997.

61. Dunagan DP, Baker AM, Hurd DD: Bronchoscopic evaluation of pulmonary infiltrates following bone marrow transplantation. *Chest* 111:135, 1997.

62. Zavala DC: Pulmonary hemorrhage in fiberoptic transbronchial biopsy. *Chest* 70:584, 1976.

63. Trouillet JL, Guiguet M, Gibert C, et al: Fiberoptic bronchoscopy in ventilated patients: evaluation of cardiopulmonary risk under midazolam sedation. *Chest* 97:927, 1990.

64. Pincus PS, Kallenbach JM, Hurwitz MD, et al: Transbronchial biopsy during mechanical ventilation. *Crit Care Med* 15:1136, 1987.

65. O'Brien JD, Ettinger NA, Shevlin D: Safety and yield of transbronchial biopsy in mechanically ventilated patients. *Crit Care Med* 25:440, 1997.

66. Shrader DL, Lakshminarayan S: The effect of fiberoptic bronchoscopy on cardiac rhythm. *Chest* 73:821, 1978.

67. Lundgren R, Haggmark S, Reiz S: Hemodynamic effects of flexible fiberoptic bronchoscopy performed under topical anesthesia. *Chest* 82:295, 1982.

68. Luck JC, Messeder OH, Rubenstein MJ, et al: Arrhythmias from fiberoptic bronchoscopy. *Chest* 74:139, 1978.

69. Sahn SA, Scoggin C: Fiberoptic bronchoscopy in bronchial asthma: a word of caution. *Chest* 69:39, 1976.

70. Dweik RA, Mehta AC, Meeker DP, et al: Analysis of the safety of bronchoscopy after recent acute myocardial infarction. *Chest* 110:825, 1996.

71. Dunagan DP, Burke HL, Aquino SL, et al: Fiberoptic bronchoscopy in coronary care unit patients: indications, safety and clinical implications. *Chest* 114:1660, 1998.

72. Salisbury BG, Metzger LF, Altose MD, et al: Effect of fiberoptic bronchoscopy on respiratory performance in patients with chronic airways obstruction. *Thorax* 30:441, 1975.

73. Kerwin AJ, Croce MA, Timmons SD, et al: Effects of fiberoptic bronchoscopy on intracranial pressure in patients with brain injury; a prospective clinical study. *J Trauma* 48:878, 2000.

74. Peerless JR, Snow N, Likavec MJ, et al: The effect of fiberoptic bronchoscopy on cerebral hemodynamics in patients with severe head injury. *Chest* 108:962, 1995.

75. Bajwa MK, Henein S, Kamholz SL: Fiberoptic bronchoscopy in the presence of space-occupying intracranial lesions. *Chest* 104: 101,1993.

76. Reichert WW, Hall WJ, Hyde RW: A simple disposable device for performing fiberoptic bronchoscopy on patients requiring continuous artificial ventilation. *Am Rev Respir Dis* 109:394, 1974.

77. Lindholm C-E, Ollman B, Snyder JV, et al: Cardiorespiratory effects of flexible fiberoptic bronchoscopy in critically ill patients. *Chest* 74:362, 1978.
78. Lawson RW, Peters JI, Shelledy DC: Effects of fiberoptic bronchoscopy during mechanical ventilation in a lung model. *Chest* 118:824, 2000.
79. Milman N, Laub M, Munch EP, at al: Serum concentrations of lidocaine and its metabolite monoethylglycinexylidide during fiberoptic bronchoscopy in local anesthesia. *Respir Med* 92:40, 1998.
80. Williams TJ, Bowie PE: Midazolam sedation to produce complete amnesia for bronchoscopy: 2 years' experience at a district hospital. *Respir Med* 93:361, 1999.
81. Cowl CT, Prakash UBS, Kruger BR: The role of anticholinergics in bronchoscopy: a randomized clinical trial. *Chest* 118:188, 2000.
82. Williams T, Brooks T, Ward C: The role of atropine premedication in fiberoptic bronchoscopy using intravenous midazolam sedation. *Chest* 113:1394, 1998.

13. Thoracentesis

Mark M. Wilson and Richard S. Irwin

Thoracentesis, as first described in 1852 [1], is an invasive procedure that involves the introduction of a needle, cannula, or trocar into the pleural space to remove accumulated fluid or air. Although a few prospective studies have critically evaluated the clinical value and complications associated with it [2–4], most studies concerning thoracentesis have dealt with the interpretation of the pleural fluid analyses [5].

Indications

Although history (cough, dyspnea, or pleuritic chest pain) and physical findings (dullness to percussion, decreased breath sounds, and decreased vocal fremitus) suggest that an effusion is present, chest radiography or ultrasonic examination is essential to confirm the clinical suspicion. Thoracentesis can be performed for diagnostic or therapeutic reasons and, when done for diagnostic reasons, whenever possible, the procedure should be performed before any treatment has been given to avoid confusion in interpretation. Analysis of pleural fluid has been shown to yield clinically useful information in more than 90% of cases [3]. The four commonest diagnoses for symptomatic and asymptomatic pleural effusions are malignancy, congestive heart failure, parapneumonia, and postoperative sympathetic effusions [6]. A diagnostic algorithm for evaluation of a pleural effusion of unknown etiology is presented in Figure 13-1 [6]. In patients whose pleural effusion remains undiagnosed after thoracentesis and closed pleural biopsy, thoracoscopy should be considered for visualization of the pleura and directed biopsy. Thoracoscopy has provided a positive diagnosis in more than 80% of patients with recurrent pleural effusions that are not diagnosed by repeated thoracentesis, pleural biopsy, or bronchoscopy [7].

Therapeutic thoracentesis is indicated to remove fluid or air that is causing cardiopulmonary embarrassment or for relief of severe symptoms. Definitive drainage of the pleural space with a thoracostomy tube should be considered for a tension pneumothorax, a pneumothorax that is slowly enlarging, or the instillation of a sclerosing agent after drainage of a recurrent malignant pleural effusion [8].

Contraindications

Absolute contraindications to performing a thoracentesis are an uncooperative patient, the inability to identify the top of the rib clearly under the percutaneous puncture site, a lack of expertise in performing the procedure, and the presence of a coagulation abnormality that cannot be corrected. Relative contraindications to a thoracentesis include entry into an area where known bullous lung disease exists, a patient on positive end-expiratory pressure, and a patient who has only one "functioning" lung (the other having been surgically removed or that has severe disease limiting its gas exchange function). In these settings, it may be safer to perform the thoracentesis under ultrasonic guidance.

Complications

A number of prospective studies have documented that complications associated with the procedure are not infrequent [2,3,9]. The overall complication rate has been reported to be as high as 50% to 78% and can be further categorized as major (15% to 19%) or minor (31% to 63%) [3,4]. Although death due to the procedure is infrequently reported, complications may be life threatening [2].

Major complications include pneumothorax, hemopneumothorax, hemorrhage, hypotension, and reexpansion pulmonary edema. The reported incidence of pneumothorax varies between 3% and 30% [2–4,10–14], with up to one-third to one-half of those with demonstrated pneumothoraces requiring subsequent intervention. Various investigators have reported associations between pneumothorax and underlying lung disease (chronic obstructive pulmonary disease, prior thoracic radiation, prior thoracic surgery, lung cancer) [9,11,12,15,16], needle size and technique [4,16], number of passes required to obtain a sample [11,16], aspiration of air during the procedure [11,15], operator experience [2,4,9,10,13,15], use of a vacuum bottle [12], size of the effusion [3,16], male gender and symptoms during or after the thoracentesis [17], and mechanical ventilation versus spontaneously breathing patients [18]. Some of the above-mentioned studies report directly contradictory findings compared to other similar studies. This is most apparent in the reported association between pneumothorax and therapeutic thoracentesis [4,9,15–17], which was not supported by subsequent large prospective trials [12,14]. The most likely explanation for this discrepancy in the literature concerning the presumed increased risk for pneumothorax for therapeutic over diagnostic procedures is the generally lower level of operator experience in the first group. Small sample sizes also limit the generalization of reported findings to allow for the delineation of a clear risk profile for the development of a pneumothorax

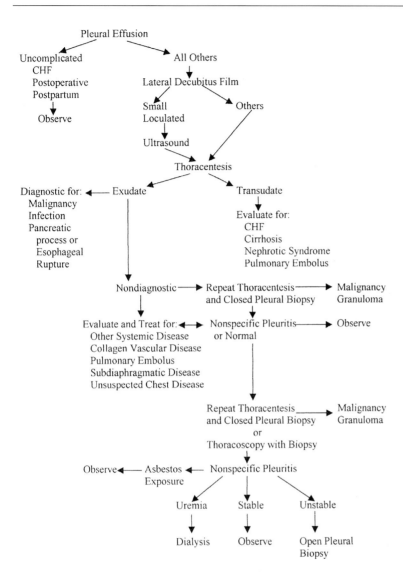

Fig. 13-1. Diagnostic algorithm for evaluation of pleural effusion. CHF, congestive heart failure. (From Smyrnios NA, Jederlinic PJ, Irwin RS: Pleural effusion in an asymptomatic patient. Spectrum and frequency of causes and management considerations. *Chest* 97:192, 1990, with permission.)

after a thoracentesis. The presence of baseline lung disease, low level of operator experience with the procedure, and the use of positive-pressure mechanical ventilation appear for now to be the best-established risk factors in the literature. Further research involving more patients is needed.

Although pneumothorax is most commonly due to laceration of lung parenchyma, room air may enter the pleural space if the thoracentesis needle is open to room air when a spontaneously breathing patient takes a deep breath (intrapleural pressure is subatmospheric). The pneumothorax may be small and asymptomatic, resolving spontaneously, or large and associated with respiratory compromise, requiring chest tube drainage. Hemorrhage can occur from laceration of an intercostal artery or inadvertent puncture of the liver or spleen, even if coagulation studies are normal. The risk of intercostal artery laceration is greatest in the elderly because of increased tortuosity of the vessels [19]. This last complication is potentially lethal, and open thoracotomy may be required to control the bleeding.

Hypotension may occur during the procedure (as part of a vasovagal reaction) or hours after the procedure (most likely due to reaccumulation of fluid into the pleural space or the pulmonary parenchyma from the intravascular space). Hypotension in the latter settings responds to volume expansion; it can usually be prevented by limiting pleural fluid drainage to 1 L or less. Other major complications are rare and include implantation of tumor along the needle tract of a previously performed

thoracentesis [20], venous and cerebral air embolism (so-called pleural shock) [21,22], and inadvertent placement of a sheared catheter into the pleural space [2].

Minor complications include dry tap or insufficient fluid, pain, subcutaneous hematoma or seroma, anxiety, dyspnea, and cough [3,23]. Reported rates for these minor complications range from 16% to 63% and depend on the method used to perform the procedure, with higher rates associated with the catheter-through-needle technique [3,4]. Dry tap and insufficient fluid are technical problems and expose the patient to increased risk of morbidity because of the need to perform a repeat thoracentesis. Under these circumstances, it is recommended that the procedure be repeated under direct sonographic guidance. Pain may originate from parietal pleural nerve endings from inadequate local anesthesia, inadvertent scraping of rib periosteum, or piercing an intercostal nerve during a misdirected needle thrust. Coughing may occur when a large effusion is evacuated, perhaps because of stimulation of airway cough receptors [23].

Procedures

GENERAL CONSIDERATIONS. The most common techniques for performing thoracentesis are catheter-over-needle, needle

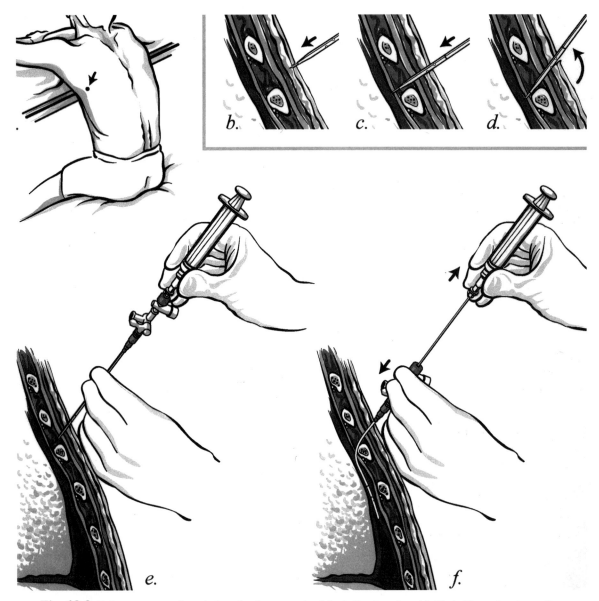

Fig. 13-2. Catheter-over-needle technique for thoracentesis of freely flowing pleural field. **A:** The patient is comfortably positioned, sitting up and leaning forward over a pillow-draped, height-adjusted, bedside table. The arms are crossed in front of the patient to elevate and spread the scapulae. The preferred entry site is along the posterior axillary line. **B:** The catheter apparatus is gently advanced through the skin and across the upper surface of the rib. The needle is advanced several millimeters at a time while continuously aspirating through the syringe. **C:** As soon as the parietal pleura has been punctured, fluid will appear in the syringe. **D:** Before the catheter is advanced any farther, the apparatus is directed downward. **E,F:** In rapid sequence, the catheter is advanced fully to the chest wall and the needle withdrawn from the apparatus. The one-way valve in the apparatus maintains a closed system until the operator manually changes the position of the stopcock to allow drainage of the pleural fluid.

only, and needle under direct sonographic guidance. The catheter-through-needle technique has been used much less frequently over the last decade.

TECHNIQUE FOR DIAGNOSTIC (NEEDLE-ONLY OR CATHETER-OVER-NEEDLE) REMOVAL OF FREELY FLOWING FLUID

1. Obtain a lateral decubitus chest radiograph to confirm a free-flowing pleural effusion.
2. Describe the procedure to the patient and obtain written informed consent. Operators should be thoroughly familiar with the procedure they will be performing and should receive appropriate supervision from an experienced operator before performing thoracentesis on their own.
3. With the patient sitting, arms at sides, mark the inferior tip of the scapula on the side to be tapped. This approximates the eighth intercostal space and should be the lowest interspace punctured, unless it has been previously determined by sonography that a lower interspace can be safely entered or chest radiographs and sonography show the diaphragm to be higher than the eighth intercostal space.
4. Position the patient sitting at the edge of the bed, comfortably leaning forward over a pillow-draped, height-adjusted, bedside table (Fig. 13-2). The patient's arms should be crossed in front to elevate and spread the scapulae. An assistant should stand in front of the patient to prevent any unexpected movements.

5. Percuss the patient's posterior chest to determine the highest point of the effusion. The interspace below this point should be entered in the posterior axillary line, unless it is below the eighth intercostal space. Gently mark the superior aspect of the rib in the chosen interspace with your fingernail. (The inferior portion of each rib contains an intercostal artery and should be avoided.)

6. Cleanse the area with iodophor and allow it to dry. Using sterile technique, drape the area surrounding the puncture site.

7. Anesthetize the superficial skin with 2% lidocaine using a 25-gauge needle. Change to an 18- to 22-gauge needle, 2 in. long, and generously anesthetize the deeper soft tissues, aiming for the top of the rib. Always aspirate through the syringe as the needle is advanced and before instilling lidocaine to ensure that the needle is not in a vessel or the pleural space. Carefully aspirate through the syringe as the pleura is approached (the rib is 1–2 cm thick). Fluid enters the syringe on reaching the pleural space. The patient may experience discomfort as the needle penetrates the well-innervated parietal pleura. Be careful not to instill anesthetic into the pleural space; it is bactericidal for most organisms, including *Mycobacterium tuberculosis*. Place a gloved finger at the point on the needle where it exits the skin (to estimate the required depth of insertion) and remove the needle.

8. Attach a three-way stopcock to a 20-gauge, 1.5-in. needle and to a 50-mL syringe. The valve on the stopcock should be open to the needle to allow aspiration of fluid during needle insertion.

9. Insert the 20-gauge needle (or the catheter-over-needle apparatus) into the anesthetic tract with the bevel of the needle down and always aspirate through the syringe as the needle/catheter-over-needle is slowly advanced. When pleural fluid is obtained using the needle-only technique, stabilize the needle by attaching a clamp to the needle where it exits the skin, to prevent further advancement of the needle into the pleural space. Once pleural fluid is obtained with the catheter-over-needle technique, direct the needle-catheter apparatus downward to ensure that the catheter descends to the most dependent area of the pleural space. Advance the catheter forward in a single smooth motion as the inner needle is simultaneously pulled back out of the chest.

10. Once pleural fluid can easily be obtained, fill a heparinized blood gas syringe from the side port of the three-way stopcock. Express all air bubbles from the sample, cap it, and place it in a bag containing iced slush for immediate transport to the laboratory.

11. Fill the 50-mL syringe and transfer its contents into the appropriate collection tubes and containers. Always maintain a closed system during the procedure to prevent room air from entering the pleural space. For most diagnostic studies, 100 mL should be ample fluid. Always ensure that the three-way stopcock has the valve closed toward the patient when changing syringes.

12. When the thoracentesis is completed, remove the needle (or catheter) from the patient's chest. Apply pressure to the wound for several minutes, and then apply a sterile bandage.

13. Obtain a postprocedure upright end-expiratory chest radiograph if a pneumothorax is suspected.

14. Immediately after the procedure, draw venous blood for total protein and lactate dehydrogenase (LDH) determinations. These studies are necessary to interpret pleural fluid values (see the section Interpretation of Pleural Fluid Analysis).

TECHNIQUE FOR THERAPEUTIC REMOVAL OF FREELY FLOWING FLUID. Steps 1 to 7 should be followed as described previously. Removal of more than 100 mL pleural fluid generally involves placement of a catheter into the pleural space to minimize the risk of pneumothorax from a needle during this longer procedure. Commercially available kits generally use a catheter-over-needle system, although catheter-through-needle systems are still available in some locations. Each different kit may have a specific set of instructions for performing this procedure. Operators should be thoroughly familiar with the recommended procedure for the catheter system that they will be using and should receive appropriate supervision from an experienced operator before performing thoracentesis on their own.

TECHNIQUE FOR DIRECTED GUIDANCE THORACENTESIS. A dynamic (real-time) sonographic scanner or computed tomography may be useful for the removal of freely flowing fluid (especially when present in small quantities) or in removal of loculated fluid. They are first used to document the pleural effusion fluid level and the depth of needle insertion necessary to enter the pleural space and will ideally minimize the risk for pneumothorax. The protocol is similar to that described for the needle-only technique, but the needle can be inserted under direct guidance after localization of the effusion. The use of a catheter is optional in this setting.

TECHNIQUE FOR REMOVAL OF FREELY MOVING PNEUMOTHORAX

1. Follow the same catheter-over-needle protocol described for removing freely moving fluid, but position the patient supine with the head of the bed elevated 30 to 45 degrees.

2. Prepare the second or third intercostal space in the anterior midclavicular line (this avoids hitting the more medial internal mammary artery) for the needle and catheter insertion.

3. Have the bevel of the needle facing up and direct the needle upward so that the catheter can be guided toward the superior aspect of the hemithorax.

4. Air can be actively withdrawn by syringe or pushed out when intrapleural pressure is supraatmospheric (e.g., during a cough), as long as the catheter is intermittently open to the atmosphere. In the latter setting, air can leave but not reenter if the catheter is attached to a one-way check-valve apparatus (Heimlich valve) or if it is put to underwater seal.

5. When local anesthesia and skin cleansing are not possible because a tension pneumothorax is life threatening, perform the procedure without them. If a tension pneumothorax is known to be present and a chest tube is not readily available, quickly insert a 14-gauge needle into the second anterior intercostal space. If a tension pneumothorax is suspected and a 14-gauge needle and 16-gauge catheter are handy, place the catheter according to the above technique to avoid puncturing the lung. If a tension pneumothorax is present, air escapes under pressure. When the situation has stabilized and the tension pneumothorax has been diagnosed, leave the needle or catheter in place until a sterile chest tube can be inserted.

Interpretation of Pleural Fluid Analysis

To determine the etiology of a pleural effusion, a number of tests on pleural fluid are helpful. A two-stage laboratory approach to the evaluation of pleural effusion should be used [24]. The initial determination should be to classify the effusion as a transudate or an exudate using the following criteria.

Table 13-1. Causes of Pleural Effusions

Etiologies of effusions that are virtually always transudates
Congestive heart failure
Nephrotic syndrome
Hypoalbuminemia
Urinothorax
Trapped lung

Etiologies of effusions that are typically exudates
Infections
Parapneumonic
Tuberculous pleurisy
Parasites (amebiasis, paragonimiasis, echinococcosis)
Fungal disease
Atypical pneumonias (virus, *Mycoplasma*, Q fever, *Legionella*)
Nocardia, Actinomyces
Subphrenic abscess
Hepatic abscess
Splenic abscess
Hepatitis
Spontaneous esophageal rupture
Noninfectious inflammations
Pancreatitis
Benign asbestos pleural effusion
Pulmonary embolism
Radiation therapy
Uremic pleurisy
Sarcoidosis
Postcardiac injury syndrome
Hemothorax
Acute respiratory distress syndrome
Malignancies
Carcinoma
Lymphoma
Mesothelioma
Leukemia
Chylothorax
Chronically increased negative intrapleural pressure
Atelectasis
Trapped lung
Cholesterol effusion

Cirrhosis
Atelectasis
Peritoneal dialysis
Constrictive pericarditis
Superior vena caval obstruction

Iatrogenic
Drug-induced (nitrofurantoin, methotrexate)
Esophageal perforation
Esophageal sclerotherapy
Central venous catheter misplacement or migration
Enteral feeding tube in space
Connective tissue disease
Lupus pleuritis
Rheumatoid pleurisy
Mixed connective tissue disease
Churg-Strauss syndrome
Wegener's granulomatosis
Familial Mediterranean fever
Endocrine disorders
Hypothyroidism
Ovarian hyperstimulation syndrome
Lymphatic disorders
Malignancy
Yellow nail syndrome
Lymphangioleiomyomatosis
Movement of fluid from abdomen to pleural space
Pancreatitis
Pancreatic pseudocyst
Meigs' syndrome
Carcinoma
Chylous ascites

Adapted from Sahn SA: The pleura. *Am Rev Respir Dis* 138:184, 1988.

Additional studies can then be ordered to help establish a final diagnosis for the etiology of the pleural effusion, especially in the setting of an exudate.

TRANSUDATES VERSUS EXUDATES. A transudate is biochemically defined by meeting all of the following criteria: pleural fluid–serum total protein ratio of less than 0.5, pleural fluid–serum LDH ratio of less than 0.6, and absolute pleural fluid LDH of less than 200 IU [25] or less than two-thirds the normal serum level. The former diagnostic criteria of pleural fluid specific gravity of less than 1.015 or total protein of less than 3.0 g/dL are no longer used.

An exudate is present when any of the foregoing criteria for transudates are not met. If a transudate is present, generally no further tests on pleural fluid are indicated [24] (Table 13-1). The one exception to this is the transudative pleural effusion due to urinothorax. Unless it is suspected and a creatinine level from the pleural fluid is measured and compared to serum levels, this etiology may be missed. If an exudate is present, further laboratory evaluation is warranted (Fig. 13-1). If subsequent testing does not narrow the differential diagnosis, a percutaneous pleural biopsy should be considered [6]. Thoracoscopy-guided pleural biopsy should be considered in patients with pleural effusion of unknown etiology despite the above-listed evaluation [7].

SELECTED TESTS THAT ARE POTENTIALLY HELPFUL TO ESTABLISH ETIOLOGY FOR A PLEURAL EFFUSION

pH. Pleural fluid pH determinations may have diagnostic and therapeutic implications [26–28]. For instance, the differential diagnosis associated with a pleural fluid pH of less than 7.2 is consistent with systemic acidemia, bacterially infected effusion (empyema), malignant effusion, rheumatoid or lupus effusion, tuberculous effusion, ruptured esophagus, noninfected parapneumonic effusion that needs drainage, and urinothorax. Pleural effusions with a pH of less than 7.2 are potentially sclerotic and require consideration for chest tube drainage to aid resolution.

Amylase. A pleural fluid amylase level that is twice the normal serum level or with an absolute value of greater than 160 Somogyi units may be seen in patients with acute and chronic pancreatitis, pancreatic pseudocyst that has dissected or ruptured into the pleural space, primary and metastatic cancer, and esophageal rupture [29].

Glucose. A low pleural fluid glucose value is defined as less than 50% of the normal serum value [5]. In this situation, the differential diagnosis includes rheumatoid and lupus effusion, bacterial empyema, malignancy, tuberculosis, and esophageal rupture [5,30].

Triglyceride and Cholesterol. Chylous pleural effusions are biochemically defined by a triglyceride level greater than 110 mg/dL and the presence of chylomicrons on a pleural fluid lipoprotein electrophoresis [31]. The usual appearance of a chylous effusion is milky, but an effusion with elevated triglycerides may also appear serous. The measurement of a triglyceride level is therefore important. Chylous effusions occur when the thoracic duct has been disrupted somewhere along its course. The most common causes are trauma and malignancy (e.g., lymphoma) [31]. A pseudochylous effusion appears grossly milky because of an elevated cholesterol level; the triglyceride level is normal. Chronic effusions, especially those associated with rheumatoid and tuberculous pleuritis, are characteristically pseudochylous [31].

Cell Counts and Differential. Although pleural fluid white blood cell count and differential are never diagnostic of any disease, it would be distinctly unusual for an effusion other than one associated with bacterial pneumonia to have a white blood cell count exceeding 50,000 per mm^3 [31]. In an exudative pleural effusion of acute origin, polymorphonuclear leukocytes predominate early, whereas mononuclear cells predominate in chronic exudative effusions. Although pleural fluid lymphocytosis is nonspecific, severe lymphocytosis (>80% of cells) is suggestive of tuberculosis or malignancy. Finally, pleural fluid eosinophilia is nonspecific.

A red blood cell count of 5,000 to 10,000 cells per mm^3 must be present for fluid to appear pinkish. Grossly bloody effusions containing more than 100,000 red blood cells per mm^3 are most consistent with trauma, malignancy, or pulmonary infarction [32]. To distinguish a traumatic thoracentesis from a preexisting hemothorax, several observations are helpful [5]. First, because a preexisting hemothorax has been defibrinated, it does not form a clot on standing. Secondly, a hemothorax is suggested when a pleural fluid hematocrit value is 50% or more of the serum hematocrit value.

Cultures and Stains. To maximize the yield from pleural fluid cultures, anaerobic and aerobic cultures should be obtained. If the sample of pleural fluid sent for culture is transported in an oxygen-free atmosphere (a capped glass syringe with all bubbles squirted out is all that is necessary), the microbiology laboratory can perform all necessary anaerobic, aerobic, fungal, and mycobacterial cultures and smears. Because acid-fast stains may be positive in 20% of tuberculous effusions [5], they should always be performed in addition to Gram's smears. By submitting pleural biopsy pieces to the pathology and microbiology laboratories, it is possible to diagnose up to 90% of tuberculous effusions percutaneously [25].

Cytology. Malignancies can produce pleural effusions by implantation of malignant cells on the pleura or impairment of lymphatic drainage secondary to tumor obstruction. The tumors that most commonly cause pleural effusions are lung, breast, and lymphoma. Pleural fluid cytology should be performed for an exudative effusion of unknown etiology, using at least 100 to 200 mL fluid. If initial cytology results are negative and strong clinical suspicion exists, additional samples of fluid can increase the chance of a positive result. In patients who are ultimately shown to have a malignancy as an etiology of their effusion, 59% have positive cytology on a single sample, 65% on the second sample, and 70% on the third sample [33]. The addition of a pleural biopsy increases the positive results to 81% [34]. In addition to malignancy, cytologic examination can definitively diagnose

rheumatoid pleuritis [35,36]. The pathognomonic picture consists of slender, elongated macrophages and giant, round, multinucleated macrophages, accompanied by amorphous granular background material.

References

1. Bowditch HI: Paracentesis thoracis. *Am J Med Sci* 23:105, 1852.
2. Seneff MG, Corwin RW, Gold LH, et al: Complications associated with thoracentesis. *Chest* 89:97, 1986.
3. Collins TR, Sahn SA: Thoracentesis: clinical value, complications, technical problems, and patient experience. *Chest* 91: 817, 1987.
4. Grogan D, Irwin RS, Channick R, et al: Complications associated with thoracentesis: a prospective randomized study comparing three different methods. *Arch Intern Med* 150:873, 1990.
5. Sahn SA: The differential diagnosis of pleural effusions. *West J Med* 137:99, 1982.
6. Smyrnios NA, Jederlinic PJ, Irwin RS: Pleural effusion in an asymptomatic patient. Spectrum and frequency of causes and management considerations. *Chest* 97:192, 1990.
7. Kendall SWH, Bryan AJ, Large SR, et al: Pleural effusions: is thoracoscopy a reliable investigation? A retrospective review. *Respir Med* 86:437, 1992.
8. Walker-Renard PB, Vaughan LM, Sahn SA: Chemical pleurodesis for malignant pleural effusions. *Ann Intern Med* 120:56, 1994.
9. Branstetter RD, Karetsky M, Rastogi R, et al: Pneumothorax after thoracentesis in chronic obstructive pulmonary disease. *Heart Lung* 23:67, 1994.
10. Bartter T, Mayo PD, Pratter MR, et al: Lower risk and higher yield for thoracentesis when performed by experimental operators. *Chest* 103:1873, 1993.
11. Doyle JJ, Hnatiuk OW, Torrington KG, et al: Necessity of routine chest roentgenography after thoracentesis. *Ann Intern Med* 124: 816, 1996.
12. Petersen WG, Zimmerman R: Limited utility of chest radiograph after thoracentesis. *Chest* 117:1038, 2000.
13. Swinburne AJ, Bixby K, Fedullo AJ, et al: Pneumothorax after thoracentesis. *Arch Intern Med* 151:2095, 1991.
14. Colt HG, Brewer N, Barbur E: Evaluation of patient-related and procedure-related factors contributing to pneumothorax following thoracentesis. *Chest* 116:134, 1999.
15. Gerardi D, Scalise P, Lahiri B: The utility of the routine post-thoracentesis chest radiograph (abstract). *Chest* 106:83S, 1994.
16. Raptopoulos V, Davis LM, Lee G, et al: Factors affecting the development of pneumothorax associated with thoracentesis. *AJR Am J Roentgenol* 156:917, 1991.
17. Aleman C, Alegre J, Armadans L, et al: The value of chest roentgenography in the diagnosis of pneumothorax after thoracentesis. *Am J Med* 107:340, 1999.
18. Gervais DA, Petersein A, Lee MJ: US-guided thoracentesis requirement for postprocedure chest radiography in patients who receive mechanical ventilation versus patients who breathe spontaneously. *Radiology* 204:503, 1997.
19. Carney PA, Ravin CE: Intercostal artery laceration during thoracentesis. *Chest* 75:520, 1979.
20. Stewart BN, Block AJ: Subcutaneous implantation of cancer following thoracentesis. *Chest* 66:456, 1974.
21. Wilson MM, Curley FJ: Gas embolism (Pt I). Venous gas emboli. *J Intensive Care Med* 11:182, 1996.
22. Wilson MM, Curley FJ: Gas embolism (Pt II). Arterial gas embolism and decompression sickness. *J Intensive Care Med* 11:261, 1996.
23. Irwin RS, Rosen MJ: Cough: a comprehensive review. *Arch Intern Med* 137:1186, 1977.
24. Peterman TA, Speicher CE: Evaluating pleural effusions: a two stage laboratory approach. *JAMA* 252:1051, 1984.
25. Light RW, MacGregor MI, Luchsinger PC, et al: Pleural effusions: the diagnostic separation of transudates and exudates. *Ann Intern Med* 77:507, 1972.

26. Potts DE, Levin DC, Sahn SA: Pleural fluid pH in parapneumonic effusions. *Chest* 70:328, 1976.
27. Light R, Girard WM, Jenkinson SG, et al: Parapneumonic effusions. *Am J Med* 69:507, 1980.
28. Good JT, Taryle DA, Maulitz RM, et al: The diagnostic value of pleural fluid pH. *Chest* 78:55, 1980.
29. Light RW, Ball WC: Glucose and amylase in pleural effusions. *JAMA* 225:257, 1973.
30. Potts DE, Taryle DA, Sahn SA: The glucose-pH relationship in parapneumonic effusions. *Arch Intern Med* 138:1378, 1978.
31. Staats BA, Ellefson RD, Budahn LL, et al: The lipoprotein profile of chylous and nonchylous pleural effusions. *Mayo Clin Proc* 55:700, 1980.
32. Light RS, Erozan YS, Ball WC: Cells in pleural fluid. *Arch Intern Med* 132:854, 1973.
33. Hausheer FH, Yarbro IW: Diagnosis and treatment of malignant pleural effusion. *Semin Oncol* 12:54, 1985.
34. Winkelman M, Pfitzer P: Blind pleural biopsy in combination with cytology of pleural effusions. *Acta Cytol* 25:373, 1981.
35. Sahn SA: The pleura. *Am Rev Respir Dis* 138:184, 1988.
36. Naylor B: The pathognomonic cytologic picture of rheumatoid pleuritis. *J Clin Cytol Cytopathol* 34:465, 1990.

14. Arterial Puncture for Blood Gas Analysis

Deborah H. Markowitz and
Richard S. Irwin

Analysis of a sample of arterial blood for pH_a, partial arterial carbon dioxide pressure ($PaCO_2$), partial arterial oxygen pressure (PaO_2), bicarbonate, and percent oxyhemoglobin saturation is performed with an arterial blood gas (ABG) analysis. Because an ABG can be safely and easily obtained and furnishes rapid and accurate information on how well the lungs and kidneys are working [1–3], it is the single most useful laboratory test in managing patients with respiratory and metabolic disorders. One should not rely on oximetry alone to evaluate arterial oxygen saturation (SaO_2) fully. Given the shape of the oxyhemoglobin saturation curve, there must be a substantial fall in PaO_2 before SaO_2 is altered to any appreciable degree. Moreover, it is not possible to predict the level of PaO_2 and $PaCO_2$ reliably using physical signs such as cyanosis [4] and depth of breathing, respectively [5]. Also, a discrepancy between SaO_2 measured by pulse oximetry and that calculated by the ABG can aid in the diagnosis of carboxyhemoglobinemia and methemoglobinemia (see Chapter 26).

Unsuspected hypoxemia or hypercapnia (acidemia) can cause a constellation of central nervous system and cardiovascular signs and symptoms. The clinician should have a high index of suspicion that a respiratory or metabolic disorder, or both, is present in patients with these findings and is most appropriately evaluated by obtaining an ABG. Although acute hypercapnia to 70 mm Hg (pH 7.16) and hypoxemia to less than 30 mm Hg may lead to coma and circulatory collapse, chronic exposures permit adaptation with more subtle effects [6]. Thus, the ABG provides the most important way of making a diagnostic assessment of the nature and severity of a respiratory or metabolic disturbance and following its progression or resolution over time.

The normal range of values for pH_a is 7.35 to 7.45 and 35 to 45 mm Hg for $PaCO_2$ [7]. For PaO_2, the accepted predictive regression equation in nonsmoking, upright, normal individuals aged 40 to 90 years is [8]: PaO_2 = 108.75 (0.39 × age in years).

Drawing the Arterial Blood Gas Specimen

PERCUTANEOUS ARTERIAL PUNCTURE. The conventional technique of sampling arterial blood using a glass syringe is described in detail, because it is the standard to which all other methods are compared. The pulsatile arterial vessel is easily palpated in most cases. If a large enough needle is used, entry is apparent as the syringe fills spontaneously by the pressurized arterial flow of blood, without the need for applying a vacuum or using a vacuum-sealed collecting tube. It is logical to preferentially enter arteries that have the best collateral circulation so that, if spasm or clotting occurs, the distal tissue is not deprived of perfusion. Logic also dictates that puncture of a site where the artery is superficial is preferable, because entry is easiest and pain is minimized. The radial artery best fulfills the above criteria; it is very superficial at the wrist, and the collateral circulation to the hand by the ulnar artery provides sufficient collateral blood flow in approximately 92% of normal adults in the event of total occlusion of the radial artery [9].

The absence of a report of total occlusion of the radial artery after puncture for ABG in an adult with normal hemostasis attests to the safety of the percutaneous arterial puncture. It also suggests that determining the adequacy of collateral flow to the superficial palmar arch by Allen's test [10], a modification of Allen's test [11] (see Chapter 3), or Doppler ultrasound [9] before puncture is not routinely necessary. If radial artery sites are not accessible, dorsalis pedis, posterior tibial, superficial temporal (in infants), brachial, and femoral arteries are alternatives (see Chapter 3).

CONTRAINDICATIONS. Brachial and especially femoral artery punctures are not advised in patients with abnormal hemostatic mechanisms, because adequate vessel tamponade may not be possible in that these vessels are not located superficially, risking greater chance of complications [12]. If frequent sampling of superficial arteries in the same situation becomes necessary, arterial cannulation is recommended (see Chapter 3). Moreover, any vessel that has been reconstructed surgically should not be punctured for fear of forming a pseudoaneurysm, compromising the integrity of an artificial graft site or seeding the foreign body that could become a nidus for infection.

The conventional recommended radial artery technique is as follows:

1. Put on protective gloves and sit in a comfortable position facing the patient.
2. With the patient's palm up, slightly hyperextend the wrist and palpate the radial artery. Severe hyperextension may obliterate the pulse.
3. Cleanse the skin with an alcohol swab.
4. With a 25-gauge needle, inject enough 1% lidocaine intradermally to raise a small wheal at the point where the skin puncture is to be made. The local anesthetic makes subsequent needle puncture with a 22-gauge needle less painful and often painless [13]. If local anesthesia is not given, however, the potential pain and anxiety, if associated with breath holding, may cause substantial blood gas changes. Thirty-five seconds of breath holding in normal subjects has been associated with a fall in Pao_2 of 50 mm Hg and a pH of 0.07 and a rise in $Paco_2$ of 10 mm Hg [14].
5. Attach a needle no smaller than 22 gauge to a glass syringe that can accept 5 mL blood.
6. Wet the needle and syringe with a sodium heparin solution (1,000 units per mL). Express all excess solution.
7. With the needle, enter the artery at an angle of approximately 30 degrees to the long axis of the vessel. This insertion angle minimizes the pain due to inadvertently scraping the periosteum below the artery.
8. As soon as the artery is entered, blood appears in the syringe. Allow the arterial pressure to fill the syringe with at least 3 mL blood [15]. Do not apply suction by pulling on the syringe plunger.
9. Immediately after obtaining the specimen, expel any tiny air bubbles to ensure that the specimen will be anaerobic; then cap the syringe.
10. Roll the blood sample between both palms for 5 to 15 seconds to mix the heparin and blood. Apply pressure to the puncture site for 5 minutes or longer, depending on the presence of a coagulopathy. If the arterial sample was obtained from the brachial artery, compress this vessel so that the radial pulse cannot be palpated.
11. Immerse the capped sample in a bag of ice and water (slush) and immediately transport it to the blood gas laboratory.
12. Write on the ABG slip the time of the drawing and the conditions under which it was drawn (e.g., fraction of inspired oxygen, ventilator settings, position of the patient).

Deviations from these recommended techniques may introduce the following errors:

1. The syringe material may influence the results of Pao_2 [16–18]. The most accurate results have been consistently obtained using a glass syringe. If plastic is used, the following errors may occur: (a) Falsely low Pao_2 values may be obtained because plastic allows oxygen to diffuse to the atmosphere from the sample whenever the Po_2 exceeds 221 mm Hg. (b) Plastic syringes with high surface area to volume ratios (e.g., 1-mL tuberculin syringes) worsen gas permeability errors as compared to standard 3-mL syringes. For this reason, butterfly infusion kits with their long thin tubing should not be used [19]. (c) Plastic syringes tenaciously retain air bubbles, and extra effort is necessary to remove them [17]. (d) Plastic impedes smooth movement of the plunger, which could have an impact on the clinician's confidence that arterial rather than venous blood has been sampled.
2. If suction is applied for plunger assistance, gas bubbles may be pulled out of the solution. If they are expelled, measured Pao_2 and $Paco_2$ tensions may be falsely lowered [20].
3. Although liquid heparin is a weak acid, plasma pH is not altered because it is well buffered by hemoglobin. Mixing liquid heparin with blood dilutes dissolved gasses, shifting their concentration to that of heparin (Po_2 approximately 150 mm Hg, Pco_2 less than 0.3 mm Hg at sea level and room temperature). The degree of alteration depends on the amount of heparin relative to blood and the hemoglobin concentration [20–22]. The dilution error is no greater than 4% if a glass syringe and 22-gauge needle are only wetted with approximately 0.2 mL heparin and 3 to 5 mL blood collected. Any less heparin risks a clotted and unusable sample. Dilutional errors are avoided with the use of crystalline heparin, but this preparation is difficult to mix, which risks clotting of the specimen.
4. If an ABG specimen is not analyzed within 1 minute of being drawn or not immediately cooled to 2°C, the Po_2 and pH fall and Pco_2 rises because of cellular respiration and consumption of oxygen by leukocytes, platelets, and reticulocytes [23]. This is of particular concern in patients with leukemia (leukocytes greater than 40×10^9 per L) or thrombocytosis ($1,000 \times 10^9$ per L) [24].
5. Inadvertent sampling of a vein normally causes a falsely low Pao_2. A venous Po_2 greater than 50 mm Hg can be obtained if the sampling area is warmed. The Po_2 of "arterialized" venous blood can approximate Pao_2 when blood flow is greatly increased by warming, compromising the time for peripheral oxygen extraction.

COMPLICATIONS. Using the conventional radial artery technique described previously, complications are unusual. They include a rare vasovagal episode, local pain, and limited hematomas, occurring no more than 0.58% of the time [1–3]. An expanding aneurysm of the radial artery and reflex sympathetic dystrophy [25] have been reported even more rarely after frequent punctures [26].

Measurements from the Arterial Blood Gas Specimen

Although pH, Pco_2, Po_2, bicarbonate, and Sao_2 are all usually reported, it is important to understand that the bicarbonate and Sao_2 are calculated, not directly measured. Although the calculated bicarbonate value is as reliable as the measured pH and Pco_2 values given their immutable relationship through the Henderson-Hasselbalch equation, the calculated Sao_2 is often inaccurate because of the many variables that cannot be corrected for (e.g., 2,3-diphosphoglycerate, binding characteristics of hemoglobin).

The patient in the intensive care unit often requires serial ABG measurements to follow the progression of critical illness and guide therapy accordingly. It is understandable to interpret fluctuations in the ABG data as signs of the patient's condition worsening or improving, depending on the trend. However, even in 26 hemodynamically stable ventilator-dependent trauma patients, PaO_2 and $PaCO_2$ varied significantly when the mean difference of four ABG samples was analyzed from each patient within a 1-hour period (13 ± 18 mm Hg and 2.5 ± 4.0 mm Hg, respectively) [27]. Whether this variability was due to deviations in the collector's technique or inherent error in the ABG analyzer, or both, is unclear. Nevertheless, routine monitoring of ABGs without an associated change in patient status may not be warranted and may lead to an unproductive, lengthy, and expensive search for the cause.

When electrolytes and other blood values are measured from the unused portion of an ABG sample, clinicians should be aware of the following: Traditional liquid and crystalline heparins for ABG sampling are sodium-heparin salts, which artificially increase plasma sodium concentrations. Calcium and potassium bind to the negatively charged heparins, spuriously lowering their values. Lithium or electrolyte-balanced heparin is now available that contains physiologic concentrations of sodium and potassium, which should be used whenever sodium, potassium, ionized magnesium, ionized calcium, chloride, glucose, and lactate are measured in an ABG specimen [28–30]. Although lithium or balanced heparin minimizes the errors in electrolyte concentrations, dilutional error may still exist if excessive amounts are used for anticoagulation.

By convention, ABG specimens are analyzed at 37°C. Although no studies have demonstrated that correction for the patient's temperature is clinically necessary, blood gases drawn at temperatures greater than 39°C should probably be corrected for temperature [31]. Because the solubility of oxygen and carbon dioxide increases as blood is cooled to 37°C, the hyperthermic patient is more acidotic and less hypoxemic than uncorrected values indicate. Therefore, for each 1°C that the patient's temperature is greater than 37°C, PaO_2 should be increased 7.2%, $PaCO_2$ increased 4.4%, and pH decreased 0.015. It is not necessary to correct the $PaCO_2$ and pH in the hypothermic patient [32], because acid-base changes *in vivo* parallel the changes of blood *in vitro*. However, PaO_2 values must be corrected for temperature lest significant hypoxemia be overlooked. The PaO_2 at 37°C is decreased by 7.2% for each degree that the patient's temperature is less than 37°C.

Physician Responsibility

Even when the ABG values of pH, PCO_2, PO_2, and bicarbonate appear consistently reliable, the clinician should periodically check the accuracy of the blood gas samples because the bicarbonate is calculated, not directly measured. Aliquots of arterial blood can be sent simultaneously for ABG analysis and to the chemistry laboratory for a total $(T)CO_2$ content. Accuracy of the blood gas laboratory's values can be checked using Henderson's simple mathematical equation, which is a rearrangement of the Henderson-Hasselbalch equation [33]: $[H^+] = 25 \times PaCO_2/HCO_3^-$. $[H^+]$ is

Table 14-1. Relation between $[H^+]$ and pH over a Normal Range of pH Values[a]

pH	$[H^+]$ (nM/L)
7.36	44
7.37	43
7.38	42
7.39	41
7.40	40
—	—
7.41	39
7.42	38
7.43	37
7.44	36

[a]Note that pH 7.40 corresponds to hydrogen ion concentration of 40 nM/L and that, over the small range shown, each deviation in pH of 0.01 units corresponds to opposite deviation in $[H^+]$ of 1 nM/L. For pH values between 7.28 and 7.45, $[H^+]$ calculated empirically in this fashion agrees with the actual value obtained by means of logarithms to the nearest nM/L (nearest 0.01 pH unit). However, in the extremes of pH values, below pH 7.28 and above pH 7.45, the estimated $[H^+]$ is always lower than the actual value, with the discrepancy reaching 11% at pH 7.10 and 5% at pH 7.50.
Modified from Kassirer J, Bleich H: Rapid estimation of plasma carbon dioxide tension from pH and total carbon dioxide content. *N Engl J Med* 171:1067, 1965.

solved by using the pH measured in the blood gas laboratory (Table 14-1). Measured TCO_2 should be close to the calculated bicarbonate value. Venous TCO_2 should not be used in this exercise because it is often greater than arterial TCO_2.

Alternatives

Although little progress has been made in noninvasive pH measurement, there have been four important areas of technologic development: oximetry, transcutaneous PO_2 and PCO_2 gas measurements, expired PCO_2, and indwelling intravascular electrode systems. (See Chapter 26 for further discussion.)

Many situations may arise whereby arterial blood samples are not available. For example, severe peripheral vascular disease makes radial arterial puncture difficult, or the patient refuses arterial blood sampling or cannulation. In general, in the absence of circulatory failure or limb ischemia, central and peripheral venous blood may substitute for arterial when monitoring acid-base and ventilatory status. In hemodynamically stable patients, pH_a is, on average, 0.03 units higher than central venous pH (pH_{cv}) and $PaCO_2$ is lower than central venous carbon dioxide ($P_{cv}CO_2$) by 5 mm Hg [34], and changes in each are tightly correlated [35]. Regression analysis reveals $pH_a = (1.027 \times pH_{cv}) - 0.156$ and $PaCO_2 = (0.754 \times P_{cv}CO_2) + 2.75$. In shock, the accentuated discrepancy may be due to increased carbon dioxide generated by the buffering of acids in conditions characterized by increased lactic acid production.

It must be made clear that, in the absence of warming a sampling area to collect "arterialized" venous blood, an arterial sample is still necessary for evaluation of accurate oxygenation status for precise measurements of PO_2 and alveolar-arterial oxygen gradient determination. Once the oxygenation and acid-base status have been identified, pulse oximetry can be used to follow trends in SaO$_2$ in stable or improving patients because serial ABGs are costly and risk vessel injury with repeated arterial punctures.

References

1. Fleming W, Bowen J: Complications of arterial puncture. *Milit Med* 139:307, 1974.
2. Petty T, Bigelow B, Levine B: The simplicity and safety of arterial puncture. *JAMA* 195:181, 1966.
3. Sackner M, Avery W, Sokolowski J: Arterial punctures by nurses. *Chest* 59:97, 1971.
4. Comoroe J, Botelho S: The unreliability of cyanosis in the recognition of arterial anoxemia. *Am J Med Sci* 214:1, 1947.
5. Mithoefer J, Bossman O, Thibeault D, et al: The clinical estimation of alveolar ventilation. *Am Rev Respir Dis* 98:868, 1968.
6. Weiss E, Faling L, Mintz S, et al: Acute respiratory failure in chronic obstructive pulmonary disease I. Pathophysiology. *Disease-a-Month* 1, October 1969.
7. Raffin T: Indications for arterial blood gas analysis. *Ann Intern Med* 105:390, 1986.
8. Cerveri I, Zoia M, Fanfulla F, et al: Reference values of arterial oxygen tension in the middle-aged and elderly. *Am J Respir Crit Care* 152:934, 1995.
9. Felix WJ, Sigel B, Popky G: Doppler ultrasound in the diagnosis of peripheral vascular disease. *Semin Roentgenol* 4:315, 1975.
10. Allen E: Thromboangiitis obliterans: methods of diagnosis of chronic occlusive arterial lesions distal to the wrist, with illustrative cases. *Am J Med Sci* 178:237, 1929.
11. Bedford R: Radial arterial function following percutaneous cannulation with 18- and 20-gauge catheters. *Anesthesiology* 47:37, 1977.
12. Macon WI, Futrell J: Median-nerve neuropathy after percutaneous puncture of the brachial artery in patients receiving anticoagulants. *N Engl J Med* 288:1396, 1973.
13. Giner J, Casan P, Belda J, et al: Pain during arterial puncture. *Chest* 110:1143, 1996.
14. Sasse S, Berry R, Nguyen T: Arterial blood gas changes during breath-holding from functional residual capacity. *Chest* 110:958, 1996.
15. Bloom S, Canzanello V, Strom J, et al: Spurious assessment of acid-base status due to dilutional effect of heparin. *Am J Med* 79:528, 1985.
16. Janis K, Gletcher G: Oxygen tension measurements in small samples: sampling errors. *Am Rev Respir Dis* 106:914, 1972.
17. Winkler J, Huntington C, Wells D, et al: Influence of syringe material on arterial blood gas determinations. *Chest* 66:518, 1974.
18. Ansel G, Douce F: Effects of syringe material and needle size on the minimum plunger-displacement pressure of arterial blood gas syringes. *Respir Care* 27:147, 1982.
19. Thelin O, Karanth S, Pourcyrous M, et al: Overestimation of neonatal PO$_2$ by collection of arterial blood gas values with the butterfly infusion set. *J Perinatol* 13:65, 1993.
20. Adams A, Morgan-Hughes J, Sykes M: pH and blood gas analysis: methods of measurement and sources of error using electrode systems. *Anaesthesia* 22:575, 1967.
21. Bloom S, Canzanello V, Strom J, et al: Spurious assessment of acid-base status due to dilutional effect of heparin. *Am J Med* 79:528, 1985.
22. Hansen J, Simmons D: A systematic error in the determination of blood PCO$_2$. *Am Rev Respir Dis* 115:1061, 1977.
23. Eldridge F, Fretwell L: Change in oxygen tension of shed blood at various temperatures. *J Appl Physiol* 20:790, 1965.
24. Schmidt C, Mullert-Plathe O: Stability of PO$_2$, PCO$_2$ and pH in heparinized whole blood samples: influence of storage temperature with regard to leukocyte count and syringe material. *Eur J Clin Chem Clin Biochem* 30:767, 1992.
25. Criscuolo C, Nepper G, Buchalter S: Reflex sympathetic dystrophy following arterial blood gas sampling in the intensive care unit. *Chest* 108:578, 1995.
26. Mathieu A, Dalton B, Fischer J, et al: Expanding aneurysm of the radial artery after frequent puncture. *Anesthesiology* 38:401, 1973.
27. Hess D, Agarwal N: Variability of blood gases, pulse oximeter saturation, and end-tidal carbon dioxide pressure in stable, mechanically ventilated trauma patients. *J Clin Monit* 8:111, 1992.
28. Burnett R, Covington A, Fogh-Anderson N: Approved IFCC recommendations on whole blood sampling, transport and storage for simultaneous determination of pH, blood gases and electrolytes. *Eur J Clin Chem Clin Biochem* 33:247, 1995.
29. Lyon M, Bremner D, Laha T, et al: Specific heparin preparations interfere with the simultaneous measurement of ionized magnesium and ionized calcium. *Clin Biochem* 28:79, 1995.
30. Toffaletti J, Thompson T: Effects of blended lithium-zinc heparin on ionized calcium and general clinical chemistry tests. *Clin Chem* 41:328, 1995.
31. Curley F, Irwin R: Disorders of temperature control, I: Hyperthermia. *J Intens Care Med* 1:5, 1986.
32. Curley F, Irwin R: Disorders of temperature control, III: Hypothermia. *J Intens Care Med* 1:270, 1986.
33. Kassirer J, Bleich H: Rapid estimation of plasma carbon dioxide tension from pH and total carbon dioxide content. *N Engl J Med* 272:1067, 1965.
34. Adrogue H, Rashad M, Gorin A, et al: Assessing acid-base status in circulatory failure; differences between arterial and central venous blood. *N Engl J Med* 320:1312, 1989.
35. Philips B, Peretz D: A comparison of central venous and arterial blood gas values in the critically ill. *Ann Intern Med* 70:745, 1969.

15. Tracheostomy

A. Alan Conlan, Scott E. Kopec,
and Wayne E. Silva

The terms *tracheotomy* and *tracheostomy* are interchangeable. Derived from the Greek words *tracheia arteria* (rough artery) and *tome* (incision), *tracheotomy* refers to the operation that opens the trachea, whereas *tracheostomy* results in the formation of a tracheostoma, or the opening itself. Although tracheostomy is referred to intermittently from the first century BC [1–3], it was not performed regularly until the 1800s, when used by Trousseau and Bretonneau in the management of diphtheria. In the early 1900s, Chevalier Jackson [4], describing refinements to the operation, warned against tracheostomy involving the cricothyroid membrane or first tracheal ring because of the risk of injury to the cricoid cartilage and subsequent subglottic stenosis. During this period, the procedure was used to treat difficult cases of respiratory paralysis from poliomyelitis. Largely because of improvements in tubes and advances in clinical care, endotracheal intubation gradually has become the treatment of choice for short-term airway management [3,5].

Although tracheostomy is occasionally required in critically ill and injured patients who cannot be intubated for various reasons (e.g., cervical spine injury, upper airway obstruction, laryngeal injury, anatomic considerations), the most common use of this procedure today is to provide long-term access to the airway in patients who are dependent on mechanical ventilation. With improvements in critical care medicine, more patients are surviving initial episodes of acute respiratory failure, trauma, and extensive surgeries and are requiring prolonged periods of mechanical ventilation. It is now common practice to convert these patients expeditiously from translaryngeal intubation to tracheostomy. Tracheostomy is becoming a very common procedure in the intensive care unit (ICU). A survey reported the prevalence of tracheostomies in ICU patients to be 10% [6].

In this chapter, we review the indications, contraindications, complications, and techniques associated with tracheostomy. We also discuss the timing of converting an orally intubated patient to tracheostomy and the use of percutaneously placed tracheostomies versus the classic open technique.

Indications

The indications for tracheostomy can be divided into three general categories: to bypass obstruction of the upper airway, to provide an avenue for tracheal toilet and removal of retained secretions, and to provide a means for ventilatory support. These indications are summarized in Table 15-1 [7–12].

Anticipated prolonged ventilatory support, especially in patients who are receiving mechanical ventilation via translaryngeal intubation, is the most common indication for placing a tracheostomy in the ICU. Translaryngeal intubation and tracheostomy have several advantages and disadvantages in patients who require prolonged ventilator support [13], and these are summarized in Table 15-2. Most authors believe that, when the procedure is performed by a skilled

surgical group, the potential benefits of tracheostomy over translaryngeal intubation for most patients justify the application despite its potential risks. However, there are no detailed clinical trials that consistently confirm the advantages of tracheostomy in patients who require prolonged mechanical ventilation.

Contraindications

Tracheostomy has no absolute contraindications. Certain conditions, however, warrant special attention before anesthesia and surgery. In patients undergoing conversion from translaryngeal intubation to a tracheostomy for prolonged ventilatory support, the procedure should be viewed as elective or semielective. Therefore, the patient should be as medically stable as possible, and all attempts should be made to correct existing coagulopathies. For obvious reasons, emergent tracheostomies for upper airway obstruction may need to be performed when the patient is unstable or has a coagulopathy.

Timing of Tracheostomy

When to perform a tracheostomy on an intubated, critically ill patient has been very controversial. Several reviews have addressed this topic [13–16]. In 1987, the National Association of Medical Directors of Respiratory Care issued a consensus statement that tracheostomy was preferred in patients requiring an artificial airway for more than 21 days [17]. In part, this recommendation was based on reports of high complication rates for open tracheostomy; hence, the consensus statement reported that the risks of earlier tracheostomy were outweighed by the benefits. However, other studies [18–21] and the reported low morbidity and mortality of bedside percutaneous tracheostomies [16,22–24] confirm that it does not appear justified to avoid tracheostomy based solely on the risk of operative complications. The lower morbidity and mortality of the procedure shift the risk-benefit ratio to more of a benefit in the majority of patients who require prolonged ventilator support.

A more up-to-date approach regarding the timing of converting an intubated patient to a tracheostomy has been suggested by Heffner [13]. This recommendation takes into account the very low mortality and morbidity associated with placing a tracheostomy, plus the advantages and disadvantages of translaryngeal intubation and tracheostomy. In summary, if a stabilized patient has minimal barriers to weaning, and appears likely to be successfully weaned and extubated within 7 to 10 days, tracheostomy should be avoided. In patients who appear unlikely to be successfully weaned and extubated in 7 to 10 days, tracheostomy should be strongly considered. For patients whose ability to wean and be extubated is unclear, their status should be readdressed daily.

Table 15-1. Indications for Tracheostomy

Upper airway obstruction
  Laryngeal dysfunction: vocal cord paralysis
  Trauma: upper airway obstruction due to hemorrhage, edema, or crush injury; unstable mandibular fractures; injury to the larynx; cervical spine injuries
  Burns and corrosives: hot smoke; caustic gases; corrosives
  Foreign bodies
  Congenital anomalies: stenosis of the glottic or subglottic area
  Infections: croup; epiglottitis, Ludwig's angina; deep neck space infections
  Neoplasms: laryngeal cancer
  Postoperative: surgeries of the base of the tongue and hypopharynx; rigid fixation of the mandibular
  Obstructive sleep apnea [7,10–12]
Tracheal toilet
  Inability to clear secretions: generalized weakness; altered mental status; excess secretions
  Neuromuscular disease
Ventilatory support: prolonged or chronic

Adapted from Bjure J: Tracheostomy: a satisfactory method in the treatment of acute epiglottis. A clinical and functional follow-up study. *Int J Pediatr Otorhinolaryngol* 3:37, 1981; Hanline MH Jr: Tracheostomy in upper airway obstruction. *South Med J* 74:899, 1981; Taicher S, Givol M, Peleg M, et al: Changing indications for tracheostomy in maxillofacial trauma. *J Oral Maxillofac Surg* 54:292, 1996; Guilleminault C, Simmons FB, Motta J, et al: Obstructive sleep apnea syndrome and tracheostomy. *Arch Intern Med* 141:985, 1981; Burwell C, Robin E, Whaley R, et al: Extreme obesity associated with alveolar hypoventilation. *Am J Med* 141:985, 1981; Yung MW, Snowdon SL: Respiratory resistance of tracheostomy tubes. *Arch Otolaryngol* 110:591, 1984.

Table 15-2. Advantages and Disadvantages of Intubation and Tracheostomy

Advantages	Disadvantages
Translaryngeal intubation	
Reliable airway during urgent intubation	Bacterial airway colonization
	Inadvertent extubation
	Laryngeal injury
	Tracheal stenosis
	Purulent sinusitis (nasotracheal intubations)
	Patient discomfort
Tracheostomies	
Avoids direct injury to the larynx	Complications (see Table 15-3)
Facilitates nursing care	Bacterial airway colonization
Enhances patient mobility	Cost
More secure airway	Surgical scar
Improved patient comfort	Tracheal and stomal stenosis
Permits speech	
Provides psychological benefit	

From Heffner JE: Timing of tracheostomy in ventilator-dependent patients. *Clin Chest Med* 13:137,1992, with permission.

Some studies have suggested that early tracheostomy may be beneficial in some specific instances. A prospective observational study of medical ICU patients demonstrated an advantage to early tracheostomy. Patients had shorter hospital lengths of stay and lower hospital cost if they received a tracheostomy early (within an average of 6 days of admission) as opposed to late (within an average of 17 days after admission) [25]. Patients with blunt, multiple organ trauma have a shorter duration of mechanical ventilation, fewer episodes of nosocomial pneumonia [26], and a significant reduction in hospital costs [27] when the tracheostomy is performed within 1 week of their injuries. Similar benefits have been reported in patients with head trauma and poor Glasgow Coma Score [28–30] and patients with thermal injury [31], if a tracheostomy is performed within a week after the injury.

Emergency Tracheostomy

Emergency tracheostomy is a moderately difficult procedure, requiring training and skill; experience; adequate assistance, time, and lighting; and proper equipment and instrumentation. When time is short, the patient uncooperative, the anatomy distorted, and the aforementioned requirements not met, tracheostomy can be very hazardous. Emergency tracheostomy can pose significant risk to nearby neurovascular structures, particularly in small children in whom the trachea is small and not well defined. The risk of complications for emergency tracheostomy is two to five times higher than for elective tracheostomy [19,32,33]. Nonetheless, there are occasional indications for emergency tracheostomy [34], including transected trachea, anterior neck trauma with crushed larynx [35], and pediatric (younger than 12 years) patients requiring an emergency surgical airway in whom cricothyrotomy is generally not advised.

Tracheostomy in the Intensive Care Unit

PERCUTANEOUS DILATATIONAL TRACHEOSTOMY. Percutaneous dilatational tracheostomy (PDT) has surpassed open surgical tracheostomy as the procedure of choice in the ICU in a majority of cases. The concept of a tracheostomy by percutaneous dilatation was described by Toye and Weinstein in 1969 and again in 1986 [36]. Seldinger's wire-guided insertion technique for intravascular catheters has been adapted to many tube and catheter placement procedures [37]. Several modifications and variations of the Seldinger technique resulted in development of percutaneous techniques for tracheostomy and cricothyrotomy and in commercially available kits for performing these procedures. The minitracheostomy through the cricothyroid membrane has found particular favor in Great Britain, where it is used as suction access to the trachea [38,39].

The advantages of PDT over the standard open procedure are many. These advantages are summarized below:

1. In experienced hands, PDT can be performed routinely and safely in intubated ICU patients.
2. PDT can be performed bedside, whereas most open procedures are preformed in an operating room. Therefore, PDT offers a substantial cost saving of $1,000 to $1,500 per patient [40–42].
3. Performing the procedure eliminates the need to move a critically ill patient from an ICU to the operating room. Studies have shown that as many as 33% of critically ill ICU patients who are moved to other areas of the hospital for tests or procedures have significant and potentially dangerous physiologic changes [22,43,44]. This risk is avoided by performing the procedure bedside.
4. PDT avoids an open tracheostomy wound, which in turn provides improved healing and decreases the risk of wound infection [36,45].
5. The PDT technique also preserves soft tissue around the tracheostomy tube, allowing for the tube to fit snugly with less movement and angulation. This decreased movement minimizes pressure, erosions, and ischemic damage to the anterior tracheal cartilage rings.

6. Because the direction of the tube is controlled by a pre-placed wire and entry into the trachea is confirmed before the tube is placed, the risk of perforation of the posterior trachea and esophagus is lessened [46]. Placement of the wire should be monitored by fiberoptic tracheoscopy.
7. The smaller skin incision and stoma result in a more cosmetically acceptable scar [36].
8. The risk of tracheal stenosis is markedly reduced [21].

Several studies have compared PDT with standard, open tracheostomy [41–45]. These studies confirm the cost-saving advantage of PDT. Although overall short-term complication rates appear equal, PDT is associated with less perioperative bleeding and fewer stomal infections [45].

A bedside PDT has some hazards that are not commonly seen with standard open tracheostomies. The most important of these to consider are loss of airway due to bleeding, mucous, or tracheal collapse; accidental extubation; and false passage of the tracheostomy tube. These hazards can be minimized by maintaining stable endotracheal intubation during the procedure and performing the procedure with flexible fiberoptic bronchoscopic guidance. Not only does endotracheal intubation provide a secure airway during the procedure, but it also serves as a tracheal stent to prevent collapse of the trachea. An unstented trachea can collapse during insertion of a PDT, allowing through-and-through anteroposterior passage of needles and dilators to create false passages, extratracheal placement of the tube, and esophageal injury. Video tracheoscopic inspection of the trachea during the procedure also helps to assure against incorrect placement of the tube. Video tracheoscopy is mandatory if difficulties occur with dilation.

Several studies have confirmed the early and long-term safety of bedside PDT in critically ill ICU patients [21,22,24,25]. Our prospective experience of more than 300 patients at the University of Massachusetts Memorial Health Center demonstrated no mortalities and no major complications such as extratracheal tube placement, tracheal laceration, tracheolaryngeal injury, or loss of airway/accidental extubation. Our complications were limited to minimal bleeding and the development of subcutaneous emphysema in one patient who received high levels of positive end-expiratory pressure (PEEP).

In some patients who require a tracheostomy, we recommend an open surgical tracheostomy as opposed to a bedside PDT. These include patients who are not intubated, those on very high levels of PEEP, and those with large thyroid masses, laryngeal cancer, or other neck abnormalities that deny upper airway landmarks. Although lack of cervical spine clearance and the inability to extend the neck have been assumed to be relative contraindications to placing a PDT, one study refutes this assumption [47]. Similarly, morbid obesity has been assumed to be a relative contraindication, although we have reported success in placing PDTs in patients who weigh up to 500 lb [16].

OPEN SURGICAL TRACHEOSTOMY. Although PDT has several advantages over an open surgical tracheostomy, the open procedure should be considered as the procedure of choice in some clinical scenarios. For example, patients who require emergent airway access because of upper airway obstruction should undergo an open procedure. In the ICU setting, an open tracheostomy is favored in patients who are not orally or nasally intubated, those with severe respiratory failure who require high levels of PEEP, and those with anatomic or pathologic abnormalities of the neck. If for some reason a PDT cannot be performed, an open surgical procedure should be considered. The exact technique, including the Bjork flap

to prevent stenosis, is described in standard surgical texts and in the literature [48–52].

Techniques and Instruments of Percutaneous Dilatational Tracheostomy

Several percutaneous tracheostomy and cricothyrotomy techniques and instruments [53–56] have been developed. All used some form of the Seldinger artery cannulation technique with various adaptations for cutting (using a tracheostome) or dilating the pretracheal tissues and trachea. Percutaneous airways are performed at the cricothyroid membrane, subcricoid space (between the cricoid and the first tracheal ring) [57], or the level of the second to fourth tracheal rings. The cricothyroid membrane is more difficult to puncture and dilate than the trachea; considerable force must be used. All techniques require a skin incision, but it should be no larger than the tracheostomy tube that is to be placed. Although lower complication rates are cited for the dilatational technique, methods using a cutting instrument (tracheostome) have their advocates. Advantages of tracheostome techniques are that they can be used in emergencies, tracheostomy tubes with balloon cuffs are more easily advanced, and larger tubes can be inserted than with techniques that use sequential dilators [39,55,56]. Percutaneous airway procedures should be done with an endotracheal tube in place. Despite their attractiveness as methods for the unskilled, considerable training and practice are necessary for both techniques if significant, even lethal, complications are to be avoided [58–60]. The mandatory need for this procedure to be performed by a highly skilled and trained physician cannot be overemphasized.

The technique of percutaneous dilatational guidewire elective tracheostomy and procedural guidelines for numerous operators are described in the literature [61–64]. Briefly, the procedure is as follows:

1. Intubate the trachea and monitor oxygen saturation. Adjust the fraction of inspired oxygen, tidal volume, respiratory rate, and PEEP as needed to compensate for necessary air leak during the procedure.
2. Loosen the tapes fixing the endotracheal tube in place and secure the tube by hand throughout the procedure. Identify neck landmarks (Fig. 15-1A).
3. With the patient under local anesthesia and intravenous sedation, insert a needle and cannula between the first and second tracheal rings. Obtain free aspiration of air (Fig. 15-1B). If the needle impales the endotracheal tube, withdraw the tube a bit farther. A flexible fiberoptic bronchoscope should be used to confirm placement of the wire in the trachea.
4. Remove the needle, insert a J guidewire through the cannula and then remove the cannula (Fig. 15-1C). Make an incision around the guidewire (Fig. 15-1D).
5. Place a silicone guiding catheter over the guidewire and perform all dilations over this double guide (wire and silicone catheter) to prevent any kinking (Fig. 15-1E).
6. Insert and remove dilators of increasing size, up to a 36 French (Fr) for an 8-mm internal diameter cannula tracheostomy tube. Slightly overdilate the tracheostomy (Fig. 15-1F, G). Any difficulty during dilation must be evaluated by bronchoscopic examination of the upper trachea.
7. Lubricate a proper-sized dilator and preload it with the tracheostomy tube (Fig. 15-1H).
8. Thread the dilator carrying the tracheostomy tube over the silicone guide and insert it into the trachea. Positioning

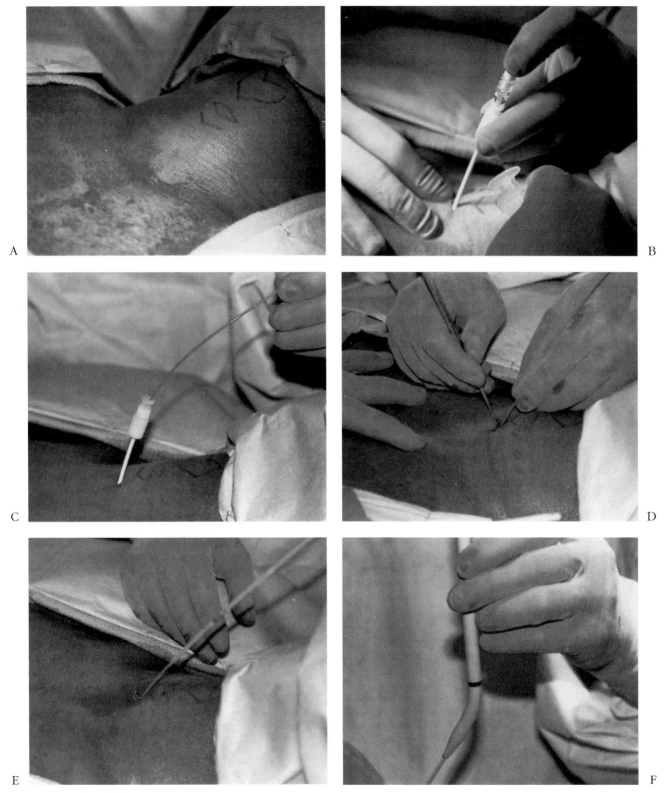

Fig. 15-1. A–I. Percutaneous dilatational tracheostomy technique (see text for details) (*continued*).

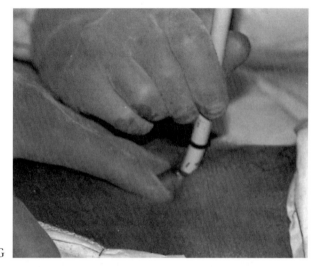

G

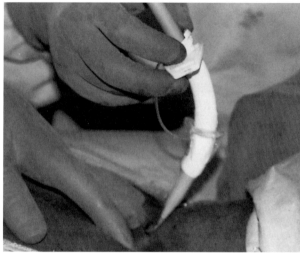

H

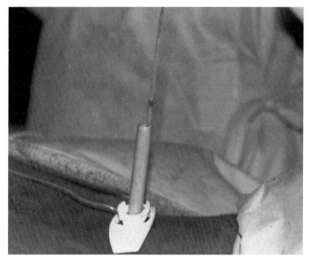

I

Fig. 15-1. (continued)

marks on the silicone guide and dilators assist in positioning (Fig. 15–1I).

9. Remove the dilator, silicone guide, and J guidewire. Fix the tracheostomy tube in place and remove the endotracheal tube. Dilatation of some tracheas can be extremely difficult; numerous tips and techniques are reported.

Tubes and Cannulas

Characteristics of a good tracheostomy tube are flexibility to accommodate varying patient anatomies, inert material, wide internal diameter, the smallest external diameter possible, a smooth surface to allow easy insertion and removal, and sufficient length to be secure once placed but not so long as to impinge the carina or other tracheal parts [14]. Until the late 1960s, when surgeons began to experiment with silicone and other synthetic materials, tracheostomy tubes and cannulas were made of metal. At present, almost all tracheostomy tubes are made of synthetic material. One disadvantage of a silicone tube over a metal one is the increased thickness of the tube wall, resulting in a larger outer diameter. Silicone tubes are available with or without a cuff. The cuff allows occlusion of the airway around the tube, which is necessary for positive-pressure ventilation. It also minimizes aspiration. In the past, cuffs were asso-

ciated with a fairly high incidence of tracheal stenosis caused by ischemia and necrosis of the mucous membrane and subsequent cicatricial contracture at the cuff site [65,66]. High-volume, low-pressure cuffs diminish pressure on the wall of the trachea, thereby minimizing (but not eliminating) problems due to focal areas of pressure necrosis [67]. If the only purpose of the tube is to secure the airway (sleep apnea) or to provide access for suctioning secretions, a tube without a cuff can be placed.

Postoperative Care

The care of a tracheostomy tube after surgery is of paramount importance. Highlighted in this section are specific issues that all intensivists need to be knowledgeable of when caring for patients with tracheostomies.

DRESSING CARE. When changing dressings and tapes, special care is needed to avoid accidental dislodging of the tracheostomy tube.

INNER CANNULAS. The inner cannulas should be used at all times in the ICU. They serve to extend the life of the tracheostomy tubes by preventing buildup of secretions within the tracheostomy. The inner cannulas can be easily removed and either cleaned or replaced with a sterile, disposable one. Disposable inner cannulas have the advantage of quick and efficient changing, a decrease in nursing time, decreased risk of cross-contamination, and guaranteed sterility [68]. The obturator should be kept at the bedside at all times, in the event that reinsertion of the tracheostomy is necessary.

HUMIDIFICATION. The upper airway moistens and humidifies inspired air. Because tracheostomies bypass the upper airway, it is vital to provide warm, humidified air to patients with tracheostomies. Humidification of inspired gases is vital in preventing complications in patients with tracheostomies. Failure to humidify the inspired gases can result in obstruction of the tube by inspissated secretions and causing increased secretions, impaired mucociliary clearance, and decreased cough [69,70].

TRACHEOSTOMY TUBE CHANGES. Tracheostomy tubes do not require routine changing. In general, the tube only needs to be changed when there is a functional problem with it, such as an air leak in the balloon, when the lumen is narrowed due to the buildup of dried secretions, or when downsizing the tube before decannulations. Ideally, a tracheostomy tube should not be changed until 7 to 10 days after its initial placement. The reason for this is to allow the tracheal stoma and the tract to mature. Patients who have their tracheostomy tube changed before the tract is fully mature risk having the tube misplaced into the soft tissue of the neck. If the tracheostomy tube needs to be replaced before the tract has had time to mature, the tube should be changed over a guide, such as a suction catheter [71,72].

ORAL FEEDING AND SWALLOWING DYSFUNCTION ASSOCIATED WITH TRACHEOSTOMIES. Great caution should be exercised before initiating oral feedings in patients with tracheostomy. Numerous studies have demonstrated that patients are at a significantly increased risk for aspiration when a tracheostomy is in place.

Physiologically, patients with tracheostomies are more like to aspirate because the tracheostomy tube tethers the larynx, preventing its normal upward movement, which is needed to assist in glottic closure and cricopharyngeal relaxation [73,74]. Tracheostomy tubes also disrupt normal swallowing by compressing the esophagus and interfering with deglutition [75], decreasing the duration of vocal cord closure [76], and resulting in uncoordinated laryngeal closure [77]. In addition, prolonged orotracheal intubation can result in prolonged swallowing disorders even after the endotracheal tube is converted to a tracheostomy [78]. It is therefore not surprising that more than 65% of patients with tracheostomies aspirate when swallowing [79–81].

Before one attempts to initial oral feedings in a patient with a tracheostomy, several objective criteria must be met. The patient must be consistently alert, appropriate, and able to follow complex commands. He or she should also have adequate cough and swallowing reflexes, adequate oral motor strength, and a significant respiratory reserve [82]. These criteria are probably best assessed by a certified speech therapist. However, clinical assessment may only identify 34% of the patients at high risk for aspiration [83]. Augmenting the bedside swallowing evaluation by coloring feedings or measuring the glucose in tracheal secretions may not increase the sensitivity in detecting the risk of aspiration [84,85]. A video barium swallow may allow the identification of 50% to 80% of patients with tracheostomies who are at a high risk to aspi-

rate oral feeding [83,86]. A direct laryngoscopy to directly observe a patient's swallowing mechanics coupled with a video barium swallow may be more sensitive in predicting which patients are at risk for aspiration [83]. Scintigraphic studies may be the most sensitive tests to determine which patients are aspirating [87] and are much easier to perform than endoscopy. Plugging of the tracheostomy [87] or using a Passy-Muir valve [88] may reduce aspiration in patients with tracheostomies who are taking oral feedings, but this is not a universal finding [89].

Because of the high risk for aspiration and the difficulty in assessing which patients are at high risk to aspirate, we do not institute oral feedings in patients with tracheostomy in the ICU. We believe that the potential risks of placing a percutaneous endoscopically placed gastrostomy feeding tube are much less than the risks of aspiration of oral feedings and their complications (i.e., recurrent pneumonia, acute respiratory distress syndrome, and prolonging and inhibiting weaning). However, we are unaware of any prospective studies addressing the complications between these two methods of providing enteric nutritional support in patients with tracheostomies.

Complications

Tracheostomies, whether inserted by percutaneous dilatation or by the open surgical procedure, are associated with a variety of complications. These complications are best grouped by the time of occurrence after the placement and are divided into immediate, intermediate, and late complications [16] (Table 15-3). The reported incidence of complications varies from 3% to 13% [6,21,47,90] and mortality from 0.03% to 0.6%

Table 15-3. Complications of Tracheostomies

Immediate complications (0–24 h)
    Cardiorespiratory arrest
    Major hemorrhage
    Tracheolaryngeal injury
    Crushed airway from dilational tracheostomy
    Loss of airway control
    Pneumothorax
    Pneumomediastinum
    Acute surgical emphysema
    Esophageal injury
    Tube displacement
    Arrhythmia
    Hypotension
    Hypoxia/hypercapnia
    Bacteremia
Intermediate complications (from day 1 to day 7)
    Persistent bleeding
    Tube displacement
    Tube obstruction (mucus, blood)
    Major atelectasis
    Wound infection/cellulitis
Late complications (after day 7)
    Tracheoinnominate artery fistula
    Tracheomalacia
    Tracheal stenosis
    Necrosis and loss of anterior tracheal cartilage
    Tracheoesophageal fistula
    Major aspiration
    Chronic speech and swallowing deficits
    Tracheocutaneous fistula

From Conlan AA, Kopec SC: Tracheostomy in the ICU. *J Intensive Care* 15:1, 2000, with permission.

[21,90]. Posttracheostomy mortality and morbidity are caused by iatrogenic tracheal laceration [91], hemorrhage, tube dislodgment, infection, and obstruction. Neurosurgical patients have a higher posttracheostomy complication rate than do other patients [92,93]. Tracheostomy is more hazardous in children than in adults and carries special risks in the very young, often related to the experience of the surgeon [94]. We discuss some of these complications. A comprehensive understanding of immediate, intermediate, and late complications of tracheostomy and their management is essential for the intensivist.

OBSTRUCTION. Occasionally, a tube becomes plugged with clotted blood or inspissated secretions. In this case, the inner cannula should be removed immediately and the patient suctioned. Should that fail, it may be necessary to remove the outer cannula also, a decision that must take into consideration the reason the tube was placed and the length of time it has been in place. Obstruction also may be due to angulation of the distal end of the tube against the anterior or posterior tracheal wall. An undivided thyroid isthmus pressing against the angled tracheostomy tube can force the tip against the anterior tracheal wall, whereas a low superior transverse skin edge can force the tip of the tracheostomy tube against the posterior tracheal wall. An indication of this type of obstruction is an expiratory wheeze. Division of the thyroid isthmus and proper placement of transverse skin incisions prevent anterior or posterior tube angulation and obstruction [95].

TUBE DISPLACEMENT/DISLODGMENT. Dislodgment of a tracheostomy tube that has been in place for 2 weeks or longer is managed simply by replacing the tube. If it cannot be immediately replaced or if it is replaced and the patient cannot be ventilated (indicating that the tube is not in the trachea), orotracheal intubation should be performed. Immediate postoperative displacement can be fatal if the tube cannot be promptly replaced and the patient cannot be reintubated.

Dislodgment in the early postoperative period is usually caused by one of several technical problems. Failure to divide the thyroid isthmus may permit the intact isthmus to ride up against the tracheostomy tube and thus displace it [95]. Excessively low placement of the stoma (i.e., below the second and third rings) can occur when the thoracic trachea is brought into the neck by overextending the neck or by excessive traction on the trachea. When the normal anatomic relationships are restored, the trachea recedes below the suprasternal notch, causing the tube to be dislodged from the trachea [95,96]. The risk of dislodgment of the tracheostomy tube, a potentially lethal complication, can be minimized by (a) transection of the thyroid isthmus at surgery, if indicated; (b) proper placement of the stoma; (c) avoidance of excessive neck hyperextension or tracheal traction, or both; (d) application of sufficiently tight tracheostomy tube retention tapes; and (e) suture of the tracheostomy tube flange to the skin in patients with short necks. Some surgeons apply retaining sutures to the trachea for use in the early postoperative period in case the tube becomes dislodged, allowing the trachea to be pulled into the wound for reintubation. Making a Bjork flap involves suturing the inferior edge of the trachea stoma to the skin, thus allowing a sure pathway for tube placement. Bjork flaps, however, tend to interfere with swallowing and promote aspiration [97]. Reintubation of a tracheostomy can be accomplished using a smaller, beveled endotracheal tube and then applying a tracheostomy tube over the smaller tube, using the Seldinger technique [98]. Using a nasogastric tube as a guidewire has also been described [99].

If a tracheostomy becomes dislodged within 7 to 10 days of surgery, we recommend translaryngeal endotracheal intuba-tion to establish a safe airway. The tracheostomy tube can then be replaced under less urgent conditions and with fiberoptic guidance if needed.

SUBCUTANEOUS EMPHYSEMA. In approximately 5% of patients, subcutaneous emphysema develops after tracheostomy [98]. It is most likely to occur when dissection is extensive or the wound is closed tightly, or both. Partial closure of the skin wound is appropriate, but the underlying tissues should be allowed to approximate naturally. Subcutaneous emphysema generally resolves over the 48 hours after tracheostomy, but when the wound is closed tightly and the patient is coughing or on positive-pressure ventilation, pneumomediastinum, pneumopericardium, and/or tension pneumothorax may occur [95].

PNEUMOTHORAX AND PNEUMOMEDIASTINUM. The cupola of the pleura extends well into the neck, especially in patients with emphysema; thus, the pleura can be damaged during tracheostomy. This complication is more common in the pediatric age group because the pleural dome extends more cephalad in children [1]. The incidence of pneumothorax after tracheostomy is approximately 5% [1,98]. Many surgeons routinely obtain a postoperative chest radiograph.

HEMORRHAGE. Minor postoperative fresh tracheostomy bleeding occurs in up to 37% of cases [1] and is probably the most common complication of this procedure. Postoperative coughing and straining can cause venous bleeding by dislodging a clot or ligature. Elevating the head of the bed, packing the wound, and/or using homeostatic materials usually control minor bleeding. Major bleeding occurs in 5% of tracheotomies and is due to hemorrhage from the isthmus of the thyroid gland, loss of a ligature from one of the anterior jugular veins, or injury to the transverse jugular vein that crosses the midline just above the jugular notch [100]. Persistent bleeding may require a return to the operating room for management. Techniques to decrease the likelihood of early posttracheostomy hemorrhage include (a) use of a vertical incision; (b) careful dissection in the midline, with care to pick up each layer of tissue with instruments rather than simply spreading tissues apart; (c) liberal use of ligatures rather than electrocautery; and (d) careful division and suture ligation of the thyroid isthmus. Late hemorrhage after tracheostomy is usually due to bleeding granulation tissue or another relatively minor cause. However, in these late cases, a tracheoinnominate artery fistula needs to be ruled out.

TRACHEOINNOMINATE ARTERY FISTULA. At one point, it had been reported that 50% of all tracheostomy bleeding occurring more than 48 hours after the procedure is due to an often fatal complication of rupture of the innominate artery caused by erosion of the tracheostomy tube at its tip or cuff into the vessel [98]. However, since the advent of the low-pressure cuff, the incidence of this complication has decreased considerably and occurs less than 1% of the time [101].

Eighty-five percent of tracheoinnominate fistulas occur within the first month after tracheostomy [102], although they have been reported as late as 7 months after operation. Other sites of delayed exsanguinating posttracheostomy hemorrhage include the common carotid artery, superior and inferior thyroid arteries, aortic arch, and innominate vein [102]. Rupture and fistula formation are caused by erosion through the trachea into the artery due to excessive cuff pressure or by angulation of the tube tip against the anterior trachea. Infection and other factors that weaken local tissues, such as malnourishment and steroids, also seem to play a role [103]. The innominate artery rises to approximately the level of the sixth ring anterior to the trachea, and low placement of the stoma can also create close proximity of the tube tip or cuff to the innominate artery. Rarely, an anomaly of the innominate, occurring with an incidence of 1% to 2% [102], is responsible for this disastrous complication. Pulsation of the tracheostomy tube is an indication of potentially fatal positioning [102]. Initially, hemorrhage from a tracheoinnominate fistula is usually not exsanguinating. Herald bleeds must be investigated promptly using fiberoptic tracheoscopy. If a tracheoinnominate fistula seems probable (minimal tracheitis, anterior pulsating erosions), the patient should be taken to the operating room for evaluation. Definitive management involves resection of the artery [104]. The mortality is greater than 50%. Sudden exsanguinating hemorrhage can be managed by hyperinflation of the tracheostomy cuff tube or reintubation with an endotracheal tube through the stoma, attempting to place the cuff at the level of the fistula. A lower neck incision with blind digital compression on the artery may be part of a critical resuscitative effort [105].

MISPLACEMENT OF TUBE. Misplacement of tube is a technical error that occurs at the time of surgery or when the tube is changed or replaced through a fresh stoma. If it is not recognized, associated mediastinal emphysema and tension pneumothorax can occur, along with alveolar hypoventilation. Injury to neurovascular structures, including the recurrent laryngeal nerve, is possible [96]. The patient must be orally intubated or the tracheostoma recannulated. Some advise placing retaining sutures in the trachea at the time of surgery. The availability of a tracheostomy set at the bedside after tracheostomy facilitates emergency reintubation.

STOMAL INFECTIONS. An 8% to 12% incidence of cellulitis or purulent exudate is reported [1,20,98]. Attention to the details of good stoma care and early use of antibiotics are advised. The use of the PDT technique has virtually eliminated infection.

TRACHEOESOPHAGEAL FISTULA. Tracheoesophageal fistula caused by injury to the posterior tracheal wall and cervical esophagus occurs in fewer than 1% of patients, more commonly in the pediatric age group. Early postoperative fistula is a result of iatrogenic injury during the procedure [98,105]. The chances of creating a fistula can be minimized by entering the trachea initially with a horizontal incision between two tracheal rings (the second and third), thereby eliminating the initial cut into a hard cartilaginous ring [95]. A late tracheoesophageal fistula may be due to tracheal necrosis caused by tube movement or angulation, as in neck hyperflexion, or excessive cuff pressure [96,98,105]. A tracheoesophageal fistula should be suspected in patients with cuff leaks, abdominal distention, recurrent aspiration pneumonia, and reflux of gastric fluids through the tracheostomy site. It may be demonstrated on endoscopy and contrast studies. Tracheoesophageal fistulas require surgical repair.

SUBGLOTTIC EDEMA AND TRACHEAL STENOSIS. Placement of the tracheostomy tube in close proximity to the glottic area (cricothyrotomy or first tracheal ring tracheostomy) may lead to edema and eventual subglottic stenosis. This is more likely to occur if there is mucosal injury from a previous endotracheal intubation or infection at the stoma site, or both [106,107]. Meticulous care of tracheostomy stomas and prompt treatment of upper airway infections can help to prevent this complication. Removal of a button of cartilage during tracheostomy in adults is acceptable, but in an infant or young child, this maneuver may result in tracheal stenosis. Subglottic edema is a significant cause of decannulation problems.

DYSPHAGIA AND ASPIRATION. The major swallowing disorder associated with tracheostomy is aspiration. Some patients with tracheostomy tubes complain of the sensation of a mass in the lower neck. This may lead to dysphagia and aspiration [107], particularly if the cuff is left inflated while the patient is eating [108]. The presence of a gag reflex does not confer protection against aspiration of pharyngeal contents. The defects reported are delayed triggering of the swallow response and pharyngeal pooling of contrast materials [109]. The causes include decreased laryngeal elevation and anterior movement during deglutition, because the tube itself or a Bjork flap fixes the trachea to the skin; esophageal compression by an inflated cuff; and desensitization of the larynx, leading to loss of protective reflexes and uncoordinated laryngeal closure. For these reasons, we do not recommend oral feeding in ICU patients with tracheostomies.

TRACHEOCUTANEOUS FISTULA. Although the tracheostoma generally closes rapidly after decannulation, a persistent fistula occasionally remains, particularly when the tracheostomy tube is present for a prolonged period. If this occurs, the fistula tract can be excised and the wound closed primarily, under local anesthesia [110].

Cricothyrotomy

Cricothyrotomy (cricothyroidotomy) [111] was condemned in Jackson's 1921 article [4] on high tracheostomies because of excessive complications, particularly subglottic stenoses [112,113]. He emphasized the importance of the cricoid cartilage as an encircling support for the larynx and trachea. However, the favorable report by Brantigan and Grow [114] evaluating 655 cricothyrotomies, with a complication rate of only 6.1% and no cases of subglottic stenosis, prompted reevaluation of cricothyrotomy for elective and emergency airway access. Further reports emphasized the advantages of cricothyrotomy over tracheostomy, which included technical simplicity, speed of performance, low complication rate [113,115–118], suitability as a bedside procedure, usefulness for isolation of the airway from median sternotomy [117,119] and radical neck dissection incisions [120], lack of need to hyperextend the neck, and formation of a smaller scar. Also, because cricothyrotomy results in less encroachment on the mediastinum, there is less chance of esophageal injury and virtually no chance of pneumothorax or tracheoarterial fistula [113].

Despite these considerations, many authorities currently recommend that cricothyrotomy should be used as an elective long-term method of airway access only in highly selected patients [112,113,120–122]. Use of cricothyrotomy in the emergency setting, particularly for managing trauma, is not controversial [111,123,124].

EMERGENCY CRICOTHYROTOMY. Because cricothyrotomy requires a small number of instruments and less training than tracheostomy and can be performed quickly, it is indicated as a means for controlling the airway in an emergency when oral or nasotracheal intubation is unsuccessful or contraindicated. In emergency situations, translaryngeal intubations fail because of massive oronasal hemorrhage or regurgitation, structural deformities of the upper airway, muscle spasm and clenched teeth, and obstruction by foreign bodies of the upper airway [111]. Cricothyrotomy finds its greatest use in trauma management. Actual or suspected cervical spine injury, alone or in combination with severe facial trauma, makes nasotracheal and orotracheal intubation difficult and hazardous. Thus, cricothyrotomy has an important role in emergency airway management [123].

CONTRAINDICATIONS. Cricothyrotomy should not be used to manage airway obstruction that occurs immediately after endotracheal extubation, because the obstruction may be found below the larynx [4,113,123]. Likewise, with primary laryngeal trauma or disease such as tumor and infection, cricothyrotomy may prove useless. It is contraindicated in infants and in children younger than 10 to 12 years under all circumstances [123]. In this age group, percutaneous transtracheal jet ventilation may be a temporizing procedure until tracheostomy can be performed.

ANATOMY. The cricothyroid space is no larger than 7 to 9 mm in its vertical dimension, smaller than the outside diameter of most tracheostomy tubes (No. 6 Shiley outside diameter is 10 mm). The cricothyroid artery runs across the midline in the upper portion, and the membrane fuses vertically in the midline. The anterosuperior edge of the thyroid cartilage is the laryngeal prominence. The cricothyroid membrane is approximately 2 to 3 cm below this laryngeal prominence and can be identified as an indentation immediately below the thyroid cartilage. The lower border of the cricothyroid membrane is the cricoid cartilage [117,118,122,125,126]. A description of the procedure is contained in standard surgical texts.

COMPLICATIONS. The reported incidence of short- and long-term complications of cricothyrotomy ranges from 6.1% [114] for procedures performed in elective, well-controlled, carefully selected cases to greater than 50% [111,112,124,127] for procedures performed under emergency or other suboptimal conditions.

The incidence of subglottic stenosis after cricothyrotomy is 2% to 3% [112,113]. This major complication occurs at the tracheostomy or cricothyrotomy site but not at the cuff site [128]. Necrosis of cartilage due to iatrogenic injury to the cricoid cartilage or pressure from the tube on the cartilage may play a role [123]. Possible reasons that subglottic stenosis may occur more commonly with cricothyrotomy than with tracheostomy are as follows: The larynx is the narrowest part of the laryngotracheal airway; subglottic tissues, especially in children, are intolerant of contact; and division of the cricothyroid membrane and the cricoid cartilage destroy the only complete ring supporting the airway [3,112]. Prior laryngotracheal injury, as with prolonged translaryngeal intubation, is a major risk factor for the development of subglottic stenosis after cricothyrotomy [112,113].

Conclusions

Tracheostomy is one of the most common surgical procedures performed in the ICU and is the airway of choice for patients who require mechanical ventilation for more than 2 weeks.

Because the exact timing for converting patients to tracheostomy is not entirely clear, the physician must weigh the risks and benefits of tracheostomy versus translaryngeal intubation and estimate the expected length of need of mechanical ventilation for each individual patient. Percutaneous dilatation tracheostomy is safe and offers significant advantages over an open surgical tracheostomy. PDT should now be the procedure of choice for surgical airway access in most ICU patients. However, PDT should only be performed by experienced and skilled physicians.

References

1. Goldstein SI, Breda SD, Schneider KL: Surgical complications of bedside tracheotomy in an otolaryngology residency program. *Laryngoscope* 97:1407, 1987.
2. Heffner JE, Miller KS, Sahn SA: Tracheostomy in the intensive care unit, 1: indication, techniques, management. *Chest* 90:269, 1986.
3. Goodall EW: The story of tracheotomy. *Br J Child Dis* 31:167, 1934.
4. Jackson C: High tracheotomy and other errors. The chief causes of chronic laryngeal stenosis. *Surg Gynecol Obstet* 32:392, 1921.
5. McClelland RMA: Tracheostomy: its management and alternatives. *Proc R Soc Med* 65:401, 1972.
6. Fischler L, Erhart S, Kleger GR, et al: Prevalence of tracheostomy in ICU patients. *Intensive Care Med* 26:1428, 2000.
7. Bjure J: Tracheotomy: a satisfactory method in the treatment of acute epiglottis. A clinical and functional follow-up study. *Int J Pediatr Otorhinolaryngol* 3:37, 1981.
8. Hanline MH Jr: Tracheotomy in upper airway obstruction. *South Med J* 74:899, 1981.
9. Taicher S, Givol M, Peleg M, et al: Changing indications for tracheostomy in maxillofacial trauma. *J Oral Maxillofac Surg* 54:292, 1996.
10. Guilleminault C, Simmons FB, Motta J, et al: Obstructive sleep apnea syndrome and tracheostomy. *Arch Intern Med* 141:985, 1981.
11. Burwell C, Robin E, Whaley R, et al: Extreme obesity associated with alveolar hypoventilation. *Am J Med* 141:985, 1981.
12. Yung MW, Snowdon SL: Respiratory resistance of tracheostomy tubes. *Arch Otolaryngol* 110:591, 1984.
13. Heffner JE: Timing of tracheostomy in ventilator-dependent patients. *Clin Chest Med* 12:611, 1991.
14. Lewis RJ: Tracheostomies: indications, timing, and complications. *Clin Chest Med* 13:137, 1992.
15. Heffner JE: Timing of tracheostomy in mechanical ventilated patients. *Am Rev Respir Dis* 147:768, 1993.
16. Conlan AA, Kopec SE: Tracheostomy in the ICU. *J Intensive Care Med* 15:1, 2000.
17. Marsh HM, Gillespie DJ, Baumgartner AE: Timing of tracheostomy in the critically ill patient. *Chest* 96:190, 1989.
18. Astrachan DI, Kirchner JC, Goodwin JW Jr: Prolonged intubation vs tracheotomy: complications, practical and psychological considerations. *Laryngoscope* 98:1165, 1988.
19. Stock CM, Woodward CG, Shapiro BA, et al: Perioperative complications of elective tracheostomy in critically ill patients. *Crit Care Med* 14:861, 1986.
20. Dayal VS, Masri WE: Tracheostomy in the intensive care setting. *Laryngoscope* 96:58, 1986.
21. Walz MK, Peitgen K, Thurauf N, et al: Percutaneous dilatational tracheostomy—early results and long-term outcome. *Intensive Care Med* 24:685, 1998.
22. Friedman Y, Fildes J, Mizock B, et al: Comparison of percutaneous and surgical tracheostomies. *Chest* 110:480, 1996.
23. Rosenbower TJ, Morris JA, Eddy VA, et al: The long-term complications of percutaneous dilatational tracheostomy. *Am Surg* 64:82, 1998.
24. Moe KS, Stoeckli SJ, Schmid S, et al: Percutaneous tracheostomy: a comprehensive evaluation. *Ann Otol Rhinol Laryngol* 108:384, 1999.
25. Brook AD, Sherman G, Malen J, et al: Early versus late tracheostomy in patients who require prolonged mechanical ventilation. *Am J Crit Care* 9:352, 2000.
26. Lesnik I, Rappaport W, Fulginiti J, et al: The role of early tracheostomy in blunt, multiple organ trauma. *Am Surg* 58:346, 1992.

27. Armstrong PA, McCarthy MC, Peoples JB: Reduced use of resources by early tracheostomy in ventilator-dependent patients with blunt trauma. *Surgery* 124:763, 1998.

28. Teoh WH, Goh KY, Chan C: The role of early tracheostomy in critically ill neurosurgical patients. *Ann Acad Med Singapore* 30:234, 2001.

29. Koh WY, Lew TWK, Chin NM, et al: Tracheostomy in a neuro-intensive care setting: indications and timing. *Anaesth Intensive Care* 25:365, 1997.

30. D'Amelio LF, Hammond JS, Spain DA, et al: Tracheostomy and percutaneous endoscopic gastrostomy in the management of the head-injured patient. *Am Surg* 60:180, 1994.

31. Sellers BJ, Davis BL, Larkin PW, et al: Early predictors of prolonged ventilator dependence in thermally injured patients. *J Trauma* 43:899, 1997.

32. Seid AB, Thomas GK: Tracheostomy, in Paparela MM, Shumrick DA (eds): *Otolaryngology.* 2nd ed. Philadelphia, WB Saunders, 1980, p 3004 (vol 3).

33. Skaggs JA, Cogbill CL: Tracheostomy: management, mortality, complications. *Am Surg* 35:393, 1969.

34. American College of Surgeons Committee on Trauma: *Advanced Trauma Life Support Course for Physicians, Instructor Manual.* Chicago, American College of Surgeons, 1985, p 159.

35. Kline SN: Maxillofacial trauma, in Kreis DJ, Gomez GA (eds): *Trauma Management.* Boston, Little, Brown, and Company 1989.

36. Toye FJ, Weinstein JD: Clinical experience with percutaneous tracheostomy and cricothyroidotomy in 100 patients. *J Trauma* 26:1034, 1986.

37. Hazard PB, Garrett HE Jr, Adams JW, et al: Bedside percutaneous tracheostomy: experience with 55 elective procedures. *Ann Thorac Surg* 46:63, 1988.

38. Av J, Walker WS, Inglis D, et al: Percutaneous cricothyroidostomy (minitracheostomy) for bronchial toilet: results of therapeutic and prophylactic use. *Ann Thorac Surg* 48:850, 1989.

39. Fisher EW, Howard DJ: Percutaneous tracheostomy in a head and neck unit. *J Laryngol Otol* 106:625, 1992.

40. Cobean R, Beals M, Moss C, et al: Percutaneous dilatational tracheostomy: a safe cost-effective bedside procedure. *Arch Surg* 131:265, 1996.

41. Freeman BD, Isabella K, Cobb JP, et al: A prospective, randomized study comparing percutaneous with surgical tracheostomy in critically ill patients. *Crit Care Med* 29:926, 2001.

42. Bowen CP, Whitney LR, Truwit JD, et al: Comparison of safety and cost of percutaneous versus surgical tracheostomy. *Am Surg* 67:54, 2001.

43. Indeck M, Peterson S, Brotman S: Risk, cost and benefit of transporting patients from the ICU for special studies. *Crit Care Med* 15:350, 1987.

44. Henrich DE, Blythe WR, Weissler MC, et al: Tracheostomy and the intensive care unit. *Laryngoscope* 107:844, 1997.

45. Freeman BD, Isabella K, Lin N, et al: A meta-analysis of prospective trials comparing percutaneous and surgical tracheostomy in critically ill patients. *Chest* 118:1412, 2000.

46. Helms U, Heilman K: Ein neues Krikothyreoidotomie-Besteck für den Notfall. *Anaesthetist* 34:47, 1985.

47. Mayberry JC, Wu IC, Goldman RK, et al: Cervical spine clearance and neck extension during percutaneous tracheostomy in trauma patients. *Crit Care Med* 28:3566, 2000.

48. Upadhtay A, Maurer J, Turner J, et al: Elective bedside tracheostomy in the intensive care unit. *J Am Coll Surg* 183:51, 1996.

49. Eliachar I, Goldsher M, Joachims HZ, et al: Superiorly based tracheostomal flap to counteract tracheal stenosis: experimental study. *Laryngoscope* 91:976, 1981.

50. Orringer MB: Endotracheal intubation and tracheostomy: indications, techniques, and complications. *Surg Clin North Am* 60:1447, 1980.

51. Montgomery WW: Surgery of the trachea, in Montgomery WW (ed): *Surgery of the Upper Respiratory Tract.* 2nd ed. Philadelphia, Lea & Febiger, 1979, p 365 (vol 2).

52. Seid AB, Thomas GK: Tracheostomy, in Paparela MM, Shumrick DA (eds): *Otolaryngology.* Philadelphia, WB Saunders, 1980, p 3004 (vol 3).

53. Wain JC, Wilson DJ, Mathisen DJ: Clinical experience with minitracheotomy. *Ann Thorac Surg* 49:881, 1990.

54. Weiss S: A new instrument for pediatric emergency cricothyrotomy. *Natl Pediatr Trade J* 11(Winter):9, 1987.

55. Schachner A, Ovil J, Sidi J, et al: Rapid percutaneous tracheostomy. *Chest* 98:1266, 1990.

56. Ivatury R, Siegel JH, Stahl WM, et al: Percutaneous tracheostomy after trauma and critical illness. *J Trauma* 32:133, 1992.

57. Ciaglia P, Firsching R, Suniec C: Elective percutaneous dilatational tracheostomy: a new simple bedside procedure. Preliminary report. *Chest* 6:715, 1985.

58. Ravlo O, Bach V, Lybecker H, et al: A comparison between two emergency cricothyroidotomy instruments. *Acta Anaesthesiol Scand* 31:317, 1987.

59. Bjoraker DG, Kumar NB, Brown ACD: Evaluation of an emergency cricothyrotomy instrument. *Crit Care Med* 15:157, 1987.

60. Wang MB, Berke GS, Ward PH, et al: Early experience with percutaneous tracheotomy. *Laparoscope* 102:157, 1992.

61. Wease GL, Frikker M, Villalba M, et al: Bedside tracheostomy in the intensive care unit. *Arch Surg* 131:552, 1996.

62. Ciaglia P, Graniero KD: Percutaneous dilatational tracheostomy: results and long-term follow-up. *Chest* 101:464, 1992.

63. Anderson HL, Bartlett RH: Elective tracheotomy for mechanical ventilation by the percutaneous technique. *Clin Chest Med* 12:555, 1991.

64. Marx WH, Ciaglia P, Graniero KD: Some important details in the technique of percutaneous dilatational tracheostomy via the modified Seldinger technique. *Chest* 110:762, 1996.

65. Cooper JD, Grillo HC: The evolution of tracheal injury due to ventilatory assistance through cuffed tubes: a pathologic study. *Ann Surg* 169:334, 1969.

66. Stool SE, Campbell JR, Johnson DG: Tracheostomy in children: the use of plastic tubes. *J Pediatr Surg* 3:402, 1968.

67. Grillo HZ, Cooper JD, Geffin B, et al: A low pressured cuff for tracheostomy tubes to minimize tracheal inner injury. *J Thorac Cardiovasc Surg* 62:898, 1971.

68. Crow S: Disposable tracheostomy inner cannula. *Infect Control* 7:285, 1986.

69. Forbes AR: Temperature, humidity and mucous flow in the intubated trachea. *Br J Anaesth* 46:29, 1974.

70. Chalon J, Patel C, Ali M, et al: Humidity and the anaesthetized patient. *Anesthesiology* 50:195, 1979.

71. Gilsdorf JR: Facilitated endotracheal and tracheostomy tube replacement. *Surg Gynecol Obstet* 159:587, 1984.

72. Young JS, Brady WJ, Kesser B, et al: A novel method for replacement of a dislodged tracheostomy tube: the nasogastric tube guidewire technique. *J Emerg Med* 14:205, 1996.

73. Bonanno PC: Swallowing dysfunction after tracheostomy. *Ann Surg* 174:29, 1971.

74. Shelly R: The post-insertion protocol for management of the Olympic tracheostomy button in neurosurgical patients. *J Neurosurg Nurs* 13:294, 1981.

75. Betts RH: Posttracheostomy aspiration. *N Engl J Med* 273:155, 1965.

76. Shaker R, Dodds WJ, Dantas EO: Coordination of deglutitive glottic closure with oropharyngeal swallowing. *Gastroenterology* 98:1478, 1990.

77. Buckwater JA, Sasaki CT: Effect of tracheostomy on laryngeal function. *Otolaryngol Clin North Am* 21:701, 1988.

78. Devita MA, Spierer-Rundback MS: Swallowing disorders in patients with prolonged intubation or tracheostomy tubes. *Crit Care Med* 18:1328, 1990.

79. Cameron JL, Reynolds J, Zuidema GD: Aspiration in patients with tracheostomies. *Surg Gynecol Obstet* 136:68, 1973.

80. Bone DK, Davis JL, Zuidema GD, et al: Aspiration pneumonia. *Ann Thorac Surg* 18:30, 1974.

81. Muz J, Mathog RH, Nelson R, et al: Aspiration in patients with head and neck cancer and tracheostomy. *Am J Otolaryngol* 10:282, 1989.

82. Godwin JE, Heffner JE: Special critical care considerations in tracheostomy management. *Clin Chest Med* 12:573, 1991.

83. Tolep K, Getch CL, Criner GJ: Swallowing dysfunction in patients receiving prolonged mechanical ventilation. *Chest* 109:167, 1996.

84. Metheny NA, Clouse RE: Bedside methods for detecting aspiration in tube-fed patients. *Chest* 111:724, 1997.

85. Thompson-Henry S, Braddock B: The modified Evan's blue dye procedure fails to detect aspiration in the tracheostomized patient: five case reports. *Dysphagia* 10:172, 1995.

86. Elpern EH, Scott MG, Petro L, et al: Pulmonary aspiration in mechanically ventilated patients with tracheostomies. *Chest* 105:563, 1994.

87. Muz J, Hamlet S, Mathog R, et al: Scintigraphic assessment of aspiration in head and neck cancer patients with tracheostomy. *Head Neck* 16:17, 1994.
88. Dettelbach MA, Gross RD, Mahlmann J, et al: Effect of the Passy-Muir valve on aspiration in patients with tracheostomy. *Head Neck* 17:297, 1995.
89. Leder SB, Tarro JM, Burell MI: Effect of occlusion of a tracheostomy tube on aspiration. *Dysphagia* 11:254, 1996.
90. Dulguerov P, Gysin C, Perneger TV, et al: Percutaneous or surgical tracheostomy: a meta-analysis. *Crit Care Med* 27:1617, 1999.
91. Massard G, Rouge C, Dabbagh A, et al: Tracheobronchial lacerations after intubation and tracheostomy. *Ann Thorac Surg* 61:1483, 1996.
92. Dunham CM, LaMonica C: Prolonged tracheal intubation in the trauma patient. *J Trauma* 24:120, 1984.
93. Miller JD, Kapp JP: Complications of tracheostomies in neurosurgical patients. *Surg Neurol* 22:186, 1984.
94. Shinkwin CA, Gibbin KP: Tracheostomy in children. *J R Soc Med* 89:188, 1996.
95. Kirchner JA: Avoiding problems in tracheotomy. *Laryngoscope* 96:55, 1986.
96. Kenan PD: Complications associated with tracheotomy: prevention and treatment. *Otolaryngol Clin North Am* 12:807, 1979.
97. Malata CM, Foo IT, Simpson KH, et al: An audit of Bjork flap tracheostomies in head and neck plastic surgery. *Br J Oral Maxillofac Surg* 34:42, 1996.
98. Heffner JE, Miller KS, Sahn SA: Tracheostomy in the intensive care unit, 2: complications. *Chest* 90:430, 1986.
99. Young JS, Brady WJ, Kesser B, et al: A novel method for replacement of the dislodged tracheostomy tube: the nasogastric tube guidewire technique. *J Emerg Med* 14:205, 1996.
100. Muhammad JK, Major E, Wood A, et al: Percutaneous dilatational tracheostomy: hemorrhagic complications and the vascular anatomy of the anterior neck. *Int J Oral Maxillofac Surg* 29:217, 2000.
101. Schaefer OP, Irwin RS: Tracheoarterial fistula: an unusual complication of tracheostomy. *J Intensive Care Med* 10:64, 1995.
102. Mamikunian C: Prevention of delayed hemorrhage after tracheotomy. *Ear Nose Throat J* 67:881, 1988.
103. Oshinsky AE, Rubin JS, Gwozdz CS: The anatomical basis for posttracheotomy innominate artery rupture. *Laryngoscope* 98:1061, 1988.
104. Keceligil HT, Erk MK, Kolbakir F, et al: Tracheoinnominate artery fistula following tracheostomy. *Cardiovasc Surg* 3:509, 1995.
105. Thomas AN: The diagnosis and treatment of tracheoesophageal fistula caused by cuffed tracheal tubes. *J Thorac Cardiovasc Surg* 65:612, 1973.
106. El-Naggar M, Sadogopan S, Levine H, et al: Factors influencing choice between tracheostomy and prolonged translaryngeal intubation in acute respiratory failure: a prospective study. *Anesth Analg* 55:195, 1976.

107. Burns HP, Dayar VS, Scott A, et al: Laryngotracheal trauma: observations on its pathogenesis and its prevention following prolonged orotracheal intubation in the adult. *Laryngoscope* 89:1316, 1979.
108. Bonanno PC: Swallowing dysfunction after tracheotomy. *Ann Surg* 174:29, 1971.
109. DeVita MA, Spierer-Rundback L: Swallowing disorders in patients with prolonged orotracheal intubation or tracheostomy tubes. *Crit Care Med* 18:1328, 1990.
110. Hughes M, Kirchner JA, Branson RJ: A skin-lined tube as a complication of tracheostomy. *Arch Otolaryngol* 94:568, 1971.
111. Mace SE: Cricothyrotomy. *Emerg Med* 6:309, 1988.
112. Esses BA, Jafek BW: Cricothyroidotomy: a decade of experience in Denver. *Ann Otol Rhinol Laryngol* 96:519, 1987.
113. Cole RR, Aguilar EA: Cricothyroidotomy versus tracheotomy: an otolaryngologist's perspective. *Laryngoscope* 98:131, 1988.
114. Brantigan CO, Grow JB: Cricothyroidotomy: elective use in respiratory problems requiring tracheotomy. *J Thorac Cardiovasc Surg* 71:72, 1976.
115. Boyd AD, Romita MC, Conlan AA, et al: A clinical evaluation of cricothyroidotomy. *Surg Gynecol Obstet* 149:365, 1979.
116. Sise MJ, Shacksord SR, Cruickshank JC, et al: Cricothyroidotomy for long term tracheal access. *Ann Surg* 200:13, 1984.
117. O'Connor JV, Reddy K, Ergin MA, et al: Cricothyroidotomy for prolonged ventilatory support after cardiac operations. *Ann Thorac Surg* 39:353, 1985.
118. Lewis GA, Hopkinson RB, Matthews HR: Minitracheotomy: a report of its use in intensive therapy. *Anesthesia* 41:931, 1986.
119. Pierce WS, Tyers FO, Waldhausen JA: Effective isolation of a tracheostomy from a median sternotomy wound. *J Thorac Cardiovasc Surg* 66:841, 1973.
120. Morain WD: Cricothyroidotomy in head and neck surgery. *Plast Reconstr Surg* 65:424, 1980.
121. Kuriloff DB, Setzen M, Portnoy W, et al: Laryngotracheal injury following cricothyroidotomy. *Laryngoscope* 99:125, 1989.
122. Hawkins ML, Shapiro MB, Cue JI, et al: Emergency cricothyrotomy: a reassessment. *Am Surg* 61:52, 1995.
123. Jorden RC, Rosen P: Airway management in the acutely injured, in Moore EE, Eiseman B, Van Way CW (eds): *Critical Decisions in Trauma*. St. Louis, Mosby, 1984, p 30.
124. McGill J, Clinton JE, Ruiz E: Cricothyrotomy in the emergency department. *Ann Emerg Med* 11:361, 1982.
125. Terry RM, Cook P: Hemorrhage during minitracheostomy: reduction of risk by altered incision. *J Laryngol Otol* 103:207, 1989.
126. Cutler BS: Cricothyroidotomy for emergency airway, in Vander Salm TJ, Cutler BS, Wheeler HB (eds): *Atlas of Bedside Procedures*. Boston, Little, Brown, 1988, p 231.
127. Erlandson MJ, Clinton JE, Ruiz E, et al: Cricothyrotomy in the emergency department revisited. *J Emerg Med* 7:115, 1989.
128. Brantigan CO, Grow JB: Subglottic stenosis after cricothyroidotomy. *Surgery* 91:217, 1982.

16. Gastrointestinal Endoscopy

Bernard D. Clifford and Peter E. Krims

Over the past 30 years, continuing improvements in endoscope technology have led to dramatic changes in the practice of gastrointestinal endoscopy in critically ill patients. From the development of the first widely used semiflexible gastroscope popularized by Schindler in the 1940s to the current generation of video endoscope technology, gastrointestinal endoscopy has moved from an esoteric elective diagnostic procedure to routine therapy in intensive care units (ICUs) worldwide [1]. This chapter reviews the indications for, contraindications to, techniques for, and complications of endoscopy in critically ill patients.

Endoscopes

Current fiberoptic gastrointestinal endoscopes are slim, flexible, and capable of viewing more than 90% of the upper gastrointestinal tract (esophagus, stomach, duodenum) and colon. Enteroscopes can visualize portions of the small intestine, and the terminal ileum can be examined with a standard colonoscope [2]. Charged couple device chip technology and video monitors have replaced fiberoptic bundles on newer instruments, allowing digital storage of

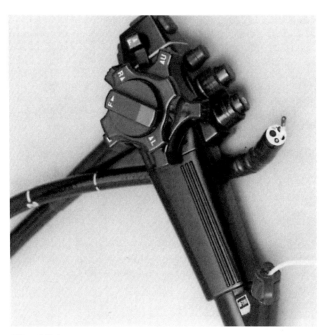

Fig. 16-1. Video upper endoscope. Note the control knobs controlling tip deflection, buttons controlling suction and air and water insufflation, and the tip of the insertion tube with a heater probe catheter protruding through the operating channel.

images for documentation and teaching and improving teamwork during difficult therapeutic procedures. The endoscopes are equipped with a fiberoptic bundle for light delivery; a charged couple device chip (video endoscope) or a fiberoptic bundle (fiberscope) for image delivery; operating channels for suctioning, biopsies, and various therapies; and a separate channel for insufflation of air and water. Wheels and buttons on the handle of the instrument control tip deflection, suction, and air and water insufflation (Fig. 16-1).

Indications

The indications for elective gastrointestinal endoscopy in the ICU are similar to those for other hospitalized patients (Table 16-1); however, it is usually delayed until the patient's cardiopulmonary status has been stabilized. Although cardiopulmonary complications of gastrointestinal endoscopy are infrequent, it should be performed only when the likely benefits clearly outweigh the risks. Gastrointestinal endoscopy in patients with clinically insignificant bleeding or minimally troublesome gastrointestinal complaints should be postponed

Table 16-1. Indications for Gastrointestinal (GI) Endoscopy

Upper GI endoscopy
  GI bleeding
  Caustic ingestion
  Foreign body ingestion
Endoscopic retrograde cholangiopancreatography
  Severe gallstone pancreatitis with cholangitis or jaundice
  Severe cholangitis
Lower GI endoscopy
  GI bleeding
  Acute adynamic ileus

until their medical-surgical illnesses improve. Endoscopy is sometimes indicated in patients with occult blood loss, when anticoagulation or thrombolytic therapy is contemplated. Generally, it should be performed only when the results will alter plans for therapy.

Some authors distinguish between indications for diagnostic and therapeutic endoscopic procedures. However, it cannot always be predicted when therapy may be needed during a procedure that is anticipated to be diagnostic. Therefore, all endoscopists who perform gastrointestinal procedures should be competent in endoscopic therapy. This recommendation is bolstered by randomized trials in upper gastrointestinal bleeding showing that patient outcome is improved only if endoscopic therapy is provided [3,4].

UPPER GASTROINTESTINAL ENDOSCOPY. The indications for upper gastrointestinal endoscopy in ICU patients, listed in Table 16-1, include upper gastrointestinal bleeding, caustic ingestion, and foreign body ingestion. In patients with upper gastrointestinal bleeding, those with severe or recurrent bleeding and significant underlying cardiopulmonary disease have the highest morbidity and mortality and may benefit the most from therapeutic endoscopy directed toward hemostasis [5,6]. Therefore, patients with upper gastrointestinal bleeding, evidence of hemodynamic instability, and a continuing need for transfusions should undergo urgent upper endoscopy with plans for appropriate endoscopic therapy (see below).

Endoscopic placement of gastrostomy feeding tubes is increasingly used in ICUs for enteral nutrition. Percutaneous endoscopic gastrostomy (PEG) tubes can be inserted at the bedside under intravenous and local sedation (see Chapter 25). During PEG placement, small-bore jejunal tubes can be advanced endoscopically through the PEG tube into the small intestine to provide postpyloric feeding and minimize the risk of aspiration of gastric contents. PEG tubes are less easily dislodged than nasogastric tubes and are usually better tolerated. Severe, life-threatening complications are rarely associated with PEG placement [7].

ENDOSCOPIC RETROGRADE CHOLANGIOPANCREATOGRAPHY. Endoscopic retrograde cholangiopancreatography (ERCP) is used only occasionally in the ICU and is therefore discussed only briefly here. It is indicated in ICU patients with cholangitis that is unresponsive to medical therapy and with acute gallstone pancreatitis complicated by cholangitis or jaundice (Table 16-1). A number of retrospective and prospective controlled trials have shown that ERCP combined with sphincterotomy and stone extraction reduces complications in patients with cholangitis. In acute gallstone pancreatitis, early ERCP may be beneficial in selected patients, but it carries with it the risks of bleeding, perforation, and worsening pancreatitis [8–10]. Emergent ERCP can be performed safely on the day of admission to the ICU when appropriate.

LOWER GASTROINTESTINAL ENDOSCOPY. Lower gastrointestinal endoscopy can be performed for acute lower gastrointestinal bleeding (Table 16-1), but it is technically difficult in the setting of active bleeding, and the diagnostic accuracy may therefore be lower. Colonoscopy appears to have the highest yield in diagnosing and sometimes treating lower gastrointestinal bleeding. It is safe when appropriate resuscitation has been performed. Technetium-labeled erythrocyte scanning or angiography, or both, are other methods that are commonly used for localizing a bleeding site [11,12].

Table 16-2. Contraindications to Endoscopy

Suspected/impending perforated viscus
Severe diverticulitis or severe inflammatory bowel disease
Refractory hypotension or hypoxemia (unstable patient)
Uncooperative patient
Unprotected airway in a confused or stuporous patient with acute
   upper gastrointestinal bleeding

Endoscopic colonic decompression has been advised in critically ill patients with acute adynamic ileus. Anecdotal reports and small uncontrolled series suggest that when the diameter of the right colon exceeds 12 cm, perforation is imminent and decompression is necessary. Other studies suggest that the colonic dilation may not progress to life-threatening complications and that decompression is unnecessary [13–16].

Contraindications

Table 16-2 lists contraindications to endoscopy. In general, endoscopy (and the associated air insufflation) should be avoided in patients with known or suspected gastrointestinal perforation and those known to be at high risk for perforation. Hemodynamic instability is a relative contraindication for endoscopy, but the benefits of therapeutic endoscopy may outweigh the risks in some critically ill patients. For example, patients with severe cholangitis are likely to benefit from therapeutic ERCP even in the presence of refractory hypotension or hypoxemia. The risk of a bleeding complication from endoscopic sphincterotomy is higher in patients with a coagulopathy or thrombocytopenia, and ERCP may be delayed while the underlying condition is corrected. Patients who are unable to cooperate should have endoscopy delayed; otherwise, endotracheal intubation and heavy sedation or general anesthesia may be necessary to facilitate the procedure. Finally, patients with acute upper gastrointestinal bleeding who are confused or stuporous should have their airway protected with an endotracheal tube before endoscopy. This is especially applicable to patients with variceal hemorrhage.

Complications

The principal risks of any endoscopic procedure are bleeding and perforation. These and other complications are outlined in Table 16-3. Bleeding can occur after biopsy, polypectomy, endoscopic sphincterotomy, and therapeutic treatment of bleeding sites (varices, ulcers, arteriovenous malformations). Most bleeding is minimal and self-limited, but repeat endoscopy and surgery may be necessary to control recurrent bleeding. Angiography can assist in localizing the bleeding source in postendoscopy bleeding.

Perforation of the lumen may result from direct pressure of the endoscope, catheters, or guidewires on the wall. In

Table 16-3. Complications of Endoscopy

Bleeding
Perforation of the gastrointestinal tract lumen by endoscope, catheters, or guidewires
Aspiration
Reaction to sedative medication

the setting of severe infectious or inflammatory colitis, simple air insufflation or instrumentation can cause rupture of the intestinal lumen. Broad-spectrum antibiotics and intravenous fluids should be given, and surgery may be required. If duodenal perforation is encountered after endoscopic sphincterotomy, early medical therapy and stabilization of the patient may preclude the need for surgery [17]. Aspiration of stomach contents and blood in upper gastrointestinal bleeding can be minimized by protecting the airway with endotracheal intubation in patients with severe bleeding or altered mental states. A history of medication allergies and reactions should be obtained before sedative drugs are administered. Sedative medications have their own complications, usually cardiopulmonary, as a consequence of medication-induced hypoxemia (2 to 5 per 1,000 cases). Other complications can occur, including apnea, hypotension, and, rarely, death (0.3 to 0.5 per 1,000 cases) [18]. Patients with a history of alcohol abuse can have paradoxic reactions to benzodiazepine medications; caution should be used in sedating these patients. In our experience, sedation with relatively high-dose narcotics has been successful in patients who abuse alcohol.

Techniques

UPPER GASTROINTESTINAL ENDOSCOPY. Proper patient preparation is crucial for a safe and complete endoscopic examination. The patient (or legal representative) should understand the nature, indications, and complications of the procedure. Fluid resuscitation and optimal treatment of hypoxemia should precede all endoscopic examinations. Obtunded patients with gastrointestinal bleeding should be intubated to prevent aspiration, and intubation should be considered in nonobtunded patients with severe bleeding and those undergoing foreign body removal. Nasogastric or orogastric lavage with a large-bore tube (greater than 40 French) should be performed to evacuate blood and clots from the stomach before endoscopy in acute gastrointestinal bleeding.

Proper patient selection optimizes outcome and minimizes risk. Upper gastrointestinal bleeding is the commonest condition for upper endoscopy in the ICU. Patients with continued or recurrent upper gastrointestinal bleeding as seen by red blood in the nasogastric aspirate should have urgent upper endoscopy as early as possible, usually within 6 to 8 hours after presentation. In patients with massive hemorrhage, endoscopy can be performed in the operating room in anticipation of surgical therapy.

A team approach is required to perform endoscopy in critically ill patients. The team consists of an experienced endoscopist, a specially trained endoscopy technician, and a nurse skilled in monitoring patients undergoing endoscopy. For complex procedures, the nurse is situated at the patient's head, ensuring airway patency and administering intravenous sedation as needed, and the technician provides assistance to the endoscopist. The procedure is generally performed under intravenous (conscious) sedation. A topical anesthetic is applied to the pharynx to reduce the gag reflex. Intravenous benzodiazepines (diazepam, midazolam) with or without narcotics (meperidine, fentanyl) are commonly used. We prefer midazolam and fentanyl because of their amnestic effect and short half-life, respectively. For longer procedures, the use of droperidol may augment the effects of the benzodiazepine/narcotic combination. Proper patient monitoring is needed, with frequent (every 5 minutes) blood pressure measurement and continuous heart rate and oxygen saturation by pulse oximetry. Supplemental oxygen by nasal prongs is generally administered to minimize the risk of hypoxemia.

Endoscopy is performed with a "therapeutic" instrument equipped with a large operating channel to allow suctioning of blood and hemostatic therapy. The endoscope is passed into the patient's mouth to the posterior pharynx under direct visualization. Gentle pressure on the upper esophageal sphincter allows passage of the instrument into the esophagus. If the patient is awake, voluntary swallow may facilitate passage of the endoscope into the esophagus. The upper gastrointestinal tract is rapidly surveyed to locate the site of bleeding. If an active bleeding site is found, hemostatic therapy can be attempted immediately. Frequently, a large clot remains in the fundus or the body of the stomach, obscuring the mucosa in this area. If the examination is otherwise negative, moving or removing the clot should be attempted. In patients with significant recent bleeding and endoscopic evidence of recent hemorrhage (a visible vessel or adherent clot on an ulcer), hemostatic therapy to prevent rebleeding should be strongly considered [19].

HEMOSTATIC THERAPY IN UPPER GASTROINTESTINAL ENDOSCOPY.
Actively bleeding lesions in the upper gastrointestinal tract can be effectively treated with laser photocoagulation, heater probe therapy, mono- and bipolar electrocoagulation (bicap), or injection therapy. Laser photocoagulation is cumbersome and expensive and rarely used. Injection sclerotherapy is simple and inexpensive, requiring only a needle catheter and a liquid medium. Medications that are often used include absolute ethanol, epinephrine (a vasoconstrictor), and sodium morrhuate (a sclerosant). Injection therapy alone may be less effective in briskly bleeding ulcers and can be combined with cauterization. Treatment of bleeding esophageal varices by applying small rubber bands with or without injection sclerotherapy appears more effective than injection sclerotherapy alone. Fewer treatment sessions and complications, less rebleeding, and decreased mortality are benefits of esophageal variceal ligation [20–24].

The precise method of hemostasis of bleeding lesions of the gastrointestinal tract varies depending on the hemostatic method used. Heater probe, bipolar electrocautery probe, and injection therapy are widely available and commonly used for treatment of ulcers or vascular lesions. Heater probes generate heat using electrical current delivered to the tip of the catheter, whereas bipolar electrocautery delivers electrical current directly to the tissue, causing coagulation necrosis. Both techniques work best using the stiff catheter to compress the bleeding site directly and provide energy (heat or electrical current) to "weld" the vessel shut. Because therapy with heater probe or bicap equipment requires an *en face* view, lesions seen tangentially may be difficult to treat with these methods. Injection therapy allows treatment of such lesions and can be combined with probe therapy. Injection therapy for ulcers generally begins on the periphery of the lesion with an injection in all four quadrants, with injection of the vessel or clot as needed to complete hemostasis.

For therapy of bleeding esophageal varices with esophageal variceal ligation, initial assessment of the bleeding source with the endoscope is performed. The number of varices, location of the bleeding site, and severity or grade of the varices are noted. The endoscope is removed from the patient, and an adapter that allows placement of multiple bands is attached to the endoscope. Because the banding adapter limits the field of view, the initial survey is important. Next, the endoscope is reinserted, and the varices are banded to effect hemostasis or obliteration. Variceal sclerotherapy involves the injection of 1 to 4 mL sclerosant directly into or next to the varix. This technique can be used when banding is unavailable or in combination with banding at the initial bleeding episode or for subsequent treatment.

LOWER GASTROINTESTINAL ENDOSCOPY.
Lower gastrointestinal endoscopy, which is technically difficult at times in well-prepared, healthy outpatients, can be extremely challenging in critically ill patients with colonic hemorrhage. Also, the colon tends to act as a reservoir for blood, making even identification of the relative source for hemorrhage (left vs. right colon), which is most useful to the surgeon, almost impossible unless the colon has been well prepared.

Instruments that are available for examination of the lower gastrointestinal tract include the anoscope, sigmoidoscopes (rigid and flexible), and the colonoscope. Anoscopes can be used to evaluate for sources of anorectal bleeding such as fissures or hemorrhoids. Rigid sigmoidoscopes are rarely used outside of operating rooms due to the discomfort associated with their use. Flexible sigmoidoscopes can be easily inserted to 65 cm without sedation in most patients. Colonoscopes of 140 to 180 cm in length are used to examine beyond the splenic flexure.

Patient preparation for colonoscopy is more intensive than for upper gastrointestinal endoscopy. Usually, a gallon of nonabsorbed polyethylene glycol is given by mouth or nasogastric tube 4 to 12 hours before the examination. Magnesium citrate can be used over 24 to 48 hours in patients who have been taking clear liquids. Any oral iron preparations should be discontinued several days before the examination. The examination is similar to that of upper gastrointestinal endoscopy with respect to support staff, sedation, and monitoring of the patient (see above). Abdominal pressure applied by an assistant during colonoscopy may help in advancing the colonoscope.

Colonoscopy has been reported as therapy for pseudoobstruction [13–16]. Decompression by colonoscopy should not be first-line therapy for pseudoobstruction. Nasogastric and rectal tube placement, discontinuation of offending medications (narcotics and phenothiazines), treatment of underlying illness, and frequent repositioning (every 2 hours) of debilitated ICU patients often allow resolution of pseudoobstruction.

References

1. Hirschowitz BI: Development and application of endoscopy. *Gastroenterology* 104:337, 1993.
2. Wayne JD: Small-intestinal endoscopy. *Endoscopy* 33:24, 2001.
3. Peterson WL, Barnett CC, Smith HJ, et al: Routine early endoscopy in upper gastrointestinal tract bleeding. *N Engl J Med* 304:925, 1981.
4. Laine L: Multipolar electrocoagulation in the treatment of active upper gastrointestinal tract hemorrhage: a prospective controlled trial. *N Engl J Med* 316:1613, 1987.
5. NIH Consensus Conference: Therapeutic endoscopy and bleeding ulcers. *JAMA* 262:1369, 1989.
6. Savides TJ, Jensen DM: Therapeutic endoscopy for nonvariceal gastrointestinal bleeding. *Gastroenterol Clin North Am* 29:465, 2000.
7. Safidi BY, Marks JM, Ponsky JL: Percutaneous endoscopic gastrostomy: an update. *Endoscopy* 30:781, 1998.

8. Folsch UR, Nitsche R, Ludtke R, et al: Early ERCP and papillotomy compared with conservative treatment for acute biliary pancreatitis. *N Engl J Med* 336:237, 1997.

9. Sharma VK, Howden CW: Metaanalysis of randomized controlled trials of endoscopic retrograde cholangiography and endoscopic sphincterotomy for the treatment of acute biliary pancreatitis. *Am J Gastroenterol* 94:3211, 1999.

10. Soetikino RM, Carr-Locke DL: Endoscopic management of acute gallstone pancreatitis. *Gastrointest Endosc Clin North Am* 8:1, 1998.

11. Richter JM, Christensen MR, Kaplan LM, et al: Effectiveness of current technology in the diagnosis and management of lower gastrointestinal hemorrhage. *Gastrointest Endosc* 41:93, 1995.

12. Jensen DM: Current management of severe lower gastrointestinal bleeding. *Gastrointest Endosc* 41:171, 1995.

13. Dorudi S, Berry AR, Kerrelewell MGW: Acute colonic pseudoobstruction. *Br J Surg* 79:99, 1992.

14. Sloyer AF, Panella VS, Demas BE, et al: Olgivie's syndrome: successful management without colonoscopy. *Dig Dis Sci* 33:1391, 1988.

15. Harig JM, Fumo DE, Loo FD, et al: Treatment of acute nontoxic megacolon during colonoscopy: tube placement versus simple decompression. *Gastrointest Endosc* 34:23, 1988.

16. Burke G, Shellito PC: Treatment of recurrent colonic pseudoobstruction by endoscopic placement of a fenestrated overtube. *Dis Colon Rectum* 30:615, 1987.

17. Chung RS, Sviak MV, Ferguson DR: Surgical decisions in the management of duodenal perforation complicating endoscopic sphincterotomy. *Am J Surg* 165:700, 1993.

18. Benjamin SB: Complications of conscious sedation. *Gastrointest Endosc Clin North Am* 6:277, 1996.

19. Laine L: Refining the prognostic value of endoscopy in patients presenting with bleeding ulcers. *Gastrointest Endosc* 39:461, 1993.

20. Lin H, Perng C, Lee F, et al: Endoscopic injection for the arrest of peptic ulcer hemorrhage: final results of a prospective, randomized, comparative trial. *Gastrointest Endosc* 39:15, 1993.

21. Steigmann GV, Goff JS, Michaletz-Onody PA, et al. Endoscopic sclerotherapy as compared with endoscopic ligation for bleeding esophageal varices. *N Engl J Med* 326:1527, 1992.

22. Laine L, Cook C: Endoscopic ligation compared with sclerotherapy for treatment of esophageal variceal bleeding. A meta-analysis. *Ann Intern Med* 123:280, 1995.

23. Woods KL, Qureshi WA: Long-term management of variceal bleeding. *Gastrointest Endosc Clin North Am* 9:253, 1999.

24. Saltzman JR, Aurora S: Complications of esophageal variceal band ligation. *Gastrointest Endosc* 39:185, 1993.

17. Paracentesis and Diagnostic Peritoneal Lavage

Lena M. Napolitano

Abdominal Paracentesis

INDICATIONS. Abdominal paracentesis is a simple procedure that can be easily performed at the bedside in the intensive care unit and may provide important diagnostic information or therapy in critically ill patients with ascites. Diagnostic abdominal paracentesis is usually performed to determine the exact etiology of the accumulated ascites or to ascertain whether infection is present, as in spontaneous bacterial peritonitis. It can also be used in any clinical situation in which the analysis of a sample of peritoneal fluid might be useful in ascertaining a diagnosis and guiding therapy [1]. The evaluation of ascites should therefore include a diagnostic paracentesis with ascitic fluid analysis.

As a therapeutic intervention, abdominal paracentesis is usually performed to drain large volumes of abdominal ascites [2]. Ascites is the most common presentation of decompensated cirrhosis, and its development heralds a poor prognosis, with a 50% 2-year survival rate. Effective first-line therapy for ascites includes sodium restriction (2 g per day), use of diuretics, and large-volume paracentesis. Ideally, a combination of a loop diuretic and aldosterone antagonist is used. When tense or refractory ascites is present, large-volume paracentesis is safe and effective and has the advantage of producing immediate relief from ascites and its associated symptoms [3]. Paracentesis has also recently been used to manage the development of acute tense ascites resulting in abdominal compartment syndrome in critically ill patients. Therapeutic abdominal paracentesis can be palliative by diminishing abdominal pain from abdominal distention or improving pulmonary function by allowing better diaphragmatic excursion in patients who have ascites refractory to aggressive medical management. One study documented that large-volume paracentesis decreases esophageal variceal pressure, size, and wall tension in cirrhotics and may be an effective adjunct in the treatment of esophageal variceal bleeding [4] (see Chapter 93). Transjugular intrahepatic portocaval shunt (TIPS) has emerged as the treatment of choice for selected patients with refractory ascites, although serial large-volume paracenteses should be attempted first [5,6]. A randomized prospective trial compared large-volume paracentesis and TIPS in 60 patients with cirrhosis and refractory ascites, and multivariate analysis confirmed that TIPS was independently associated with survival without the need for transplantation (p = .02), with a mean follow-up of 45 months [7]. At 3 months, 61% of the TIPS patients had no ascites, compared to 18% of the paracentesis group (p = .006). TIPS, however, may hasten death in those with advanced liver failure.

TECHNIQUES. Before abdominal paracentesis is initiated, a catheter must be inserted to drain the urinary bladder, and any underlying coagulopathy or thrombocytopenia should be corrected. The patient must be positioned correctly. If he or she is critically ill, the procedure is performed in the supine position. If the patient is clinically stable and abdominal paracentesis is being performed for therapeutic volume removal of ascites, the patient can be placed in the sitting position, leaning slightly forward, to increase the total volume of ascites removed.

The site for paracentesis on the anterior abdominal wall is then chosen (Fig. 17-1). The preferred site is in the lower

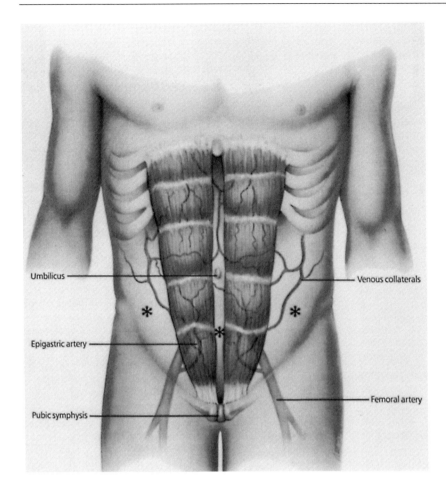

Fig. 17-1. Suggested sites for paracentesis.

Labels on figure: Umbilicus, Venous collaterals, Epigastric artery, Femoral artery, Pubic symphysis

abdomen, just lateral to the rectus abdominis muscle and infe-rior to the umbilicus. It is important to stay lateral to the rectus abdominis muscle to avoid injury to the inferior epigastric artery and vein. In patients with chronic cirrhosis and caput medusae (engorged anterior abdominal wall veins), these vis-ible vascular structures must be avoided. Injury to these veins can cause significant bleeding because of underlying portal hypertension and may result in hemoperitoneum. The left lower quadrant of the abdominal wall is preferred over the right lower quadrant for abdominal paracentesis because crit-ically ill patients often have cecal distention. The ideal site is therefore in the left lower quadrant of the abdomen, lateral to the rectus abdominis muscle in the midclavicular line and inferior to the umbilicus. If the patient had previous abdomi-nal surgery limited to the lower abdomen, it may be difficult to perform a paracentesis in the lower abdomen, and the upper abdomen may be chosen. The point of entry, however, remains lateral to the rectus abdominis muscle in the midclav-icular line. If there is concern that the ascites is loculated because of previous abdominal surgery or peritonitis, abdom-inal paracentesis should be performed under ultrasound guid-ance to prevent iatrogenic complications.

Abdominal paracentesis can be performed by the needle technique, the catheter technique, or with ultrasound guid-ance. Diagnostic paracentesis usually requires 20 to 50 mL peritoneal fluid and is commonly performed using the needle technique. However, if large volumes of peritoneal fluid are required (i.e., for cytologic examination), the catheter tech-nique is used because it is associated with a lower incidence of complications. Therapeutic paracentesis, as in the removal of large volumes of ascites, should always be performed with the catheter technique. Ultrasound guidance can be helpful in

diagnostic paracentesis using the needle technique or in ther-apeutic paracentesis with large volume removal using the catheter technique.

Needle Technique. With the patient in the appropriate posi-tion and the access site for paracentesis determined, the patient's abdomen is prepared with 10% povidone-iodine solu-tion and sterilely draped. If necessary, intravenous sedation is administered to prevent the patient from moving excessively during the procedure (see Chapter 25). Local anesthesia, using 1% or 2% lidocaine with 1 to 200,000 epinephrine, is infiltrated into the site. A skin wheal is created with the local anesthetic, using a short 25- or 27-gauge needle. Then, using a 22-gauge, 1.5-in. needle, the local anesthetic is infiltrated into the subcuta-neous tissues and anterior abdominal wall, with the needle per-pendicular to the skin. Before the anterior abdominal wall and peritoneum are infiltrated, the skin is pulled taut inferiorly, allowing the peritoneal cavity to be entered at a different loca-tion than the skin entrance site, thereby decreasing the chance of ascitic leak. This is known as the *Z-track technique*. While tension is maintained inferiorly on the abdominal skin, the nee-dle is advanced through the abdominal wall fascia and perito-neum, and local anesthetic is injected. Intermittent aspiration identifies when the peritoneal cavity is entered, with return of ascitic fluid into the syringe. The needle is held securely in this position with the left hand, and the right hand is used to with-draw approximately 20 to 50 mL ascitic fluid into the syringe for a diagnostic paracentesis.

Once adequate fluid is withdrawn, the needle and syringe are withdrawn from the anterior abdominal wall and the para-centesis site is covered with a sterile dressing. The needle is removed from the syringe, because it may be contaminated with skin organisms. A small amount of peritoneal fluid is sent in a sterile container for Gram's stain and culture and sensitivity testing. The remainder of the fluid is sent for appropriate studies, which may include cytology, cell count and differential, protein, specific gravity, amylase, pH, lactate dehydrogenase, bilirubin, triglycerides, and albumin. A serum to ascites albumin gradient greater than 1.1 g per dL is indicative of portal hypertension and cirrhosis [8,9]. Peritoneal fluid can be sent for smear and culture for acid-fast bacilli if tuberculous peritonitis is in the differential diagnosis.

Catheter Technique. The patient is placed in the proper position, and the anterior abdominal wall site for paracentesis is prepared and draped in the usual sterile fashion. Aseptic technique is used throughout the procedure. The site is anesthetized with local anesthetic as described for the needle technique. A 22-gauge, 1.5-in. needle attached to a 10-mL syringe is used to document the free return of peritoneal fluid into the syringe at the chosen site. This needle is removed from the peritoneal cavity and a catheter-over-needle assembly is used to gain access to the peritoneal cavity. If the anterior abdominal wall is thin, an 18- or 20-gauge angiocath can be used as the catheter-over-needle assembly. If the anterior abdominal wall is quite thick, as in obese patients, it may be necessary to use a long (5.25-in.) catheter-over-needle assembly (18- or 20-gauge) or a percutaneous single-lumen central venous catheter (18- or 20-gauge) and gain access to the peritoneal cavity using the Seldinger technique.

The peritoneal cavity is entered as for the needle technique. The catheter-over-needle assembly is inserted perpendicular to the anterior abdominal wall using the Z-track technique; once peritoneal fluid returns into the syringe barrel, the catheter is advanced over the needle, the needle is removed, and a 20- or 50-mL syringe is connected to the catheter. The tip of the catheter is now in the peritoneal cavity and can be left in place until the appropriate amount of peritoneal fluid is removed. This technique, rather than the needle technique, should be used when large volumes of peritoneal fluid must be removed, because complications (e.g., intestinal perforation) may occur if a needle is left in the peritoneal space for an extended period.

When the Seldinger technique is used in patients with a large anterior abdominal wall, access to the peritoneal cavity is initially gained with a needle or catheter-over-needle assembly. A guidewire is then inserted through the needle and an 18- or 20-gauge single-lumen central venous catheter threaded over the guidewire. It is very important to use the Z-track method for the catheter technique to prevent development of an ascitic leak, which may be difficult to control and may predispose the patient to peritoneal infection.

Ultrasound Guidance Technique. Patients who have had previous abdominal surgery or peritonitis are predisposed to abdominal adhesions, and it may be quite difficult to gain free access into the peritoneal cavity for diagnostic or therapeutic paracentesis. Ultrasound-guided paracentesis can be very helpful in this population by providing accurate localization of the peritoneal fluid collection and determining the best abdominal access site. This procedure can be performed using the needle or catheter technique as described above, depending on the volume of peritoneal fluid to be drained. Once the fluid collection is localized by the ultrasound probe, the abdomen is prepared and draped in the usual sterile fashion. A sterile sleeve can be placed over the ultrasound probe so that there is direct ultrasound visualization of the needle or catheter as it enters the peritoneal cavity. The needle or catheter is thus directed to the area to be drained, and the appropriate amount of peritoneal or ascitic fluid is removed. If continued drainage of a loculated peritoneal fluid collection is desired, the radiologist can place a chronic indwelling peritoneal catheter using a percutaneous guidewire technique (see Chapter 28).

The use of ultrasound guidance for drainage of loculated peritoneal fluid collections has markedly decreased the incidence of iatrogenic complications related to abdominal paracentesis. If the radiologist does not identify loculated ascites on the initial ultrasound evaluation and documents a large amount of peritoneal fluid that is free in the abdominal cavity, he or she can then indicate the best access site by marking the anterior abdominal wall with an indelible marker. The paracentesis can then be performed by the clinician and repeated whenever necessary. This study can be performed at the bedside in the intensive care unit with a portable ultrasound unit.

COMPLICATIONS. The most common complications related to abdominal paracentesis are bleeding and persistent ascitic leak. Because most patients in whom ascites have developed also have some component of chronic liver disease with associated coagulopathies, it is very important to correct any underlying coagulopathy before proceeding with abdominal paracentesis. In addition, it is very important to select an avascular access site on the anterior abdominal wall. The Z-track technique is very helpful in minimizing persistent ascitic leak and should always be used. Another complication associated with abdominal paracentesis is intestinal or urinary bladder perforation, with associated peritonitis and infection. Intestinal injury is more common when the needle technique is used. Because the needle is free in the peritoneal cavity, iatrogenic intestinal perforation may occur if the patient moves or if intraabdominal pressure increases with Valsalva maneuver or coughing. Urinary bladder injury is less common and underscores the importance of draining the urinary bladder with a catheter before the procedure. This injury is more common when the abdominal access site is in the suprapubic location; therefore, this access site is not recommended. Careful adherence to proper technique of paracentesis minimizes associated complications.

In patients who have large-volume chronic abdominal ascites, such as that secondary to hepatic cirrhosis or ovarian carcinoma, transient hypotension and a circulatory dysfunction syndrome may develop when a considerable amount of ascitic fluid is removed during therapeutic abdominal paracentesis. A significant inverse correlation between changes in plasma renin activity and systemic vascular resistance has been demonstrated in those patients following paracentesis, suggesting that peripheral arterial vasodilation may be responsible for this circulatory dysfunction. A study has documented that early hemodynamic changes after paracentesis are avoided if intraabdominal pressure is maintained at its original level with a pneumatic girdle [10]. It is very important to obtain reliable peripheral or central venous access in these patients so that fluid resuscitation can be performed if transient hypotension develops during the procedure. Wang et al. [11] reported a 31% (13 of 42 patients) incidence of severe hypotension in posthepatitic cirrhotic patients with massive ascites who underwent large-volume paracentesis (4.8 to 15.5 L). This study determined two factors (withdrawn ascitic fluid greater than 7.5 L and the absence of peripheral edema) that reached statistical significance to predict the occurrence of severe clinical hypotension. More recently, Peltekian et al. [12] documented that a single large-volume (5 L) paracentesis without albumin replacement caused no disturbance in systemic or renal hemodynamics in 12 patients with biopsy-proven cirrhosis and tense, diuretic-resistant ascites.

Large-volume ascites removal in such patients is only transiently therapeutic; the underlying chronic disease induces reaccumulation of the ascites. Percutaneous placement of a tunneled catheter is a viable and safe technique to consider in patients who have symptomatic malignant ascites that require frequent therapeutic paracentesis for relief of symptoms [13,14]. A novel technique developed for treatment of resistant ascites in patients with cirrhosis is the saphenous-peritoneal anastomosis as a peritoneal-venous shunt [15]. It requires further investigation as a durable option in the chronic management of ascites.

Diagnostic Peritoneal Lavage

Before the introduction of diagnostic peritoneal lavage (DPL) by Root et al. in 1965 [16], nonoperative evaluation of the injured abdomen was limited to standard four-quadrant abdominal paracentesis. Abdominal paracentesis for evaluation of hemoperitoneum was associated with a high false-negative rate. This clinical suspicion was confirmed by Giacobine and Siler [17] in an experimental animal model of hemoperitoneum documenting that a 500-mL blood volume in the peritoneal cavity yielded a positive paracentesis rate of only 78%. The initial study by Root et al. [16] reported 100% accuracy in identification of hemoperitoneum using 1 L peritoneal lavage fluid. Many subsequent clinical studies confirmed these findings, with the largest series reported by Fischer et al. in 1978 [18]. They reviewed 2,586 cases of DPL and reported a false-positive rate of 0.2%, false-negative rate of 1.2%, and overall accuracy of 98.5%. Since its introduction in 1965, DPL has become a cornerstone in the evaluation of blunt and penetrating abdominal injuries. However, it is nonspecific for determination of type or extent of organ injury. Recent advances have led to the use of ultrasound and rapid helical computed tomography in the emergent evaluation of abdominal trauma [19–21] and have significantly decreased the use of DPL in the evaluation of abdominal trauma [22].

INDICATIONS. The primary indication for DPL is evaluation of blunt abdominal trauma in patients with associated hypotension or altered level of consciousness. Altered neurologic status in trauma patients may be secondary to drug or alcohol ingestion or due to traumatic brain injury. Such findings make abdominal physical examination unreliable, necessitating definitive evaluation for traumatic abdominal injury. If the patient is hemodynamically stable and can be transported safely, computed tomographic scan of the abdomen and pelvis is the diagnostic method of choice. If the patient is hemodynamically unstable or requires emergent surgical intervention for a craniotomy, thoracotomy, or vascular procedure, it is imperative to determine whether there is a coexisting intraperitoneal source of hemorrhage to prioritize treatment of life-threatening injuries. DPL is therefore used to diagnose the extent of abdominal trauma in patients with multisystem injury or those who require general anesthesia for treatment of associated traumatic injuries. Patients with associated thoracic or pelvic injuries should also have definitive evaluation for abdominal trauma, and DPL can be used in these individuals.

DPL can be used to evaluate penetrating abdominal trauma [23,24]. Thal [25,26] evaluated the utility of DPL in patients with stab wounds to the lower thorax and abdomen. DPL had a false-positive rate of 2.4% and a false-negative rate of 4.9%, defining a positive lavage as a red blood cell count greater than 100,000 cells per mm³ of lavage fluid. Boyle et al. [27] recommend DPL as the initial diagnostic study in stable patients with penetrating trauma to the back and flank, defining a red blood cell count greater than 1,000 mm³ as a positive test. Implemen-

tation of this protocol decreased the total celiotomy rate from 100% to 24%, and the therapeutic celiotomy rate increased from 15% to 80%. DPL has also been evaluated as a tool for determining intraabdominal injury in patients with gunshot wounds to the lower thorax and abdomen. These clinical studies [24,28] documented high false-positive and false-negative rates; therefore, DPL is not recommended in patients with gunshot wounds to the thorax or abdomen, and mandatory exploratory laparotomy or thoracotomy is indicated.

DPL may prove useful in evaluation for possible peritonitis or ruptured viscus in patients with an altered level of consciousness but no evidence of traumatic injury. DPL can be considered in critically ill patients with sepsis to determine whether intraabdominal infection is the underlying source. When DPL is used to evaluate intraabdominal infection, a white blood cell count greater than 500 cells per mm³ of lavage fluid is considered positive. DPL can also serve a therapeutic role. It is very effective in rewarming patients with significant hypothermia. It may potentially be used therapeutically in pancreatitis, fecal peritonitis, and bile pancreatitis, but multiple clinical studies have not documented its efficacy in these cases.

DPL should not be performed in patients with clear signs of significant abdominal trauma and hemoperitoneum associated with hemodynamic instability. These patients should be transported to the operating room immediately and undergo emergent celiotomy. Pregnancy is a relative contraindication to DPL; it may be technically difficult to perform because of the gravid uterus and is associated with a higher risk of complications. Bedside ultrasound evaluation of the abdomen in the pregnant trauma patient is associated with least risk to woman and to fetus. An additional relative contraindication to DPL is multiple previous abdominal surgeries. These patients commonly have multiple abdominal adhesions, and it may be very difficult to gain access to the free peritoneal cavity. If DPL is indicated, it must be performed by the open technique to prevent iatrogenic complications such as intestinal injury.

TECHNIQUES. Three techniques can be used to perform DPL: the closed percutaneous technique, the semiclosed technique, and the open technique. The closed percutaneous technique, introduced by Lazarus and Nelson in 1979 [29], is easy to perform, can be done rapidly, is associated with a low complication rate, and is as accurate as the open technique. It should not be used in patients who have had previous abdominal surgery or a history of abdominal adhesions. The open technique entails the placement of the peritoneal lavage catheter into the peritoneal cavity under direct visualization. It is more time consuming than the closed percutaneous technique. The semiclosed technique requires a smaller incision than the open technique and uses a peritoneal lavage catheter with a metal stylet to gain entrance into the peritoneal cavity. It has become less popular as clinicians have become more familiar and skilled with the Lazarus-Nelson closed technique.

The patient must be placed in the supine position for all three techniques. A catheter is placed into the urinary bladder, and a nasogastric tube is inserted into the stomach to prevent iatrogenic bladder or gastric injury. The nasogastric tube is placed on continuous suction for gastric decompression. The skin of the anterior abdominal wall is prepared with 10% povidone-iodine solution and sterilely draped, leaving the periumbilical area exposed. Standard aseptic technique is used throughout the procedure. Local anesthesia with 1% or 2% lidocaine with 1 to 200,000 epinephrine is used as necessary throughout the procedure. The infraumbilical site is used unless there is clinical concern of possible pelvic fracture and retroperitoneal or pelvic hematoma, in which case the supraumbilical site is optimal.

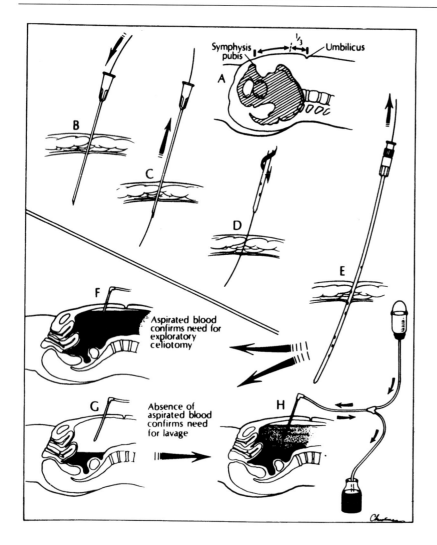

Fig. 17-2. The closed percutaneous technique for diagnostic peritoneal lavage, using a Seldinger guidewire method.

Closed Percutaneous Technique. With the closed percutaneous technique (Fig. 17-2), local anesthesia is infiltrated inferior to the umbilicus and a 5-mm skin incision is made just at the inferior umbilical edge. An 18-gauge needle is inserted through this incision and into the peritoneal cavity, angled toward the pelvis at approximately a 45-degree angle with the skin. The penetration through the linea alba and then through the peritoneum is felt as two separate "pops." A J-tipped guidewire is passed through the needle and into the peritoneal cavity, again directing the wire toward the pelvis by maintaining the needle at a 45-degree angle to the skin. The 18-gauge needle is then removed and the peritoneal lavage catheter inserted over the guidewire into the peritoneal cavity, using a twisting motion and guided inferiorly toward the pelvis. The guidewire is then removed, and a 10-mL syringe is attached to the catheter for aspiration. If free blood returns from the peritoneal catheter before the syringe is attached, or if gross blood returns in the syringe barrel, hemoperitoneum has been documented; the catheter is removed, and the patient is transported quickly to the operating room for emergent celiotomy. If no gross blood returns on aspiration through the catheter, peritoneal lavage is performed using 1 L Ringer's lactate solution or normal saline that has been previously warmed to prevent hypothermia. The fluid is instilled into the peritoneal cavity through the peritoneal lavage catheter; afterward, the peritoneal fluid is allowed to drain out of the peritoneal cavity by gravity until the fluid return slows. A minimum of 250 mL lavage fluid is considered a representa-

tive sample of the peritoneal fluid [30]. A sample is sent to the laboratory for determination of red blood cell count, white blood cell count, amylase concentration, and presence of bile, bacteria, or particulate matter. When the lavage is completed, the catheter is removed and a sterile dressing applied over the site. Suture approximation of the skin edges is not necessary when the closed technique is used for DPL.

Semiclosed Technique. Local anesthetic is infiltrated in the area of the planned incision and a 2- to 3-cm vertical incision made in the infraumbilical or supraumbilical area. The incision is continued sharply down through the subcutaneous tissue and linea alba, and the peritoneum is then visualized. Forceps, hemostats, or Allis clamps are used to grasp the edges of the linea alba and elevate the fascial edges to prevent injury to underlying abdominal structures. The peritoneal lavage catheter with a metal inner stylet is inserted through the closed peritoneum into the peritoneal cavity at a 45-degree angle to the anterior abdominal wall, directed toward the pelvis. When the catheter–metal stylet assembly is in the peritoneal cavity, the peritoneal lavage catheter is advanced into the pelvis and the metal stylet removed. A 10-mL syringe is attached to the catheter, and aspiration is conducted as previously described. When the lavage is completed, the fascia must be reapproximated with sutures, the skin closed, and a sterile dressing applied.

Open Technique. After the administration of appropriate local anesthetic, a vertical midline incision approximately 3 to

5 cm long is made. This incision is commonly made in the infraumbilical location, but in patients with presumed pelvic fractures or retroperitoneal hematomas or in pregnant patients, a supraumbilical location is preferred. The vertical midline incision is carried down through the skin, subcutaneous tissue, and linea alba under direct vision. The linea alba is grasped on either side using forceps, hemostats, or Allis clamps, and the fascia is elevated to prevent injury to the underlying abdominal structures. The peritoneum is identified, and a small vertical peritoneal incision is made to gain entrance into the peritoneal cavity. The peritoneal lavage catheter is then inserted into the peritoneal cavity under direct visualization and advanced inferiorly toward the pelvis. It is inserted without the stylet or metal trocar. When in position, a 10-mL syringe is attached for aspiration. If aspiration of the peritoneal cavity is negative (i.e., no gross blood returns), peritoneal lavage is performed as described above. As in the semiclosed technique, the fascia and skin must be reapproximated to prevent dehiscence or evisceration, or both.

A prospective randomized study documented that the Lazarus-Nelson technique of closed percutaneous DPL can be performed faster than the open procedure [31]. The procedure times with the closed technique varied from 1 to 3 minutes, compared with 5 to 24 minutes for the open technique. In addition, it was documented that the closed percutaneous technique is as accurate as the open procedure and was associated with a lower incidence of wound infections and complications. The closed percutaneous technique, using the Seldinger technique, should therefore be used initially in all patients except those who have had previous abdominal surgery or in pregnant patients. This has been confirmed in a study of 2,501 DPLs performed over a 75-month period for blunt or penetrating abdominal trauma [32]. The majority (2,409, or 96%) were performed using the percutaneous or "closed" technique, and 92 (4%) were done open because of pelvic fractures, previous scars, and pregnancy. Open DPL was less sensitive than closed DPL in patients who sustained blunt trauma (90% vs. 95%) but slightly more sensitive in determining penetration (100% vs. 96%). Overall, there were few (21, or 0.8%) complications, and the overall sensitivity, specificity, and accuracy were 95%, 99%, and 98% using a red blood cell count of 100,000 per mm^3 in blunt trauma and 10,000 per mm^3 in penetrating trauma as the positive threshold.

Cotter et al. [33] reported a modification of DPL that allows more rapid infusion and drainage of lavage fluid. This modification uses cystoscopy irrigation tubing for instillation and drainage of the peritoneal lavage fluid. The cystoscopy irrigation system dramatically reduced influx and efflux times, saving an average of 19 minutes per patient for the completion of peritoneal lavage. This modification can be applied to the closed percutaneous or open technique for DPL to decrease the procedure time in critically ill patients.

INTERPRETATION OF RESULTS. The current guidelines for interpretation of positive and negative results of DPL are listed in Table 17-1. A positive result can be estimated by the inability to read newsprint or typewritten print through the lavage fluid as it returns through clear plastic tubing. This test is not reliable, however, and a quantitative red blood cell count in a sample of the peritoneal lavage fluid must be performed [34]. For patients with nonpenetrating abdominal trauma, a red blood cell count greater than 100,000 cells per mm^3 of lavage fluid is considered positive and requires emergent celiotomy, and fewer than 50,000 cells per mm^3 is considered negative. Red blood cell counts in the range of 50,000 to 100,000 per mm^3 are considered indeterminate.

Table 17-1. Interpretation of Diagnostic Peritoneal Lavage Results

Positive
  Nonpenetrating abdominal trauma
    Immediate gross blood return via catheter
    Immediate return of intestinal contents or food particles
    Aspiration of 10 mL blood via catheter
    Return of lavage fluid via chest tube or urinary catheter
    Red blood cell (RBC) count >100,000/mm^3
    White blood cell (WBC) count >500/mm^3
    Amylase >175 U/100 mL
  Penetrating abdominal trauma
    Immediate gross blood return via catheter
    Immediate return of intestinal contents or food particles
    Aspiration of 10 mL blood via catheter
    Return of lavage fluid via chest tube or Foley catheter
    RBC count used is variable, from >1,000/mm^3 to >100,000/mm^3
    WBC count >500/mm^3
    Amylase >175 U/100 mL
Negative
  Nonpenetrating abdominal trauma
    RBC count <50,000/mm^3
    WBC count <100/mm^3
    Amylase <75 U/100 mL
  Penetrating abdominal trauma
    RBC count used is variable, from <1,000/mm^3 to <50,000/mm^3
    WBC count <100/mm^3
    Amylase <75 U/100 mL

The guidelines for patients with penetrating abdominal trauma are much less clear. Feliciano et al. [35] support the use of the same criteria established for blunt abdominal trauma and reported an overall accuracy of 91.2% using these guidelines in penetrating abdominal trauma. Thal [25,26] reported a false-positive rate of 2.4% and false-negative rate of 4.9% in patients who had DPL using the standard guidelines for blunt abdominal trauma in individuals with thoracoabdominal stab wounds. Other clinical studies used a red blood cell count of greater than 2,000 cells per mm^3 or greater than 10,000 cells per mm^3 as the criterion for a positive DPL in patients with penetrating thoracic or abdominal trauma [23,24]; this leads to a higher false-positive rate and a lower false-negative rate. Future clinical studies with a large trauma patient population are required to establish the guidelines clearly for positive and negative DPL results in patients with penetrating thoracoabdominal injury.

Determination of hollow viscus injury by DPL is much more difficult. A white blood cell count greater than 500 cells per mm^3 of lavage fluid or an amylase concentration greater than 175 units per dL of lavage fluid is usually considered positive. These studies, however, are not as accurate as the use of red blood cell count in the lavage fluid to determine the presence of hemoperitoneum [36]. One study in patients with blunt abdominal trauma determined that the white blood cell count in lavage fluid has a positive predictive value of only 23% and probably should not be used as an indicator of a positive DPL [37]. Other studies analyzed alkaline phosphatase levels in DPL fluid to determine whether this assay is helpful in the diagnosis of hollow viscus injuries [38,39]. The results have been variable. One study of 545 patients who sustained blunt or penetrating abdominal injury determined that alkaline phosphatase levels greater than ten in the DPL effluent were predictive of hollow visceral injury with a specificity of 99.4% and a sensitivity of 93.3% [39]. Additional studies are required to confirm these results and establish the use of alkaline phosphatase levels as a positive indicator of significant intraabdominal injury.

It must be stressed that DPL is not accurate for determination of retroperitoneal visceral injuries or diaphragmatic injuries [40].

The incidence of false-negative DPL results is approximately 30% in patients who sustained traumatic diaphragmatic rupture. In addition, DPL is insensitive in detecting subcapsular hematomas of the spleen or liver that are contained, with no evidence of hemoperitoneum. Although DPL is now used in the evaluation of nontraumatic intraabdominal pathology, the criteria for positive lavage in these patients have not yet been established. Additional clinical studies are needed.

COMPLICATIONS. Complications of DPL by the techniques described here include malposition of the lavage catheter, injury to the intraabdominal organs or vessels, iatrogenic hemoperitoneum, wound infection or dehiscence, evisceration, and possible unnecessary laparotomy. DPL is a very valuable technique, however, and if it is performed carefully, with attention to detail, these complications are minimized. Wound infection, dehiscence, and evisceration are more common with the open technique; therefore, the closed percutaneous technique is recommended in all patients who do not have a contraindication to this technique. Knowledge of all techniques is necessary, however, because the choice of technique should be based on the individual patient's presentation.

References

1. Gerber DR, Bekes CE: Peritoneal catheterization. *Crit Care Clin* 8: 727, 1992.
2. Garcia N, Sanyal AJ: Ascites. *Curr Treat Options Gastroenterol* 4:527, 2001.
3. Inturri P, Graziotto A, Roxxaro L: Treatment of ascites: old and new remedies. *Dig Dis* 14:145, 1996.
4. Kravetz D, Romero G, Argonz J, et al: Total volume paracentesis decreases variceal pressure, size, and variceal wall tension in cirrhotic patients. *Hepatology* 25:59, 1997.
5. Yu AS, Hu KQ: Management of ascites. *Clin Liver Dis* 5:541, 2001.
6. Zervos EE, Rosemurgy AS: Management of medically refractory ascites. *Am J Surg* 181:256, 2001.
7. Rossle M, Ochs A, Gulberg V, et al: A comparison of paracentesis and transjugular intrahepatic portosystemic shunting in patients with ascites. *N Engl J Med* 342:1701, 2000.
8. Sartori M, Andorno S, Gambaro M, et al: Diagnostic paracentesis: a two-step approach. *Ital J Gastroenterol* 28:81, 1996.
9. Dittrich S, Yordi LM, DeMattos AA: The value of serum-ascites albumin gradient for the determination of portal hypertension in the diagnosis of ascites. *Hepatogastroenterology* 48:166, 2001.
10. Cabrera J, Falcon L, Gorriz E, et al: Abdominal decompression plays a major role in early postparacentesis hemodynamic changes in cirrhotic patients with tense ascites. *Gut* 48:384, 2001.
11. Wang SS, Chen CC, Chao Y, et al: Sequential hemodynamic changes for large volume paracentesis in post-hepatitic cirrhotic patients with massive ascites. *Proc Natl Sci Counc Repub China B* 20:117, 1996.
12. Peltekian KM, Wong F, Liu PP, et al: Cardiovascular, renal and neurohumoral responses to single large-volume paracentesis in patients with cirrhosis and diuretic-resistant ascites. *Am J Gastroenterol* 92:394, 1997.
13. O'Neill MJ, Weissleder R, Gervais DA, et al: Tunneled peritoneal catheter placement under sonographic and fluoroscopic guidance in the palliative treatment of malignant ascites. *AJR Am J Roentgenol* 177:615, 2001.
14. Richard HM III, Coldwell DM, Boyd-Kranis RL, et al: Pleurx tunneled catheter in the management of malignant ascites. *J Vasc Interv Radiol* 12:373, 2001.
15. Deen KI, deSilva AP, Jayakody M, et al: Saphenoperitoneal anastomosis for resistant ascites in patients with cirrhosis. *Am J Surg* 181:145, 2001.
16. Root H, Hauser C, McKinley C, et al: Diagnostic peritoneal lavage. *Surgery* 57:633, 1965.
17. Giacobine JW, Siler VE: Evaluation of diagnostic abdominal paracentesis with experimental and clinical studies. *Eur Gynecol Obstet* 110:676, 1960.
18. Fischer R, Beverlin B, Engrav L, et al: Diagnostic peritoneal lavage 14 years and 2586 patients later. *Am J Surg* 136:701, 1978.
19. Wherrett LJ, Boulanger BR, McLellan BA, et al: Hypotension after blunt abdominal trauma: the role of emergent abdominal sonography in surgical triage. *J Trauma* 41:815, 1996.
20. McKenney MG, Martin L, Lentz K, et al: 1,000 consecutive ultrasounds for blunt abdominal trauma. *J Trauma* 40:607, 1996.
21. Catre MG: Diagnostic peritoneal lavage versus abdominal computed tomography in blunt abdominal trauma: a review of prospective studies. *Can J Surg* 38:117, 1995.
22. Branney SW, Moore EE, Cantrill SV, et al: Ultrasound based key clinical pathway reduces the use of hospital resources for the evaluation of blunt abdominal trauma. *J Trauma* 42:1086, 1997.
23. Merlotti GJ, Marcet E, Sheaff CM, et al: Use of peritoneal lavage to evaluate abdominal penetration. *J Trauma* 25:228, 1985.
24. Gruenberg JC, Brown RS, Talbert JG, et al: The diagnostic usefulness of peritoneal lavage in penetrating trauma. *Am Surg* 48:401, 1982.
25. Thal ER: Evaluation of peritoneal lavage and local exploration in lower chest and abdominal stab wounds. *J Trauma* 17:642, 1977.
26. Thal ER: Peritoneal lavage: reliability of RBC count in patients with stab wounds to chest and abdomen. *Arch Surg* 119:579, 1984.
27. Boyle EM, Maier RV, Salazar JD, et al: Diagnosis of injuries after stab wounds to the back and flank. *J Trauma* 42:260, 1997.
28. Thal ER, May RA, Beesinger D: Peritoneal lavage: its unreliability in gunshot wounds of the lower chest and abdomen. *Arch Surg* 115:430, 1980.
29. Lazarus HM, Nelson JA: A technique for peritoneal lavage without risk or complication. *Surg Gynecol Obstet* 149:889, 1979.
30. Sweeney JF, Albrink MH, Bischof E, et al: Diagnostic peritoneal lavage: volume of lavage effluent needed for accurate determination of a negative lavage. *Injury* 25:659, 1994.
31. Howdieshell TR, Osler RM, Demarest GB: Open versus closed peritoneal lavage with particular attention to time, accuracy and cost. *Am J Emerg Med* 7:367, 1989.
32. Nagy KK, Roberts RR, Joseph KT, et al: Experience with over 2500 diagnostic peritoneal lavages. *Injury* 31:479, 2000.
33. Cotter CP, Hawkins ML, Kent RB, et al: Ultrarapid diagnostic peritoneal lavage. *J Trauma* 29:615, 1989.
34. Gow KW, Haley LP, Phang PT: Validity of visual inspection of diagnostic peritoneal lavage fluid. *Can J Surg* 39:114, 1996.
35. Feliciano D, Bitondo C, Steed G, et al: Five hundred open taps or lavages in patients with abdominal stab wounds. *Am J Surg* 148:772, 1984.
36. Feliciano DV, Bitondo Dyer CG: Vagaries of the lavage white blood cell count in evaluating abdominal stab wounds. *Am J Surg* 168:680, 1994.
37. Soyka J, Martin M, Sloan E, et al: Diagnostic peritoneal lavage: is an isolated WBC count greater than or equal to 500/mm^3 predictive of intra-abdominal trauma requiring celiotomy in blunt trauma patients? *J Trauma* 30:874, 1990.
38. Megison SM, Weigelt JA: The value of alkaline phosphatase in peritoneal lavage. *Ann Emerg Med* 19:5, 1990.
39. Jaffin JH, Ochsner G, Cole FJ, et al: Alkaline phosphatase levels in diagnostic peritoneal lavage as a predictor of hollow visceral injury. *J Trauma* 34:829, 1993.
40. Fischer RP, Freeman T: The inadequacy of peritoneal lavage in diagnosing acute diaphragmatic rupture. *J Trauma* 16:538, 1976.

18. Management of Acute Esophageal Variceal Hemorrhage with Gastroesophageal Balloon Tamponade

Marie T. Pavini and Juan Carlos Puyana

Esophageal variceal hemorrhage is an acute, severe, dramatic complication of the patient with portal hypertension that carries a high mortality and significant incidence of recurrence [1]. Whereas urgent endoscopy, sclerotherapy [2–4] and band ligation [5] are considered first-line treatment, balloon tamponade remains a valuable intervention in the treatment of bleeding esophageal varices (Fig. 18-1).

Historical Development

In 1930, Westphal described the use of an esophageal sound as a means of controlling variceal hemorrhage [6]. In 1947, successful control of hemorrhage by balloon tamponade was achieved by attaching an inflatable latex bag to the end of a Miller-Abbot tube [7]. In 1949, a two-balloon tube was described by Patton and Johnson [8]. A triple-lumen tube with gastric and esophageal balloons (one lumen for gastric aspiration and the other two for balloon inflation) was described by Sengstaken and Blakemore in 1950 [9]. In 1953, Linton proposed a single gastric balloon tube with a suction lumen below the balloon as a diagnostic tool to differentiate between gastric and esophageal bleed and a larger balloon (800 mL) capable of compressing the submucosal veins in the cardia, thereby minimizing flow to the esophageal veins [10,11]. An additional suction port above Linton's gastric balloon was introduced by Nachlas in 1955 [12]. The Minnesota tube was described in 1968 [12a] as a modification of the Sengstaken-Blakemore tube, incorporating the esophageal suction port described later.

Role of Balloon Tamponade in the Management of Bleeding Esophageal Varices

Extensive clinical experience on the use of balloon tamponade has been accumulated since 1950, when it was described by Sengstaken and Blakemore [9]. However, some controversy remains regarding the safety and effectiveness of these techniques. There is a wide range in the incidence of rebleeding and mortality, with the discrepancy explained in part by the diversity of techniques used. In some instances, the tube was used after prolonged unsuccessful pharmacologic therapy, usually in patients with severe hemodynamic compromise. Independent predictors of mortality in intensive care unit patients with bleeding esophageal varices were recently described by Lee et al. [13] and include total volume of sclerosing agent (ethanolamine), blood transfusion of greater than ten units of red cells, Glasgow Coma Scale, coagulopathy reflected by an average 2.6 ± 1.6 international normalized ratio for prothrombin test, and presence of shock.

A number of studies comparing the efficacy of balloon tamponade against sclerotherapy have shown that the incidence and severity of complications and success in controlling bleeding favor the use of sclerotherapy or band ligation as the first line of treatment [14,15]. The decision to use other therapeutic alternatives depends on the response to the initial therapy, the severity of the hemorrhage, and the patient's underlying condition. Combined pharmacologic therapy with vasoactive drugs and balloon tamponade can control the hemorrhage in 90% of cases [16]. Octreotide or combination vasopressin and nitroglycerin diminish portal vein pressure while emergency endoscopy is performed to confirm the diagnosis [17,18]. Pourriat et al. advocate administration of octreotide by emergency medical personnel before a patient is transferred to the hospital [19]. Other alternatives include percutaneous transhepatic embolization, which is recommended in poor-risk patients who do not stop bleeding despite other measures; esophagogastric devascularization with gastroesophageal stapling for patients without cirrhosis as well as for low-risk patients with cirrhosis [20]; portosystemic shunt [21,22]; and esophageal transection [23].

Indications and Contraindications

A Sengstaken-Blakemore tube is indicated in patients with a diagnosis of esophageal variceal hemorrhage in which neither band ligation nor sclerotherapy is technically possible, readily available, or has failed [25]. An adequate anatomic diagnosis is imperative before any of these balloon tubes are inserted. Severe upper gastrointestinal bleeding attributed to esophageal varices in patients with clinical evidence of chronic liver disease results from other causes in 40% of cases. The tube is contraindicated in patients with recent esophageal surgery or esophageal stricture [26]. Some authors do not recommend balloon tamponade when a hiatal hernia is present, but there are reports of successful hemorrhage control in some of these patients [27].

Technical and Practical Considerations

AIRWAY CONTROL. Endotracheal intubation is imperative in patients with hemodynamic compromise, encephalopathy, or both. The incidence of aspiration pneumonia is directly related to the presence of encephalopathy or impaired mental status [28,29]. Suctioning of pulmonary secretions and blood accumulated in the hypopharynx is facilitated in patients with endotracheal intubation. Sedatives and analgesics are more readily administered in intubated patients and may be required often because these tubes are poorly tolerated in

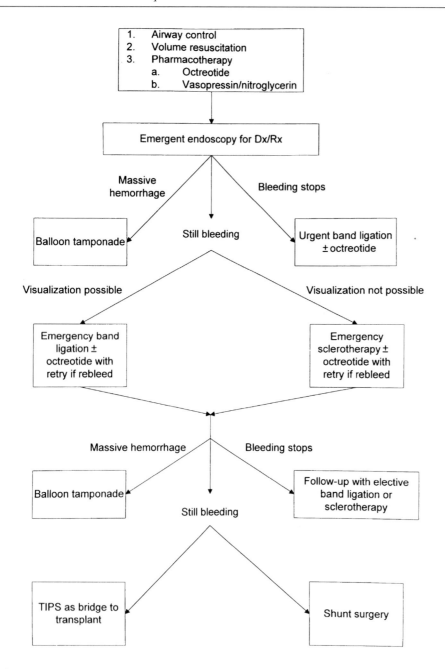

Fig. 18-1. Management of esophageal variceal hemorrhage. Dx, diagnosis; Rx, therapy; TIPS, transjugular intrahepatic portosystemic shunt.

most patients. Sedatives must be used cautiously, however, because a number of these patients have impaired liver metabolism. We recommend inserting an endotracheal tube (see Chapter 1) in any patient who will have balloon tamponade. The incidence of pulmonary complications is significantly lower when endotracheal intubation is routinely used [28].

HYPOVOLEMIA, SHOCK, AND COAGULOPATHY. Adequate intravenous access should be obtained with large-bore venous catheters and fluid resuscitation undertaken with crystalloids and colloids. A central venous catheter or pulmonary artery catheter may be required to monitor intravascular filling pressures, especially in patients with severe cirrhosis, advanced age, or underlying cardiac and pulmonary disease. The hematocrit should be maintained above 28%, and coagulopathy should be treated with fresh-frozen plasma and platelets. Four to six units of packed red cells should always be available in case of severe recurrent bleeding, which commonly occurs in these patients [16].

CLOTS AND GASTRIC DECOMPRESSION. Placement of an Ewald tube and aggressive lavage and suctioning of the stomach and duodenum facilitates endoscopy, diminishes the risk of aspiration, and may help control hemorrhage from causes other than esophageal varices.

The diagnostic endoscopic procedure should be done as soon as the patient is stabilized after basic resuscitation. Endoscopy is performed in the intensive care unit or operating room under controlled monitoring and with adequate equipment and personnel. An endoscope with a large suction channel should be used. Octreotide [30] or combination vasopressin and nitroglycerin should be administered as part of initial resuscitation.

TUBE, PORTS, AND BALLOONS. Several studies have published combined experience with tubes such as the Linton and Nachlas tube [16,31–33]. The techniques described here are limited to the use of the Minnesota (Fig. 18-2) and inserted Sengstaken-Blakemore (Fig. 18-3) tubes. All lumens

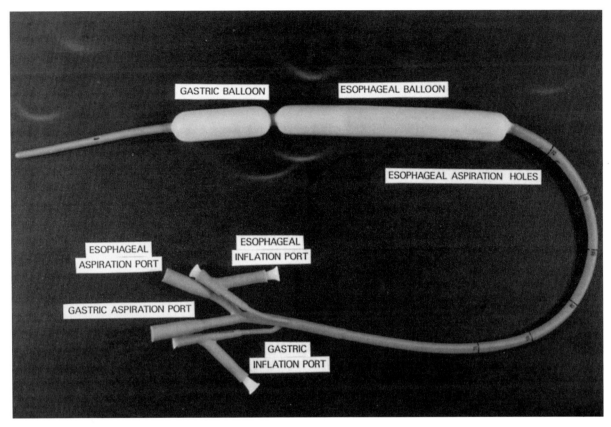

Fig. 18-2. Minnesota tube.

should be patent, and the balloons should be inflated and checked for leaks. The Minnesota tube has a fourth lumen that allows intermittent suctioning above the esophageal balloon, facilitating suctioning of saliva, blood, and pulmonary secretions in the hypopharynx [29] (Fig. 18-4). When using a standard Sengstaken-Blakemore tube, a No. 18 Salem sump with surgical ties is attached above the esophageal balloon as originally described by Boyce [33a] and through the mouth. Suctioning above the esophageal balloon and hypopharynx diminishes, but does not eliminate, the risk of aspiration pneumonia.

INSERTION AND PLACEMENT OF THE TUBE. The tube should be generously lubricated with lidocaine jelly. It can be inserted through the nose or mouth, but the nasal route is not recommended in patients with coagulopathy. The tube is passed into the stomach. Auscultation in the epigastrium while air is injected through the gastric lumen verifies the position of the tube, but the position of the gastric balloon must be confirmed radiologically at this time. The gastric balloon is inflated with no more than 80 mL of air, and a (portable) radiograph is obtained that includes the upper abdomen and lower chest (Fig. 18-5). When it is documented that the gastric balloon is below the diaphragm, it should be further inflated with air, slowly, to a volume of 250 to 300 mL [34]. The gastric balloon of the Minnesota tube can be inflated to 450 mL. Tube balloon inlets should be clamped with rubber shod hemostats after insufflation. Hemorrhage is frequently controlled with insufflation of the gastric balloon alone without applying traction [35], but in patients with torrential hemorrhage, it is necessary to apply traction (*vide infra*). If the bleeding continues, the esophageal balloon should be inflated to a pressure of approxi-

mately 45 mm Hg (bedside manometer). This pressure should be monitored and maintained. Some authors inflate the esophageal balloon in all patients immediately after insertion [16].

FIXATION AND TRACTION TECHNIQUES. Fixation and traction on the tube depend on the route of insertion. When the nasal route is used, traction should not be applied against the nostril, because this can easily cause skin and cartilage necrosis. When traction is required, the tube should be attached to a cord that is passed over a pulley in a bed with an overhead orthopedic frame and aligned directly as it comes out of the nose to avoid contact with the nostril. This system allows maintenance of traction with a known weight (500 to 1,500 g) that is easily measured and constant. When the tube is inserted through the mouth, traction is better applied by placing a football helmet on the patient and attaching the tube to the face mask of the helmet after a similar weight is applied for tension. Pressure sores can occur in the head and forehead when the helmet does not fit properly or when it is used for a prolonged period of time. Several authors recommend overhead traction for oral and nasal insertion [36].

MAINTENANCE AND MONITORING. The gastric lumen is placed on intermittent suction. The Minnesota tube has an esophageal lumen that can also be placed on low, intermittent suction. If the Salem sump has been used as previously described, then continuous suction can be used on the sump tube. The tautness and inflation of balloons should be checked an hour after insertion and periodically by experienced personnel. The tube should be left in place a minimum of 24 hours. The gastric balloon tamponade can be maintained con-

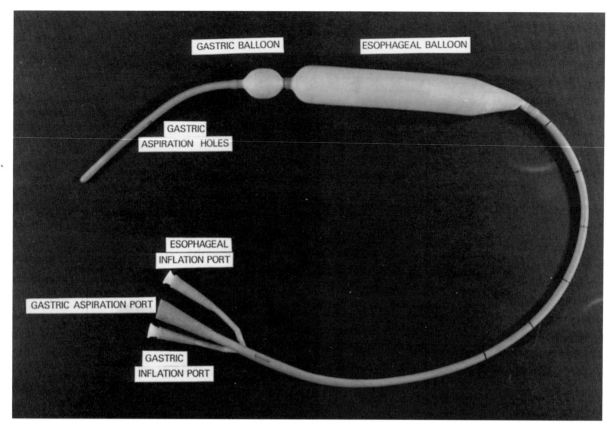

Fig. 18-3. Sengstaken-Blakemore tube.

tinuously up to 48 hours. The esophageal balloon, however, must be deflated for 30 minutes every 8 hours [28]. The position of the tube should be monitored radiologically every 24 hours or sooner if there is any indication of tube displacement. A pair of scissors should be at the bedside in case the balloon ports need to be cut for rapid decompression, because the balloon can migrate and acutely obstruct the airway.

REMOVAL OF THE TUBE. Once hemorrhage is controlled, the esophageal balloon is deflated first; the gastric balloon is left inflated for an additional 24 to 48 hours. If there is no evidence of bleeding, the gastric balloon is deflated, and the tube is left in place 24 hours longer. If bleeding recurs, the appropriate balloon is reinflated. The tube is removed if no further bleeding occurs.

Complications

Aspiration pneumonia is the most common complication of balloon tamponade. The severity and fatality rate is related to the presence of impaired mental status and encephalopathy in patients with poor control of the airway. The incidence ranges from 0% to 12%. Acute laryngeal obstruction and tracheal rupture are the most severe of all complications and the worst examples of tube migration. Migration of the tube occurs when the gastric balloon is not inflated properly after adequate positioning in the stomach or when excessive traction (greater than 1.5 kg) is used, causing migration to the esophagus or hypopharynx. Mucosal ulceration of the gastroesophageal junction is common and is directly related to prolonged traction time (greater than 36 hours). Perforation of the esophagus is reported as a result of misplacing the gastric balloon above the diaphragm (Fig. 18-6). It is imperative that the position be confirmed radiologically immediately after passing the tube and before the gastric balloon is inflated with more than 80 mL of air. Rupture of the esophagus carries a high mortality, especially in patients with severe hemorrhage who already have serious physiologic impairment. The incidence of complications that are a direct cause of death ranges from 0% to 20%.

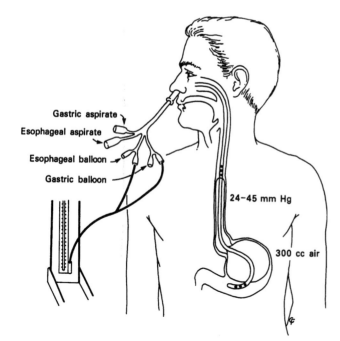

Fig. 18-4. Proper positioning of the Minnesota tube.

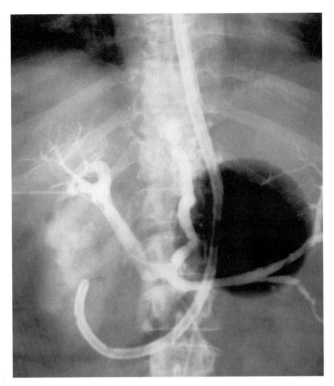

Fig. 18-5. Radiograph showing correct position of the tube; the gastric balloon is seen below the diaphragm. Note the Salem sump above the gastric balloon and adjacent to the tube. (Courtesy of Ashley Davidoff, MD.)

Unusual complications, such as impaction, result from obstruction of the balloon ports making it impossible to deflate the balloon. Occasionally, surgery is required to remove the tube [24]. Other complications include necrosis of the nostrils and nasopharyngeal bleeding.

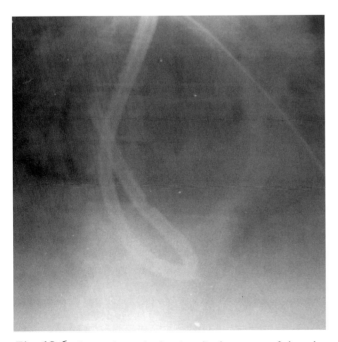

Fig. 18-6. Chest radiograph showing distal segment of the tube coiled in the chest and the gastric balloon inflated above the diaphragm in the esophagus. (Courtesy of Ashley Davidoff, MD.)

Acknowledgments

The authors thank Charles F. Foltz and Susan A. Bright, Medical Media Service, West Roxbury Veterans' Administration Medical Center, West Roxbury, MA; and Susan St. Martin, UMass Memorial Medical Center, Worcester, MA.

References

1. Terblanche J, Krige JE, Bornman PC: The treatment of esophageal varices. *Annu Rev Med* 43:69, 1992.
2. Lo GH, Lai KH, Ng WW, et al: Injection sclerotherapy preceded by esophageal tamponade versus immediate sclerotherapy in arresting active variceal bleeding: a prospective randomized trial. *Gastrointest Endosc* 38:421, 1992.
3. Llach J, Bordas JM, Nieto I, et al: Endoscopic sclerotherapy to arrest uncontrolled variceal bleeding in cirrhotic patients with high surgical risk. *Hepatogastroenterology* 45:2181, 1998.
4. Navarro VJ, Garcia-Tsao G: Variceal hemorrhage. *Crit Care Clin* 11:391, 1995.
5. Cipolletta L, Bianco MA, Rotondano G, et al: Emergency endoscopic ligation of actively bleeding gastric varices with a detachable snare. *Gastrointest Endosc* 47:400, 1998.
6. Westphal K: Uber eine Kompressions Behandlung der Blutungen aus Oesophagusvarizen. *Dtsch Med Wochenschr* 56:1135, 1930.
7. Rowentree LG, Zimmerman EF, Todd MH, et al: Intraesophageal venous tamponade: Its use in case of variceal hemorrhage from the esophagus. *JAMA* 13:630, 1947.
8. Patton TB, Johnson CG: Method for control of bleeding from esophageal varices. *Arch Surg* 59:502, 1949.
9. Sengstaken RW, Blakemore AH: Balloon tamponade for the control of hemorrhage from esophageal varices. *Ann Surg* 131:781, 1950.
10. Linton RR: The emergency and definitive treatment of bleeding esophageal varices. *Gastroenterology* 21:1, 1953.
11. Linton RR: The treatment of esophageal varices. *Surg Clin North Am* 46:485, 1966.
12. Nachlas MN: A new triple-lumen tube for diagnosis and treatment of upper gastrointestinal hemorrhage. *N Engl J Med* 252:720, 1955.
12a. Edlich RF, Lande AJ, Goodale RL, Wangensteen OH: Prevention of aspiration pneumonia by continuous esophageal aspiration during esophagogastric tamponade and gastric cooling. *Surgery* 64:405,1968.
13. Lee H, Hawker FH, Selby W, et al: Intensive care treatment of patients with bleeding esophageal varices: results, predictors of mortality, and predictors of the adult respiratory distress syndrome. *Crit Care Med* 20:1555, 1992.
14. Idezuki Y, Sanjo K, Bandai Y, et al: Current strategy for esophageal varices in Japan. *Am J Surg* 160:98, 1990.
15. Moreto M, Zaballa M, Bernal A, et al: A randomized trial of tamponade or sclerotherapy as immediate treatment for bleeding esophageal varices. *Surg Gynecol Obstet* 167:331, 1988.
16. Panes J, Teres J, Bosch J: Efficacy of balloon tamponade in treatment of bleeding gastric and esophageal varices: results in 151 consecutive episodes. *Dig Dis Sci* 33:454, 1988.
17. Sandford NL, Kerlin P: Current management of oesophageal varices. *Aust N Z Med J* 25:528, 1995.
18. Stein C, Korula J: Variceal bleeding: what are the options? *Postgrad Med* 98(6):143, 1995.
19. Pourriat JL, Leyacher S, Letoumelin P, et al: Early administration of the association terlipressin-nitroglycerin (TER-NTG) in cirrhotic active digestive bleeding (ADB). *Hepatology* 19:1151, 1994.
20. Mathur SK, Shah SR, Soonawala ZF, et al: Transabdominal extensive oesophagastric devascularization with gastro-oesophageal stapling in the management of acute variceal bleeding. *Br J Surg* 84:413, 1997.
21. Sanyal AJ, Freedman AM, Luketic VA, et al: Transjugular intrahepatic portosystemic shunts for patients with active variceal hemorrhage unresponsive to sclerotherapy. *Gastroenterology* 111:138, 1996.
22. Banares R, Casado M, Rodriquez-Laiz JM, et al: Urgent transjugular intrahepatic portosystemic shunt for control of acute variceal bleeding. *Am J Gastroenterol* 93:75, 1998.

23. Lewis JJ, Basson MD, Modlin IM: Surgical therapy of acute esophageal variceal hemorrhage. *Dig Dis Sci* 10[Suppl 1]:46, 1992.
24. Gossat D, Bolin TD: An unusual complication of balloon tamponade in the treatment of esophageal varices: a case report and brief review of the literature. *Am J Gastroenterol* 80:600, 1985.
25. Burnett DA, Rikkers LF: Nonoperative emergency treatment of variceal hemorrhage. *Surg Clin North Am* 70:291,1990.
26. McCormick PA, Burroughs AK, McIntyre N: How to insert a Sengstaken-Blakemore tube. *Br J Hosp Med* 43:274, 1990.
27. Minocha A, Richards RJ: Sengstaken-Blakemore tube for control of massive bleeding from gastric varices in hiatal hernia. *J Clin Gastroenterol* 14:36, 1992.
28. Cello JP, Crass RA, Grendell JH, et al: Management of the patient with hemorrhaging esophageal varices. *JAMA* 256:1480, 1986.
29. Pasquale MD, Cerra FB: Sengstaken-Blakemore tube placement. *Crit Care Clin* 8:743, 1992.
30. Erstad B: Octreotide for acute variceal bleeding. *Ann Pharmacother* 35:618, 2001.
31. Cook D, Laine L: Indications, technique and complications of

32. balloon tamponade for variceal gastrointestinal bleeding. *J Intensive Care Med* 7:212, 1992.
33. Teres J, Cecilia A, Bordas JM, et al: Esophageal tamponade for bleeding varices: controlled trial between the Sengstaken-Blakemore tube and the Linton-Nachlas tube. *Gastroenterology* 75:566, 1978.
33. Avgerinos A, Armonis A: Balloon tamponade technique and efficacy in variceal haemorrhage. *Scand J Gastroenterol* 29[Suppl 207]:11, 1994.
33a. Boyce HW: Modification of the Sengstaken-Blackmore balloon tube. *N Engl J Med* 267:195, 1962.
34. Duarte B: Technique for the placement of the Sengstaken-Blakemore tube. *Surg Gynecol Obstet* 168:449, 1989.
35. Pinto Correia J, Martins Alves M, Alexandrino P, et al: Controlled trial of vasopressin and balloon tamponade in bleeding esophageal varices. *Hepatology* 4:885, 1984.
36. Hunt PS, Korman MG, Hansky J, et al: An 8-year prospective experience with balloon tamponade in emergency control of bleeding esophageal varices. *Dig Dis Sci* 27:413, 1982.

19. Endoscopic Placement of Feeding Tubes

Lena M. Napolitano

Indications for Enteral Feeding

Nutritional support is an essential component of intensive care medicine (see Chapters 197–199) [1–4]. It has become increasingly evident that nutritional support administered via the enteral route is far superior to total parenteral nutrition [5,6]. Although there are absolute or relative contraindications to enteral feeding in selected cases, most critically ill patients can receive some or all of their nutritional requirements via the gastrointestinal tract. Even when some component of nutritional support must be provided intravenously, feeding via the gut is desirable.

Provision of nutrition through the enteral route aids in prevention of gastrointestinal mucosal atrophy, thereby maintaining the integrity of the gastrointestinal mucosal barrier. Derangements in the barrier function of the gastrointestinal tract may permit the systemic absorption of gut-derived microbes and microbial products (bacterial translocation), which has been implicated as important in the pathophysiology of syndromes of sepsis and multiple organ system failure [7–9]. Other advantages of enteral nutrition are preservation of immunologic gut function and normal gut flora, improved use of nutrients, and reduced cost. Some studies suggest that clinical outcome is improved and infectious complications are decreased in patients who receive enteral nutrition compared with parenteral nutrition [10–12]. Additional clinical studies suggest that immune-enhancing enteral diets containing specialty nutrients (e.g., arginine, glutamine, nucleotides, and omega-3 fatty acids) may also reduce septic complications [13–16].

Several developments, including new techniques for placement of feeding tubes, availability of smaller caliber, minimally reactive tubes, and an increasing range of enteral formulas,

have expanded the ability to provide enteral nutritional support to critically ill patients. Enteral feeding at a site proximal to the pylorus may be absolutely or relatively contraindicated in patients with increased risk of pulmonary aspiration, but feeding more distally (particularly distal to the ligament of Treitz) decreases the likelihood of aspiration. Other relative or absolute contraindications to enteral feeding include fistulas, intestinal obstruction, upper gastrointestinal hemorrhage, and severe inflammatory bowel disease. Enteral feeding is not recommended in patients with severe malabsorption or early in the course of severe short-gut syndrome.

Access to the Gastrointestinal Tract

After deciding to provide enteral nutrition, the clinician must decide whether to deliver the formula into the stomach, duodenum, or jejunum, and determine the optimal method for accessing the site, based on the function of the patient's gastrointestinal tract, duration of enteral nutritional support required, and risk of pulmonary aspiration. Gastric feeding provides the most normal route for enteral nutrition, but it is commonly poorly tolerated in the critically ill patient because of gastric dysmotility with delayed emptying [17]. Enteral nutrition infusion into the duodenum or jejunum may decrease the incidence of aspiration because of the protection afforded by a competent pyloric sphincter; however, the risk of aspiration is not completely eliminated by feeding distal to the pylorus [18,19]. Infusion into the jejunum is associated with the lowest risk of pulmonary aspiration. An advantage of this site of administration is that enteral feeding can be initiated early in the postoperative period, because postoperative ileus primarily affects the colon and stomach and only rarely involves the small intestine.

Techniques

Enteral feeding tubes can be placed via the transnasal, transoral, or percutaneous transgastric routes. If these procedures are contraindicated or unsuccessful, the tube may be placed by endoscopy using endoscopic and laparoscopic technique or surgically via a laparotomy [20,21].

NASOENTERIC ROUTE. Nasoenteric tubes are the most commonly used means of providing enteral nutritional support in critically ill patients. This route is preferred for short- to intermediate-term enteral support when eventual resumption of oral feeding is anticipated. It is possible to infuse enteral formulas into the stomach using a conventional 16 or 18 French (Fr) polyvinyl chloride nasogastric tube, but patients are usually much more comfortable if a small-diameter silicone or polyurethane feeding tube is used. Nasoenteric tubes vary in luminal diameter (6 to 14 Fr) and length, depending on the desired location of the distal orifice: stomach, 30 to 36 in.; duodenum, 43 in.; jejunum, at least 48 in. Some tubes have tungsten-weighted tips designed to facilitate passage into the duodenum via normal peristalsis; others have a stylet. Most are radiopaque. Newer tubes permit gastric decompression while delivering formula into the jejunum.

Nasoenteric feeding tubes should be placed with the patient in a semi-Fowler's or sitting position [22]. The tip of the tube should be lubricated, placed in the patient's nose, and advanced to the posterior pharynx. If possible, the patient should be permitted to sip water as the tube is slowly advanced into the stomach. Once in position, air should be insufflated through the tube while auscultating over the stomach with a stethoscope. The presence of a gurgling sound suggests, but does not prove, that the tube is in the gastric lumen. A chest radiograph should be obtained to confirm the position of the tube before initiating feeding. Capnography may be used to prevent inadvertent placement of small-bore feeding tubes into the lungs [23,24]. The tube should be securely taped to the forehead or cheek without tension. If the tube is placed for duodenal or jejunal feeding, a loop 6 to 8 in. long may be left extending from the nose and the tube advanced 1 to 2 in. every hour. Placing the patient in a right lateral decubitus position may facilitate passage through the pylorus.

Delayed gastric emptying has been confirmed in critically ill patients [16] and may contribute to gastric feeding intolerance. One study randomized 80 critically ill patients to gastric feeding with erythromycin (200 mg IV every 8 hours as a prokinetic agent) or through a transpyloric feeding tube, and identified that the two were equivalent in achieving goal caloric requirements [25]. Spontaneous transpyloric passage of enteral feeding tubes in critically ill patients is commonly unsuccessful secondary to the preponderance of gastric atony. The addition of a tungsten weight to the end of enteral feeding tubes and the development of wire or metal stylets in enteral feeding tubes are aimed at improving the success rate for spontaneous transpyloric passage. Various bedside techniques, including air insufflation, pH-assisted, magnet-guided [26], and spontaneous passage with or without motility agents are available to facilitate transpyloric feeding passage. Intravenous metoclopramide and erythromycin have been recommended as prokinetic agents. A randomized prospective trial in critically ill patients compared the success rate of transpyloric passage of weighted versus unweighted enteral feeding tubes, both with inner stylets. This study demonstrated that the combination of preinsertion metoclopramide and a tapered, unweighted feeding tube with inner stylet achieved transpyloric position in 84% of patients at 4 hours after placement compared with 36% with the weighted enteral feeding tubes (p <.002) [27]. Another randomized study [28] determined that erythromycin (200 mg IV) administered 30 minutes before insertion of an enteral feeding tube with a weighted tip and inner stylet resulted in successful postpyloric placement in 61% of intensive care unit patients, significantly better than a 35% success rate in patients receiving placebo (p <.05). Nasoenteral feeding tubes with inner stylets are therefore recommended for use in critically ill patients. However, these tubes must be inserted by skilled practitioners using defined techniques [29,30].

If the tube does not pass into the duodenum on the first attempt, placement can be attempted under endoscopic assistance or fluoroscopic guidance. Endoscopic placement of nasoenteral feeding tubes is easily accomplished in the critically ill patient and can be performed at the bedside using portable equipment [31–35]. Transnasal or transoral endoscopy can be used for placement of nasoenteral feeding tubes in critically ill patients [36]. The patient is sedated appropriately, and topical anesthetic is applied to the posterior pharynx with lidocaine or benzocaine spray. A nasoenteric feeding tube 43 to 48 in. long with an inner wire stylet is passed transnasally into the stomach. The endoscope is inserted and advanced through the esophagus into the gastric lumen. An endoscopy forceps is passed through the biopsy channel of the endoscope and used to grasp the tip of the enteral feeding tube. The endoscope, along with the enteral feeding tube, is advanced distally into the duodenum as far as possible (Fig. 19-1).

The endoscopy forceps and feeding tube remain in position in the distal duodenum as the endoscope is withdrawn back into the gastric lumen. The endoscopy forceps is opened, the feeding tube released, and the endoscopy forceps withdrawn carefully back into the stomach. On first pass, the feeding tube is usually lodged in the second portion of the duodenum. The portion of the feeding tube that is redundant in the stomach is advanced slowly into the duodenum using the endoscopy forceps to achieve a final position distal to the ligament of Treitz (Fig. 19-2). An abdominal radiograph is obtained at the completion of the procedure to document the final position of the nasoenteral feeding tube. Endoscopic placement of postpyloric

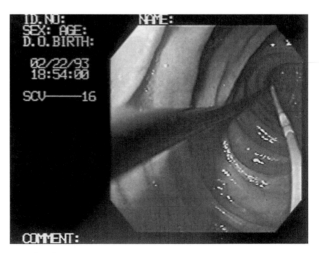

Fig. 19-1. Endoscopic placement of nasoenteral feeding tube. Endoscopy forceps and gastroscope advance the feeding tube in the duodenum.

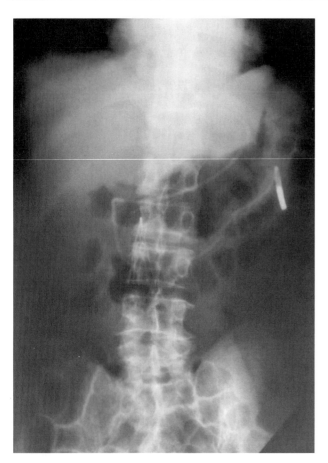

Fig. 19-2. Abdominal radiograph documenting the optimal position of an endoscopically placed nasoenteral feeding tube, past the ligament of Treitz.

enteral feeding tubes is highly successful, eliminates the risk of transporting the patient to radiology for fluoroscopic placement, and allows prompt achievement of nutritional goals, because enteral feeding can be initiated immediately after the procedure.

PERCUTANEOUS ROUTE. Percutaneous endoscopic gastrostomy (PEG) tube placement, introduced by Ponsky in 1990, has become the procedure of choice for patients requiring prolonged enteral nutritional support [37–39]. PEG tubes range in size from 20 to 28 Fr. PEG rapidly replaced open gastrostomy as the method of choice for enteral nutrition. Unlike surgical gastrostomy, PEG does not require general anesthesia and laparotomy and eliminates the discomfort associated with chronic nasoenteric tubes. This procedure can be considered in patients who have normal gastric emptying and low risk for pulmonary aspiration and can be performed in the operating room, an endoscopy unit, or at the bedside in the intensive care unit with portable endoscopy equipment.

PEG should not be performed in patients with near or total obstruction of the pharynx or esophagus, in the presence of coagulopathy, or when transillumination is inadequate. Relative contraindications are ascites, gastric cancer, and gastric ulcer. Previous abdominal surgery is not a contraindication. The original method for PEG was the pull technique; more recent modifications are the push and introducer techniques.

Pull Technique. The pull technique is performed with the patient in the supine position. The abdomen is prepared and draped. The posterior pharynx is anesthetized with a topical spray or solution (e.g., benzocaine spray or viscous lidocaine),

and IV sedation (e.g., 1 to 2 mg of midazolam) is administered. A prophylactic antibiotic, usually a first-generation cephalosporin, is administered before the procedure. The fiberoptic gastroscope is inserted into the stomach, which is then insufflated with air. The lights are dimmed, and the assistant applies digital pressure to the anterior abdominal wall in the left subcostal area approximately 2 cm below the costal margin, looking for the brightest transillumination. The endoscopist should be able to clearly identify the indentation in the stomach created by the assistant's digital pressure on the anterior abdominal wall; otherwise, another site should be chosen. When the correct spot has been identified, the assistant anesthetizes the anterior abdominal wall. The endoscopist then introduces a polypectomy snare through the endoscope. A small incision is made in the skin, and the assistant introduces a large-bore catheter-needle stylet assembly into the stomach and through the snare. The snare is then tightened securely around the catheter. The inner stylet is removed, and a looped insertion wire is introduced through the catheter and into the stomach. The cannula is slowly withdrawn so the snare grasps the wire. The gastroscope is then pulled out of the patient's mouth with the wire firmly grasped by the snare. The end of the transgastric wire exiting the patient's mouth is then tied to a prepared gastrostomy tube. The assistant pulls on the end of the wire exiting from the abdominal wall while the endoscopist guides the lubricated gastrostomy tube into the posterior pharynx and the esophagus. With continued traction, the gastrostomy tube is pulled into the stomach so that it exits on the anterior abdominal wall. The gastroscope is reinserted into the stomach to confirm adequate placement of the gastrostomy tube against the gastric mucosa and to document that no bleeding has occurred. The intraluminal portion of the tube should contact the mucosa, but excessive tension on the tube should be avoided because this can lead to ischemic necrosis of the gastric wall. The tube is secured to the abdominal wall using sutures. Feedings may be initiated immediately after the procedure or 24 hours later.

Push Technique. The push technique method is similar to the pull technique. The gastroscope is inserted and a point on the anterior abdominal wall localized, as for the pull technique. Rather than introducing a looped insertion wire, however, a straight guidewire is snared and brought out through the patient's mouth by withdrawing the endoscope and snare together. A commercially developed gastrostomy tube (Sachs-Vine) with a tapered end is then passed in an aboral direction over the wire, which is held taut. The tube is grasped and pulled the rest of the way out. The gastroscope is reinserted to check the position and tension on the tube.

Introducer Technique. The introducer technique method uses a peel-away introducer technique originally developed for the placement of cardiac pacemakers and central venous catheters. The gastroscope is inserted into the stomach, and an appropriate position for placement of the tube is identified. After infiltration of the skin with local anesthetic, a 16- or 18-gauge needle is introduced into the stomach. A J-tipped guidewire is inserted through the needle into the stomach and the needle is withdrawn. Using a twisting motion, a 16-Fr introducer with a peel-away sheath is passed over the guidewire into the gastric lumen [40,41]. The guidewire and introducer are removed, leaving in place the sheath that allows placement of a 14-Fr Foley catheter. The sheath is peeled away after the balloon is inflated with 10 mL of normal saline.

Percutaneous Endoscopic Gastrostomy/Jejunostomy. If postpyloric feeding is desired (especially in patients at high risk for pulmonary aspiration), a percutaneous endoscopic gastrostomy (PEG)/jejunostomy may be performed. The tube allows simultaneous gastric decompression and duodenal/jejunal enteral feeding [42–45]. A second smaller feeding tube can be attached and passed through the gastrostomy tube and advanced endoscopically into the duodenum or jejunum. When the PEG is in position, a guidewire is passed through it and grasped using endoscopy forceps. The guidewire and endoscope are passed into the duodenum as distally as possible. The jejunal tube is then passed over the guidewire through the PEG into the distal duodenum and advanced into the jejunum, and the endoscope is withdrawn. An alternative method is to grasp a suture at the tip of the feeding tube or the distal tip of the tube itself and pass the tube into the duodenum using forceps advanced through the biopsy channel of the endoscope. This obviates the need to pass the gastroscope into the duodenum, which may result in dislodgment of the tube when the endoscope is withdrawn.

Fluoroscopic Technique. Percutaneous gastrostomy and gastrojejunostomy can also be performed using fluoroscopy [46,47]. The stomach is insufflated with air using a nasogastric tube or a skinny needle if the patient is obstructed proximally. Once the stomach is distended and position is checked again with fluoroscopy, the stomach is punctured with an 18-gauge needle. A heavy-duty wire is passed and the tract is dilated to 7 Fr. A gastrostomy tube may then be inserted into the stomach. An angiographic catheter is introduced and manipulated through the pylorus. The percutaneous tract is then further dilated, and the gastrojejunostomy tube is advanced as far as possible.

Complications. The most common complication after percutaneous placement of enteral feeding tubes is infection, usually involving the cutaneous exit site and surrounding tissue [48]. Gastrointestinal hemorrhage has been reported but is usually due to excessive tension on the tube, leading to necrosis of the stomach wall. Gastrocolic fistulas, which develop if the colon is interposed between the anterior abdominal wall and stomach when the needle is introduced, have been reported. Adequate transillumination aids in avoiding this complication. Separation of the stomach from the anterior abdominal wall can occur, resulting in peritonitis when enteral feeding is initiated. In most instances, this complication is caused by excessive tension on the gastrostomy tube. Another potential complication is pneumoperitoneum, secondary to air escaping after puncture of the stomach during the procedure, and is usually clinically insignificant. If the patient develops fever and abdominal tenderness, a Gastrografin study should be obtained to exclude the presence of a leak.

All percutaneous gastrostomy and jejunostomy procedures described above have been established as safe and effective. The method is selected based on the endoscopist's experience and training and the patient's nutritional needs.

SURGICAL PROCEDURES. Since the advent of PEG, surgical placement of enteral feeding tubes is usually performed as a concomitant procedure as the last phase of a laparotomy performed for another indication. Occasionally, an operation solely for tube placement is performed in patients requiring permanent tube feedings when a percutaneous approach is contraindicated or unsuccessful. In these cases, the laparoscopic approach to enteral access should be considered [49]. Laparoscopic gastrostomy was introduced in 2000, 10 years after the PEG. Patients who are not candidates for PEG, due to head and neck cancer, esophageal obstruction, large hiatal hernia, gastric volvulus, or overlying intestine or liver, should be considered for laparoscopic gastrostomy or jejunostomy.

Gastrostomy. Gastrostomy is a simple procedure when performed as part of another intraabdominal operation. It should be considered when prolonged enteral nutritional support is anticipated after surgery.

Complications are quite common after surgical gastrostomy. This may reflect the poor nutritional status and associated medical problems in many patients who undergo this proce-

dure. Potential complications include wound infection, dehiscence, gastrostomy disruption, internal or external leakage, gastric hemorrhage, and tube migration.

Needle-Catheter Jejunostomy. The needle-catheter jejunostomy procedure consists of the insertion of a small (5-Fr) polyethylene catheter into the small intestine at the time of laparotomy for another indication. Kits containing the necessary equipment for the procedure are available from commercial suppliers (e.g., Vivonex). A needle is used to create a submucosal tunnel from the serosa to the mucosa on the antimesenteric border of the jejunum. A catheter is inserted through the needle, and then the needle is removed. The catheter is brought out through the anterior abdominal wall, and the limb of jejunum is secured to the anterior abdominal wall with sutures. The tube can be used for feeding immediately after the operation. The potential complications are similar to those associated with gastrostomy, but patients may have a higher incidence of diarrhea. Occlusion of the needle-catheter jejunostomy is common because of its small luminal diameter, and elemental nutritional formulas are preferentially used.

Transgastric Jejunostomy. Critically ill patients who undergo laparotomy commonly require gastric decompression and a surgically placed tube for enteral nutritional support. Routine placement of separate gastrostomy and jejunostomy tubes is common in this patient population and achieves the objective of chronic gastric decompression and early initiation of enteral nutritional support through the jejunostomy. Technical advances in surgically placed enteral feeding tubes led to the development of transgastric jejunostomy [50] and duodenostomy tubes, which allow simultaneous decompression of the stomach and distal feeding into the duodenum or jejunum. The advantage of these tubes is that only one enterotomy into the stomach is needed, eliminating the possible complications associated with open jejunostomy tube placement. In addition, only one tube is necessary for gastric decompression and jejunal feeding, eliminating the potential complications of two separate tubes for this purpose. The transgastric jejunostomy tube is placed surgically in the same manner as a gastrostomy tube, and the distal portion of the tube is advanced manually through the pylorus into the duodenum, with its final tip resting as far distally as possible in the duodenum or jejunum (Fig. 19-3). The transgastric jejunostomy tube is preferred to transgastric duodenostomy tubes because it is associated with less reflux of feedings into the stomach and a decreased risk of aspiration pneumonia. Surgical placement of transgastric jejunostomy tubes at the time of lap-

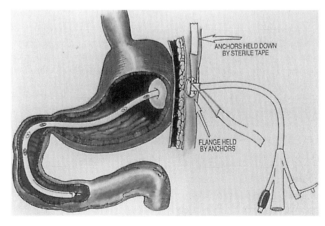

Fig. 19-3. Transgastric duodenal feeding tube, which allows simultaneous gastric decompression and duodenal feeding, can be placed percutaneously (with endoscopic or fluoroscopic assistance) or surgically.

arotomy is recommended for patients who will likely require prolonged gastric decompression and enteral feeding.

Delivering the Tube Feeding Formula

The enteral formula can be delivered by intermittent bolus feeding, gravity infusion, or continuous pump infusion.

In the intermittent bolus method, the patient receives 300 to 400 mL of formula every 4 to 6 hours. The bolus is usually delivered with the aid of a catheter-tipped, large-volume (60-mL) syringe. The main advantage of bolus feeding is simplicity. This approach is often used for patients requiring prolonged supplemental enteral nutritional support after discharge from the hospital. Bolus feeding can be associated with serious side effects, however. Bolus enteral feeding into the stomach can cause gastric distention, nausea, cramping, and aspiration. The intermittent bolus method should not be used when feeding into the duodenum or jejunum because boluses of formula can cause distention, cramping, and diarrhea.

Gravity-infusion systems allow the formula to drip continuously over 16 to 24 hours or intermittently over 20 to 30 minutes, four to six times per day. This method requires constant monitoring because the flow rate can be extremely irregular. The main advantages of this approach are simplicity, low cost, and close simulation of a normal feeding pattern.

Continuous pump infusion is the preferred method for the delivery of enteral nutrition in the critically ill patient. A peristaltic pump can be used to provide a continuous infusion of formula at a precisely controlled flow rate: This decreases problems with distention and diarrhea. Gastric residuals tend to be smaller with continuous pump-fed infusions, and the risk of aspiration may be decreased. In adult burn patients, continuous feedings are associated with less stool frequency and shorter time to achieve nutritional goals [51].

Medications

When medications are administered via an enteric feeding tube, it is important to be certain the drugs are compatible with each other and with the enteral formula. In general, medications should be delivered separately rather than as a combined bolus. For medications that are better absorbed in an empty stomach, tube feedings should be suspended for 30 to 60 minutes before administration.

Medications should be administered in an elixir formulation via enteral feeding tubes whenever possible to prevent occlusion of the tube. Enteral tubes should always be flushed with 20 mL of saline after medications are administered. To use an enteral feeding tube to administer medications dispensed in tablet form, often the pills must be crushed and delivered as slurry mixed with water. This is inappropriate for some medications, however, such as those absorbed sublingually or formulated as a sustained-released tablet or capsule.

Complications

Enteral tube placement is associated with few complications if physicians adhere to appropriate protocols and pay close attention to the details of the procedures.

NASOPULMONARY INTUBATION. Passage of an enteral feeding tube into the tracheobronchial tree most commonly occurs in patients with diminished cough or gag reflexes due to obtundation, altered mental status, or other causes [52]. The presence of a tracheostomy or endotracheal tube does not guarantee proper placement. A chest (or upper abdominal) radiograph should always be obtained before initiating tube 'feedings with a new tube to ensure that the tube is properly positioned. Endotracheal or transpulmonary placement of a feeding tube can be associated with pneumothorax, hydrothorax, pneumonia, and abscess formation. Capnography should be considered to prevent inadvertent placement of small-bore feeding tubes into the lungs [23,24].

ASPIRATION. Pulmonary aspiration is a serious and potentially fatal complication of enteral nutritional support [53,54]. The incidence of this complication is variable and depends on the patient population studied. The two most common bedside tests for detecting aspiration in tube-fed patients include adding dye to the formula and observing for its appearance in tracheobronchial secretions, and using glucose oxidase reagent strips to test tracheobronchial secretions for glucose-containing enteral formula [55]. Several studies indicate that the dye method is far less sensitive than the glucose method, but the glucose method lacks specificity. A patented technique for adding color to nutritional formulas without pouring, mixing, or injecting dye is now available (Colormark, Ross Products, Columbus, OH, http://www.ross.com). This dye set contains a total of 250 mg of blue dye, of which approximately 220 mg is released, at a rate of 10 mg per hour of feeding, and can be used for patients weighing 25 kg or more. It also prevents inadvertent bacterial contamination of enteral feeds that can occur with multi-use bottles of blue dye.

Major risk factors for aspiration include obtundation or altered mental status, absence of cough or gag reflexes, delayed gastric emptying, gastroesophageal reflux, and feeding in the supine position. The risk of pulmonary aspiration is minimized when the enteral feeding tube is positioned in the jejunum past the ligament of Treitz.

GASTROINTESTINAL INTOLERANCE. Delayed gastric emptying is sometimes improved by administering the prokinetic agents metoclopramide (10 to 20 mg IV) or erythromycin (200 mg IV). Dumping syndrome (i.e., diarrhea, distention, and abdominal cramping) can limit the use of enteral feeding. Dumping may be caused by delivering a hyperosmotic load into the small intestine.

Diarrhea in critically ill patients should not be attributed to intolerance of enteral feeding until other causes are excluded. Other possible etiologies for diarrhea include medications (e.g., magnesium-containing antacids, quinidine), alterations in gut microflora due to prolonged antibiotic therapy, antibiotic-associated colitis, ischemic colitis, viral or bacterial enteric infection, electrolyte abnormalities, and excessive delivery of bile salts into the colon. Diarrhea can also be a manifestation of intestinal malabsorption because of enzyme deficiencies or villous atrophy [56].

Even if diarrhea is caused by enteral feeding, it can be controlled in nearly 50% of cases by instituting a continuous infusion of formula (if bolus feedings are used), slowing the rate of infusion, changing the formula, adding fiber to the enteral formula, or adding antidiarrheal agents (e.g., tincture of opium) [57].

METABOLIC COMPLICATIONS. Prerenal azotemia and hypernatremia can develop in patients fed with hyperosmolar solutions. The administration of free water, either added to the formula or as separate boluses to replace obligatory losses, can avert this situation. Deficiencies of essential fatty acids and fat-soluble vitamins can develop after prolonged support with enteral solutions that contain minimal amounts of fat. Periodic enteral supplementation with linoleic acid or IV supplementation with emulsified fat (Intralipid) can prevent this [58]. The amount of linoleic acid necessary to prevent chemical and clinical fatty acid deficiency has been estimated to be 2.5 to 20.0 g per day.

BACTERIAL CONTAMINATION. Bacterial contamination of enteral solutions [59–61] occurs when commercial packages are opened and mixed with other substances. The risk of contamination also depends on the duration of feeding. Tube feeding formulas have been implicated in causing *Pseudomonas* and *Enterobacter* sepsis [62]. Contaminated formula also appears to play a significant role in the etiology of diarrhea in patients receiving enteral nutrition [61].

OCCLUDED FEEDING TUBES. Precipitation of certain proteins when exposed to an acid pH may be an important factor leading to the solidifying of formulas [63]. Most premixed intact protein formulas solidify when acidified to a pH less than 5. To prevent occlusion of feeding tubes, the tube should be flushed with saline before and after checking residuals. Small-caliber nasoenteric feeding tubes should be flushed with 20 mL of saline every 4 to 6 hours to prevent tube occlusion, even when enteral feedings are administered by continuous infusion.

Medications are a frequent cause of clogging. When administering medications enterally, liquid elixirs should be used, if available, because even tiny particles of crushed tablets can occlude the distal orifice of small-caliber feeding tubes. If tablets are used, it is important to crush them to a fine powder and solubilize them in liquid before administration. In addition, tubes should be flushed with saline before and after the administration of any medications.

Several maneuvers are useful for clearing a clogged feeding tube. The tube can be irrigated with warm saline, a carbonated liquid, cranberry juice, or an enzyme solution (e.g., Viokase). Commonly, a mixture of lipase, amylase, and protease (Pancrease) dissolved in sodium bicarbonate solution (for enzyme activation) is instilled into the tube with a syringe and the tube clamped for approximately 30 minutes to allow enzymatic degradation of precipitated enteral feedings. The tube is then vigorously flushed with saline. The pancreatic enzyme solution was successful in restoring tube patency in 96% of cases where formula clotting was the likely cause of occlusion and use of Coke or water had failed [64]. Prevention of tube clogging with flushes and pancreatic enzyme are therefore the methods of choice in maintenance of chronic enteral feeding tubes.

References

1. Koruda MJ, Guenter P, Rombeau JL: Enteral nutrition in the critically ill. *Crit Care Clin* 3:133, 1987.
2. Baker JP, Lemoyne M: Nutritional support in the critically ill patient: if, when, how, and what. *Crit Care Clin* 3:97, 1987.
3. McCarthy MC: Nutritional support in the critically ill surgical patient. *Surg Clin North Am* 71:831, 1991.
4. Koretz RL: Nutritional supplementation in the ICU: how critical is nutrition for the critically ill? *Am J Respir Crit Care Med* 151:570, 1995.
5. DeLegge MH: Enteral access—the foundation of feeding. *JPEN J Parenter Enteral Nutr* 25;(2 Suppl):S8, 2001.
6. Napolitano LM, Bochicchio G: Enteral feeding in the critically ill. *Curr Opin Crit Care* 6:1, 2000.
7. Napolitano LM, Baker CC: Bacterial translocation: fact or fancy? *Adv Trauma Crit Care* 7:79, 1992.
8. Alverdy JC, Aoys E, Moss G: Total parenteral nutrition promotes bacterial translocation from the gut. *Surgery* 104:185, 1988.
9. Li J, Kudsk KA, Gocinski B, et al: Effects of parenteral and enteral nutrition on gut-associated lymphoid tissue. *J Trauma* 39:44, 1995.
10. Moore FA, Moore EE, Jones TN, et al: TEN versus TPN following major abdominal trauma—reduced septic morbidity. *J Trauma* 29:916, 1989.
11. Moore FA, Feliciano DV, Andrassy RJ, et al: Early enteral feeding, compared with parenteral, reduces postoperative septic complications: the results of a meta-analysis. *Ann Surg* 216:172, 1992.
12. Kudsk KA, Croce MA, Fabian TC, et al: Enteral vs. parenteral feeding: effects on septic morbidity following blunt and penetrating abdominal trauma. *Ann Surg* 215:503, 1992.
12a. Edlich RT, Lande AJ, Goodale RL, et al: Prevention of aspiration pneumonia by continuous esophageal aspiration during esophagogastric tamponade and gastric cooling. *Surgery* 64:405, 1968.
13. Beale RJ, Bryg DJ, Bihari DJ: Immunonutrition in the critically ill: a systematic review of clinical outcome. *Crit Care Med* 27:2799, 1999.
14. Heys SD, Walker LG, Smith I, et al: Enteral nutritional supplementation with key nutrients in patients with critical illness and cancer: a meta-analysis of randomized controlled clinical trials. *Ann Surg* 299:467, 1999.
15. Heyland DK, Novak F, Drover JW, et al: Should immunonutrition become routine in critically ill patients? A systematic review of the evidence. *JAMA* 286:944, 2001.
16. Galban C, Montejo JC, Mesejo A, et al: An immune-enhancing enteral diet reduces mortality rate and episodes of bacteremia in septic intensive care unit patients. *Crit Care Med* 28:643, 2000.
17. Ritz MA, Fraser R, Edwards N, et al: Delayed gastric emptying in ventilated critically ill patients: measurement by 13 C-octanoic acid breath test. *Crit Care Med* 29:1744, 2001.
18. Esparza J, Boivin MA, Hartshorne MF, et al: Equal aspiration rates in gastrically and transpylorically fed critically ill patients. *Intensive Care Med* 27:660, 2001.
19. Montecalvo MA, Steger KA, Farber HW, et al: Nutritional outcome and pneumonia in critical care patients randomized to gastric versus jejunal tube feedings. The Critical Care Research Team. *Crit Care Med* 20:1377, 1992.
20. Gauderer MWL, Stellato TA: Gastrostomies: evolution, techniques, indications and complications. *Curr Probl Surg* 23:657, 1986.
21. Raakow R, Hintze R, Schmidt S, et al: The laparoscopic Janeway gastrostomy. An alternative technique when percutaneous endoscopic gastrostomy is impractical. *Endoscopy* 33:610, 2001.
22. Boyes RJ, Kruse JA: Nasogastric and nasoenteric intubation. *Crit Care Clin* 8:865, 1992.
23. Bruns SM, Carpenter R, Truwit JD: Report on the development of a procedure to prevent placement of feeding tubes into the lungs using end-tidal CO₂ measurements. *Crit Care Med* 29:936, 2001.
24. Kindopp AS, Drover JW, Heyland DK: Capnography confirms correct feeding tube placement in intensive care unit patients. *Can J Anesth* 48:705, 2001.
25. Boivin MA, Levy H: Gastric feeding with erythromycin is equivalent to transpyloric feeding in the critically ill. *Crit Care Med* 29:1916, 2001.
26. Boivin M, Levy H, Hayes J: A multicenter, prospective study of the placement of transpyloric feeding tubes with assistance of a magnetic device. The Magnet-Guided Enteral Feeding Tube Study Group. *JPEN J Parenter Enteral Nutr* 24:304, 2000.
27. Lord LM, Weiser-Maimone A, Pulhamus M, et al: Comparison of weighted vs unweighted enteral feeding tubes for efficacy of transpyloric intubation. *JPEN J Parenter Enteral Nutr* 17:271, 1993.
28. Kalliafas S, Choban PS, Ziegler D, et al: Erythromycin facilitates postpyloric placement of nasoduodenal feeding tubes in intensive care unit patients: randomized, double-blinded, placebo-controlled trial. *JPEN J Parenter Enteral Nutr* 20:385, 1996.
29. Zaloga GP: Bedside method for placing small bowel feeding tubes in critically ill patients. A prospective study. *Chest* 100:1643, 1991.

30. Paz HL, Weinar M, Sherman MS: Motility agents for the placement of weighted and unweighted feeding tubes in critically ill patients. *Intensive Care Med* 22:301, 1996.

31. Pleatman MA, Naunheim KS: Endoscopic placement of feeding tubes in the critically ill patient. *Surg Gynecol Obstet* 165:69, 1987.

32. Mathus-Vliegen EM, Tytgat GN, Merkus MP: Feeding tubes in endoscopic and clinical practice: the longer the better? *Gastrointest Endosc* 39:537, 1993.

33. Hudspeth DA, Thorne MT, Meredith JW: A simple endoscopic technique for nasoenteric feeding tube placement. *J Am Coll Surg* 180:229, 1995.

34. Vaswani SK, Clarkston WK: Endoscopic nasoenteral feeding tube placement following cardiothoracic surgery. *Am Surg* 62:421, 1996.

35. Napolitano LM, Wagel M, Heard SO: Endoscopic placement of nasoenteric feeding tubes in critically ill patients: a reliable alternative. *J Laparoendosc Adv Surg Tech* 8:395, 1998.

36. Kulling D, Bauerfeind P, Fried M: Transnasal versus transoral endoscopy for the placement of nasoenteral feeding tubes in critically ill patients. *Gastrointest Endosc* 52:506, 2000.

37. Ponsky JL, Gauderer MWL, Stellato TA, et al: Percutaneous approaches to enteral alimentation. *Am J Surg* 149:102, 1985.

38. Kozarek RA, Ball RJ, Ryan JA: When push comes to shove: a comparison between two methods of percutaneous endoscopic gastrostomy. *Am J Gastroenterol* 81:642, 1986.

39. De Vivo P, Mastronardi P, Ciritella P, et al: Early percutaneous endoscopic gastrostomy (PEG). A safe and effective enteral feeding technique in neurologic intensive care unit. *Minerva Anestesiol* 62:197, 1996.

40. Dormann AJ, Glosemeyer R, Leistner U, et al: Modified percutaneous endoscopic gastrostomy (PEG) with gastropexy—early experience with a new introducer technique. *Z Gastroenterol* 38:933, 2000.

41. Deitel M, Bendago M, Spratt EH, et al: Percutaneous endoscopic gastrostomy by the "pull" and "introducer" methods. *Can J Surg* 31:102, 1988.

42. Duckworth PF Jr, Kirby DF, McHenry L: Percutaneous endoscopic gastrojejunostomy made easy: a simplified endoscopic technique. *Gastrointest Endosc* 37:241, 1991.

43. Baskin WN: Advances in enteral nutrition techniques: clinical review. *Am J Gastroenterol* 87:1547, 1992.

44. Stellato TA: Endoscopic intervention for enteral access. *World J Surg* 16:1042, 1992.

45. Henderson JM, Strodel WE, Gilinsky NH: Limitations of percutaneous endoscopic jejunostomy. *JPEN J Parenter Enteral Nutr* 17:546, 1993.

46. Ho SG, Marchinkow LO, Legiehn GM, et al: Radiological percutaneous gastrostomy. *Clin Radiol* 56:902, 2001.

47. Giuliano AW, Yoon HC, Lomis NN, et al: Fluoroscopically guided percutaneous placement of large-bore gastrostomy and gastrojejunostomy tubes: review of 109 cases. *J Vasc Interv Radiol* 11:239, 2001.

48. Schurink CA, Tuynman H, Scholten P, et al: Percutaneous endoscopic gastrostomy: complications and suggestion to avoid them. *Eur J Gastroenterol Hepatol* 13:819, 2001.

49. Edelman DS: Laparoendoscopic approaches to enteral access. *Semin Laparosc Surg* 8:195, 2001.

50. Shapiro T, Minard G, Kudsk KA: Transgastric jejunal feeding tubes in critically ill patients. *Nutr Clin Pract* 12:164, 1997.

51. Hiebert J, Brown A, Anderson R, et al: Comparison of continuous vs intermittent tube feedings in adult burn patients. *JPEN J Parenter Enteral Nutr* 5:73, 1981.

52. Rassias AJ, Ball PA, Corwin HL: A prospective study of tracheopulmonary complications associated with the placement of narrow-bore enteral feeding tubes. *Crit Care* 2:25, 1998.

53. Mullan H, Roubenoff RA, Roubenoff R: Risk of pulmonary aspiration among patients receiving enteral nutrition support. *JPEN J Parenter Enteral Nutr* 16:160, 1992.

54. Olivares L, Segovia A, Revuelta R: Tube feeding and lethal aspiration in neurological patients: a review of 720 autopsy cases. *Stroke* 5:654, 1974.

55. Metheny NA, Clouse RE: Bedside methods for detecting aspiration in tube-fed patients. *Chest* 111:724, 1997.

56. Ringel AF, Jameson GL, Foster ES: Diarrhea in the intensive care patient. *Crit Care Clin* 11:465, 1995.

57. Niemiec PN, Vanderveen TW, Morrison JT, et al: Gastrointestinal disorders caused by medication and electrolytes solution osmolarity during enteral nutrition. *JPEN J Parenter Enteral Nutr* 7:387, 1983.

58. Dodge JA, Yassa JG: Essential fatty acids deficiency after prolonged treatment with elemental diet. *Lancet* 2:192, 1975.

59. Beattie TK, Anderton A: Decanting versus sterile pre-filled nutrient containers—the microbiological risks in enteral feeding. *Int J Environ Health Res* 11:81, 2001.

60. McKinlay J, Wildgoose A, Wood W, et al: The effect of system design on bacterial contamination of enteral tube feeds. *J Hosp Infect* 47:138, 2001.

61. Okuma T, Nakamura M, Totake H, et al: Microbial contamination of enteral feeding formulas and diarrhea. *Nutrition* 16:719, 2000.

62. Casewell M, Cooper J, Webster M: Enteral feeds contamination with Enterobacter cloacae as a cause of septicemia. *BMJ* 282:973, 1981.

63. Perkins AM, Marcuard SP: Clogging of feeding tubes. *JPEN J Parenter Enteral Nutr* 12:403, 1988.

64. Marcuard SP, Stegall KS: Unclogging feeding tubes with pancreatic enzyme. *JPEN J Parenter Enteral Nutr* 14:198, 1990.

20. *Therapeutic Hemapheresis*

Irma O. Szymanski and Brian E. Moore

The usefulness of hemapheresis, or selective removal of a specific blood component, first became apparent in the 1960s, when it was demonstrated that the hyperviscosity syndrome of Waldenström's macroglobulinemia could be effectively treated with removal of a patient's plasma [1]. Subsequently, the removal of a cellular component was developed as a therapeutic modality, including erythrocytapheresis, plateletpheresis, and leukapheresis. Our understanding of the usefulness of therapeutic hemapheresis has improved greatly in recent years. This chapter focuses on the latest concepts regarding the mechanism, indications, and adverse effects of hemapheresis.

Mechanism

The principle behind hemapheresis is simple: Relief is obtained by reduction of the blood component causing the symptoms. *Cytapheresis* involves partial removal of a cellular blood compo-

Table 20-1. Indications for Therapeutic Cytapheresis

Procedure	Disease	Indications
Erythrocytapheresis	Sickle cell disease	Unrelenting crises, pregnancy, acute pulmonary syndromes, renal artery occlusions, intrahepatic cholestasis, priapism
Leukapheresis	Acute myelogenous leukemia	To relieve leukostasis when blast count is >100,000/mm^3
	Chronic myelogenous leukemia	To relieve leukostasis when white blood cell count is >200,000/mm^3
Plateletpheresis	Thrombocytosis	To prevent thrombosis or hemorrhage when platelet count is >1,000,000/mm^3

nent. *Erythrocytapheresis* during sickle cell crisis relieves symptoms by replacing sickled cells with normal donor red blood cells. *Leukapheresis* provides symptomatic relief for patients with acute myelogenous leukemia by reducing the excessive numbers of blast cells (greater than or equal to 100,000 per mm^3), which cause sludging of blood flow. In chronic myelogenous leukemia, it is desirable to keep the white blood cell count below 200,000 per mm^3. Plateletpheresis in cases of thrombocytosis (platelet count greater than 1 million per mm^3) significantly reduces the chance of thrombosis (Table 20-1). Because a large volume of plasma is removed in therapeutic plasma exchange, it must be replaced with appropriate fluid to maintain a constant blood volume. To avoid allogenic, plasma-induced adverse effects, 5% albumin is the usual replacement fluid during most plasma exchange procedures. When the disease is associated with a deficiency of a certain plasma protein, as in thrombotic thrombocytopenic purpura TTP), allogenic plasma must be used as a replacement fluid.

Centrifugation is the most common technique used to separate a specific blood component from others, but plasma can also be isolated from whole blood by filtration. The latter method is not used commonly in the United States, although it is popular in Western Europe and Japan [2].

Although the first hemapheresis treatments were done by manual methods, now most institutions use automated blood processing machines for this purpose. The most commonly used device, the Cobe Spectra apheresis system (Gambro BCT, Lakewood, CO), uses a 180-mL separation channel resembling a hollow belt. As the belt turns in the centrifuge, anticoagulated whole blood flows into one end. During the centrifugal journey, the blood components settle into layers according to their specific gravity. Red blood cells, being the densest, settle at the outer wall of the belt, with white blood cells, platelets, and plasma forming the other successive layers toward the center. The components are harvested through segments of tubing that join the belt at right angles to the inner wall. Each procedure is automated and individualized according to the size of a patient's blood and plasma volume, quantity of the blood component to be removed, and type of replacement fluid used. Because the extracorporeal volume is small, this machine allows for hemapheresis to be performed safely in children and small adults and is generally preferred for less-stable intensive care unit patients.

REMOVAL OF A SPECIFIC PLASMA COMPONENT. Removal of only the pathologic plasma constituent, rather than whole plasma, theoretically would be the most efficient way of performing therapeutic plasma exchange. With the aid of various devices it is possible to remove immune complexes, immunoglobulins, specific antibodies, or low-density lipoprotein (LDL) from separated plasma and return the processed plasma to the patient, without a need to administer other replacement fluids.

The Prosorba column (Cypress Bioscience, Inc., San Diego, CA), designed to remove circulating immune complexes and immunoglobulin G from plasma, has been approved by the U.S. Food and Drug Administration for treatment of intractable idiopathic thrombocytopenic purpura, including that induced by the human immunodeficiency virus [3]. A column contains 200 mg of purified staphylococcal protein A, covalently coupled to an inert silica matrix. Protein A has a high avidity for the Fc portion of immunoglobulin G, particularly in the immune-complexed state. Plasma flowing through the column is therefore largely purified of immune complexes. It is believed that circulating immune complexes suppress the development of antiidiotypes, which blunt the formation of harmful autoantibodies. Data show that after Prosorba treatment, titers of autoantibody (idiotype) decreased and those of antiidiotype increased in plasma of patients with idiopathic thrombocytopenic purpura [3]. Therefore, this treatment is thought to modulate and normalize the immune response.

Excorim AB (Lund, Sweden) developed a device that removes large amounts of circulating immune complexes and immunoglobulin G from plasma. It consists of a set of two small columns that can be regenerated after use. While the patient's plasma is passed through one column to absorb immunoglobulins, the other is regenerated using a special elution procedure. The system is now manufactured in the United States by Fresenius Medical Care North America (Lexington, MA) for use in the treatment of patients with hemophilia A and B who have factor VIII or factor IX antibody titers above 10 Bethesda units per mL.

LDL apheresis is designed to remove apolipoprotein B–containing lipoproteins from the plasma of patients with familial hypercholesterolemia. Available methods include heparin-induced extracorporeal LDL precipitation, heparin-agarose adsorption, columns containing immobilized antibodies to LDL, and columns containing dextran sulfate cellulose [4]. LDL apheresis is effective in reducing atherosclerosis, but owing to the prolonged regimen, the therapy is quite expensive.

VASCULAR ACCESS. Good vascular access is essential for hemapheresis. At least one good antecubital vein is required to draw whole blood through a 17-gauge cannula. The processed blood can be returned to a smaller vein in the opposite arm through an indwelling catheter. If peripheral access cannot be obtained, a femoral or subclavian catheter may be used. The selection of an appropriate catheter is important to permit rapid, continuous blood flow, as thin, pliable catheters tend to collapse during blood withdrawal. We have had good experience with the Mahurkar dual-lumen polyurethane catheter (11.5 French, 19.5 cm in length; Quinton, Mansfield, MA) inserted into the subclavian vein. The subclavian catheter can be left in place for up to 4 weeks. Acu Flex-FSN (Gambro BCT), a 5.5-in., double-lumen catheter, is excellent for femoral vein blood access and can be left in place for 3 to 4 days.

Indications

The efficacy of hemapheresis in treating various diseases may be demonstrated by means of randomized, controlled clinical trials or by showing that removal of a blood component is associated with improvement in the patient's condition. However, reduction in the concentration of a pathogenic protein is not always associated with clinical improvement. This could have many explanations; for example, the damage done by an antibody could have been irreversible, or the avidity of an antibody to its target tissue may be high even when its plasma concentration is low. Finally, decrease in the concentration of specific antibodies by plasma removal is thought to cause a rebound phenomenon in antibody synthesis [5]. Orlin and Berkman [6] showed that although the concentration of immunoglobulins was 40% of the initial value on the tenth day after plasmapheresis, anti-A at that time had 100% agglutinating activity, indicating either enhanced synthesis or production of anti-A of high avidity.

Because it is expensive, invasive, and time-consuming, hemapheresis should only be used in conditions for which it has an established benefit. Indications for therapeutic cytapheresis are listed in Table 20-1 [7]. These procedures should be repeated as necessary to relieve symptoms or to reach a target cell value. Diseases in which therapeutic plasma exchange is considered either primary or supplemental therapy are shown in Table 20-2 [8]. The following section addresses the uses of therapeutic plasma exchange in disorders encountered in the intensive care unit. The recommended schedules and therapeutic end-points in some of those diseases are shown in Table 20-3.

ACUTE GUILLAIN-BARRÉ SYNDROME. Guillain-Barré syndrome (GBS) is an acute ascending polyneuropathy thought to be caused by an antibody to myelin. A controlled clinical trial comparing plasma exchange to standard therapy for GBS appeared in 1985 [9]. This study of 245 patients found statistically significant differences favoring plasma exchange in the following recovery parameters: improvement at 4 weeks, time to improve one clinical grade, time to independent walking, and outcome at 6 months. In general, patients treated with plasma exchange spent less time in the intensive care unit and hospital. Patients who were treated within 7 days of onset of the symptoms fared better than patients whose treatment was started later. The replacement fluid, as a rule, was 5% albumin. A French study published in 1987 confirmed the beneficial effects of plasma exchange, although the volume of plasma exchanged was slightly greater and the composition of the replacement solution was different (including intravenous immunoglobulin) [10]. In some patients, fresh-frozen plasma was used, and this was associated with more complications (e.g., fever, skin rash, hepatitis) [10]. A report from the Netherlands indicated that intravenous immunoglobulin is as effective as plasma exchange in the treatment of GBS [11]. Although initially the symptoms of some patients in the United States worsened after immunoglobulin infusions [12], currently most neurologists use intravenous immunoglobulin as first-line therapy for acute GBS [13]. According to the literature and in the authors' experience, plasma exchange is also effective in ameliorating symptoms of the Miller-Fisher variant (ophthalmoplegia) of GBS [14].

MYASTHENIA GRAVIS. Myasthenia gravis is a fluctuating weakness of voluntary muscles caused by an antibody to the

Table 20-2. Effectiveness of Plasma Exchange Therapy in Various Diseases

Standard, primary therapy
  Thrombotic thrombocytopenic purpura
  Posttransfusion purpura
  Acute Guillain-Barré syndrome
  Chronic idiopathic demyelinating polyradiculopathy
  Myasthenia gravis in crisis
  Goodpasture's syndrome
  Refsum's disease (phytanic acid storage disease)
  Familial hypercholesterolemia (via selective adsorption)
Adjunctive therapy
  Hyperviscosity syndrome
  Hemolytic uremic syndrome
  Cold agglutinin disease
  Cryoglobulinemia (antineutrophil cytoplasmic antibody–positive)
  Coagulation factor inhibitors, refractory to other therapy
  HELLP (*h*emolysis, *e*levated *l*iver enzymes, and *l*ow *p*latelet count) syndrome, postpartum
  Renal failure with myeloma
  Pemphigus vulgaris
  Eaton-Lambert myasthenic syndrome
  Pediatric autoimmune neuropsychiatric disorders associated with streptococcal infections
  Sydenham's chorea

Based in part on McLeod BC: Introduction to the third special issue: clinical applications of therapeutic apheresis. *J Clin Apheresis* 15:1, 2000.

postsynaptic anticholinesterase receptor. Plasma exchange therapy is indicated in myasthenic crises, rapidly progressive disease (especially with uncontrolled bulbar or respiratory muscle compromise), preparation for thymectomy or a worsening condition after thymectomy, as an alternative therapy in cases in which corticosteroid therapy is contraindicated, as a means to decrease the dose of corticosteroids in patients having unacceptable side effects, and in patients who are refractory to other treatment modalities [15]. When therapeutic plasma exchange is used for these indications, improvement is usually rapid. Patients may require administration of their usual medication (e.g., pyridostigmine or neostigmine) during the procedure to maintain therapeutic drug concentrations.

Acetylcholine esterase receptor antibodies can be removed by passing plasma over a polyvinyl alcohol gel, to which either tryptophane or phenylalanine has been linked covalently (Immunosorba TR-350-Asahi). This device is not currently available in the United States.

THROMBOTIC THROMBOCYTOPENIC PURPURA. TTP is a consumptive thrombocytopenia, associated with neurologic and renal symptoms owing to microvascular thrombosis. It is caused by platelet aggregation by von Willebrand factor (VWF) multimers. These patients are thought to have either a congenital deficiency of a metalloprotease that cleaves VWF multimers or autoantibodies to this protease [16]. The effectiveness of therapeutic plasma exchange is owing to removal of the VWF multimer, removal of an antibody to the cleaving metalloprotease, or both, and infusing normal plasma containing the metalloprotease [16]. Other conditions (e.g., systemic lupus erythematosus, bone marrow transplant, metastatic cancer, and medication-induced syndromes) can also cause a TTP-like clinical picture, but may respond better to a more specific therapy. A Canadian multicenter-controlled clinical trial compared plasma exchange to plasma infusion in 102 patients with TTP. The

Table 20-3. Treatment Schedules and Therapeutic End-Points of Diseases Treated with Plasma Exchange in the Intensive Care Unit

Disease	Total amount of plasma removed	Replacement fluid	Therapeutic end-point
Acute Guillain-Barré syndrome	200 to 250 mg/kg within 2 wk	Albumin	Not applicable
Acute myasthenia gravis crisis	150 mL/kg within 3 exchanges	Albumin	Amelioration of symptoms
Thrombotic thrombocytopenic purpura	1.5 plasma volume removal daily for at least 3 d, then 1 plasma volume removal until therapeutic end-point	Fresh-frozen plasma, cryo-poor fresh-frozen plasma, or PLAS+^{R}SD	Normal platelet count for 2 to 3 d and normal lactic dehydrogenase
Goodpasture's syndrome	1 plasma volume removal daily or every other d	Albumin, IV immunoglobulin when IgG <200 mg/dL	Disease stabilization

IgG, immunoglobulin G; PLAS+^{R}SD, pooled plasma, solvent/detergent treated (VI Technologies, Inc., Watertown, MA).

results, published in 1991, showed plasma exchange to be the more effective treatment, with a mortality rate of 21.5% compared with 37.2% in the plasma infusion group [17]. The authors' protocol for treatment of TTP involves daily plasma exchanges (at least three, with removal of 1.5 plasma volumes per procedure). The replacement fluid is a combination of 5% albumin during the first half of the procedure, followed by a plasma product during the latter half. The therapy is continued until platelet count and LDH level normalize and may be followed with one or two additional procedures. In the authors' experience, it is beneficial to include corticosteroids from the start of therapy, especially if it is likely that an autoantibody to the metalloprotease is present. It has been reported that resistant cases have responded to Prosorba column treatment [18]. Although vincristine is sometimes added to the therapeutic regimen, it does not seem to be effective, whereas splenectomy may be beneficial in some cases. It appears that "cryo-poor" plasma (fresh-frozen plasma from which cryoprecipitate has been removed) might be a more desirable replacement fluid than fresh-frozen plasma [19]. The authors have had good experience in using pooled, solvent/ detergent-treated plasma, as it lacks large VWF multimers and is also associated with a low incidence of allergic reactions.

RAPIDLY PROGRESSIVE GLOMERULONEPHRITIS. Therapeutic plasma exchange is currently the primary line of therapy for only one type of rapidly progressive glomerulonephritis, the antiglomerular basement membrane–positive Goodpasture's syndrome, particularly when there is moderate or severe renal disease with pulmonary hemorrhage. Because pulmonary hemorrhage can be fatal, it constitutes a medical emergency, and plasma exchange must be performed without delay [20–22]. The role of plasma exchange is only secondary for patients who have rapidly progressive glomerulonephritis associated with antineutrophil cytoplasm antibodies (i.e., systemic vasculitis owing to Wegener's granulomatosis or polyarteritis nodosa) [23]. Plasma exchange is not thought to be beneficial in patients with immune complex–mediated rapidly progressive glomerulonephritis [22]. Currently plasma exchange is considered experimental therapy for recurrent focal glomerulosclerosis.

DRUG OVERDOSE AND POISONING. Theoretically, plasma exchange is effective in removing protein-bound toxins and drugs that have been given in overdose. Case reports have confirmed the beneficial effect of this approach when treating patients poisoned with the mushroom toxin amanitin [24] and the nephrotoxic herbicide paraquat [25].

CONTRAINDICATIONS. For treatment of appropriate disorders, there are only relative contraindications for performance of therapeutic hemapheresis. Patients with severe cardiac failure or those who are otherwise hemodynamically unstable might not tolerate the blood volume changes during the procedure. Patients receiving intravenous heparin therapy should not undergo plasma exchange unless subcutaneous heparin can be substituted. Patients with thrombotic events should not undergo treatment with Prosorba columns because the complement activation can aggravate thrombotic tendencies. Finally, patients receiving angiotensin-converting enzyme (ACE) inhibitors should not undergo plasmapheresis, with or without Prosorba columns.

Adverse Effects

EFFECTS OF TRANSIENT HYPOCALCEMIA AND HYPOMAGNESEMIA. The citrate anticoagulant given during the procedure lowers plasma-ionized calcium and magnesium levels [26]. Not uncommonly, this effect can cause the patient to feel a perioral tingling sensation. Other effects include paresthesias, twitching, muscle cramping, tetany, nausea, vomiting, abdominal pain, chills, fever, hypotension, increase in cQT interval, and hemodynamic depression. Symptoms owing to hypocalcemia have been observed in 7.7% of procedures [27,28]. The reactions are usually mild and respond to slowing down the reinfusion rate. During the procedure, however, some patients require a slow intravenous infusion of calcium gluconate (1 g added to 250 mL of 0.9% saline solution) to relieve the symptoms. Droperidol, when used in combination with apheresis, prolongs the QT interval [29,30].

ALLERGIC REACTIONS. An allergic or anaphylactic reaction may occur in a sensitized patient. Because solvent/ detergent-treated plasma is derived from a pool of up to 6,000 different donor units, it contains only a small amount of any individual "allergenic" plasma and therefore reduces the likelihood of an allergic reaction. To prevent allergic reactions, the authors usually premedicate patients with diphenhydramine hydrochloride (Benadryl) and sometimes give hydrocortisone as an intravenous push approximately 30 minutes before giving plasma. Anaphylactic reactions are rare, occurring in immunoglobulin A–deficient patients who have formed anti–immunoglobulin A antibodies.

These reactions should be treated with intravenous fluids and epinephrine.

ANGIOTENSIN-CONVERTING ENZYME INHIBITOR-ASSOCIATED EFFECTS. Patients receiving ACE inhibitors may have life-threatening anaphylactoid reactions when undergoing hemodialysis, LDL removal from plasma using dextran sulfate columns, or treatment of plasma with Prosorba columns [31–33]. Because of the potential to induce atypical reactions, ACE inhibitors should be withheld for 24 to 48 hours before plasmapheresis [28,34]. The symptoms are thought to be mediated by generation of bradykinin during the procedure. Because kininase II (identical to ACE) contributes to inactivation of bradykinin, this function is impaired in patients receiving ACE inhibitors. If bradykinin reaches toxic levels, the patient may have severe flushing, dyspnea, hypotension, and bradycardia. In such cases, the procedure must be discontinued immediately and the patient treated with intravenous fluids and possibly epinephrine.

APNEA AFTER SUXAMETHONIUM ANESTHESIA. Plasma cholinesterase, which is necessary for degradation of suxamethonium anesthetic, is reduced by extensive plasma removal [35]. To avoid prolonged apnea after suxamethonium anesthesia, it is prudent to allow at least 72 hours between plasma exchange and anesthesia. As a less desirable alternative, fresh-frozen plasma infusions may be given.

MEDICATION DEPLETION. Removal of large volumes of plasma may lower the concentration of medications. It may be advisable to administer intravenous medications after the procedure has been completed. It has been reported, however, that vancomycin, gentamicin, and digoxin do not show clinically significant reduction in total body stores during plasmapheresis [36].

HYPOTENSIVE EPISODES. Patients undergoing hemapheresis may have vasovagal reactions or hypotensive episodes. Hypotension has been reported to account for 18% of all complications and is particularly likely to occur in patients whose disease impairs the ability to maintain vascular tone (e.g., GBS, diabetes) [27]. Hypotensive episodes respond readily to crystalloid or colloid infusion.

FLU-LIKE SYMPTOMS. If a Prosorba column is used in the hemapheresis process, complement can be activated, causing a variety of flu-like symptoms. Symptoms such as chills, fever, muscle and joint pain, nausea, respiratory difficulties, hypotension, and hypertension have been noted in approximately 35% of procedures performed [3]. Because the usual course of therapy often requires several procedures, approximately 70% of patients experience some of these symptoms. Although these adverse effects are usually minor, some have been fatal [37,38]. To reduce complications, the authors medicate the patient with acetaminophen (Tylenol) and diphenhydramine hydrochloride before giving the treated plasma. It has also been reported that patients receiving small doses of prednisone during treatment have a lower incidence of adverse reactions [3].

CATHETER EFFECTS. When catheters are used, they may become clotted or infected, requiring removal to avoid sys-temic complications. The rigid catheters may perforate the great vessels, the pleural cavity, and the pericardium. The result may be hemothorax or pericardial effusion, even several days after insertion of the catheter, causing hemodynamic instability [39]. The use of catheters requires strict adherence to protocols to maintain patency and sterility.

Summary

Therapeutic hemapheresis is useful in ameliorating symptoms by virtue of decreasing the concentration of pathologic cells or plasma constituents. It is quite effective, even life-saving, in certain disease processes that are of limited duration. The role of plasma exchange in the treatment of chronic disease is less clear cut. Development and licensing of newer devices capable of selectively removing specific abnormal plasma proteins will add to the sophistication of hemapheresis therapy.

References

1. Solomon A, Fahey JL: Plasmapheresis therapy in macroglobulinemia. *Ann Intern Med* 58:789, 1963.
2. Gurland HJ: Therapeutic apheresis update. *Adv Exp Med Biol* 260: 193, 1989.
3. Snyder HW Jr, Cochran SK, Balint JP Jr, et al: Experience with protein A-immunoadsorption in treatment-resistant adult immune thrombocytopenic purpura. *Blood* 79:2237, 1992.
4. Gordon BR, Saal SD: Low-density lipoprotein apheresis using the Liposorber dextran sulfate cellulose system for patients with hypercholesterolemia refractory to medical therapy. *J Clin Apheresis* 11:128, 1996.
5. Schlansky R, DeHoratius RJ, Pincus T, et al: Plasmapheresis in systemic lupus erythematosus: a cautionary note. *Arthritis Rheum* 24:49, 1981.
6. Orlin JB, Berkman EM: Partial plasma exchange using albumin replacement: removal and recovery of normal plasma constituents. *Blood* 56:1055, 1980.
7. Berkman EM: Therapeutic apheresis: what it can and can't do. *Diagn Med* 7:55, 1984.
8. McLeod BC: Introduction to the third special issue: clinical applications of therapeutic apheresis. *J Clin Apheresis* 15:1, 2000.
9. The Guillain-Barré Syndrome Study Group: Plasmapheresis and acute Guillain-Barré syndrome. *Neurology* 35:1096, 1985.
10. French Cooperative Group on Plasma Exchange in Guillain-Barré Syndrome: Efficiency of plasma exchange in Guillain-Barré syndrome: role of replacement fluids. *Ann Neurol* 22:753, 1987.
11. van der Meché FGA, Schmitz PIM, the Dutch Guillain-Barré Study Group: A randomized trial comparing intravenous immune globulin and plasma exchange in Guillain-Barré syndrome. *N Engl J Med* 326:1123, 1992.
12. Castro LHM, Ropper AH: Human immune globulin infusion in Guillain-Barré syndrome: worsening during and after treatment. *Neurology* 43:1034, 1993.
13. Kuwabara S, Mori M, Ogawara K, et al: Intravenous immunoglobulin therapy for Guillain-Barré syndrome with IgG and anti-GM1 antibody. *Muscle Nerve* 24:54, 2001.
14. Littlewood R, Bajada S: Successful plasmapheresis in the Miller-Fisher syndrome. *BMJ* 282:778, 1981.
15. Lisak RP: Plasma exchange in neurologic diseases. *Arch Neurol* 41:654, 1984.
16. Furlan M, Robles R, Solenthaler M, et al: Deficient activity of von Willebrand factor-cleaving protease in chronic relapsing thrombotic thrombocytopenic purpura. *Blood* 1;89(9):3097, 1997.
17. Rock GA, Shumak KH, Buskard NA, et al: Comparison of plasma

exchange with plasma infusion in the treatment of thrombotic thrombocytopenic purpura. *N Engl J Med* 325:393, 1991.

18. Gaddis T, Guthrie T, Mittelman A, et al: Protein A immunoadsorption (PAI) in classical thrombotic thrombocytopenia purpura (TTP) refractory to plasma exchange report of eleven patients. *Blood* 80[Suppl 1]:63a, 1992.

19. Rock G, Shumak KH, Sutton DM, et al: Cryosupernatant as replacement fluid for plasma exchange in thrombotic thrombocytopenic purpura. Members of the Canadian Apheresis Group. *Br J Haematol* 94:383, 1996.

20. Lockwood CM, Boulton-Jones JM, Lowenthal RM, et al: Recovery from Goodpasture's syndrome after immunosuppressive treatment and plasmapheresis. *BMJ* 2:252, 1975.

21. Johnson JP, Whitman W, Briggs WA, et al: Plasmapheresis and immunosuppressive agents in antibasement membrane antibody induced Goodpasture's syndrome. *Am J Med* 64:354, 1978.

22. Erickson SB, Kutz SB, Donadio JV Jr, et al: Use of combined plasmapheresis and immunosuppression in the treatment of Goodpasture's syndrome. *Mayo Clin Proc* 54:714, 1979.

23. Glockner WM, Sieberth HG, Wichmann HE, et al: Plasma exchange and immunosuppression in rapidly progressive glomerulonephritis: a controlled, multicenter study. *Clin Nephrol* 29:1, 1988.

24. Mercuriali F, Sirchia G: Plasma exchange for mushroom poisoning. *Transfusion* 17:644, 1977.

25. Miller J, Sanders E, Webb D: Plasmapheresis for paraquat poisoning. *Lancet* 1:875, 1978.

26. Bolan CD, Greer SE, Cecco SA, et al: Comprehensive analysis of citrate effects during plateletpheresis in normal donors. *Transfusion* 41(9):1165, 2001.

27. Sutton DM, Nair RG, Rock G: Complications of plasma exchange. *Transfusion* 29:124, 1989.

28. Strauss RG: Mechanisms of adverse effects during hemapheresis. *J Clin Apheresis* 11:160, 1996.

29. Food and Drug Administration Communication: Revised black box warning for droperidol (Akorn Pharmaceuticals), December 4, 2001.

30. Szymanski IO: Ionized calcium levels during plateletpheresis. *Transfusion* 18:701, 1978.

31. Tielemans C, Madhoun P, Lenaers M, et al: Anaphylactoid reactions during hemodialysis on AN69 membranes in patients receiving ACE inhibitors. *Kidney Int* 38:982, 1990.

32. Kojuma S, Shida M, Takano H: Effects of losartan on blood pressure and humoral factors in a patient who suffered from anaphylactoid reactions when treated with ACE ihibitors during LDL apheresis. *Hypertens Res* 24(5):595, 2001.

33. Keller C, Grutzmacher P, Bahr F, et al: LDL-apheresis with dextran sulphate and anaphylactoid reactions to ACE inhibitors. *Lancet* 341:60, 1993.

34. Owen HG, Brecher ME: Atypical reactions associated with use of angiotensin-converting enzyme inhibitors and apheresis. *Transfusion* 34:891, 1994.

35. Evans RT, Macdonald R, Robinson A: Suxamethonium apnoea associated with plasmaphoresis. *Anaesthesia* 35:198, 1980.

36. Friedberg RC, Fischer JS, McClellan SD: Plasmapheresis-mediated clearance of vancomycin, gentamicin, and digoxin. *Transfusion* 34(Suppl):35, 1994.

37. Huestis DW, Rifkin RM, Durie BGM, et al: An unexpected complication following immunoadsorption with a Staphylococcal protein in a column. *J Clin Apheresis* 7:75, 1992.

38. Smith RE, Gottschall JL, Pisciotta AV: Life-threatening reaction to staphylococcal protein A immunomodulation. *J Clin Apheresis* 7:4, 1992.

39. Quillen K, Magarace L, Flanagan J, et al: Vascular erosion caused by a double-lumen central venous catheter during therapeutic plasma exchange. *Transfusion* 35:510, 1995.

21. Cerebrospinal Fluid Aspiration

John P. Weaver, Robin I. Davidson, and Viviane Tabar

This chapter presents guidelines for safe cerebrospinal fluid (CSF) aspiration for the emergency department or the intensive care physician, and it provides a basic understanding of the indications, techniques, and potential complications of these procedures.

Most CSF aspiration procedures are routinely and safely performed and require readily accessible equipment and sterile supplies located in most hospital patient care units. The majority of CSF aspirations are performed using local anesthesia. Sedation is seldom necessary, except in the pediatric population [1]. Radiographic imaging is needed in situations in which external anatomic landmarks provide inadequate guidance for safe needle placement or when needle placement using external landmarks alone has proved unsuccessful due to anatomic variations caused by trauma, operative scar, congenital defects, or degenerative changes. Fluoroscopy may be used for lumbar puncture, C1-2 puncture, and myelography. Computed tomography (CT) or magnetic resonance imaging (MRI) is used for stereotactic placement of ventricular catheters. Clinicians should recognize the need for specialized equipment and training in certain cases.

An implanted reservoir or shunt system should not be accessed without prior consultation with a neurosurgeon, despite the apparent simplicity of the procedure itself. Violating implanted systems carries several risks, including infection, which can result in a lengthy hospital stay; a prolonged antibiotic course; and several operative procedures for shunt externalization, hardware removal, and insertion of a new shunt system.

Contraindications to lumbar puncture include skin infection at the entry site, anticoagulation or blood dyscrasias, papilledema in the presence of supratentorial masses, posterior fossa lesions, and known spinal subarachnoid block or spinal cord arteriovenous malformations.

Cerebrospinal Fluid Access

DIAGNOSTIC PURPOSES. CSF analysis continues to be a major diagnostic tool in many diseases. The most common indications for CSF sampling are the suspicion of a central nervous system (CNS) infection and subarachnoid hemorrhage (SAH). CSF access is necessary for neurodiagnostic procedures such as myelography and cisternography.

CSF pressure recording, particularly the opening pressure, is important in the diagnosis and treatment of normal pressure hydrocephalus, benign intracranial hypertension, and head injury. The diagnostic tests performed on the aspirated CSF depend on the patient's age, history, and differential diagnosis. A basic profile includes glucose and protein values, a blood cell count, Gram's stain, and cultures.

CSF glucose depends on blood glucose levels and is usually equivalent to two-thirds of the serum glucose. It is slightly higher in neonates. Glucose is transported into the CSF via carrier-facilitated diffusion, and changes in spinal fluid glucose concentration lag blood levels by approximately 2 hours. Increased CSF glucose is nonspecific and usually reflects hyperglycemia. Hypoglycorrhachia can be the result of any inflammatory or neoplastic meningeal disorder and reflects increased glucose use by nervous tissue or leukocytes and inhibited transport mechanisms. The lower glucose concentrations are usually accompanied by elevated lactate levels reflecting anaerobic glycolysis.

CSF protein content is usually less than 0.5% of that in plasma due to blood–brain barrier exclusion. Albumin constitutes up to 75% of CSF protein, and immunoglobulin G is the major component of the gamma-globulin fraction. Immunoglobulin G freely traverses a damaged blood–brain barrier. Although often nonspecific, an elevated protein level in the CSF is an indicator of CNS pathology. There is a gradient of total protein content in the spinal CSF column, with the highest level normally found in the lumbar subarachnoid space at 20 to 50 mg per dL, followed by the cisterna magna at 15 to 25 mg per dL and the ventricles at 6 to 12 mg per dL. A value exceeding 500 mg per dL is compatible with an intraspinal tumor with a complete subarachnoid block, meningitis, or bloody CSF [2]. Low protein levels are seen in healthy children younger than 2 years of age, pseudotumor cerebri, acute water intoxication, and leukemic patients.

Normal CSF cell counts include no erythrocytes and a maximum of 5 leukocytes per mm³. A greater number of cells are normally found in children (up to 10 per mm³, mostly lymphocytes). CSF cytology can be helpful in identifying cells to diagnoses CNS primary or metastatic tumors and inflammatory disorders [3].

Hemorrhage. A *nontraumatic* SAH in the adult population is commonly due to a ruptured aneurysm. A paroxysmal severe headache is the classic symptom of aneurysm rupture, but atypical headaches reminiscent of migraine are not uncommon. Up to 50% of patients with a warning "leak" headache are undiagnosed after evaluation by their physician, and 55% of patients with premonitory warning headaches had normal CT findings, but all had a positive finding of SAH on lumbar puncture [4]. Lumbar puncture is indicated after SAH if the head CT is not diagnostic and if the clinical history and presentation are atypical. A lumbar puncture should not be performed without prior CT if the patient has any focal neurologic deficits. Such deficits might indicate the presence of an intracranial hematoma, which would increase the likelihood of transtentorial herniation after a lumbar puncture. An SAH could also extend into the ventricular system, presenting as acute obstructive hydrocephalus. In such a case, CT scan would demonstrate ventriculomegaly, which is best treated by the placement of a ventricular catheter.

A traumatic lumbar puncture presents a diagnostic dilemma, especially in the context of a suspected SAH. Some of its differentiating characteristics include a decreasing red blood cell count in tubes collected serially during the procedure, the presence of a fibrinous clot in the sample obtained, and a typical ratio of approximately 1 leukocyte per 700 red blood cells. Xanthochromia is more indicative of SAH and is quickly evaluated by spinning a fresh CSF sample and comparing the color of the supernatant to that of water, or by the use of a spectrophotometer. Spinal fluid accelerates red blood cell hemolysis, and hemoglobin products are released within 2 hours of the initial hemorrhage. Associated findings, such as a slightly depressed glucose level, increased protein, and an elevated opening pressure, are also more suggestive of the presence of an SAH. Another method to differentiate between blood in CSF due to an intracranial hemorrhage and that due to a traumatic spinal tap has been demonstrated in neonates [5]. The mean corpuscular volume of erythrocytes in the CSF can be compared with that in peripheral blood. The mean corpuscular volume in CSF is lower than in venous blood in cases of SAH, but the values are similar if the hemorrhage was induced by the lumbar puncture.

Infection. CSF evaluation is the single most important aspect of the laboratory diagnosis of meningitis. It usually includes a Gram's stain, blood cell count with white cell differential, protein and glucose levels, and aerobic and anaerobic cultures with antibiotic sensitivities. With suspicion of tuberculosis or fungal meningitis, the fluid is analyzed by acid-fast stain, India ink preparation, and cryptococcal antigen, and then cultured in appropriate media. More extensive cultures are performed in the immunocompromised patient.

Immunoprecipitation tests to identify bacterial antigens for *Streptococcus pneumoniae*, *Streptococcus* group B, *Haemophilus influenzae*, and *Neisseria meningitidis* (meningococcus) allow rapid diagnosis and early specific treatment. Viral cultures or, more recently, polymerase chain reaction tests, can be performed on CSF for rapid identification of several viruses, particularly those commonly responsible for CNS infections in patients with acquired immunodeficiency syndrome. Polymerase chain reaction tests exist for herpes, varicella zoster, cytomegalovirus, and Epstein-Barr virus, as well as toxoplasmosis and *Mycobacterium tuberculosis* [6]. If the clinical suspicion is high for meningitis, antibiotic therapy should be initiated without delay after CSF collection [7].

Rodewaid et al. proposed an argument to perform a limited CSF analysis in the pediatric population to save time and money [8]. In their study, the decision to analyze CSF for protein or glucose was based on initial analysis of the nucleated blood cell count. A negative screening test was defined as a nucleated blood cell count less than 6 per mm³. The results demonstrated that the screening test was much more sensitive and specific than other routine tests in predicting the presence of an infection. These results provided the basis for a strategy for sequential testing of CSF.

In the neonatal population, Schewerenski et al. reported that lumbar puncture and CSF analysis might be more useful after 1 week of age than in the first week of life [9]. This prospective study assessed the frequency and diagnostic use of lumbar punctures as part of an evaluation for congenital or postnatal infection in the neonate. It showed rare positive CSF cultures during the first week of life. Of these, only one had a simultaneous positive blood culture and clinically evident meningitis. The yield after the first week of life was approximately five times higher [9].

Shunt System Failure. A ventriculoperitoneal shunt is the most commonly encountered system. The hardware varies, but commonly consists of a ventricular catheter connected to a reservoir and valve complex at the skull and a subcutaneous catheter in the neck and anterior chest wall to the peritoneum. The distal tubing may also have been inserted in the jugular vein, the pleura, or even the urinary bladder. A shunt failure is often due to obstruction of the ventricular catheter or an infection of the shunt system. Shunts can also become disconnected or obstructed distally due to poor CSF absorption or formation of an intraabdominal pseudocyst.

Clinical presentation of an obstructed shunt is highly variable; it may be slowly progressive or intermittent, or there may be a rapid decline in mentation progressing into a coma. A CT scan should be performed immediately and compared with previous studies. Ventriculomegaly is a good indicator of a malfunctioning shunt, but noncompliant ventricles may remain small and not vary significantly in size, and the ventricular system in a shunted patient is often congenitally or chronically abnormal.

Aspiration from the reservoir or valve system of a shunt can be performed to determine patency and to collect CSF to rule out an infectious process. One should remember, however, that shunt aspiration is an invasive procedure that carries a risk of contaminating the system with skin flora. A shunt infection often requires a lengthy hospital stay with shunt externalization, antibiotic treatment, and replacement of all hardware. Therefore, shunts should be tapped very selectively and after all potential sources of infection have been evaluated. When shunt failure is due to distal obstruction, aspiration of CSF may temper neurologic impairment and even be life saving until formal shunt revision can be performed. The determination of the need for a shunt tap, as well as the procedure, is best left to a neurosurgeon.

Normal Pressure Hydrocephalus. Serial lumbar punctures or continuous CSF drainage via a lumbar subarachnoid catheter can be used as a provocative diagnostic test to select patients who would benefit from a shunt for CSF diversion. The results have a positive predictive value if the patient's gait improves. Lumbar CSF access may also be used for infusion tests, measurement of CSF production rate, pressure-volume index, and outflow resistance or absorption. Some studies suggest that these values are also predictive of therapeutic CSF diversion [10–12].

Benign Intracranial Hypertension (Pseudotumor Cerebri). Benign intracranial hypertension occurs in young persons, often obese young women. Intracranial pressure (ICP) is elevated without focal deficits and in the absence of ventriculomegaly or mass lesions. Etiologic factors for childhood presentation include chronic middle ear infection, dural sinus thrombosis, head injury, vitamin A overdosage, tetracycline exposure, internal jugular venous thrombosis, and idiopathic causes [13]. Some authors have proposed a broader definition of the "pseudotumor cerebri syndrome" based on the underlying pathophysiologic mechanism of presumed CSF circulation disorder [14].

Symptoms of intracranial hypertension develop over several months. Headache is the most common symptom, but dizziness, blurred vision, diplopia, transient visual obscuration, and abnormal facial sensations can also occur [15]. Objective signs include visual impairment, papilledema, and sixth-nerve palsy. A lumbar puncture demonstrates an elevated ICP (up to 40 cm H_2O), and CSF dynamics demonstrate an increase in outflow resistance. Serial daily punctures can be

therapeutic, with CSF aspirated until closing pressure is within normal limits (less than 20 cm H_2O). In some cases, this can restore the balance between CSF formation and absorption; other cases require medical therapy such as weight loss, steroids, acetazolamide, diuretics, and glycerol. When all fails, placement of a permanent shunting system may be necessary.

Neoplasms. The subarachnoid space can be infiltrated by various primary or secondary tumors, giving rise to symptoms of meningeal irritation. CSF cytology can determine the presence of neoplastic cells, although their complete identification is not always possible. A generous amount of CSF or multiple samples may be required. Systemic neoplasms such as melanoma or breast cancer have a greater propensity to metastasize into the CSF spaces than do primary CNS tumors and may even present primarily as meningeal carcinomatosis. Ependymoma, medulloblastoma or primitive neuroectodermal tumor, germinoma, and high-grade glioma are the most commonly disseminated primary tumors. Hematopoietic cancers such as leukemia and lymphoma also frequently infiltrate the subarachnoid spaces with little or no parenchymal involvement. CSF sampling is useful for an initial diagnostic and screening tool in the neurologically intact patient who harbors a tumor type with high risk of CNS relapse. Cisternal puncture may enhance the diagnosis if the lumbar CSF is nondiagnostic [16]. Acute leukemias that tend to invade the CNS include acute lymphocytic leukemia, acute nonlymphocytic leukemia, acute myelogenous leukemia, acute myelomonocytic leukemia, and acute undifferentiated leukemia [17]. Individual proliferating T- and B-lymphocytes can also be detected in the CSF and may aid in the differentiation of an opportunistic infection from a leukemic infiltration [18].

CSF analysis for autoantibodies could play a role in the diagnosis of some paraneoplastic syndromes (e.g., anti-Yo titers in paraneoplastic cerebellar degeneration) [19]. A contrast-enhanced MRI of the brain and spine may detect tumor seeding in the subarachnoid space, obviating the need for a lumbar puncture.

Myelography. Lumbar puncture is the most common means of access for lumbar and cervical myelography because the density of contrast material is higher than CSF and may be directed by gravity to the area of interest. Cervical C1-2 puncture may be the usual access route for cervical myelography but is often reserved for patients in whom a successful lumbar puncture is not possible due to extensive arachnoiditis, epidural tumor, severe spinal stenosis, or CSF block.

Other Neurologic Disorders. There is extensive literature on CSF changes in multiple sclerosis. Typical lumbar puncture findings are normal ICP, normal glucose levels, mononuclear pleocytosis, and elevated protein levels due to increased endothelial permeability. Immunoelectrophoresis reveals elevated immunoglobulin G and oligoclonal bands [20]. Antibodies against cardiolipin synthetic lecithin, a lectin protein involved in the structural stabilization of myelin, have been detected in the CSF of patients with multiple sclerosis and may constitute a very sensitive and specific diagnostic test [21].

CSF findings described in other disease states include elevated tau protein and decreased β-amyloid precursor protein in Alzheimer's disease and the presence of anti-GM1 antibodies and cytoalbumin dissociation in Guillain-Barré syndrome.

Therapeutic Intervention

FISTULAS. CSF leaks occur for a variety of reasons, including nontraumatic and traumatic etiologies. Iatrogenic postoperative CSF leaks may occur after skull base tumor resection as a result of dural or bony defects, despite intraoperative attempts at a watertight dural closure. Orthostatic headaches are a characteristic symptom, and CSF rhinorrhea may be evident. CSF fistulas after middle cranial fossa or cerebellopontine angle surgery occur infrequently, and usually the CSF leaks through the auditory tube to the nasopharynx. Dural closure in the posterior fossa after suboccipital craniectomy is often difficult and not watertight. A fistula in that area usually results in a pseudomeningocele, which is clinically apparent as subcutaneous swelling at the incision site with potential wound breakdown.

Leaks after lumbar surgery are unusual but may occur as a result of recent myelography, dural tear, or inadequate dural closure [22]. In pediatric patients, repairs of meningoceles or other spina bifida defects are more likely to present with a CSF leak because of dural or fascial defects.

The most common presentation of a CSF fistula follows trauma. Basilar skull fractures that traverse the ethmoid or frontal sinus can lead to CSF rhinorrhea. Another relatively common fracture follows the long axis of the petrous bone and usually involves the middle ear. Hemotympanum may be noted on examination, and CSF otorrhea occurs if the tympanic membrane is ruptured. Delayed leaks are not uncommon because the fistula can be occluded with adhesions, hematoma, or herniated brain tissue, which temporarily tamponades the defect.

The diagnosis of a leak is often easily made on clinical examination. At times, the nature of a "drainage fluid" is uncertain and laboratory characterization is necessary. Dipping the fluid for glucose is misleading, as nasal secretions are positive for glucose. A chloride level often shows a higher value than in peripheral blood, but identification of β_2-transferrin is the most accurate diagnostic for CSF. This protein is produced by neuraminidase in the brain and is uniquely found in the spinal fluid and perilymph [23].

Postural drainage by patient's head elevation is the primary treatment of a leak. Placement of a lumbar drainage catheter or daily lumbar punctures can be useful nonoperative approaches should conservative therapy fail. The use of a continuous lumbar drainage catheter is somewhat controversial because of the potential for intracranial contamination from the sinuses if the ICP is lowered. To help prevent such complications, the lumbar drain collection bag should be maintained no lower than the patient's shoulder level and the duration of drainage should not exceed 5 days.

Intracranial Hypertension. Intracranial hypertension (see Chapters 22 and 169) can cause significant neurologic morbidity or even death. Access to the intracranial CSF space is useful in diagnosis and treatment [24]. A ventriculostomy is commonly used as an ICP monitor and as a means to treat intracranial hypertension by CSF drainage. An ICP measuring device is often placed after traumatic brain injury for patients who exhibit a deterioration in mental status resulting in a Glasgow Coma Scale score less than 8, a motor score less than 6 (not aphasic), diffuse brain edema, hematoma (epidural, subdural, intraparenchymal), cortical contusions, or absent or compressed basal cisterns on initial CT. ICP monitoring can also be indicated in cerebrovascular diseases, including aneurysmal SAH, spontaneous cerebral hematoma, ischemic and hypoxic cerebral insults, and intraventricular hemorrhage. Obstructive hydrocephalus is another major indication for placement of a ventricular catheter for drainage and monitoring. Cerebral edema also contributes to elevated ICP; it often surrounds tumors, intracranial hematomas, ischemic brain, and traumatic contusions, or it could occur postoperatively or after cranial radiation therapy. Diffuse brain swelling also occurs in the setting of inflammatory and infectious disorders such as Reye's syndrome or meningitis, or as a result of hyperthermia, carbon dioxide retention, or intravascular congestion.

Drug Therapy. The CSF can be a route of administration for medications such as chemotherapeutic agents and antibiotics. Treatment of lymphoma and leukemia often involves intrathecal injections of various agents, which may be infused through a lumbar route or an intraventricular injection via an implant reservoir. Meningeal carcinomatosis is treated by intrathecal chemotherapy (e.g., methotrexate); serial injections of small amounts are performed in an attempt to minimize neurotoxicity [25]. Treatment of meningitis and ventriculitis may include intrathecal antibiotics in addition to systemic therapy. Careful dosage and administration are recommended, especially if the ventricular route is used, as many antibiotics can cause seizures or an inflammatory ventriculitis when given intrathecally.

Techniques of Cerebrospinal Fluid Access

There are several techniques for CSF aspiration. All procedures should be performed using sterile technique, and the skin is prepared with antiseptic washing and draped with sterile towels.

LUMBAR PUNCTURE. Lumbar puncture is a common procedure that is readily performed by the general practitioner, rarely requiring radiologic assistance. It can be performed in any hospital or outpatient setting where commercially prepared lumbar puncture trays are available. In patients with advanced degenerative changes or extensive previous lumbar surgery or congenital defects, the use of fluoroscopic needle placement may be required. C1-2 punctures are seldom required.

In adults, CSF aspirations are adequately performed under local anesthesia using 1% lidocaine without premedication. In the pediatric population, however, sedation is often required and allows for a smoother procedure. This is also true in the case of anxious, confused, or combative adult patients.

Oral or rectal chloral hydrate is often used in children, and conscious sedation using intravenous midazolam and fentanyl can be highly successful in adults and children if performed by an experienced individual under appropriate monitoring. The application of a topical anesthetic, such as EMLA cream (2.5% lidocaine and 2.5% prilocaine, Astra Pharmaceuticals, Westboro, MA), preceding injection can also be useful. It is most effective if combined with an occlusive dressing and left undisturbed for approximately 60 minutes. On the other hand, it has been demonstrated in a controlled clinical trial that in the neonatal population, injection of a local anesthetic for lumbar puncture is probably not required and does not reduce perceived stress or discomfort [26].

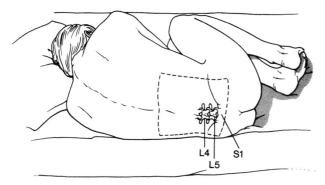

Fig. 21-1. Patient in the lateral decubitus position with back at edge of bed and knees, hips, back, and neck flexed. [From Davidson RI: Lumbar puncture, in VanderSalm TJ (ed): *Atlas of Bedside Procedures.* 2nd ed. Boston, Little, Brown and Company, 1988, with permission.]

Figures 21-1 and 21-2 depict some of the steps for lumbar puncture [27]. The patient is placed in the lateral knee–chest position or sitting while leaning forward over a bedside table. The sitting position is often preferred in obese patients, in whom adipose tissue can obscure the midline, or in elderly patients with significant lumbar degenerative disease. The local anesthetic is injected subcutaneously using a 25- or 27-gauge needle. A 1.5-in. needle is then inserted through the skin wheal and additional local anesthetic is injected along the midline, thus anesthetizing the interspinous ligaments and muscles. This small anesthetic volume is usually adequate; however, a more extensive field block is accomplished by additional injections on each side of the interspinous space near the lamina [28].

The point of skin entry is midline between the spinous processes of L3-4, at the level of the superior iliac crests. Lower needle placement at L4-5 or L5 to S1 is required in children and neonates to avoid injury to the conus medullaris, which lies more caudal than in adults. The needle is

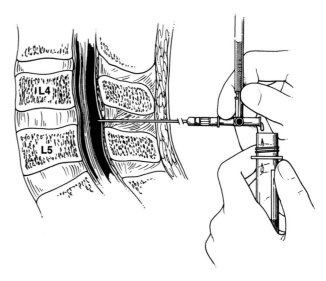

Fig. 21-3. The spinal needle is advanced to the spinal subarachnoid space and cerebrospinal fluid samples collected after opening pressure is measured. [Reprinted from Davidson RI: Lumbar puncture, in VanderSalm TJ (ed): *Atlas of Bedside Procedures.* 2nd ed. Boston, Little, Brown and Company, 1988, with permission.]

advanced with the stylet or obturator in place to maintain needle patency and prevent iatrogenic intraspinal epidermoid tumors [2]. The bevel of the needle should be parallel to the longitudinal fibers of the dura or to the spinal column. The needle should be oriented rostrally at an angle of approximately 30 degrees to the skin and virtually aiming toward the umbilicus. When properly oriented, the needle passes through the following structures before entering the subarachnoid space: skin, superficial fascia, supraspinous ligament, interspinous ligament, ligamentum flavum, epidural space with its fatty areolar tissue and internal vertebral plexus, dura, and arachnoid membrane (Fig. 21-3). The total depth varies from less than 1 in. in the very young patient to as deep as 4 in. in the obese adult. The kinesthetic sensations of passing through the ligaments into the epidural space followed by dural puncture are quite consistent and recognized with practice. Once intradural, the bevel of the needle is redirected in a cephalad direction to improve CSF flow. An 18- to 20-gauge spinal needle should be used for pressure measurement. The opening pressure is best measured with the patient's legs relaxed and extended partly from the knee-chest position. Pressure measurements may be difficult in children and may be estimated using CSF flow rate [29]. Once CSF is collected, the closing pressure is measured before needle withdrawal. It is best to replace the stylet in the needle before exiting the subarachnoid space. CSF pressure measurements are not accurate if performed in the sitting position due to the hydrostatic pressure of the CSF column above the entry point or if a significant amount of CSF was lost when the stylet is first withdrawn. If necessary, the pressure could be measured by reclining the patient to the lateral position once entry in the CSF space has been secured. A coaxial needle was found to be helpful in morbidly obese patients [30].

Although a lumbar puncture is typically safe, there are a number of potential complications and risks involved. Hemorrhage is uncommon but can be seen in association with

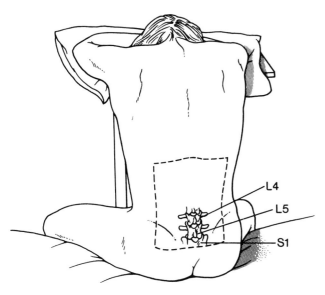

Fig. 21-2. Patient sitting on the edge of the bed, leaning on bedside stand. [From Davidson RI: Lumbar puncture, in VanderSalm TJ (ed): *Atlas of Bedside Procedures.* 2nd ed. Boston, Little, Brown and Company, 1988, with permission.]

bleeding disorders and anticoagulation therapy. Spinal SAH has been reported under such conditions, resulting in blockage of CSF outflow with subsequent back and radicular pain with sphincter disturbances and even paraparesis [31]. Spinal subdural hematoma is likewise infrequent, but it is associated with significant morbidity. Surgical intervention for subdural clot evacuation must be prompt. Infection by introduction of skin flora in the subarachnoid spaces, causing meningitis, is uncommon and preventable if aseptic techniques are used. Risks of infection are increased in serial taps or placement of lumbar catheters for the treatment of CSF fistulas.

Postdural puncture headache (PDPH) is the most common complication after lumbar puncture. Its reported frequency varies from 1% to 70% [32]. It is thought to be due to excessive leakage of CSF into the paraspinous spaces, resulting in intracranial hypotension with stretching and expansion of the pain-sensitive intracerebral veins. MRI has demonstrated a reduced CSF volume after lumbar puncture but no significant brain displacement and no correlation with PDPH [33]. Psychological factors and previous history of headaches seem to strongly influence the patient's risk of and tolerance to PDPH [34]. A smaller needle size, parallel orientation to the dural fibers, and a paramedian approach are associated with a decreased risk of PDPH. The reinsertion of the stylet before withdrawal of the spinal needle has also been reported to decrease the risk of headache after lumbar puncture [32].

The choice of needle type has been the subject of literature debate. Several needle tip designs are available, including the traditional Quincke with a beveled cutting tip; the Sprotte with a pencil point and side hole; and the Whitacre, which is similar to the Sprotte but with a smaller side hole [35]. When comparing needle types, many researchers have mixed the comparisons of size and tip designs. Therefore, it is difficult to make conclusive statements regarding the use of blunt-tipped or atraumatic needles, especially when cost issues are to be considered. The cost of a Whitacre or Sprotte atraumatic spinal needle is several times that of a Quincke needle. However, the use of an atraumatic needle seems to be adequate for the performance of a diagnostic lumbar puncture and is probably associated with a lower risk of PDPH [36].

PDPH typically develops within 72 hours and lasts 3 to 5 days. Conservative treatment consists of bed rest, hydration, and analgesics. Nonphenothiazine antiemetics are administered if the headache is associated with nausea. If the symptoms are more severe, methylxanthines (e.g., caffeine or theophylline) are prescribed orally or parenterally. These agents are successful in up to 85% of patients [37]. Several other pharmacologic agents are discussed in the literature, but none seems to be as effective as caffeine. If the headache persists or is unaffected, an epidural blood patch is then recommended, as it is one of the most effective treatments for this condition [38]. Epidural injection of other agents, such as saline, dextran, or adrenocorticotropic hormone, has also been described and may be valuable under certain conditions (e.g., sepsis, acquired immunodeficiency syndrome) [39].

Other parameters controlling needle choice include the purpose of the procedure and whether an injection is to be performed. If a pressure reading is an important part of the procedure, a larger-gauge needle is necessary, especially if an atraumatic tip is to be used. CSF flow rate is also slow in the smaller-size atraumatic needle, and a 20-gauge needle is probably required for large-volume drainage [36]. Needles as small as 26- or 27-gauge can be used for aspiration or therapeutic infusion. Injection through an atraumatic spinal needle has to be carefully performed, because the needle hole is lateral and not directly at the tip: This has disfavored the use of blunt-tipped needles in myelography to avoid subdural injection.

An uncommon sequela of lumbar puncture or continuous CSF drainage is hearing loss. Drainage decreases ICP, which is transmitted to the perilymph via the cochlear aqueduct and can cause hearing impairment [40]. The rate of occurrence of this complication is reported to be 0.4% but is probably higher, because it goes unrecognized and seems reversible. There are a few documented cases of irreversible hearing loss [41].

Transient sixth-nerve palsy has also been reported, probably due to nerve traction after significant CSF removal. Neurovascular injury can occur uncommonly in the setting of a subarachnoid block due to spinal tumors. In this situation, CSF drainage leads to significant traction and spinal coning with subsequent neurologic impairment [42,43].

LATERAL CERVICAL (C1-2) PUNCTURE. The C1-2 or lateral cervical puncture was originally developed for percutaneous cordotomy. It may be used for myelography or aspiration of CSF if the lumbar route is inaccessible. It is most safely performed by a radiologist under fluoroscopic guidance, although that is not always necessary. The puncture is performed with the patient supine, the head and neck flexed, and the lateral neck draped. The skin entry point is 1 cm caudal and 1 cm dorsal to the tip of the mastoid process. The site is infiltrated with a local anesthetic, and the spinal needle is introduced and directed toward the junction of the middle and posterior thirds of the bony canal to avoid an anomalous vertebral or posterior inferior cerebellar artery that may lie in the anterior half of the canal. The stylet should be removed frequently to check for CSF egress. When the procedure is performed under fluoroscopy, the needle is seen to be perpendicular to the neck and just under the posterior ring of C1. The same sensation is recognized when piercing the dura as in a lumbar puncture, and the bevel is then directed cephalad in a similar fashion. Complications of the lateral cervical puncture include injury to the spinal cord or the vertebral artery and irritation of a nerve root, causing local pain and headache.

CISTERNAL PUNCTURE. A cisternal puncture provides CSF access via the cisterna magna when other routes are not possible. A preoperative lateral skull radiograph is performed to ensure normal anatomy. The patient is positioned sitting with the head slightly flexed. The hair is shaved in the occipital region and the area prepared, draped, and infiltrated with lidocaine. The entry point is in the midline between the external occipital protuberance in the upper margin of the spinous process of C2 or via an imaginary line through both external auditory meati [5]. The spinal needle is directed through a slightly cephalad course and usually strikes the occipital bone. It is then redirected more caudally in a stepwise fashion until it passes through the atlantooccipital membrane and dura, producing a "popping" sensation. The cisterna magna usually lies 4 to 6 cm deep to the skin; the needle should not be introduced beyond 7.0 to 7.5 cm from the skin, to prevent injury to the medulla or the vertebral arteries. The procedure can be performed relatively safely in a cooperative patient as the cisterna magna is a large CSF space; however, it is rarely practiced due to the greater potential morbidity.

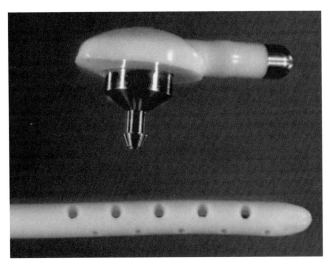

Fig. 21-4. Close-up view of Rickham reservoir in the calvarial opening, the funneled base connected directly to the proximal end of the ventricular catheter. The distal perforated end is shown.

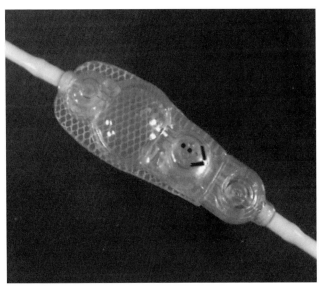

Fig. 21-5. A domed reservoir in series in one type of shunt valve. The large, clear-domed area for puncture lies immediately proximal to the one-way valve.

ASPIRATION OF RESERVOIRS AND SHUNTS. Inline subcutaneous reservoirs in ventriculoatrial or ventriculoperitoneal shunting systems are located proximal to the unidirectional valve and can be accessed percutaneously. The reservoirs are usually button-sized, measuring approximately 7 to 10 mm in diameter and 2 mm in height. They can be located in the burr hole directly connected to the ventricular catheter (Fig. 21-4) or as an integral part of the valve system (Fig. 21-5). Indications for reservoir taps have been previously discussed.

The procedure can be performed in any hospital or outpatient setting. Gloves, mask, antiseptic solution, razor, sterile drapes, 23- or 25-gauge needle (short-hub or butterfly), tuberculin syringe, and sterile collection tubes are readied. The patient can be in any comfortable position that allows access to the reservoir. Sedation may be required for toddlers but is otherwise unnecessary. Reference to a skull radiograph may be helpful in localization. The reservoir is palpated, the overlying hair is shaved, and the skin is cleansed. Local anesthesia is usually not required. The use of topical anesthetic creams is occasionally considered, but it requires shaving of a larger area of the scalp. The needle is inserted perpendicular to the skin and into the reservoir, to a total depth of 2 to 5 mm. A manometer is then connected to the needle or butterfly tubing for pressure measurement. Drug injection or CSF collection is performed. A "dry tap" usually indicates faulty placement or catheter obstruction. Occasionally, an old reservoir may have retracted into the burr hole and not be palpable or may be too calcified for needle penetration. Older shunting systems may not even have a reservoir. Risks and complications of shunt aspiration include improper insertion, contamination with skin flora, introduction of blood in the shunt system, and choroid plexus hemorrhage due to vigorous aspiration. Although the aspiration technique is quite simple, it is always best to consult a neurosurgeon.

Lumboperitoneal Shunt. Lumboperitoneal shunts are placed via percutaneous insertion of a lumbar subarachnoid catheter or through a small skin incision. They are tunneled subcutaneously around the patient's flank to the abdomen, where the distal catheter enters the peritoneal

cavity through a separate abdominal incision. A reservoir, valve, or both may be used and are located on the lateral aspect of the flank. Careful palpation between the two incisions usually reveals the tubing path and reservoir placement in the nonobese patient. Aspiration is simple after the patient is placed in lateral decubitus position. A pillow under the dependent flank may be of assistance. The same technique as described for a ventricular shunt is then performed. Fluid aspiration should be particularly gentle, because an additional risk of this procedure is nerve root irritation.

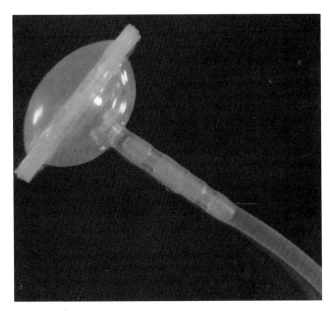

Fig. 21-6. Close-up view of an Ommaya double-domed reservoir, the caudal half of which is designed to lie within the burr hole.

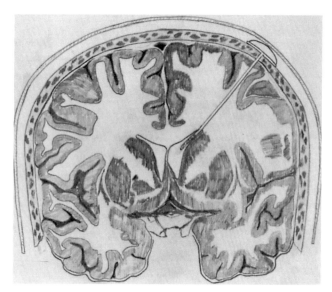

Fig. 21-7. Coronal section through the brain at the level of the frontal horns, illustrating the subgaleal/epicalvarial location at the Ommaya reservoir, with the distal perforated part of the catheter lying within the ventricle.

Ommaya and Other Reservoirs. Ommaya and other reservoirs are inserted as part of a blind system consisting of a catheter located in a CSF space, usually the lateral ventricle, and without distal runoff. Such systems are placed for CSF access purposes only, such as for instillation of antibiotics or chemotherapeutic agents or CSF aspiration for treatment and monitoring. The reservoirs do not divert or shunt CSF.

Ommaya reservoirs are dome-shaped structures (Fig. 21-6) with a diameter of 1 to 2 cm and have a connecting port placed at their base or side. They are placed subcutaneously and attached to a ventricular subarachnoid catheter (Fig. 21-7). Aspiration technique is essentially the same as from a shunt reservoir; however, the Ommaya reservoir is often larger and differs in shape from many shunt reservoirs. It is accessed, preferably, with a 25-gauge needle or butterfly. CSF is allowed to flow by gravity if possible; a volume equal to that to be instilled is removed and held for analysis or reinjection. The antibiotic or chemotherapeutic agent is injected; 1 mL of CSF or sterile saline can be used to flush the dose into the ventricle, or gentle barbotage of the reservoir may be performed to achieve the same goal. Risks and complications are essentially the same as in shunt aspirations (i.e., infection, bleeding, improper insertion), with the addition of chemical ventriculitis or arachnoiditis.

VENTRICULOSTOMY. A ventriculostomy is a catheter placed in the lateral ventricle for CSF drainage or ICP monitoring and treatment. It is performed by a neurosurgeon in the operating room, at the bedside in the intensive care unit, or in the emergency department. It is usually performed through the nondominant hemisphere and into the frontal horn of the lateral ventricle. An alternate approach is to cannulate the occipital horn or trigone through an occipital entry point located 6 cm superior to the inion and 4 cm from the midline. Premedication is not necessary unless the patient is very anxious or combative. Radiographic guidance

is typically not required unless the procedure is being performed stereotactically. CT or MRI stereotaxy is needed if the ventricles are small, as in diffuse brain swelling or slit-ventricle syndrome. Complications of ventriculostomy placement include meningitis or ventriculitis, scalp wound infection, intracranial hematoma or cortical injury, and failure to cannulate the ventricle.

LUMBAR DRAINAGE. Continuous CSF drainage via a lumbar catheter is useful in the treatment of CSF fistulas and as a provocative test to demonstrate the potential effects of shunting in normal pressure hydrocephalus or ventriculomegaly of various etiologies. Commercially available lumbar drainage kits are closed sterile systems that drain into a replaceable collection bag. Catheter placement is performed just as in lumbar puncture, but a large-bore Tuohy needle is used, through which the catheter is threaded once CSF return has been confirmed. Needle orientation follows the same guidelines as discussed for a lumbar puncture and is even more important in the case of this large-gauge needle. Epidural catheter kits could also be used, although the catheters tend to be slightly stiffer and have a narrower diameter.

Complications include hemorrhage in the epidural or subarachnoid space, infection, inability to aspirate CSF, CSF leak, nerve root irritation, and most ominously, a supratentorial subdural hematoma secondary to overdrainage. This complication tends to be more common in elderly individuals. The potential for overdrainage is significant because of the large diameter of the catheter, and because the amount of drainage depends on the cooperation of the patient and the nursing staff.

Summary

Of the various techniques available for CSF access, lumbar puncture is the procedure most commonly and safely performed by the general practitioner. Other techniques are described that may require the assistance of a radiologist, neurologist, anesthesiologist, or neurosurgeon.

References

1. Friedman AG, Mulhern RK, Fairclough D, et al: Midazolam premedication for pediatric bone marrow aspiration and lumbar puncture. *Med Pediatr Oncol* 19:499, 1992.
2. Wood J: Cerebrospinal fluid: techniques of access and analytical interpretation, in Wilkins R, Rengachary S (eds): *Neurosurgery.* 2nd ed. New York, McGraw-Hill, 1996, p 165.
3. Bigner SH: Cerebrospinal fluid cytology: current status and diagnostic applications. *J Neuropathol Exp Neurol* 51:235, 1992.
4. Leblanc R: The minor leak preceding subarachnoid hemorrhage. *J Neurosurg* 66:35, 1981.
5. Yurdakok M, Kocabas CN: CSF erythrocyte volume analysis: a simple method for the diagnosis of traumatic tap in newborn infants. *Pediatr Neurosurg* 17:199, 1991–1992.
6. D'Arminio-Monteforte A, Cinque P, Vago L, et al: A comparison of brain biopsy and CSF PCR in the diagnosis of CNS lesions in AIDS patients. *J Neurol* 244:35, 1997.
7. Greenlee JE: Approach to diagnosis of meningitis: cerebrospinal fluid evaluation. *Infect Dis Clin North Am* 4:583, 1990.

8. Rodewald LE, Woodin KA, Szilagyi PG, et al: Relevance of common tests of cerebrospinal fluid in screening for bacterial meningitis. *J Pediatr* 119:363, 1991.

9. Schewerenski J, McIntyre L, Bauer CR: Lumbar puncture frequency and cerebrospinal fluid analysis in the neonate. *Am J Dis Child* 145:54, 1991.

10. Albeck MJ, Borgesen SE, Gjerris F, et al: Intracranial pressure and cerebrospinal fluid outflow conductance in healthy subjects. *J Neurosurg* 74:597, 1991.

11. Lundar T, Nornes H: Determination of ventricular fluid outflow resistance in patients with ventriculomegaly. *J Neurol Neurosurg Psychiatry* 53:896, 1990.

12. Tans JT, Poortvliet DC: Reduction of ventricular size after shunting for normal pressure hydrocephalus related to CSF dynamics before shunting. *J Neurol Neurosurg Psychiatry* 51:521, 1988.

13. Dhiravibulya K, Ouvrier R, Johnston I, et al: Benign intracranial hypertension in childhood: a review of 23 patients. *J Paediatr Child Health* 27:304, 1991.

14. Johnston I, Hawke S, Halmagyi J, et al: The pseudotumor syndrome: disorders of cerebrospinal fluid circulation causing intracranial hypertension without ventriculomegaly. *Arch Neurol* 48:740, 1991.

15. Adams RD, Victor M: *Principles of Neurology.* 3rd ed. New York, McGraw-Hill, 1985.

16. Rogers LR, Duchesneau PM, Nunez C, et al: Comparison of cisternal and lumbar CSF examination in leptomeningeal metastasis. *J Neurol* 42:1239, 1992.

17. Bigner SH, Johnston WWW: The cytopathology of cerebrospinal fluid, I. Non-neoplastic condition, lymphoma and leukemia. *Acta Cytol* 25:335, 1981.

18. Thomas RS, Beuche W, Felgenhauer K: The proliferation rate of T and B lymphocytes in cerebrospinal fluid. *J Neurol* 238:27, 1991.

19. Furneaux HM, Rosenblum MK, Dalmau J, et al: Selective expression of Purkinje cell antigens in tumor tissue in patients with paraneoplastic cerebellar degeneration. *N Engl J Med* 322:1844, 1990.

20. Fishman RA: *Cerebrospinal Fluid in Diseases of the Nervous System.* 2nd ed. Philadelphia, WB Saunders, 1992.

21. Zanetta JP, Tranchant C, Kuchler-Bopp S, et al: Presence of anti-CSL antibodies in the cerebrospinal fluid of patients: a sensitive and specific test in the diagnosis of multiple sclerosis. *J Neuroimmuol* 52:175, 1994.

22. Agrillo U, Simonetti G, Martino V: Postoperative CSF problems after spinal and lumbar surgery: general review. *J Neurosurg Sci* 35:93, 1991.

23. Nandapalan V, Watson ID, Swift AC: β_2-Transferrin and CSF rhinorrhea. *Clin Otolaryngol* 21:259, 1996.

24. Lyons MK, Meyer FB: Cerebrospinal fluid physiology and the management of increased intracranial pressure. *Mayo Clin Proc* 65:684, 1990.

25. Nakagawa H, Murasawa A, Kubo S, et al: Diagnosis and treatment of patients with meningeal carcinomatosis. *J Neurooncol* 13:81, 1992.

26. Porter FL, Miller JP, Cole FS, et al: A controlled clinical trial of local anesthesia for lumbar punctures in newborns. *Pediatrics* 88:663, 1991.

27. Davidson RI: Lumbar puncture, in VanderSalm TJ (ed): *Atlas of Bedside Procedures.* 2nd ed. Boston, Little, Brown and Company, 1988.

28. Wilkinson HA: Technical note: anesthesia for lumbar puncture. *JAMA* 249:2177, 1983.

29. Ellis RW III, Strauss LC, Wiley JM, et al: A simple method of estimating cerebrospinal fluid pressure during lumbar puncture. *Pediatrics* 89:895, 1992.

30. Johnson JC, Deeb ZL: Coaxial needle technique for lumbar puncture in the morbidly obese patient. *Radiology* 179:874, 1991.

31. Scott EW, Cazenave CR, Virapongse C: Spinal subarachnoid hematoma complicating lumbar puncture: diagnosis and management. *Neurosurgery* 25:287, 1989.

32. Strupp M, Brandt T: Should one reinsert the stylet during lumbar puncture? *N Engl J Med* 336:1190, 1997.

33. Grant F, Condon B, Hart I, et al: Changes in intracranial CSF volume after lumbar puncture and their relationship to post-LP headache. *J Neurol Neurosurg Psychiatry* 54:440, 1991.

34. Lee T, Maynard N, Anslow P, et al: Post-myelogram headache: physiological or psychological? *Neuroradiology* 33:155, 1991.

35. Peterman S: Post myelography headache: a review. *Radiology* 200:765, 1996.

36. Carson D, Serpell M: Choosing the best needle for diagnostic lumbar puncture. *Neurology* 47:33, 1996.

37. Leibold RA, Yealy DM, Coppola M, et al: Post-dural puncture headache: characteristics, management and prevention. *Ann Emerg Med* 22:1863, 1993.

38. Choi A, Laurito CE, Cunningham FE: Pharmacologic management of post-dural headache. *Ann Pharmacother* 30:831, 1996.

39. Barrios-Alarcon J, Aldrete JA, Paragas-Tapia D: Relief of post-lumbar puncture headache with epidural dextran 40: a preliminary report. *Reg Anesth* 14:78, 1989.

40. Walsted A, Salomon G, Thomsen J: Hearing decrease after loss of cerebrospinal fluid: a new hydrops model? *Acta Otolaryngol* 111:468, 1991.

41. Michel O, Brusis T: Hearing loss as a sequel of lumbar puncture. *Ann Otol Rhinol Laryngol* 101:390, 1992.

42. Wong MC, Krol G, Rosenblum MK: Occult epidural chloroma complicated by acute paraplegia following lumbar puncture. *Ann Neurol* 31:110, 1992.

43. Mutoh S, Aikou I, Ueda S: Spinal coning after lumbar puncture in prostate cancer with asymptomatic vertebral metastasis: a case report. *J Urol* 145:834, 1991.

22. Neurologic and Intracranial Pressure Monitoring

Eric A. Bedell, Donald J. Deyo, and Donald S. Prough

Physiologic monitoring, both systemic and neurologic, is routinely used in the management of critically ill patients with neurologic diseases such as traumatic brain injury (TBI), subarachnoid hemorrhage (SAH), stroke, and ischemic encephalopathy after cardiac arrest. When choosing monitors, the risks of each monitoring technique must be weighed against the benefits (whether proven or inferred) that are conferred by the information generated. Other important characteristics include the ability of a technique to detect abnormalities (sensitivity), differentiate between dissimilar disease states (specificity), and to alter long-term prognosis (Table 22-1). The design of a monitoring device necessitates tradeoffs between various performance characteristics. For instance, a monitor with high positive predictive value (i.e., that falls outside threshold values only when cerebral ischemia is unequivocally present) is unlikely to detect less-profound ischemia. A monitor that is highly sensitive to changes in cerebral oxygenation frequently warns of small changes that are unlikely to produce brain injury.

The importance of brain monitoring is based on the high vulnerability of the brain to ischemic injury. The brain uses more oxygen and glucose per 100 g of tissue than any large organ, yet has no appreciable reserves of oxygen or glucose and is thus completely dependent upon uninterrupted cerebral blood flow (CBF) to supply the metabolic substrates required for continued function and survival. Even transient interruptions in CBF, whether local or global, can injure or kill neural cells. Therefore, clinical monitoring of neuronal well-being emphasizes early detection and reversal of potentially dangerous conditions. Although no compelling data demonstrate that morbidity and mortality are altered by the information gathered from current neurologic monitoring techniques, most clinicians caring for patients with critical neurologic illness have confidence that their use improves management. In this chapter, we will review currently available techniques, emphasizing the following questions:

1. Under what circumstances do simple measurements of systemic variables, such as blood pressure, the partial pressures of carbon dioxide ($PaCO_2$) and oxygen (PaO_2), and body temperature fail to provide sufficient information about the adequacy of cerebral oxygen delivery?
2. Under what circumstances does more precise information about the adequacy of cerebral oxygen delivery direct therapeutic interventions that improve outcome of patients at risk?
3. In what situations is the proportion of patients that develop avoidable injury sufficiently large to justify the risk and cost of the application of the neurologic monitoring device?

Goals of Brain Monitoring

Monitoring devices cannot independently improve outcome. Instead, they contribute physiologic data that can be integrated into a care plan that, despite adding any risks that are entailed by the monitoring devices, may lead to an overall decrease in morbidity and mortality. The risks inherent in the monitoring technique cannot be overemphasized. Consider the flow-directed, pulmonary arterial catheter as a paradigm of risk versus benefit. The pulmonary arterial catheter provides real-time hemodynamic data in critically ill patients and can readily be used to guide fluid replacement and inotropic infusions, yet has failed to improve overall morbidity and mortality [1]. Perhaps the potential benefits of the monitor are counterbalanced by inadequate physician training, poor data interpretation, and the inherent risks of central catheterization. As a result, improved patient selection, clinician education, and ongoing research are required to improve results [2,3]. Similar concerns, less extensively studied, apply to neurologic monitoring.

Neurologic monitoring falls into two general categories: qualitative measurements [e.g., electroencephalographic (EEG) and evoked-potential (EP) monitoring] and quantitative/semiquantitative monitors [e.g., intracranial pressure (ICP), transcranial Doppler ultrasonography, jugular bulb venous oxygen saturation ($SjvO_2$), and brain tissue oxygen tension ($PbtO_2$)]. Qualitative monitoring provides information as to the integrated functioning of the brain/nervous system, whereas quantitative monitoring provides specific measurements that may be useful in directing specific therapeutic interventions and gauging therapeutic effectiveness.

Nonneurologic examples of qualitative and quantitative monitors include peripheral nerve stimulation for assessing neuromuscular blockade and continuous electrocardiography (ECG), respectively. Peripheral nerve stimulation assesses the qualitative function of the neuromuscular junction by depolarizing a peripheral nerve and evaluating the muscle response. It provides information about overall function, but does not uniquely identify or quantify the nature of abnormalities. Continuous ECG provides specific and quantitative information about heart rate and rhythm and facilitates evaluation of interventions, such as beta-blocker administration for the treatment of sinus tachycardia, but does not provide information about the adequacy of cardiac function with respect to systemic needs. For each example, the limitations of the device are well known and information can be interpreted within the context of the monitor. Failure to appreciate these limitations can interfere with patient management. Indeed, few clinicians would assess cardiac well being based only on the ECG. In the same way, care must be taken when applying information gathered from neurologic monitoring.

Cerebral Ischemia

Virtually all neurologic monitors detect actual or possible cerebral ischemia, defined as cerebral delivery of oxygen (CDO_2) insufficient to meet metabolic needs. Cerebral ischemia is traditionally characterized as global or focal and

Table 22-1. Glossary of Neurologic Monitor Characteristics

Term	Definition
Bias	Average difference (positive or negative) between monitored values and "gold standard" values
Precision	Standard deviation of the differences (bias) between measurements
Sensitivity	Probability that the monitor demonstrates cerebral ischemia when cerebral ischemia is present
Positive predictive value	Probability that cerebral ischemia is present when the monitor suggests cerebral ischemia
Specificity	Probability that the monitor will not demonstrate cerebral ischemia when cerebral ischemia is not present
Negative predictive value	Probability that cerebral ischemia is not present when the monitor reflects no cerebral ischemia
Threshold value	The value used to separate acceptable (i.e., no ischemia present) from unacceptable (i.e., ischemia present)
Speed	The time elapsed from the onset of actual ischemia or the risk of ischemia until the monitor provides evidence

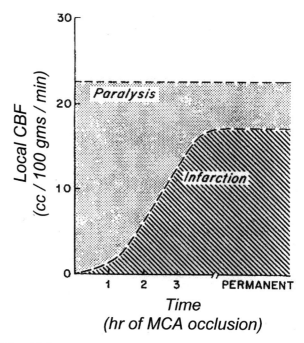

Fig. 22-1. Schematic representation of ischemic thresholds in awake monkeys. The threshold for reversible paralysis occurs at local cerebral blood flow of approximately 23 mL • 100g^{-1} • min^{-1}. Irreversible injury (infarction) is a function of the magnitude of blood flow reduction and the duration of that reduction. Relatively severe ischemia is potentially reversible if the duration is sufficiently short. MCA, middle cerebral artery. (From Jones TH, Morawetz RB, Crowell RM, et al: Thresholds of focal cerebral ischemia in awake monkeys. *J Neurosurg* 54:773–782, 1981, with permission.)

complete or incomplete (Table 22-2). Systemic monitors readily detect most global cerebral insults, such as hypotension, hypoxemia, and cardiac arrest. Therefore, brain-specific monitors can provide additional information primarily in situations, such as stroke, SAH with vasospasm, and TBI, in which focal cerebral oxygenation may be impaired despite adequate systemic oxygenation and perfusion.

The severity of ischemic brain damage is proportional to the magnitude and duration of reduced CDo_2. For monitoring to affect long-term patient morbidity and mortality, recognition of reversible cerebral ischemia is one of the primary goals. In monkeys, potentially reversible paralysis develops if regional CBF declines below about 23 mL • 100g^{-1} • min^{-1}; whereas infarction of brain tissue generally requires that CBF remain below 18 mL • 100g^{-1} • min^{-1} [4]. The tolerable duration of more profound ischemia is inversely proportional to the severity of CBF reduction (Fig. 22-1).

When a cerebral monitor detects ischemia, the results must be carefully interpreted. Often, all that is known is that cerebral oxygenation in the region of brain that is assessed by that monitor has fallen below a critical threshold. Such information does not imply that ischemia will progress to infarction. Because more severe ischemia produces neurologic injury in less time than less severe ischemia, a time and dose effect must be considered. Therefore, it is impossible to use a threshold monitor to predict with certainty whether changes in neurologic function will be followed by irreversible cerebral injury. In addition, if regional ischemia involves structures that are not components of the monitored variable, then infarction could develop without warning.

Table 22-2. Characteristics of Types of Cerebral Ischemic Insults

Characteristics	Examples
Global, incomplete	Hypotension, hypoxemia, cardiopulmonary resuscitation
Global, complete	Cardiac arrest
Focal, incomplete	Stroke, subarachnoid hemorrhage with vasospasm

In healthy persons, CBF is tightly regulated through multiple pathways such that CDo_2 is adjusted to meet the metabolic requirements of the brain. In the normal, "coupled" relationship, CBF is dependent on the cerebral metabolic rate for oxygen ($CMRo_2$), which varies directly with body temperature and with the level of brain activation (Fig. 22-2A). As $CMRo_2$ increases or decreases, CBF increases or decreases to match oxygen requirements with oxygen delivery. Pressure autoregulation maintains CBF at a constant rate (assuming unchanged metabolic needs) over a wide range of systemic blood pressures (Fig. 22-2B). If pressure autoregulation is intact, changes of cerebral perfusion pressure (CPP) do not alter CBF over a range of pressures of 50 to 130 mm Hg [5]. CPP is described by the equation:

$$CPP = MAP - ICP$$

where MAP = mean arterial pressure.

After neurologic insults such as TBI, the cerebral vasculature may have an impaired ability to increase CBF in response to decreasing CPP [6–8]. This failure to maintain adequate CDo_2 can lead to ischemia and add to preexisting brain injury.

Normally, $Paco_2$ powerfully regulates cerebral vascular resistance over a range of $Paco_2$ of 20 to 80 mm Hg (Fig. 22-2C). CBF is acutely halved if $Paco_2$ is halved, and doubled if $Paco_2$ is doubled. However, in healthy brain, there are limits to maximal cerebral vasodilation and vasoconstriction, such that decreases in CBF to the point of inadequate CDo_2 are countered by local vasodilatory mechanisms to restore flow and CDo_2. In healthy brain, hyperventilation does not produce severe cerebral ischemia; however, after TBI, hypocapnia can result in inadequate CDo_2 as reflected in decreased $Pbto_2$ and $Sjvo_2$ [9,10]. Thus, one indication for cerebral oxygenation monitoring includes the intent to use therapeutic hyperventilation, in which case monitoring can influ-

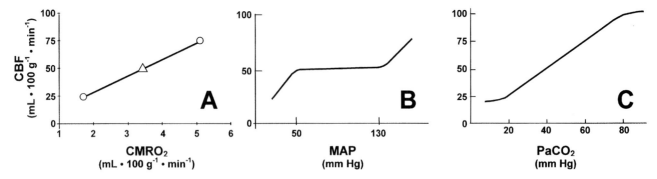

Fig. 22-2. **A:** The normal relationship between the cerebral metabolic rate of oxygen consumption ($CMRO_2$) and cerebral blood flow (CBF) is characterized by closely coupled changes in both variables. Normally, CBF is 50 mL per 100 g per minute in adults (*open triangle*). As $CMRO_2$ increases or decreases, CBF changes in a parallel fashion (*solid line*). **B:** Effect of mean arterial pressure (MAP) on CBF. Note that changes in MAP produce little change in CBF over a broad range of pressures. If intracranial pressure exceeds normal limits, substitute cerebral perfusion pressure on the horizontal axis. **C:** Effect of partial pressure of carbon dioxide ($PaCO_2$) on CBF. Changes in $PaCO_2$ exert powerful effects on cerebral vascular resistance across the entire clinically applicable range of values.

ence the endpoint of hyperventilation [11–13]. If hyperventilation is required to acutely reduce ICP, administration of an increased inspired oxygen concentration can markedly increase $SjvO_2$ (Fig. 22-3) [13]. In response to decreasing arterial oxygen content (CaO_2), whether the reduction is secondary to a decrease of hemoglobin concentration ([Hgb]) or of arterial oxygen saturation (SaO_2), CBF normally increases, although injured brain tissue has impaired ability to increase CBF [14–16].

Techniques of Neurologic Monitoring

Frequent, accurately recorded neurologic examinations are an essential aspect of neurologic monitoring. Neurologic examination quantifies three key characteristics: level of consciousness, focal brain dysfunction, and trends in neurologic function. Recognition of changing consciousness may warn of a variety of treatable conditions such as progression of intracranial hypertension, and systemic complications of intracranial pathology such as hyponatremia. Focal neurologic findings suggest a localized lesion. Comparable levels of consciousness imply better prognoses in patients who are improving than in those who are deteriorating. When the condition of a patient deteriorates, or when techniques such as deep sedation or use of muscle relaxants are used, neurologic examination becomes less informative, and other monitoring techniques must be used. Even so, changes in the neurologic examination over time remain an important aspect of medical care.

The Glasgow Coma Scale (GCS), originally developed as a prognostic tool for patients with TBI [17], has become popular as a quick, reproducible estimate of level of consciousness (Table 22-3). The scale, which includes eye opening, motor responses in the best functioning limb, and verbal responses,

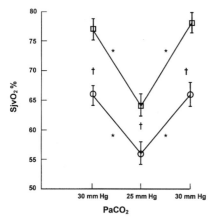

Fig. 22-3. The effect of hyperoxia on percent oxygen saturation of jugular venous blood ($SjvO_2$) at two levels of partial pressure of carbon dioxide ($PaCO_2$). Stars indicate $p < .001$ for $SjvO_2$ at $PaCO_2$, 25 to 30 mm Hg at each partial arterial pressure of oxygen (PaO_2). The daggers indicate $p < .001$ for $SjvO_2$ between PaO_2 at each $PaCO_2$ level. Circles indicate PaO_2 of 100 to 150 mm Hg. Squares indicate PaO_2 of 200 to 250 mm Hg. (From Thiagarajan A, Goverdhan PD, Chari P et al: The effect of hyperventilation and hyperoxia on cerebral venous oxygen saturation in patients with traumatic brain injury. *Anesth Analg* 87:850–853, 1998, with permission.)

Table 22-3. Glasgow Coma Scale

Component	Response	Score
Eye opening	Spontaneously	4
	To verbal command	3
	To pain	2
	None	1
		Subtotal: 1–4
Motor response (best extremity)	Obeys verbal command	6
	Localizes pain	5
	Flexion-withdrawal	4
	Flexor (decorticate posturing)	3
	Extensor (decerebrate posturing)	2
	No response (flaccid)	1
		Subtotal: 1–6
Best verbal response	Oriented and converses	5
	Disoriented and converses	4
	Inappropriate words	3
	Incomprehensible sounds	2
	No verbal response	1
		Subtotal: 1–5
		Total: 3–15

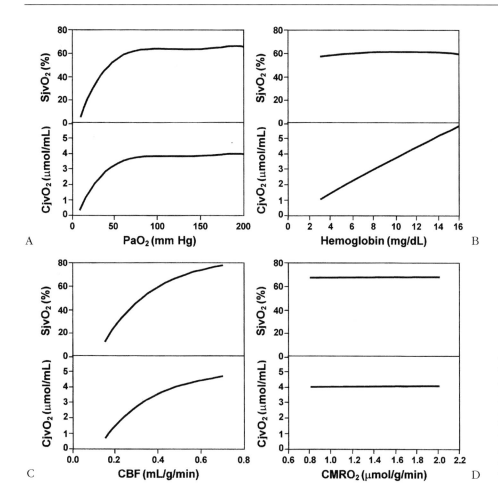

Fig. 22-4. Changes in jugular venous saturation (SjvO$_2$) and jugular venous oxygen content (CjvO$_2$) in a normal subject in response to hypoxia **(A)**, normovolemic anemia **(B)**, reduced cerebral blood flow (CBF) **(C)**, and increased cerebral metabolic rate of oxygen (CMRO$_2$) **(D)**. (From Feldman Z, Robertson CS: Monitoring of cerebral hemodynamics with jugular bulb catheters. *Crit Care Clin* 13:51–77, 1997, with permission.)

should be supplemented by recording pupillary size and reactivity and the status of focal neurologic findings. The scale is used to characterize the severity of TBI, with severe TBI defined as a GCS score less than or equal to 8, moderate TBI as a GCS score of 9 to 12, and mild TBI as that associated with a GCS score greater than 12 [18]. Lower GCS scores are associated with poorer long-term outcomes [9].

Systemic Monitoring

Monitoring of blood pressure, SaO$_2$, and body temperature provides important data about the adequacy of global brain oxygenation and the vulnerability of the brain to ischemic injury. Perhaps the most important systemic monitor is blood pressure, because CPP is a determinant of outcome, especially in head-injured patients. Chesnut et al. reported that even brief periods of hypotension (systolic blood pressure less than 90 mm Hg) worsened outcome after TBI [19,20], although ideal blood pressure management after TBI has yet to be defined [21]. Proposed treatment protocols include CPP greater than 70 mm Hg [22], CPP greater than 60 mm Hg [23], or CPP greater than 50 mm Hg, based on assumptions regarding cerebral perfusion maintenance [22,23] or aggravation of cerebral edema [21].

Another essential step in insuring adequate CDO$_2$ is the maintenance of adequate CaO$_2$, which in turn is dependent on [Hgb] and SaO$_2$; therefore, hypoxemia and anemia can reduce CDO$_2$, which may result in compensatory increases in CBF. However, there is a limit to this compensatory mechanism. As SaO$_2$ (or PaO$_2$) decreases below the compensatory threshold, SjvO$_2$, a measure of the ability of CDO$_2$ to supply CMRO$_2$, and jugular venous oxygen content (CjvO$_2$) decrease (Fig. 22-4A) [24]. The correlation is most evident below a PaO$_2$ of approximately 60 mm Hg, the PaO$_2$ at which SaO$_2$ is 90% and below which SaO$_2$ rapidly decreases. In contrast, as [Hgb] is reduced by normovolemic hemodilution, SjvO$_2$ remains relatively constant (Fig. 22-4B) [24].

Monitoring of body temperature is a fundamental aspect of care of critically ill neurologic and neurosurgical patients, primarily because of experimental evidence that mild hyperthermia worsens and mild hypothermia attenuates ischemic injury. The relationship between brain temperature and CMRO$_2$ is expressed as the Q$_{10}$, or change in CMRO$_2$ per 10°C change in temperature, as follows:

$$Q_{10} = (R1/R2)^{10/(T1-T2)}$$

where R1 and R2 describe CMRO$_2$ at temperatures T1 and T2, respectively. The average Q$_{10}$ value is 2, which predicts a 7% change in CMRO$_2$ per degree Celsius. However, hypothermia (34°C) decreases the basal component of CMRO$_2$ more than the active component by reducing membrane permeability to Na$^+$–K$^+$ leak [25].

Table 22-4. Outcome at Discharge in Relation to Intracranial Diagnosis (% of Patients)

Outcome	DI I	DI II	DI III	DI IV	Evacuated mass	Nonevacuated mass
Good recovery	27.0	8.5	3.3	3.1	5.1	2.8
Moderate disability	34.6	26.0	13.1	3.1	17.7	8.3
Severe disability	19.2	40.7	26.8	18.8	26.0	19.4
Persistent vegetative state	9.6	11.2	22.9	18.8	12.3	16.7
Death	9.6	13.5	34.0	56.2	38.8	52.8
Total	100	100	100	100	100	100

DI, diffuse injury. DI categories I through IV represent increasingly severe classes of diffuse brain injury.
From Marshall LF, Marshall SB, Klauber MR, et al: A new classification of head injury based on computerized tomography. *J Neurosurg* 75:S14–S20, 1991, with permission.

The method of temperature monitoring is important. Thermal gradients exist throughout the body, and the site of measurement influences the diagnosis of hypothermia, normothermia, or hyperthermia. Measurements of systemic temperature may underestimate brain temperature. In the future, direct brain temperature monitoring may be preferable in some patients [31–33].

Brain protection was once considered to be a dose-dependent function of body temperature, with substantial benefit obtained only from reduction to temperatures of 26° to 28°C, such as have been commonly used during cardiopulmonary bypass. In rats subjected to global ischemic [26] or traumatic insults [27], however, mild hypothermia (30° to 33°C) provided substantial protection, whereas increases of a few degrees above normal worsened outcome. In experimental global ischemia, mild to moderate hypothermia attenuated histopathologic damage, inhibited glutamate release during ischemia, and reduced hydroxyl radical generation during reperfusion [28]. In head-injured patients, a single-center, phase II, randomized clinical trial demonstrated that reduction of temperature to 33° to 34°C within 10 hours of TBI and continuing for 24 hours significantly improved outcome in patients with admission GCS scores of 5 to 7 [29]. However, in a subsequent multicenter trial, mild hypothermia initiated after TBI failed to improve outcome [30]. Although induction of hypothermia failed to improve outcome, a subgroup of patients who were hypothermic on hospital entry and were rewarmed after randomization to normothermic management had particularly poor outcomes.

Neuroimaging

Cranial computed tomographic (CT) scans, magnetic resonance imaging (MRI), positron emission spectroscopy (PET) scans, cerebral angiography, and radionuclide scans do not function as monitors, *per se.* Rather, they are indicated in response to suspicion of a new or progressive anatomic lesion, such as a subdural or intracerebral hematoma or cerebral arterial vasospasm, that requires altered treatment. Most neuroimaging modalities provide static, discontinuous data and require moving a critically ill patient from the intensive care unit (ICU) to a remote location. Even so, these techniques play an important role in the overall management of patients with brain injury.

CT scans obtained at the time of admission to the hospital can provide valuable prognostic information. Marshall et al. predicted outcome of head-injured patients in relation to four grades of increasingly severe diffuse brain injury and

the presence of evacuated or non-evacuated intracranial mass lesions (Table 22-4) [34]. Normal CT scans at admission in patients with GCS scores less than 8 are associated with a 10% to 15% incidence of ICP elevation [35–37]; however, the risk of ICP elevation increases in patients older than age 40 years, those with unilateral or bilateral motor posturing, or those with systolic blood pressure less than 90 mm Hg [35]. In the future, the advent of smaller, portable, bedside CT scanners may prompt greater use of imaging for monitoring.

Although MRI often provides better resolution than CT scans, powerful magnets are incompatible with ferrous metals, a ubiquitous component of life-support equipment. To address this issue, MRI-compatible ventilators and monitors have been developed [38]. Recent advances in MRI technology, such as diffusion-weighted imaging, magnetic resonance spectroscopy (carbon, phosphorus, and nitrogen-labeled), and phase-contrast angiography may provide information about brain function, oxidative metabolic pathways, cerebral blood volume, and functional CBF [39–43]. These techniques, while undergoing further evaluation and validation, may one day prove useful in evaluating brain injury and its management. Recent clinical evidence of brain mitochondrial dysfunction after TBI, despite apparently adequate CDo_2, suggests that functional cellular evaluation and associated therapy may someday be as important as maintaining CDo_2 [44].

Cerebral Blood Flow Monitoring

The first quantitative clinical method of measurement of CBF, the Kety-Schmidt technique [45], calculated global CBF from the difference between the arterial and jugular bulb concentration curves of an inhaled, inert gas as it equilibrated with blood and brain tissue. Later techniques used extracranial gamma detectors to measure regional cortical CBF from washout curves after intracarotid injection of a radioisotope such as ^{133}xenon (^{133}Xe) [46]. Carotid puncture was avoided by techniques that measured cortical CBF after inhaled [47] or intravenous administration of ^{133}Xe, using gamma counting of exhaled gas to correct clearance curves for recirculation of ^{133}Xe. Among the obstacles to wider use of ^{133}Xe clearance is technical complexity, cumbersome regulations governing radionuclides, and the sustained interval of stability (5 to 15 minutes) required to perform a single measurement.

Because Xe is radiodense, saturation of brain tissue increases radiographic density in proportion to CBF. Imaging of the brain after equilibration with stable Xe provides a regional estimate of CBF that includes deep brain structures [48].

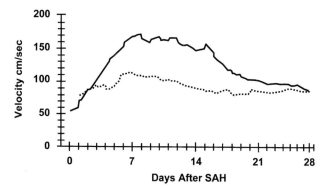

Fig. 22-5. Mean flow velocity curves of 18 patients with laterally localized aneurysms arising from the internal carotid and middle cerebral arteries. The side of the ruptured aneurysm (*continuous line*) shows a higher flow velocity than the unaffected side (*dotted line*). SAH, subarachnoid hemorrhage. (From Seiler RW, Grolimund P, Aaslid R, et al: Cerebral vasospasm evaluated by transcranial ultrasound correlated with clinical grade and CT-visualized subarachnoid hemorrhage. *J Neurosurg* 64:594–600, 1986, with permission.)

Clinical studies of CBF after TBI performed using stable Xe CT have prompted a radical revision of conventional understanding by demonstrating that one-third of patients had evidence of cerebral ischemia within 8 hours of trauma [7]. However, the requirement for an extended motionless interval in the CT scanner has inhibited wider use of this technique in critically ill patients.

In most patients, cerebral arterial flow velocity can be measured easily in intracranial vessels, especially the middle cerebral artery, using transcranial Doppler ultrasonography. Doppler flow velocity uses the frequency shift, proportional to velocity, observed when sound waves are reflected from moving red blood cells. Blood moving toward the transducer shifts the transmitted frequency to higher frequencies; blood moving away, to lower frequencies. Velocity is a function both of blood flow rate and vessel diameter. If diameter remains constant, changes in velocity are proportional to changes in CBF; however, intersubject differences in flow velocity correlate poorly with intersubject differences in CBF [49]. Entirely noninvasive, transcranial Doppler measurements can be repeated at frequent intervals or even applied continuously. The detection and monitoring of post-SAH vasospasm remains the most common use of transcranial Doppler (Fig. 22-5) [50–52]. However, further clinical research is necessary to define those situations in which the excellent capacity for rapid trend monitoring can be exploited.

Intracranial Pressure Monitoring

ICP functions as the outflow pressure for the cerebral circulation (see equation in Cerebral Ischemia section) when ICP exceeds jugular venous pressure. Because the skull is not distensible, the brain, cerebrospinal fluid (CSF), and cerebral blood volume have little room to expand without increasing ICP. Although CBF cannot be directly inferred from knowledge of MAP and ICP, severe increases in ICP reduce CPP and CBF.

The symptoms and signs of intracranial hypertension are neither sensitive nor specific. Usually, the physical findings associated with increasing ICP (e.g., Cushing's response and Cushing's triad) become apparent only when intracranial hypertension has become sufficiently severe to injure the brain. Likewise, papilledema is a late development that requires skillful ophthalmoscopy for diagnosis. Because ICP cannot otherwise be adequately assessed, direct measurement and monitoring of ICP has become a common intervention, especially in the management of TBI [53], and less commonly after critical illnesses such as SAH or stroke. ICP monitoring is recommended for the management of patients who are comatose after TBI [23]. Clinically, one of three sites—a lateral ventricle, the subdural space, or the brain parenchyma—is used for measuring ICP. Because pressure gradients may exist among various sites, it may be advantageous to monitor in or adjacent to the most severely damaged hemisphere [54], though some even recommend bilateral ICP monitoring to circumvent this problem [55].

ICP monitoring provides temporally relevant, quantitative information. Continuing debate centers on the use of this information to change patient care and reduce morbidity and mortality. The problems associated with ICP monitoring fall generally into three categories: direct morbidity (e.g., intracranial hemorrhage, cortical damage, and infection), inaccurate measurement, and misinterpretation or inappropriate use of the data. Ventricular catheterization, when performed using strict asepsis, is the method of choice for ICP monitoring and CSF drainage in patients with acute intracranial hypertension and excess CSF (i.e., acute hydrocephalus). In contrast, intraventricular catheters may be difficult to place if cerebral edema or brain swelling has compressed the ventricular system. In addition, gradual loss of calibration ("drift") is an inherent problem with hollow catheters that are fluid-coupled to external pressure transducers that must be "zeroed." Catheters also must be zeroed at the level of the external auditory meatus. Intraventricular pressure monitoring can also be performed with fiberoptic catheters that use a variable reflectance pressure sensing system (transducer tip) to measure pressure (Camino Laboratories, San Diego, CA). These fiberoptic catheters are less susceptible to short-term malfunction than conventional, fluid-filled catheters [56] but may slowly drift over days to weeks.

ICP monitoring from the subdural space uses fluid-coupled bolts (simple transcranial conduits), fluid-coupled subdural catheters (or reservoirs), or fiberoptic transducer-tipped catheters. Because subdural bolts are open tubes facing end-on against the brain surface, brain tissue may herniate into the system, obstructing the system, distorting measurements and potentially damaging the cerebral cortex. The fiberoptic system, when inserted subdurally, cannot be easily recalibrated after insertion but demonstrates low drift [56]. Of 46 patients monitored with fiberoptic catheters in the intraparenchymal (n = 43) or intraventricular (n = 3) positions, 12% developed broken components, 8.6% required repositioning for erroneous readings, and epidural hematomas complicated 3.4% [57]. Other investigators reported a rate of contamination of 13.2% and a rate of clinically significant infection 2.9% with fiberoptic ICP catheters [58]. In comparing ventriculostomy with intraparenchymal ICP devices, ventriculostomy was associated with a higher complication rate (12.4% vs. 1.2%) and, when complications occurred, was associated with a worse Glasgow Outcome Scale score [59].

In addition to revealing frankly increased ICP, monitoring can also reveal temporal information about normal and pathologic pressure waveforms. B waves, cycling at a rate of two to four per second with an amplitude of 10 mm Hg, warn of possible decompensation of intracranial compliance, whereas plateau, or A waves, consisting of cyclic increases in ICP, often 50 mm Hg or higher, and lasting as long as 15

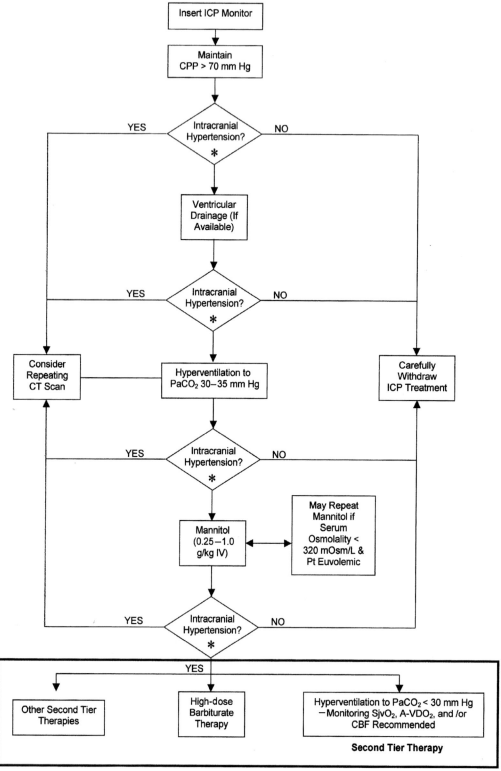

Fig. 22-6. Critical pathway for treatment of intracranial hypertension in the severe head injury patient (treatment option). A-VDo₂, arteriovenous oxygen content difference; CPP, cerebral perfusion pressure; CT, computed tomography; ICP, intracranial pressure; Paco₂, partial pressure of carbon dioxide; Sjvo₂, jugular bulb venous oxygen saturation. (From Bullock RM, Chesnut RM, Clifton GL, et al: Management and prognosis of severe traumatic brain injury. Part I. Guidelines for the management of severe traumatic brain injury. *J Neurotrauma* 17:449–553, 2000, with permission.)

to 30 minutes, suggest impending intracranial catastrophe and poor prognosis [60].

Management decisions based on ICP data are the focus of ongoing debate and study. Clinical studies after TBI have demonstrated that increased ICP is associated with worsened outcome [61]. Therefore, control of ICP has been considered

by some clinicians to be the primary focus of treatment [21]; other clinicians have considered restoration of CPP (by increasing MAP) to be the primary goal of medical management [22,62]. To date, the ideal approach has not been established by outcome trials; therefore practice patterns remain variable [63]. Clinical experience with ICP monitoring of head-injured patients has resulted in publication of clinical guide-lines that have recently been updated using an evidence-based approach (Fig. 22-6) [23].

Jugular Bulb Venous Oxygen Saturation

Several measurements of cerebral oxygenation have recently been clinically evaluated. The most extensively used is $SjvO_2$, which reflects the adequacy of CDO_2 to support $CMRO_2$. In contrast to ICP and CPP, which provide only indirect information concerning the adequacy of CDO_2 to support $CMRO_2$, $SjvO_2$ directly reflects the balance between these variables on a global or hemispheric level. CBF, $CMRO_2$, CaO_2, and $CjvO_2$ are modeled by the following equation:

$$CMRO_2 = CBF\ (CaO_2 - CjvO_2)$$

In healthy brain, if $CMRO_2$ remains constant as CBF decreases, $SjvO_2$ and $CjvO_2$ decrease (Fig. 22-4C) [24]. If flow-metabolism coupling is intact, decreases in $CMRO_2$ result in parallel decreases in CBF and $SjvO_2$ and $CjvO_2$ remain constant (Fig. 22-4D) [24].

Mixed cerebral venous blood, like mixed systemic blood, is a global average and may not reflect marked regional hypo-perfusion. Abnormally low $SjvO_2$ (i.e., less than 50%, com-pared to a normal value of 65%) suggests the possibility of cerebral ischemia; but normal or elevated $SjvO_2$ does not prove the adequacy of cerebral perfusion. Therefore, the neg-ative predictive value of a normal $SjvO_2$ is poor.

After placement, monitoring of hemoglobin saturation can be achieved through repeated blood sampling. However, repeated blood sampling yields only "snapshots" of cerebral oxygenation [12], and thus provides discontinuous data that may miss rapid changes in saturation. To achieve continuous monitoring of $SjvO_2$, indwelling fiberoptic oximetric catheters have been used. Because oxyhemoglobin and deoxyhemo-globin absorb light differently, $SjvO_2$ can be determined from differential absorbance. Oximetric jugular bulb catheters have proven somewhat challenging to maintain, requiring frequent recalibration, repositioning, and confirmation of measured saturation by analyzing blood samples in a CO-oximeter [70]. The highest frequency of confirmed desaturation episodes occurs in patients with intracerebral hematomas, closely fol-lowed by those with SAH. In patients with TBI, the number of jugular desaturations is strongly associated with poor neuro-logic outcome; even a single desaturation episode is associ-ated with a doubling of the mortality rate (Fig. 22-7) [71].

Clinical application of jugular venous bulb cannulation has been limited, perhaps in part because the technique is invasive, although the risks of cannulation injury, including hematoma and injury to the adjacent carotid, are low [64]. To insert a retro-grade jugular venous bulb catheter, the internal jugular vein can be located by ultrasound guidance or by external anatomic landmarks and use of a "seeker" needle, namely, the same tech-nique used for antegrade placement of jugular venous catheters. Once the vessel is identified, the catheter is directed cephalad, towards the mastoid process, instead of centrally. A lateral cra-nial radiograph can confirm the position just superior to the base of the skull. The decision to place a jugular bulb catheter in the left or right jugular bulb is important. Simultaneous mea-surements of $SjvO_2$ in the right and left jugular bulb demon-strates differences in saturation [65,66], suggesting that one jugular bulb frequently is dominant, carrying the greater portion of cerebral venous blood [67]. Differences in the cross-sectional areas of the vessels that form the torcula and the manner in

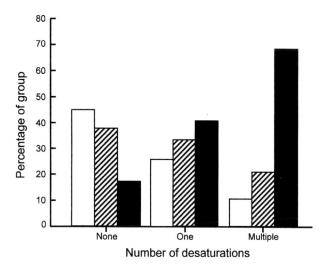

Fig. 22-7. Occurrence of jugular venous desaturation was strongly associated with a high mortality rate and a poor outcome. Three-month Glasgow Outcome Scale: white bars represent percentage of patients who had good recovery/moderate disability; striped bars rep-resent percentage of patients who had severe disability/persistent vegetative state; black bars represent percentage of patients who died. (From Gopinath SP, Robertson CS, Contant CF, et al: Jugular venous desaturation and outcome after head injury. *J Neurol Neuro-surg Psychiatry* 57:717–723, 1994, with permission.)

which blood is distributed to the right and left lateral sinus con-tribute to differences between the two jugular bulbs [67]. Ide-ally, a jugular bulb catheter should be placed on the dominant side, which can be identified as the jugular vein that, if com-pressed, produces the greater increase in ICP or as the vein on the side of the larger jugular foramen as detected by CT [68,69].

Several modifications of jugular venous oxygen monitoring have been proposed. Cerebral extraction of oxygen, which is the difference between SaO_2 and $SjvO_2$ divided by SaO_2, is less confounded by anemia than the cerebral A-VDO_2 [72]. Another concept, termed *cerebral hemodynamic reserve*, is defined as the ratio of percent change in global cerebral extraction of oxygen (reflecting the balance between $CMRO_2$ and CBF) to percent change in CPP [73]. This equation attempts to inte-grate cerebral hemodynamics and metabolism with intracra-nial compliance. Cruz et al. found that cerebral hemodynamic reserve decreased as intracranial compliance decreased, even as a consequence of minor elevations in ICP [73]. Theoreti-cally, this variable may allow more precise management of cerebral hemodynamics in patients with decreased intracranial compliance.

Brain Tissue Oxygen Tension

Another promising technique for monitoring the adequacy of CDO_2 is direct assessment of $PbtO_2$. Monitoring of $PbtO_2$ over-comes one important limitation of $SjvO_2$ monitoring, which is that the global saturation measurements provide no information about regional or focal tissue oxygenation. Only relatively pro-found focal global ischemia causes $SjvO_2$ to decrease to less than the accepted critical threshold of 50%. Even severe regional ischemia may not result in desaturation if venous effluent from other regions is normally saturated, in part because the absolute flow of poorly saturated blood returning from ischemic regions is by definition less per volume of tissue than flow from well-

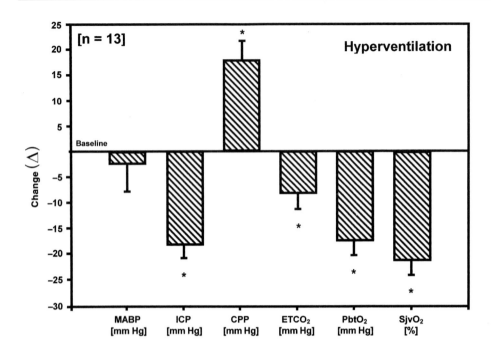

Fig. 22-8. The effect of hyperventilation-induced hypocapnia on changes in mean arterial blood pressure (MABP), intracranial pressure (ICP), cerebral perfusion pressure (CPP), end-tidal carbon dioxide (ETCO$_2$), brain tissue oxygen tension (PbtO$_2$), and jugular bulb oximetry (SjvO$_2$). *, $p <.05$ before hyperventilation versus 10 minutes later. (From Unterberg AW, Kiening KL, Härtl R, et al: Multimodal monitoring in patients with head injury: evaluation of the effects of treatment on cerebral oxygenation. *J Trauma* 42:S32–S37, 1997.)

perfused regions, resulting in a smaller percentage of poorly oxygenated to well-oxygenated blood. Intracranial, intraparenchymal probes have been developed that monitor only PbtO$_2$ or that also monitor brain tissue PCO$_2$ and pH [74]. Modified from probes designed for continuous monitoring of arterial blood gases, intraparenchymal probes can be inserted through multiple-lumen ICP monitoring bolts. Although these probes provide no information about remote regions, they nevertheless provide continuous information about the region that is contiguous to the probe. They also carry the theoretical risk of hematoma formation, infection, and direct parenchymal injury.

Evaluation of PbtO$_2$ after TBI has shown that low partial pressures (PbtO$_2$ less than 10 mm Hg for longer than 30 minutes)

powerfully predict poor outcome [75]. Both PbtO$_2$ and SjvO$_2$ may reflect changes in cerebral oxygenation secondary to alterations in CBF (Fig. 22-8) [76]. However, comparisons of simultaneous PbtO$_2$ and SjvO$_2$ monitoring suggest that each monitor detects cerebral ischemia that the other fails to detect. In 58 patients with severe TBI, the two monitors detected 52 episodes in which SjvO$_2$ decreased to less than 50% or PbtO$_2$ decreased to less than 8 mm Hg; of those 52 episodes, both monitored variables fell below the ischemic threshold in 17, only SjvO$_2$ reflected ischemia in 19, and only PbtO$_2$ reflected ischemia in 16 (Fig. 22-9) [77]. Ongoing research will determine the role of PbtO$_2$ monitoring and the relationship between PbtO$_2$ monitoring and SjvO$_2$ monitoring in critical neurologic illness.

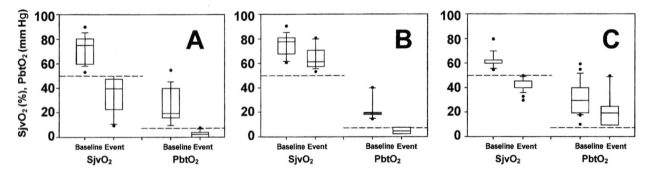

Fig. 22-9. Changes in jugular venous oxygen saturation (SjvO$_2$) and brain tissue partial pressure of oxygen (PbtO$_2$) during 52 episodes of cerebral hypoxia/ischemia. The horizontal line across the box plot represents the median, and the lower and upper ends of the box plot are the twenty-fifth and seventy-fifth percentiles, respectively. The error bars mark the 10th and 90th percentiles. The closed circles indicate any outlying points. **A:** Summary of the 17 cases in which SjvO$_2$ and PbtO$_2$ decreased to less than their respective thresholds, as defined in the text. **B:** Summary of the 16 cases in which PbtO$_2$ decreased to less than the defined threshold; but SjvO$_2$, although decreased, did not decrease to less than 50%. **C:** Summary of the 19 cases in which SjvO$_2$ decreased to less than the threshold, but PbtO$_2$ remained at greater than 10 mm Hg. (From Gopinath SP, Valadka AB, Uzura M, et al: Comparison of jugular venous oxygen saturation and brain tissue PO$_2$ as monitors of cerebral ischemia after head injury. *Crit Care Med* 27:2337–2345, 1999, with permission.)

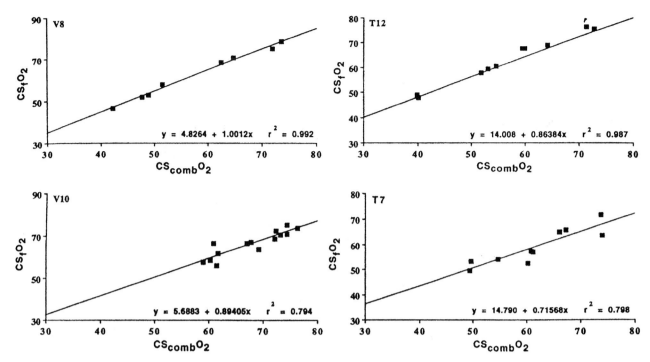

Fig. 22-10. Cerebral oximeter signal ($Cs_f O_2$) and estimated global brain oxygen saturation ($Cs_{comb}O_2$, calculated from arterial oxygen saturation and jugular venous oxygen saturation) are closely correlated for the training group (r^2 = 0.798 to 0.987) for individual subjects. The number in the upper left corner represents the individual subjects' identities. T, training set; V, validation set. The best and worst examples are represented. (From Pollard V, Prough DS, DeMelo AE, et al: Validation in volunteers of a near-infrared spectroscope for monitoring brain oxygenation *in vivo. Anesth Analg* 82:269–277, 1996, with permission.)

Near-Infrared Spectroscopy

Theoretically, the best monitor of brain oxygenation would be a noninvasive device that characterizes brain oxygenation as pulse oximeter characterizes for systemic oxygenation: Near-infrared spectroscopy (NIRS) might eventually offer the opportunity to assess the adequacy of brain oxygenation continuously and noninvasively, although to date the use of the technique has been limited. Near-infrared light penetrates the skull and, during transmission through or reflection from brain tissue, undergoes changes in intensity that are proportional to the relative concentrations of oxygenated and deoxygenated hemoglobin in the arteries,

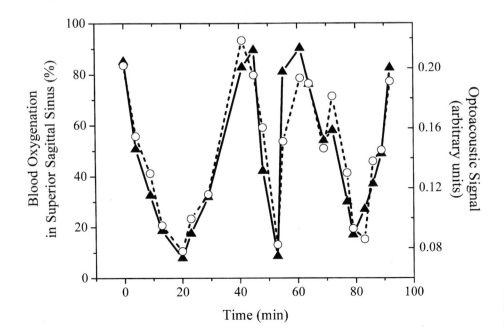

Fig. 22-11. Optoacoustic signal intensity (*dashed line*) and superior sagittal sinus hemoglobin saturation (*solid line*) as a function of time.

capillaries, and veins within the field [78]. The absorption (A) of light by a chromophore (i.e., hemoglobin) is defined by Beer's Law:

A = abc

where *a* is the absorption constant, *b* is the pathlength of the light, and *c* is the concentration of the chromophore, namely, oxygenated and deoxygenated hemoglobin.

Extensive preclinical and clinical data demonstrate that NIRS detects qualitative changes in brain oxygenation (Fig. 22-10) [79–81]. However, despite promise, many problems remain with the technology [82,83]. Brain saturation measured using NIRS correlated poorly with continuous $SjvO_2$ in patients with severe closed-head injury [84], although the technique seemed more promising for detecting desaturation during carotid endarterectomy [85] and cardiopulmonary bypass [86]. Technical challenges to quantification of the signal include inability to determine the pathlengths of reflected light of different wavelengths and inability to determine the relative proportions of arterial, capillary, and venous blood in the field. Therefore, validation studies suggest that NIRS may be more useful for qualitatively monitoring trends of brain tissue oxygenation than for actual quantification [81,87,88].

An alternative noninvasive monitor of brain oxygenation has been proposed [89]. This technique, termed *optoacoustic monitoring*, uses near-infrared light to generate miniscule acoustic waves in cerebral veins such as the superior sagittal sinus. Acoustic waves, unlike reflected light, are transmuted linearly through brain tissue and skull. Various characteristics of the acoustic signal are directly proportional to hemoglobin saturation in a targeted vein such as the superior sagittal sinus. Preliminary *in vivo* validation of this concept has been reported in sheep (Fig. 22-11) [89].

Laser Doppler Flowmetry

Laser Doppler flowmetry (LDF) uses the phase shift of laser light reflected from red blood cells to mathematically calculate blood flow through a tissue of interest. If hematocrit remains constant, the change in LDF signal is proportional to the change in blood flow. Changes in CBF in animals have been successfully measured by LDF when compared to other techniques such as hydrogen clearance and microspheres [90,91], and LDF evaluation of CBF has been used in humans with coma [92] and as a technique for evaluating autoregulation of CBF in patients with TBI [93]. LDF has been used to guide CPP management in the presence of altered CBF autoregulation [94,95]. This technique is unlikely to become a routine neurologic monitor because of difficulties with signal artifacts; small area of analysis; initial positioning of the probe; necessity for maintaining constant probe position; and provision of qualitative, not quantitative data.

Neurochemical Monitoring

Neurochemical monitoring via microdialysis allows assessment of the chemical milieu of cerebral extracellular fluid, and provides valuable information about neurochemical processes in various neuropathologic states [96,97]. In addition, microdialysate may reflect the metabolic responses to treatment modalities such as hypothermia [98], CSF drainage, and barbiturate administration. Cerebral ischemia and trauma are associated with substantial increases in energy-related metabolites such as

lactate, adenosine, inosine, and hypoxanthine; neurotransmitters such as glutamate, aspartate, dopamine, and gamma-amino butyric acid [96]; and alterations in membrane phospholipids by oxygen radicals [99]. The magnitude of release of these substances correlates with the extent of ischemic damage [100]. The lactate-pyruvate ratio in dialysate correlates with the glutamate concentration [101]. At lactate-pyruvate ratios less than 25 (normal range 15 to 20), glutamate concentrations were low, whereas at moderately elevated ratios (greater than 40), glutamate levels were increased. This suggests a threshold relationship between cerebral energy failure and release of glutamate into cerebral extracellular fluid and that the lactate-pyruvate ratio can be used as an indicator of disturbed brain energy metabolism. The use of incorporating microdialysis data in managing patients after TBI is being studied.

Electroencephalographic Monitoring

EEG has long been used in neurology for diagnosis, but has less frequently been used as a neurologic monitoring technique in critically ill patients. Rather, EEG is indicated in response to suspicion of a new or progressive abnormality such as cerebral ischemia or new onset of seizures. The cortical EEG, which is altered by mild cerebral ischemia and abolished by profound cerebral ischemia, can be used to indicate potentially damaging cerebral hypoperfusion. Likewise, the EEG can document seizures, either convulsive or non-convulsive, and provide information as to the efficacy of antiseizure therapy. Other functions include defining the depth or type of coma, documenting focal or lateral intracranial abnormalities, and the diagnosis of brain death.

If the EEG is to be used for monitoring, care must be taken and weaknesses of the technique appreciated [102]. In the ICU, electrical noise from other electrical equipment may interfere with technically adequate tracings. Continuous EEG recording is cumbersome owing to the sheer volume of data (300 pages per hour of hard copy on as many as 16 channels). Techniques of mathematical data analysis, such as rapid Fourier analysis, can be used to determine the relative amplitude in each frequency band [delta (less than 4 Hz), theta (4 to 8 Hz), alpha (8 to 13 Hz), beta (greater than 13 Hz)], which can then be displayed graphically in formats such as the compressed spectral array or density spectral array [103,104]. Recently, analytic software has been developed that processes the raw EEG signal to assess the depth of sedation, namely, the bispectral array [105–107].

Evoked Potentials

Sensory evoked potentials (EPs), which include somatosensory evoked potentials (SSEPs), brainstem auditory EPs, and visual EPs, can be used as qualitative threshold monitors to detect severe neural ischemia. Whereas the EEG records the continuous, spontaneous activity of the brain, EPs evaluate the responses of the brain to specific stimuli. To record SSEPs, stimuli are applied to a peripheral nerve, usually the median nerve at the wrist, by a low-amplitude current of approximately 20 milliseconds in duration. The resultant sensory (afferent) nerve stimulation and a measured cortical response to the stimulus are recorded at the scalp. Repeated identical stimuli are applied and signal averaging is used to remove the highly variable background EEG and other environmental electrical noise and thereby visualize reproducible evoked responses (Fig. 22-12) [108].

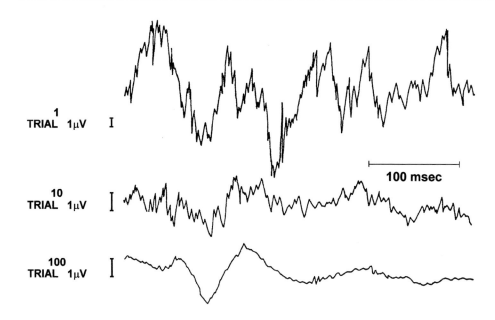

TRIAL 1 1μV I

100 msec

TRIAL 10 1μV I

TRIAL 100 1μV I

Fig. 22-12. Averaging reduces background noise. After 100 trials, this visual evoked potential is relatively noise-free. The same evoked potential is hard to distinguish after only ten trials and would be impossible to find in the original unaveraged data. (From Nuwer MR: *Evoked Potential Monitoring in the Operating Room.* New York, Raven Press, 1986, p 29, with permission.)

EPs are described in terms of the amplitude of individual peaks and the conduction delay (latency) between the stimulus and the appearance of response waveform. Because peripheral nerve stimulation can be uncomfortable, SSEPs are usually obtained on sedated or anesthetized patients. SSEPs are unaffected by neuromuscular blocking agents but are influenced by sedative, analgesic, and anesthetic agents [109–111]. In general, however, the doses of drugs required to influence EPs produced are sufficient to produce general anesthesia, and are not usually clinically important in the ICU. If a patient is undergoing EP monitoring and requires large doses of analgesic or sedative agents, potential impairment of monitoring should be considered.

Motor EPs represent a method of selectively evaluating descending motor tracts. Stimulation of proximal motor tracts (cortical or spinal) and evaluation of subsequent responses yields information that can be used for intraoperative and early postoperative neurosurgical management. Different induction strategies influence the effectiveness of the technique [116,117], and transcranial magnetic stimulation has been associated with seizure induction in susceptible populations [118]. Finally, motor EP induction and interpretation is exquisitely sensitive to sedative, analgesic, and anesthetic drugs [119], making clinical use difficult when drugs are given concurrently. Despite these limitations, motor EP evaluation has been successfully used for the management of neuro-ICU patients, and may become more common as techniques and equipment improve [120,121]. The sensitivity of EP monitoring is similar to that of EEG monitoring. EPs, especially brainstem auditory EPs, are relatively robust, although they can be modified by trauma, hypoxia, or ischemia. Because obliteration of EPs occurs only under conditions of profound cerebral ischemia or mechanical trauma, EP monitoring is one of the most specific ways in which to assess neurologic integrity in specific monitored pathways. However, as with the discussion of cerebral ischemia, there is a dose-time interaction ultimately determining the magnitude of cerebral injury. As a result, neurologic deficits occur that have not been predicted by changes in EPs [112], and severe changes in EPs may not be followed by neurologic deficits [113]. Even so, loss of cortical SSEPs remains a strong indicator of poor outcome [114,115].

Extensive use of electrophysiologic techniques in the ICU has been limited by three factors: expensive equipment, the requirement for highly trained technicians, and the need for clinical sophistication in the art of pattern recognition. Nevertheless, some research centers have used electrophysiologic monitoring as an integral part of a battery of monitors in critically ill patients with severe intracranial hypertension [122].

Summary

Appropriate use of neurologic monitoring techniques requires a thorough understanding of the indications, risks, benefits, and limitations of the techniques used. Monitoring in isolation is not associated with improved outcome after TBI and as such, represents only one component in the treatment of the patient. In the future, new modalities will undoubtedly emerge that will help guide the management of this difficult patient population.

References

1. Connors AF, Speroff T, Dawson NV, et al: The effectiveness of right heart catheterization in the initial care of critically ill patients. *JAMA* 276:889–897, 1996.
2. Bernard GR, Sopko G, Cerra F, et al: Pulmonary artery catheterization and clinical outcomes. National heart, lung, and blood institute and food and drug administration workshop report. *JAMA* 283:2568–2572, 2000.
3. Gnaegi A, Feihl F, Perret C: Intensive care physicians' insufficient knowledge of right-heart catheterization at the bedside: time to act? *Crit Care Med* 25:213–220, 1997.
4. Jones TH, Morawetz RB, Crowell RM, et al: Thresholds of focal cerebral ischemia in awake monkeys. *J Neurosurg* 54:773–782, 1981.
5. Strandgaard S, Paulson OB: Cerebral autoregulation. *Stroke* 15:413–416, 1984.
6. Bouma GJ, Muizelaar JP, Choi SC, et al: Cerebral circulation and metabolism after severe traumatic brain injury: the elusive role of ischemia. *J Neurosurg* 75:685–693, 1991.
7. Bouma GJ, Muizelaar JP, Stringer WA, et al: Ultra-early evaluation of regional cerebral blood flow in severely head-injured patients using xenon-enhanced computerized tomography. *J Neurosurg* 77:360–368, 1992.

8. DeWitt DS, Prough DS, Taylor CL, et al: Regional cerebrovascular responses to progressive hypotension after traumatic brain injury in cats. *Am J Physiol* 263:H1276–H1284, 1992.

9. Muizelaar JP, Marmarou A, Ward JD, et al: Adverse effects of prolonged hyperventilation in patients with severe head injury: a randomized clinical trial. *J Neurosurg* 75:731–739, 1991.

10. Chesnut RM: Avoidance of hypotension: condition sine qua non of successful severe head-injury management. *J Trauma* 42:S4–S9, 1997.

11. Matta BF, Lam AM, Mayberg TS: The influence of arterial oxygenation on cerebral venous oxygen saturation during hyperventilation. *Can J Anaesth* 41:1041–1046, 1994.

12. Gupta AK, Hutchinson PJ, Al-Rawi P, et al: Measuring brain tissue oxygenation compared with jugular venous oxygen saturation for monitoring cerebral oxygenation after traumatic brain injury. *Anesth Analg* 88:549–553, 1999.

13. Thiagarajan A, Goverdhan PD, Chari P, et al: The effect of hyperventilation and hyperoxia on cerebral venous oxygen saturation in patients with traumatic brain injury. *Anesth Analg* 87:850–853, 1998.

14. Phillis JW, Preston G, DeLong RE: Effects of anoxia on cerebral blood flow in the rat brain: evidence for a role of adenosine in autoregulation. *J Cereb Blood Flow Metab* 4:586–592, 1984.

15. Tommasino C, Moore S, Todd MM: Cerebral effects of isovolemic hemodilution with crystalloid or colloid solutions. *Crit Care Med* 16:862–868, 1988.

16. DeWitt DS, Prough DS, Taylor CL, et al: Reduced cerebral blood flow, oxygen delivery, and electroencephalographic activity after traumatic brain injury and mild hemorrhage in cats. *J Neurosurg* 76:812–821, 1992.

17. Teasdale G, Jennett B: Assessment of coma and impaired consciousness: a practical scale. *Lancet* 2:81–84, 1974.

18. Miller JD: Head injury. *J Neurol Neurosurg Psychiatry* 56:440–447, 1993.

19. Chesnut RM, Marshall SB, Piek J, et al: Early and late systemic hypotension as a frequent and fundamental source of cerebral ischemia following severe brain injury in the traumatic coma data bank. *Acta Neurochir* 59:121–125, 1993.

20. Chesnut RM, Ghajar J, Mass AIR, et al: Management and prognosis of severe traumatic brain injury. Part II. Early indications of prognosis in severe traumatic brain injury. *J Neurotrauma* 17:555–627, 2000.

21. Grande PO, Asgeirsson B, Nordstrom CH: Physiologic principles for volume regulation of a tissue enclosed in a rigid shell with application to the injured brain. *J Trauma* 42:S23–S31, 1997.

22. Rosner MJ, Rosner SD, Johnson AH: Cerebral perfusion pressure: management protocol and clinical results. *J Neurosurg* 83:949–962, 1995.

23. Bullock RM, Chesnut RM, Clifton GL, et al: Management and prognosis of severe traumatic brain injury. Part I. Guidelines for the management of severe traumatic brain injury. *J Neurotrauma* 17:449–553, 2000.

24. Feldman Z, Robertson CS: Monitoring of cerebral hemodynamics with jugular bulb catheters. *Crit Care Clin* 13:51–77, 1997.

25. Nemoto E, Klementavicius R, Melick J, et al: Effect of mild hypothermia on active and basal cerebral oxygen metabolism and blood flow. *Adv Exp Med Biol* 361:469–473, 1994.

26. Dietrich WD, Busto R, Alonso O, et al: Intraischemic but not postischemic brain hypothermia protects chronically following global forebrain ischemia in rats. *J Cereb Blood Flow Metab* 13:541–549, 1993.

27. Clifton GL, Jiang JY, Lyeth BG, et al: Marked protection by moderate hypothermia after experimental traumatic brain injury. *J Cereb Blood Flow Metab* 11:114–121, 1991.

28. Globus M, Alonso O, Dietrich W, et al: Glutamate release and free radical production following brain injury: effects of posttraumatic hypothermia. *J Neurochem* 65(4):1704–1711, 1995.

29. Marion DW, Penrod LE, Kelsey SF, et al: Treatment of traumatic brain injury with moderate hypothermia. *N Engl J Med* 336:540–546, 1997.

30. Clifton G: Hypothermia and severe brain injury. *J Neurosurg* 93:718–719, 2000.

31. Rumana CS, Gopinath SP, Uzura M, et al: Brain temperature exceeds systemic temperature in head-injured patients. *Crit Care Med* 26:562–567, 1998.

32. Mellergard P: Monitoring of rectal, epidural, and intraventricular temperature in neurosurgical patients. *Acta Neurochir Suppl* 60:485–487, 1994.

33. Crowder CM, Tempelhoff R, Theard MA, et al: Jugular bulb temperature: comparison with brain surface and core temperatures in neurosurgical patients during mild hypothermia. *J Neurosurg* 85:98–103, 1996.

34. Marshall LF, Marshall SB, Klauber MR, et al: A new classification of head injury based on computerized tomography. *J Neurosurg* 75:S14–S20, 1991.

35. Narayan RK, Kishore PRS, Becker DP, et al: Intracranial pressure: to monitor or not to monitor? A review of our experience with severe head injury. *J Neurosurg* 56:650–659, 1982.

36. Lobato RD, Sarabia R, Cordobes F, et al: Posttraumatic cerebral hemispheric swelling. Analysis of 55 cases studied with computerized tomography. *J Neurosurg* 68:417–423, 1988.

37. Eisenberg HM, Gary HE Jr, Aldrich EF, et al: Initial CT findings in 753 patients with severe head injury. A report from the NIH Traumatic Coma Data Bank. *J Neurosurg* 73:688–698, 1990.

38. Smith MC, Summers P, Padayachee TS: A variable pitch oxygen saturation indicator designed for use in the magnetic resonance environment. *Physiol Meas* 15:401–406, 1994.

39. Prichard JW, Rosen BR: Functional study of the brain by NMR. *J Cereb Blood Flow Metab* 14:365–372, 1994.

40. Kemp GJ: Non-invasive methods for studying brain energy metabolism: what they show and what it means. *Dev Neurosci* 22:418–428, 2000.

41. Watson NA, Beards SC, Altaf N, et al: The effect of hyperoxia on cerebral blood flow: a study in healthy volunteers using magnetic resonance phase-contrast angiography. *Eur J Anaesthesiol* 17:152–159, 2000.

42. Kolbitsch C, Schocke M, Hörmann C, et al: Effects of hyperoxia and hypocapnia on regional venous oxygen saturation in the primary visual cortex in conscious humans. *Br J Anaesth* 83:835–838, 1999.

43. Zaharchuk G, Mandeville JB, Bogdanov AA Jr, et al: Cerebrovascular dynamics of autoregulation and hypoperfusion. An MRI study of CBF and changes in total and microvascular cerebral blood volume during hemorrhagic hypotension. *Stroke* 30:2197–2205, 1999.

44. Verweij BH, Muizelaar P, Vinas FC, et al: Impaired cerebral mitochondrial function after traumatic brain injury in humans. *J Neurosurg* 93:815–820, 2000.

45. Kety SS, Schmidt CF: The nitrous oxide method for the quantitative determination of cerebral blood flow in man: theory, procedure and normal values. *J Clin Invest* 27:476–483, 1948.

46. Olesen J, Paulson OB, Lassen NA: Regional cerebral blood flow in man determined by the initial slope of the clearance of intra-arterially injected [133]Xe. Theory of the method, normal values, error of measurement, correction for remaining radioactivity, relation to other flow parameters and response to Pa_{CO_2} changes. *Stroke* 2:519–540, 1971.

47. Obrist WD, Thompson HK Jr, Wang HS, et al: Regional cerebral blood flow estimated by [133]Xenon inhalation. *Stroke* 6:245–256, 1975.

48. Tachibana H, Meyer JS, Okayasu H, et al: Changing topographic patterns of human cerebral blood flow with age measured by Xenon CT. *AJR Am J Roentgenol* 142:1027–1034, 1984.

49. Bishop CCR, Powell S, Rutt D, et al: Transcranial Doppler measurement of middle cerebral artery blood flow velocity: a validation study. *Stroke* 17:913–915, 1986.

50. Seiler RW, Grolimund P, Aaslid R, et al: Cerebral vasospasm evaluated by transcranial ultrasound correlated with clinical grade and CT-visualized subarachnoid hemorrhage. *J Neurosurg* 64:594–600, 1986.

51. Lindegaard KF: The role of transcranial Doppler in the management of patients with subarachnoid haemorrhage—a review. *Acta Neurochir Suppl* 72:59–71, 1999.

52. Qureshi AI, Sung GY, Razumovsky AY, et al: Early identification of patients at risk for symptomatic vasospasm after aneurysmal subarachnoid hemorrhage. *Crit Care Med* 28:984–990, 2000.

53. Marion DW, Spiegel TP: Changes in the management of severe traumatic brain injury: 1991–1997. *Crit Care Med* 28:16–18, 2000.

54. Sahuquillo J, Poca MA, Arribas M, et al: Interhemispheric supra–

tentorial intracranial pressure gradients in head-injured patients: are they clinically important? *J Neurosurg* 90:16–26, 1999.

55. Chambers IR, Kane PJ, Signorini DF, et al: Bilateral ICP monitoring: its importance in detecting the severity of secondary insults. *Acta Neurochir Suppl* 71:42–43, 1998.

56. Crutchfield JS, Narayan RK, Robertson CS, et al: Evaluation of a fiberoptic intracranial pressure monitor. *J Neurosurg* 72:482–487, 1990.

57. Yablon JS, Lantner HJ, McCormack TM, et al: Clinical experience with a fiberoptic intracranial pressure monitor. *J Clin Monit* 9:171–175, 1993.

58. Martinez-Manas RM, Santamarta D, de Campos JM, et al: Camino intracranial pressure monitor: prospective study of accuracy and complications. *J Neurol Neurosurg Psychiatry* 69:82–86, 2000.

59. Guyot LL, Dowling C, Diaz FG, et al: Cerebral monitoring devices: analysis of complications. *Acta Neurochir Suppl* 71:47–49, 1998.

60. Lundberg N, Troupp H, Lorin H: Continuous recording of the ventricular fluid pressure in patients with severe acute traumatic brain injury. *J Neurosurg* 22:581–590, 1965.

61. Juul N, Morris GF, Marshall SB, et al: Intracranial hypertension and cerebral perfusion pressure: influence on neurological deterioration and outcome in severe head injury. *J Neurosurg* 92:1–6, 2000.

62. Ferring M, Berre J, Vincent JL: Induced hypertension after head injury. *Int Care Med* 25:1006–1009, 1999.

63. Robertson CS, Valadka AB, Hannay HJ, et al: Prevention of secondary ischemic insults after severe head injury. *Crit Care Med* 27:2086–2095, 1999.

64. Coplin WM, O'Keefe GE, Grady MS, et al: Thrombotic, infectious, and procedural complications of the jugular bulb catheter in the intensive care unit. *Neurosurgery* 41:101–109, 1997.

65. Stocchetti N, Paparella A, Bridelli F, et al: Cerebral venous oxygen saturation studied with bilateral samples in the internal jugular veins. *Neurosurgery* 34:38–44, 1994.

66. Lam JMK, Chan MSY, Poon WS: Cerebral venous oxygen saturation monitoring: is dominant jugular bulb cannulation good enough? *Br J Neurosurg* 10:357–364, 1996.

67. Gibbs EL, Gibbs FA: The cross section areas of the vessels that form the torcula and the manner in which flow is distributed to the right and to the left lateral sinus. *Anat Rec* 59:419–426, 1934.

68. Andrews PJD, Dearden NM, Miller JD: Jugular bulb cannulation: description of a cannulation technique and validation of a new continuous monitor. *Br J Anaesth* 67:553–558, 1991.

69. Metz C, Holzschuh M, Bein T, et al: Monitoring of cerebral oxygen metabolism in the jugular bulb: reliability of unilateral measurements in severe head injury. *J Cereb Blood Flow Metab* 18:332–343, 1998.

70. Sheinberg M, Kanter MJ, Robertson CS, et al: Continuous monitoring of jugular venous oxygen saturation in head-injured patients. *J Neurosurg* 76:212–217, 1992.

71. Gopinath SP, Robertson CS, Contant CF, et al: Jugular venous desaturation and outcome after head injury. *J Neurol Neurosurg Psychiatry* 57:717–723, 1994.

72. Cruz J, Jaggi JL, Hoffstad OJ: Cerebral blood flow and oxygen consumption in acute brain injury with acute anemia: an alternative for the cerebral metabolic rate of oxygen consumption? *Crit Care Med* 21:1218–1224, 1993.

73. Cruz J: Cerebral oxygenation—monitoring and management. *Acta Neurochir* 59:86–90, 1993.

74. Zauner A, Doppenberg EMR, Woodward JJ, et al: Continuous monitoring of cerebral substrate delivery and clearance: initial experience in 24 patients with severe acute brain injuries. *Neurosurgery* 41:1082–1093, 1997.

75. van den Brink WA, van Santbrink H, Steyerberg EW, et al: Brain oxygen tension in severe head injury. *Neurosurgery* 46:868–878, 2000.

76. Unterberg AW, Kiening KL, Härtl R, et al: Multimodal monitoring in patients with head injury: evaluation of the effects of treatment on cerebral oxygenation. *J Trauma* 42:S32–S37, 1997.

77. Gopinath SP, Valadka AB, Uzura M, et al: Comparison of jugular venous oxygen saturation and brain tissue PO_2 as monitors of cerebral ischemia after head injury. *Crit Care Med* 27:2337–2345, 1999.

78. Pollard V, Prough DS: Cerebral oxygenation: near-infrared spectroscopy, in Tobin MJ (ed), *Principles and Practice of Intensive Care Monitoring*. New York, McGraw-Hill, 1998, pp 1019–1033.

79. Delpy DT, Cope M, Cady EB, et al: Cerebral monitoring in newborn infants by magnetic resonance and near infrared spectroscopy. *Scand J Clin Lab Invest Suppl* 188:9–17, 1987.

80. Delpy DT, Cope M, van der Zee P, et al: Estimation of optical path length through tissue from direct time of flight measurement. *Phys Med Biol* 33:1433–1442, 1988.

81. Pollard V, Prough DS, DeMelo AE, et al: Validation in volunteers of a near-infrared spectroscope for monitoring brain oxygenation in vivo. *Anesth Analg* 82:269–277, 1996.

82. Hirtz DG: Report of the National Institute of Neurological Disorders and Stroke workshop on near infrared spectroscopy. *Pediatrics* 91:414–417, 1993.

83. Villringer A, Planck J, Hock C, et al: Near infrared spectroscopy (NIRS): a new tool to study hemodynamic changes during activation of brain function in human adults. *Neurosci Lett* 154:101–104, 1993.

84. Unterberg A, Rosenthal A, Schneider GH, et al: Validation of monitoring of cerebral oxygenation by near-infrared spectroscopy in comatose patients, in Tsubokawa T, Marmarou A, Robertson C, et al. (eds), *Neurochemical Monitoring in the Intensive Care Unit*. New York, Springer-Verlag, 1995, pp 204–210.

85. Williams IM, Picton A, Farrell A, et al: Light-reflective cerebral oximetry and jugular bulb venous oxygen saturation during carotid endarterectomy. *Br J Surg* 81:1291–1295, 1994.

86. Konishi A, Kikuchi K: Cerebral oxygen saturation (rSO_2) during open heart surgery and postoperative brain dysfunction. *Masui* 44:1322–1326, 1995.

87. Pollard V, Prough DS, DeMelo AE, et al: The influence of carbon dioxide and body position on near-infrared spectroscopic assessment of cerebral hemoglobin oxygen saturation. *Anesth Analg* 82:278–287, 1996.

88. Henson LC, Calalang C, Temp JA, et al: Accuracy of a cerebral oximeter in healthy volunteers under conditions of isocapnic hypoxia. *Anesthesiology* 88:58–65, 1998.

89. Prough DS, Deyo DJ, Petrov YE, et al: Continuous noninvasive optoacoustic monitoring of superior sagittal sinus saturation: *in vivo* validation in sheep. *Anesthesiology* 95:A555, 2001.

90. Skarphedinsson JO, Harding H, Thoren P: Repeated measurements of cerebral blood flow in rats. Comparisons between the hydrogen clearance method and laser Doppler flowmetry. *Acta Physiol Scand* 134:133–142, 1988.

91. Eyre JA, Essex TJ, Flecknell PA, et al: A comparison of measurements of cerebral blood flow in the rabbit using laser Doppler spectroscopy and radionuclide-labeled microspheres. *Clin Phys Physiol Meas* 9:65–74, 1988.

92. Meyerson BA, Gunasekera L, Linderoth B, et al: Bedside monitoring of regional cortical blood flow in comatose patients using laser Doppler flowmetry. *Neurosurgery* 29:750–755, 1991.

93. Lam JMK, Hsiang JNK, Poon WS: Monitoring of autoregulation using laser Doppler flowmetry in patients with head injury. *J Neurosurg* 86:438–445, 1997.

94. Mascia L, Andrews PJ, McKeating EG, et al: Cerebral blood flow and metabolism in severe brain injury: the role of pressure autoregulation during cerebral perfusion pressure management. *Intensive Care Med* 26:202–205, 2000.

95. Miller JI, Chou MW, Capocelli A, et al: Continuous intracranial multimodality monitoring comparing local cerebral blood flow, cerebral perfusion pressure, and microvascular resistance. *Acta Neurochir Suppl* 71:82–84, 1998.

96. Hillered L, Persson L, Ponten U: Neurometabolic monitoring of the ischaemic human brain using microdialysis. *Acta Neurochir* 102:91–97, 1990.

97. Landolt H, Langemann H, Alessandri B: A concept for the introduction of cerebral microdialysis in neurointensive care. *Acta Neurochir Suppl* 67:31–36, 1996.

98. Hoffman WE, Charbel FT, Edelman G, et al: Brain tissue oxygen pressure, carbon dioxide pressure, and pH during hypothermic circulatory arrest. *Surg Neurol* 46:75–79, 1996.

99. Peerdeman SM, Girbes AR, Vandertop WP: Cerebral microdialysis as a new tool for neurometabolic monitoring. *Int Care Med* 26:662–669, 2000.

100. Hillered L, Persson L, Carlson H, et al: Excitatory amino acids: basic pharmacology to clinical evaluation. *Clin Neuropharmacol* 15:695–696, 1992.

101. Hillered L, Persson L: Microdialysis for neurochemical monitoring in human brain injury, in Tsubokawa T, Marmarou A, Robert-

son C, et al. (eds): *Neurochemical Monitoring in the Intensive Care Unit*. New York, Springer-Verlag, 1995, pp 59–63.

102. Nuwer M: Assessment of digital EEG, quantitative EEG, and EEG brain mapping: report of the American Academy of Neurology and the American Clinical Neurophysiology Society. *Neurology* 49:277–292, 1997.

103. Levy WJ, Shapiro HM, Maruchak G, et al: Automated EEG processing for intraoperative monitoring: a comparison of techniques. *Anesthesiology* 53:223–236, 1980.

104. Sloan TB: Electrophysiologic monitoring in head injury. *New Horiz* 3:431–438, 1995.

105. De Deyne C, Struys M, Decruyenaere J, et al: Use of continuous bispectral EEG monitoring to assess depth of sedation in ICU patients. *Int Care Med* 24:1294–1298, 1998.

106. Liu J, Singh H, White PF: Electroencephalogram bispectral analysis predicts the depth of midazolam-induced sedation. *Anesthesiology* 84:64–69, 1996.

107. Simmons LE, Riker RR, Prato BS, et al: Assessing sedation during intensive care unit mechanical ventilation with the bispectral index and the sedation-agitation scale. *Crit Care Med* 27:1499–1504, 1999.

108. Nuwer MR: *Evoked Potential Monitoring in the Operating Room*. New York, Raven, 1986.

109. Pathak KS, Amaddio MD, Scoles PV, et al: Effects of halothane, enflurane, and isoflurane in nitrous oxide on multilevel somatosensory evoked potentials. *Anesthesiology* 70:207–212, 1989.

110. Scheepstra GL, De Lange JJ, Booij LHD, et al: Median nerve evoked potentials during propofol anaesthesia. *Br J Anaesth* 62:92–94, 1989.

111. Sloan TB, Fugina ML, Toleikis JR: Effects of midazolam on median nerve somatosensory evoked potentials. *Br J Anaesth* 64:590–593, 1990.

112. Lesser RP, Raudzens P, Luders H: Postoperative neurological deficits may occur despite unchanged intraoperative somatosensory evoked potentials. *Ann Neurol* 19:22, 1986.

113. Guerit JM: Medical technology assessment EEG and evoked potentials in the intensive care unit. *Neurophysiol Clin* 29:301–317, 1999.

114. Berkhoff M, Donati F, Bassetti C: Postanoxic alpha (theta) coma: a reappraisal of its prognostic significance. *Clin Neurophysiol* 111:297–304, 2000.

115. Madl C, Kramer L, Domanovits H, et al: Improved outcome prediction in unconscious cardiac arrest survivors with sensory evoked potentials compared with clinical assessment. *Crit Care Med* 28:721–726, 2000.

116. Zentner J, Hufnagel A, Pechstein U, et al: Functional results after resective procedures involving the supplementary motor area. *J Neurosurg* 85:542–549, 1996.

117. Sala F, Krzan MJ, Jallo G, et al: Prognostic value of motor evoked potentials elicited by multipulse magnetic stimulation in a surgically induced transitory lesion of the supplementary motor area: a case report. *J Neurol Neurosurg Psychiatry* 69:828–831, 2000.

118. Fauth C, Meyer BU, Prosiegel M, et al: Seizure induction and magnetic brain stimulation after stroke. *Lancet* 339:362, 1992.

119. Taniguchi M, Nadstawek J, Langenbach U, et al: Effects of four intravenous anesthetic agents on motor evoked potentials elicited by magnetic transcranial stimulation. *Neurosurgery* 33:407–415, 1993.

120. Schwarz S, Hacke W, Schwab S: Magnetic evoked potentials in neurocritical care patients with acute brainstem lesions. *J Neurol Sci* 172:30–37, 2000.

121. Rohde V, Irle S, Hassler WE: Prediction of the post-comatose motor function by motor evoked potentials obtained in the acute phase of traumatic and non-traumatic coma. *Acta Neurochir* 141:841–848, 1999.

122. Chan KH, Dearden NM, Miller JD, et al: Multimodality monitoring as a guide to treatment of intracranial hypertension after severe brain injury. *Neurosurgery* 32:547–553, 1993.

23. *Percutaneous Suprapubic Cystostomy*

Philip J. Ayvazian

Percutaneous suprapubic cystotomy is used to divert urine from the bladder when standard urethral catheterization is impossible or undesirable [1–7]. The procedure for placement of a small diameter catheter is rapid, safe, and easily accomplished at the bedside under local anesthesia.

Urethral Catheterization

Urethral catheterization remains the principal method for bladder drainage. The indications for the catheter should be clarified, as they influence the type and size used. A history and physical examination with particular attention to the patient's genitourinary system is important.

Catheterization may be difficult with male patients in several instances. Patients with lower urinary tract symptoms (e.g., urinary urgency, frequency, nocturia, decreased stream, and hesitancy) may have hypertrophied lateral lobes of the prostate. These patients may require a larger bore catheter, such as a 20 or 22 French (Fr). Patients with a history of prior prostatic surgery such as transurethral resection of the prostate, open prostatectomy, or radical prostatectomy may have an irregular bladder neck as a result of contracture after surgery. The use of a coude-tip catheter, which has an upper

deflected tip, may help in negotiating the altered anatomy after prostate surgery. The presence of a high-riding prostate or blood at the urethral meatus suggests urethral trauma. In this situation, urethral integrity must be demonstrated by retrograde urethrogram before urethral catheterization is attempted.

Urethral catheterization for gross hematuria requires large catheters such as the 22 or 24 Fr, which have larger holes for irrigation and removal of clots. Alternatively, a three-way urethral catheter may be used to provide continuous bladder irrigation to prevent clotting. Large catheters impede excretion of urethral secretions, however, and can lead to urethritis or epididymitis if used for prolonged periods.

TECHNIQUE. In males, after the patient is prepared and draped, 10 mL of a 2% lidocaine hydrochloride jelly is injected retrograde into the urethra. Anesthesia of the urethral mucosa requires 5 to 10 minutes after occluding the urethral meatus either with a penile clamp or manually to prevent loss of the jelly. The balloon of the catheter is tested, and the catheter tip is covered with a water-soluble lubricant. After stretching the penis upward perpendicular to the body, the catheter is inserted into the urethral meatus. The catheter is advanced up to the hub to ensure its entrance into the bladder. The balloon is not inflated until urine return occurs to prevent urethral

Table 23-1. Indications for Percutaneous Cystotomy

Unsuccessful urethral catheterization in the setting of acute urinary retention
After prostatic surgery
Presence of urethral trauma
After antiincontinence procedures
Prostatic bilobar hyperplasia
Urethral stricture
Severe hypospadias
Periurethral abscess
Presence of severe urethral, epididymal, or prostate infection

trauma. Irrigation of the catheter with normal saline helps verify the position. A common site of resistance to catheter passage is the external urinary sphincter within the membranous urethra, which may contract involuntarily. Any other resistance may represent a stricture necessitating urologic consultation. In patients with prior prostate surgery, an assistant's finger placed in the rectum may elevate the urethra and allow the catheter to pass into the bladder.

In females, short, straight catheters are preferred. Typically, a smaller amount of local anesthesia is used. Difficulties in catheter placement occur after urethral surgery, vulvectomy, vaginal atrophy, or with morbid obesity. In these cases, the meatus is not visible and may be retracted under the symphysis pubis. Blind catheter placement over a finger located in the vagina at the palpated site of the urethral meatus may be successful.

When urologic consultation can be readily obtained, other techniques for urethral catheterization can be used. Filiforms and followers are useful for urethral strictures. Flexible cystoscopy may be performed to ascertain the reason for difficult catheter placement and for insertion of a guidewire. A urethral catheter then can be placed over the guidewire by a Seldinger technique.

Indications

On occasion, despite proper technique (as outlined previously), urethral catheterization is unsuccessful. These are the instances when percutaneous suprapubic cystotomy is necessary. Undoubtedly the most common indication for percutaneous suprapubic cystotomy is for the management of acute urinary retention in men. Other indications for a percutaneous suprapubic cystotomy in the intensive care unit are listed in Table 23-1.

Contradictions

The contraindications to percutaneous suprapubic cystotomy are listed in Table 23-2. An inability to palpate the bladder or

Table 23-2. Contraindications to Percutaneous Cystotomy

Nonpalpable bladder
Previous lower abdominal surgery
Coagulopathy
Known bladder tumor
Clot retention

distortion of the pelvic anatomy from previous surgery or trauma make percutaneous entry of the bladder difficult. In these situations, the risks of penetrating the peritoneal cavity become substantial. The bladder may not be palpable if the patient is in acute renal failure with oliguria or anuria, has a small contracted neurogenic bladder, or is incontinent. When the bladder is not palpable, it can be filled in a retrograde manner with saline to distend it. In men, a 14-Fr catheter is placed in the fossa navicularis just inside the urethral meatus, and the balloon is filled with 2 to 3 mL of sterile water to occlude the urethra. Saline is injected slowly into the catheter until the bladder is palpable; then, the suprapubic tube may be placed. In patients with a contracted neurogenic bladder, it is impossible to adequately distend the bladder by this approach. For these patients, ultrasonography is used to locate the bladder and allow the insertion of a 22-gauge spinal needle. Saline is instilled into the bladder via the needle to distend the bladder enough for suprapubic tube placement.

In patients with previous lower abdominal surgery, ultrasonographic guidance is often necessary before a percutaneous cystotomy can be safely performed. Previous surgery can lead to adhesions that can hold a loop of intestine in the area of insertion. Other relative contraindications include patients with coagulopathy, a known history of bladder tumors, or active hematuria and retained clots. In patients with bladder tumors, percutaneous bladder access should be avoided because tumor cell seeding can occur along the percutaneous tract. Suprapubic cystotomy tubes are a small caliber and therefore do not function effectively with severe hematuria and retained clots. Instead, open surgical placement of a large caliber tube is necessary if urethral catheterization is impossible.

Technique

There are two general types of percutaneous cystotomy tubes that range in size from 8 to 14 Fr. The first type uses an obturator with a preloaded catheter. Examples include the Stamey catheter (Cook Urological, Spencer, IN) and the Bonanno catheter (Beckton Dickinson and Co., Franklin Lakes, NJ) [8]. The Stamey device is a polyethylene malecot catheter with a luer lock hub that fits over a hollow needle obturator (Fig. 23-1A). When the obturator is locked to the hub of the catheter, the malecot flanges are pulled inward (closed), and the system is ready for use. The Bonanno catheter uses a flexible 14-Fr Teflon tube, which is inserted over a hollow 18-gauge obturator (Fig. 23-1B). The obturator locks into the catheter hub and extends beyond the catheter tip. When the obturator is withdrawn, the tube pigtails in the bladder. One advantage to the Stamey catheter is that the flanges provide a secure retaining system. The Bonanno catheter generally induces fewer bladder spasms, however, and is better tolerated.

The second type of percutaneous cystotomy tube consists of a trocar and sheath, which are used to penetrate the abdominal wall and bladder. One of the most popular systems is the Lawrence suprapubic catheter (Rusch, Dulith, GA). This system allows a standard Foley catheter to be placed after removal of the trocar (Fig. 23-1C).

The patient is placed in the supine position; a towel roll may be placed under the hips to extend the pelvis. The bladder is palpated to ensure that it is distended. The suprapubic region is shaved, prepared with 10% povidone-iodine solution, and draped with sterile towels. The insertion site is several centimeters above the symphysis pubis in the midline: This approach avoids the epigastric vessels. In obese

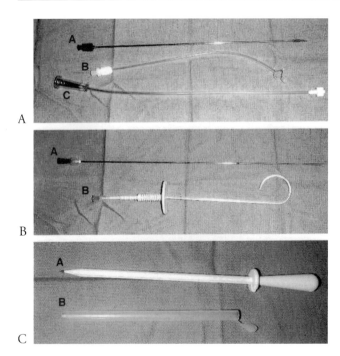

Fig. 23-1. A: Stamey suprapubic cystostomy trocar set (A is the obturator, B is the malecot catheter, and C is the drainage tube). **B:** Bonanno catheter set (A is the obturator and B is the catheter). **C:** Lawrence suprapubic catheter (A is the trocar and B is the sheath).

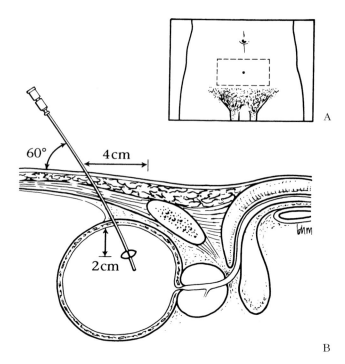

Fig. 23-2. Technique of suprapubic trocar placement. **A:** Area to be shaved, prepared, and draped before trocar placement. **B:** Position of the Stamey trocar in the bladder. The angle, distance from the pubis, and position of the catheter in relation to the bladder wall are demonstrated.

patients with a large abdominal fat pad, the fold is elevated. The needle should be introduced into the suprapubic crease, where the fat thickness is minimal. One percent lidocaine is used to anesthetize the skin, subcutaneous tissues, rectus fascia, and retropubic space. A 22-gauge spinal needle with a 5-mL syringe is directed vertically and advanced until urine is aspirated. If the bladder is smaller or if the patient had previous pelvic surgery, the needle is directed at a 60-degree caudal angle. Insertion of the cystotomy tube is predicated on the feasibility of bladder puncture and after the angle and depth of insertion is established with the spinal needle (Fig. 23-2).

At the site of bladder puncture, a small 2-mm incision is made with a No. 11 blade. The catheter mounted on the obturator is advanced in toward the bladder. Two hands are used to grasp the system to provide a forceful, but controlled, thrust through the abdominal wall. One hand can be positioned on the obturator at a site marking the depth of the bladder. A syringe attached to the end of the obturator is used to aspirate urine and confirm obturator placement. Once the bladder is penetrated, the entire system is advanced 2 to 3 cm: This prevents the catheter tip from withdrawing into the retropubic space when the bladder decompresses. After unlocking the obturator from the catheter, the obturator acts as a guide while the catheter is advanced into the bladder. When using a Stamey catheter, the catheter can be gently withdrawn until the malecot flanges meet resistance against the anterior bladder wall. The Stamey catheter is then advanced 2 cm back into the bladder to allow for movement. This maneuver pulls the catheter away from the bladder trigone and helps reduce bladder spasms.

The same general technique applies to placement of the Lawrence suprapubic catheter system. After the bladder is penetrated, urine appears at the hub of the suprapubic catheter introducer (trocar plus sheath). The trocar is then removed, and a Foley catheter is inserted. The Foley catheter balloon is inflated to secure it in the bladder. Pulling the tab at the top of the peel-away sheath allows the remaining portion of the sheath to be removed away from the catheter.

The patency of the catheter is assessed by irrigating the bladder after decompression. The catheter can be fixed with a simple nylon suture and sterile dressing. The Bonanno catheter contains a suture disc. The Lawrence suprapubic catheter does not require extra fixation, because the balloon on the Foley catheter secures it in place.

Suprapubic Catheter Care

Bladder spasms occur commonly after suprapubic catheter placement. When using a Stamey catheter or a Foley catheter, bladder spasms can be prevented by withdrawing the tube until it meets the anterior bladder wall and then advancing 2 cm back into the bladder. Persistent bladder spasms can be treated with anticholinergic therapy (e.g., oxybutynin and hyoscyamine). This medication should be discontinued before removing the suprapubic tube to prevent urinary retention.

Table 23-3. Complications of Percutaneous Cystotomy

Peritoneal and bowel perforation
Hematuria
Retained or calcified catheter
Bladder stones
Postobstructive diuresis
Hypotension
Bladder perforation

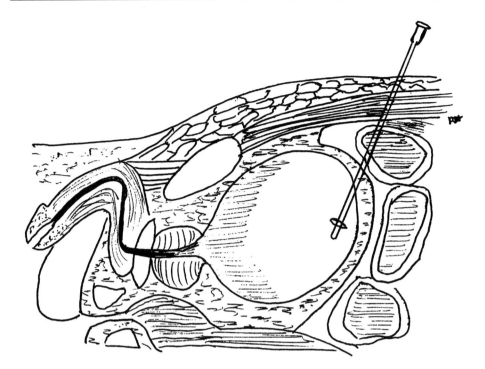

Fig. 23-3. Placement of the suprapubic tube can perforate entrapped bowel.

A suprapubic tube that ceases to drain is usually caused by kinking of the catheter or displacement of the catheter tip into the retropubic space. If necessary, suprapubic catheters may be replaced using either an exchange set (available for Stamey catheters) or by dilating the cystostomy tract. Closure of the percutaneous cystostomy tract is generally prompt after the tube is removed. Prolonged suprapubic tube use can lead to a mature tract, which may take several days to close. If the tract remains open, bladder decompression via a urethral catheter may be required.

Complications

Placement of suprapubic cystostomy tubes is generally safe with infrequent complications. Possible complications are listed in Table 23-3. Bowel complications are severe but rare with this procedure [9]. Penetration of the peritoneal cavity or bowel perforation produces peritoneal or intestinal symptoms and signs. This complication can be avoided by attempting the procedure only on well-distended bladders and using a midline approach no more than 4 cm above the pubis.

In patients who have had previous lower abdominal or pelvic surgery, an ultrasound should be used to properly place the suprapubic tube and rule out entrapped bowel (Figure 23-3). Patients who develop peritoneal symptoms and signs require a full evaluation of not only the location of the suprapubic tube (by a cystogram) but also of the cystostomy tract. A kidney-ureter-bladder and computed tomography scans may be required.

Hematuria is the most common complication after suprapubic tube placement. Rarely, it requires open cystotomy for placement of a large caliber tube for irrigation. Hematuria can occur secondary to laceration of a submucosal vessel or rapid decompression of a chemically distended bladder. It can be avoided by gradual bladder decompression.

Complications associated with the catheter include loss of a portion of the catheter in the bladder, calcification of the catheter, or bladder stone formation. These complications can be avoided

by preventing prolonged catheter use. Beyond 4 weeks, evaluation and replacement or removal must be considered.

When chronically distended bladders are decompressed, patients are at risk for postobstructive diuresis. Patients who are at greatest risk include those with azotemia, peripheral edema, congestive heart failure, and mental status changes. Patients with postobstructive diuresis (i.e., urine outputs greater then 200 mL per hour) require frequent monitoring of vital signs and intravenous fluid replacement.

Hypotension rarely occurs after suprapubic tube placement. It may be caused by a vasovagal response or relief of pelvic veins compressed by bladder distention. Fluid administration alleviates this complication.

Another rare but possible complication is a through-and-through bladder perforation. This is treated conservatively with bladder decompression.

References

1. Sethia KK, Selkon JB, Berry AR, et al: Prospective randomized controlled trial of urethral versus suprapubic catheterization. *Br J Surg* 74:624–625, 1987.
2. Carter HB: Instrumentation and endoscopy, in Walsh PC, Retnik AB, Vaughan ED, et al. (eds): *Campbell's Urology*. Philadelphia, WB Saunders, 1998.
3. Fowler JE: *Urologic Surgery*. Boston, Little, Brown and Company, 1992.
4. O'Brien WM: Percutaneous placement of a suprapubic tube with peel away sheath introducer. *J Urol* 145:1015–1016, 1991.
5. Chiou RK, Morton JJ, Engelsgjerd JS, et al: Placement of large suprapubic tube using peel-away introducer. *J Urol* 153:1179–1181, 1995.
6. Meessen S, Bruhl P, Piechota HJ: A new suprapubic cystostomy trocar system. *Urology* 56:315–316, 2000.
7. Lee MJ, Papanicolaou N, Nocks BN, et al: Fluoroscopically guided percutaneous suprapubic cystostomy for long-term bladder drainage: an alternative to surgical cystostomy. *Radiology* 188:787–789, 1993.
8. Bonanno PJ, Landers DE, Rock DE: Bladder drainage with the suprapubic catheter needle. *Obstet Gynecol* 35:807–812, 1970.
9. Hebert DB, Mitchell GW: Perforation of the ileum as a complication of suprapubic catheterization. *Obstet Gynecol* 62:662–664, 1983.

24. Aspiration of the Knee and Synovial Fluid Analysis

Eric W. Jacobson and Maria E. Abruzzo

Arthrocentesis is a safe and relatively simple procedure that involves the introduction of a needle into the joint space to remove synovial fluid. It constitutes an essential part of the evaluation of any arthritis of unknown cause, frequently with the intent to rule out a septic process [1–3].

Ropes and Bauer first categorized synovial fluid as *inflammatory* or *noninflammatory* in 1953 [4], terms that are still used today. Hollander et al. coined the term *synovianalysis* to describe the process of joint fluid analysis in 1961 [5]. Hollander et al. were instrumental in establishing the critical role of synovial fluid analysis to diagnose certain forms of arthritis [6,7]. Septic arthritis and crystalline arthritis can be diagnosed by synovial fluid analysis alone: They may present similarly but require markedly different treatments, thus necessitating early arthrocentesis and prompt synovial fluid analysis.

Indications

Arthrocentesis is performed for diagnostic and therapeutic purposes [8,9]. The main indication for arthrocentesis is to assist in the evaluation of arthritis of unknown cause. In the intensive care unit, it is most commonly performed in the setting of acute monoarthritis or oligoarthritis (presenting with one to three inflamed joints) to rule out septic arthritis. Many types of inflammatory arthritis mimic septic arthritis. Synovial fluid analysis is useful in differentiating the various causes of inflammatory arthritis [4,10] (Table 24-1). Therefore, patients presenting with monoarthritis or oligoarthritis of recent onset require prompt arthrocentesis with subsequent synovial fluid analysis, preferably before initiation of treatment.

Arthrocentesis is also used for therapeutic purposes. In a septic joint, serial joint aspirations are required to remove accumulated inflammatory or purulent fluid. This allows serial monitoring of the total white blood cell count, Gram's stain, and culture to assess response to treatment and accomplishes complete drainage of a closed space. Inflammatory fluid contains many destructive enzymes that contribute to cartilage and bony degradation; removal of the fluid may slow this destructive process [15,16]. Additionally, arthrocentesis allows for injection of long-acting corticosteroid preparations into the joint space, which may be a useful treatment for various inflammatory and noninflammatory forms of arthritis [17–19].

Before performing arthrocentesis, it must be ascertained that the true joint is inflamed and an effusion is present. This requires a meticulous physical examination to differentiate arthritis from periarticular inflammation. Bursitis, tendinitis, and cellulitis all may mimic arthritis. In the knee, the examination begins with assessment of swelling. A true effusion may cause bulging of the parapatellar gutters and the suprapatellar pouch [11]. The swelling should be confined to the joint space. To check for small effusions, the bulge test is performed [12]. Fluid is stroked from the medial joint line into the suprapatellar pouch and then from the suprapatellar pouch down along the lateral joint line. If a bulge of fluid is noted at the medial joint line, a small effusion is present (Fig. 24-1). If a large effusion is suspected, a patellar tap is performed [13]. The left hand is used to apply pressure to the suprapatellar pouch while the right hand taps the patella against the femur with sharp downward pressure. If the patella is ballottable, an effusion is probably present. Comparison with the opposite joint is helpful. Many texts describe joint examination and assessment for fluid in the knee and other joints [11–14].

Contraindications

Absolute contraindications to arthrocentesis, in general, include local infection of the overlying skin or other periarticular structures and severe coagulopathy [1–3,20]. If coagulopathy is present and septic arthritis is suspected, every effort should be made to correct the coagulopathy (with fresh-frozen plasma or alternate factors) before joint aspiration. Therapeutic anticoagulation is not an absolute contraindication, but every effort should be made to avoid excessive trauma during aspiration in this circumstance. Known bacteremia is a contraindication because inserting a needle into the joint space disrupts capillary integrity and thus allows joint space seeding [21]. If septic arthritis is strongly suspected, however, joint aspiration is indicated. The presence of articular instability (e.g., that seen with badly damaged joints) is a relative contraindication, although the presence of a large presumed inflammatory fluid may still warrant joint aspiration.

Complications

The major complications of arthrocentesis are iatrogenically induced infection and bleeding, both of which are extremely rare [1]. The risk of infection after arthrocentesis has been estimated to be less than 1 in 10,000 [22]. Hollander reported an incidence of less than 0.005% in 400,000 injections [23]. Owen reported an incidence of 0.002% to 0.004% in more than 50,000 injections [24]. Strict adherence to aseptic technique reduces the risk of postarthrocentesis infection. Significant hemorrhage is also extremely rare. Correction of prominent coagulopathy before arthrocentesis reduces this risk.

Another potential complication of arthrocentesis is direct injury to the articular cartilage by the needle. This is not quantifiable, but any injury to cartilage could be associated with degenerative change over time. To avoid cartilaginous damage, the needle should be pushed in only as far as necessary to obtain fluid; excessive movement of the needle during the procedure and aggressive complete drainage should be avoided.

A rare complication is separation of the hypodermic needle from its hub during arthrocentesis [25]. A hemostat should be available to remove a separated needle from the soft tissue if necessary.

Table 24-1. Common Causes of Noninflammatory and Inflammatory Arthritides

Noninflammatory	Inflammatory
Osteoarthritis	Rheumatoid arthritis
Trauma/internal derangement	Spondyloarthropathies
Avascular necrosis	Psoriatic arthritis
Hemarthrosis	Reiter's syndrome/reactive
Malignancy	arthritis
Benign tumors	Ankylosing spondylitis
Osteochondroma	Ulcerative colitis/regional
Pigmented villonodular syno-	enteritis
vitis	Crystal-induced arthritis
	Monosodium urate (gout)
	Calcium pyrophosphate dihy-
	drate (pseudogout)
	Hydroxyapatite
	Infectious arthritis
	Bacterial
	Mycobacterial
	Fungal
	Connective tissue diseases
	Systemic lupus erythematosus
	Vasculitis
	Scleroderma
	Polymyositis
	Hypersensitivity
	Serum sickness

Finally, other complications include discomfort from the procedure itself; allergic reactions to the skin preparation or local anesthetic [26]; and, in the case of steroid injection, local soft tissue atrophy from the glucocorticoid [14].

Technique

Joint aspiration is easily learned. A sound knowledge of the joint anatomy, including the bony and soft tissue landmarks used for joint entry, is needed. Strict aseptic technique must be followed to minimize risk of infection, and relaxation of the muscles surrounding the joint should be encouraged, because muscular contraction can impede the needle's entry into the joint.

Most physicians in the intensive care unit can aspirate the knee, as it is one of the most accessible joints. Other joints should probably be aspirated by an appropriate specialist, such as a rheumatologist or an orthopedic surgeon. Certain joints are quite difficult to enter blindly and are more appropriately entered using radiologic guidance, such as with fluoroscopy or computed tomography: These include the hip, sacroiliac, and temporomandibular joints. Many texts describe in detail the aspiration technique of other joints [3,7,14,23]. The technique for knee aspiration is as follows:

1. Describe the procedure to the patient, including the possible complications, and obtain written informed consent.
2. Collect all items needed for the procedure (Table 24-2).
3. With the patient supine and the knee fully extended, examine the knee to confirm the presence of an effusion, as described previously.
4. Identify landmarks for needle entry. The knee may be aspirated from a medial or lateral approach. The medial approach is more commonly used and is preferred when small effusions are present. Identify the superior and inferior borders of the patella. Entry should be halfway between the borders just inferior to the undersurface of the patella (Fig. 24-2). The entry site may be marked with pressure from the end of a ballpoint pen with the writing tip retracted. An indentation mark should be visible.
5. Cleanse the area with an iodine-based antiseptic solution, such as povidone-iodine (Betadine). Allow the area to dry, then wipe once with an alcohol swab. Practice universal precautions: Wear gloves at all times while handling any body fluid, although they need not be sterile for routine knee aspiration. Do not touch the targeted area once it has been cleaned.
6. Apply local anesthesia. The authors prefer ethyl chloride, which is sterile and provides superficial anesthesia. Spray ethyl chloride directly onto the designated area; stop when the first signs of freezing are evident so as not to cause any skin damage. As an alternative, a local anesthetic (1% lidocaine) may be instilled with a 25-gauge needle into the subcutaneous skin. Once numbing has occurred, deeper instillation of the local anesthetic (to the joint capsule) can be performed using a 22-gauge, 1.5-in. needle.
7. To enter the knee joint, use an 18-gauge, 1.5-inch needle with a 20- to 60-mL syringe, depending on the size of the effusion. Use a quick thrust through the skin and on through the capsule to minimize pain. Avoid hitting periosteal bone,

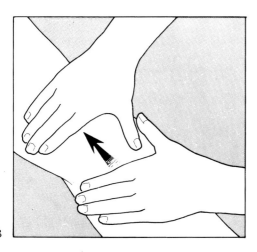
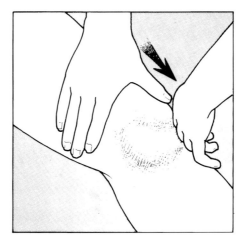

A,B

Fig. 24-1. The bulge test. **A:** Milk fluid from the suprapatellar pouch into the joint. **B:** Slide hand down the lateral aspect of the joint line and watch for a bulge medial to the joint.

Table 24-2. Arthrocentesis Equipment

Procedure	Equipment
Skin preparation and local anesthesia	Iodophor solution
	Alcohol swab
	Ethyl chloride spray
	For local anesthesia—1% lidocaine; 25-gauge, 1-in. needle; 22-gauge, 1.5-in. needle; 5-mL syringe
	Sterile sponge/cloth
Arthrocentesis	Gloves
	10- to 60-mL syringe (depending on size of effusion)
	18- to 20-gauge, 1.5-in. needle
	Sterile sponge/cloth
	Sterile clamp
	Sterile bandage
Collection	15-mL anticoagulated tube (with sodium heparin or ethylenedi-amine tetraacetic acid)
	Sterile tubes for routine cultures
	Slide, cover slip

which causes significant pain, or cartilage, which causes cartilaginous damage. Aspirate fluid to fill the syringe. If the fluid appears purulent or hemorrhagic, try to tap the joint dry, which will remove mediators of inflammation that may perpetuate an inflammatory or destructive process. If the syringe is full and more fluid remains, the sterile hemostat may be used to clamp the needle, thus stabilizing it, while switching syringes. When the syringes have been switched, more fluid can be withdrawn. The syringes must be sterile.

Conversely, effusions are sometimes difficult to aspirate. Reasons for this include increased fluid viscosity, fibrin and other debris impeding flow through the needle, too small of a needle as well as loculated fluid. Additionally, the fluid may not be accessible by the approach being used [27]. Nonetheless, if even only a drop of blood or tissue fluid is aspirated, this should be sent for crystal analysis, Gram's stain, or culture [27].

8. When the fluid has been obtained, quickly remove the needle and apply pressure to the needle site with a piece of sterile gauze. When bleeding has stopped, remove the gauze, clean the area with alcohol, and apply an adhesive bandage.

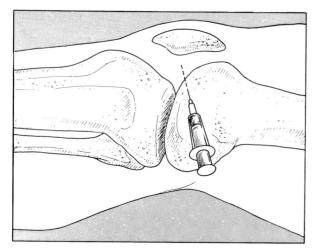

Fig. 24-2. Technique of aspirating the knee joint. The needle enters halfway between the superior and inferior borders of the patella and is directed just inferior to the patella.

If the patient is receiving anticoagulation therapy or has a bleeding diathesis, apply prolonged pressure.

9. Document the amount of fluid obtained. Perform gross examination, noting the color and clarity. A string sign may be performed at the bedside to assess fluid viscosity (see the following section). Send fluid for cell count with differential; Gram's stain; routine culture; specialized cultures for *Gonococcus, Mycobacterium,* and fungus, if indicated; and polarized microscopic examination for crystal analysis. Other tests, such as glucose and complement determinations, are generally not helpful. Use an anticoagulated tube to send fluid for cell count and crystal analysis. Sodium heparin and ethylenediamine tetraacetic acid are appropriate anticoagulants. Lithium heparin and calcium oxalate should be avoided because they can precipitate out of solution to form crystals, thus potentially giving a false-positive assessment for crystals [6,28]. Fluid may be sent for Gram's stain and culture in the syringe itself or in a sterile red-top tube.

Synovial Fluid Analysis

Synovial fluid analysis is identical for all joints and begins with bedside observation of the fluid. The color, clarity, and viscosity of the fluid are characterized. Synovial fluid is divided into noninflammatory versus inflammatory types based on the total nucleated cell count. A white blood cell count less than or equal to 2,000 per mm^3 is defined as a *noninflammatory fluid*, and a count greater than 2,000 per mm^3 is defined as an *inflammatory fluid*. Table 24-3 shows how fluid is divided into major categories based on appearance and cell count. Table 24-1 lists etiologies for noninflammatory and inflammatory effusions.

GROSS EXAMINATION

Color. Color and clarity should be tested using a clear glass tube. Translucent plastic, as used in most disposable syringes, interferes with proper assessment [1].

Normal synovial fluid is colorless. Noninflammatory and inflammatory synovial fluid appears yellow or straw-colored. Septic effusions frequently appear purulent and whitish. Depending on the number of white blood cells present, pure pus may be extracted from a septic joint. Hemorrhagic effusions appear red or brown. If the fluid looks like pure blood, the tap may have aspirated venous blood. The needle is removed, pressure applied, and the joint reentered from an alternate site. If the same bloody appearance is noted, the fluid is a hemorrhagic effusion probably not related to the trauma of the aspiration. If any question remains, the hematocrit of the effusion is compared with that of peripheral blood. The hematocrit in a hemorrhagic effusion is typically lower than that of peripheral blood. In the case of a traumatic tap, the hematocrit of the fluid should be equal to that of peripheral blood. For causes of a hemorrhagic effusion, refer to Table 24-4.

Clarity. The clarity of synovial fluid depends on the number and types of cells or particles present. Clarity is tested by reading black print on a white background through a glass tube filled with the synovial fluid. If the print is easily read, the fluid is transparent. This is typical of normal and noninflammatory synovial fluid. If the black print can be distinguished from the white background, but is not clear, the fluid is translucent: This is typical of inflammatory effusions. If nothing can be seen through the fluid, it is opaque: This occurs with grossly inflammatory, septic, and hemorrhagic fluids (Table 24-3).

Table 24-3. Joint Fluid Characteristics

Characteristic	Normal	Noninflammatory	Inflammatory	Septic
Color	Clear	Yellow	Yellow or opalescent	Variable—may be purulent
Clarity	Transparent	Transparent	Translucent	Opaque
Viscosity	Very high	High	Low	Typically low
Mucin clot	Firm	Firm	Friable	Friable
White blood cell count per mm³	200	200–2,000	2,000–100,000	>50,000, usually >100,000
Polymorphonuclear cells (%)	<25	<25	>50	>75
Culture	Negative	Negative	Negative	Usually positive

Viscosity. The viscosity of synovial fluid is a measure of the hyaluronic acid content. Hyaluronic acid is one of the major substances in synovial fluid that gives it a viscous quality. Degradative enzymes such as hyaluronidase are released in inflammatory conditions, thus destroying hyaluronic acid and other proteinaceous material, resulting in a thinner, less viscous fluid. Highly viscous fluid, on the other hand, can be seen in myxedematous effusions/hypothyroid effusions.

Viscosity can be assessed at the bedside using the string sign [1]. A drop of fluid is allowed to fall from the end of the needle or syringe and the length of the continuous string that forms estimated. Normal fluid typically forms at least a 6-cm continuous string. Inflammatory fluid does not form a string; instead, it drops off the end of the needle or syringe like water dropping from a faucet. Again, universal precautions should always be used when handling synovial fluid.

The mucin clot, another measure of viscosity, estimates the presence of intact hyaluronic acid and hyaluronic acid–protein interactions. This test is performed by placing several drops of synovial fluid in 5% acetic acid and then mixing with a stirring stick. A good mucin clot forms in normal, noninflammatory fluid. The fluid remains condensed in a clot resembling chewed gum. A poor mucin clot is seen with inflammatory fluid; the fluid disperses diffusely within the acetic acid.

CELL COUNT AND DIFFERENTIAL. The cell count should be obtained as soon as possible after arthrocentesis, as a delay of even several hours may cause an artificially low white blood cell count [29]. The total white blood cell count of synovial fluid differentiates noninflammatory from inflammatory fluid, as noted previously. In general, the higher the total white blood cell count, the more likely the joint is to be infected. This is not absolute, however, and there is considerable overlap. For instance, a total white cell count above 100,000 per mm³ may be seen in conditions other than infection [30], whereas a total white blood cell count of 50,000 per mm³ may be owing to infection, crystalline disease, or a systemic inflammatory arthropathy [26]. The technique for the cell count is identical to that used with peripheral blood. The fluid may be diluted with normal saline for a manual count, or an automated counter may be used. Viscous fluid with exces-

Table 24-4. Causes of a Hemorrhagic Effusion

Trauma (with or without fracture)
Hemophilia and other bleeding disorders
Anticoagulant therapy
Tumor (metastatic and local)
Hemangioma
Pigmented villonodular synovitis
Ehlers-Danlos syndrome
Scurvy

sive debris may clog a counter or give falsely elevated results, thus making the manual procedure somewhat more accurate.

The differential white blood cell count is also performed using the technique used for peripheral blood, typically using Wright's stain. The differential is calculated based on direct visualization. The differential count includes cells typically seen in peripheral blood, such as polymorphonuclear cells, monocytes, and lymphocytes, as well as cells localized to the synovial space. In general, the total white blood cell count and the polymorphonuclear cell count increase with inflammation and infection [30]. Septic fluid typically has a differential of greater than 75% polymorphonuclear cells (Table 24-3).

In addition to distinguishing polymorphonuclear cells from monocytes and lymphocytes. Wright's stain can detect other cells in synovial fluid that can be useful in establishing a diagnosis. For instance, iron-laden chondrocytes, which are seen in hemochromatosis, may be picked up by Wright's stain, as may be fat droplets and bone marrow spicules, which are suggestive for trauma or a fracture into the joint [27,38].

CRYSTALS. All fluid should be assessed for the presence of crystals. As with cell count, crystal analysis should be performed as soon as possible after arthrocentesis. A delay is associated with a decreased yield [29]. One drop of fluid is placed on a slide and covered with a cover slip; this is examined for crystals using a compensated polarized light microscope. The presence of intracellular monosodium urate (MSU) or calcium pyrophosphate dihydrate (CPPD) crystals confirms a diagnosis of gout or pseudogout, respectively. MSU crystals are typically long and needle shaped: They may appear to pierce through a white blood cell. The crystals are negatively birefringent, appearing yellow when parallel with the plane of reference. Typically, CPPD crystals are small and rhomboid. The crystals are weakly positively birefringent, appearing blue when oriented parallel to the plane of reference. Rotating the stage of the microscope by 90 degrees and thereby the orientation of the crystals (now perpendicular to the plane of reference) changes their color: MSU crystals turn blue and CPPD crystals yellow. Refer to Tables 24-5 and 24-6 for a classification of hyperuricemia and CPPD deposition disease.

In addition to MSU and CPPD crystals, other less common crystals may induce an inflammatory arthropathy: Basic calcium crystals (e.g., hydroxyapatite) and oxalate crystals are two such types. Hydroxyapatite crystals can incite acute articular and periarticular inflammation, much like MSU crystals in gout. Clinically, this is difficult to distinguish between septic arthritis and cellulitis, respectively [31]. On light microscopy, however, crystals appear as clumps of shiny nonbirefringent globules and with Alizarin red S stain, the clumps appear red-orange [31,32]. If hydroxyapatite is suspected, Alizarin red S stain must be requested specifically from the laboratory, as it is not a routine component of the crystal analysis. Calcium oxalate crystals can also induce an inflammatory arthritis: This

Table 24-5. Classification of Hyperuricemia

Primary hyperuricemia
    Idiopathic
    Enzymatic defects (e.g., hypoxanthine guanine phosphoribosyl-
        transferase deficiency)
Secondary hyperuricemia
    Increased production of uric acid
        Increased *de novo* purine synthesis
        Excessive dietary purine intake
        Increased nucleic acid turnover (myeloproliferative/lymphopro-
            liferative disorders, psoriasis, hemolytic anemia, ethyl alcohol
            abuse)
    Decreased renal excretion of uric acid
        Medications
            Diuretics
            Low-dose salicylates
            Pyrazinamide
            Ethambutol
            Cyclosporine
        Chronic renal failure
        Hyperacidemia (lactic acidosis, ketoacidosis, starvation, ethyl
            alcohol abuse)
        Lead nephropathy

Table 24-6. Conditions Associated with Calcium Pyrophosphate Dihydrate Deposition Disease

Hereditary
Sporadic (idiopathic)
Aging
Metabolic diseases
    Hyperparathyroidism
    Hypothyroidism
    Hypophosphatemia
    Hypomagnesemia
    Hemochromatosis
Amyloidosis
Trauma

is generally seen in patients on long-term hemodialysis [33–35] but may also be seen in young patients with primary oxalosis [31]. Clinically, arthritis secondary to calcium oxalate deposition often presents like the other crystalline arthropathies [35] and therefore can only be differentiated by synovianalysis. In this case, synovial fluid typically reveals characteristic bipyramidal crystals as well as polymorphic forms [31].

The yield for all crystals can be increased by spinning the specimen and examining the sediment. If the fluid cannot be examined immediately, it should be refrigerated to preserve the crystals. It is important to note that even in the presence of crystals, infection must be considered, since crystals can occur concomitantly with a septic joint. Other crystals include cryoimmunoglobulins in patients with multiple myeloma and essential cryoglobulinemia [36]. Cholesterol crystals may be seen in patients with chronic inflammatory arthropathies, such as rheumatoid arthritis, but this is a nonspecific finding. These crystals appear as plate-like structures with a notched corner.

GRAM'S STAIN AND CULTURE. The Gram's stain is performed as with other body fluids. It should be performed as soon as possible to screen for the presence of bacteria. It has been reported that the sensitivity of synovial fluid Gram's stain in septic arthritis ranges between 50% and 75% for nongonococcal infection and less than 10% for gonococcal infection [26]. Specificity is much higher; this suggests that a positive Gram's stain, despite a negative culture, should be considered evidence of infection [26]. In fact, it is not uncommon for only the Gram's stain to be positive in the setting of infection [26]. This being said, the absence of bacteria by Gram's stain does not rule out a septic process [27].

Synovial fluid in general should be cultured routinely for aerobic and anaerobic bacterial organisms. A positive culture confirms septic arthritis. In certain circumstances (e.g., in chronic monoarticular arthritis), fluid may be cultured for the presence of mycobacteria, fungus, and spirochetes. If disseminated gonorrhea is suspected, the laboratory must be notified, as the fluid should be plated directly onto chocolate agar or Thayer-Martin medium. Just as Gram's stain of synovial fluid in gonococcal infection is often negative, so too is synovial fluid culture [37]. Synovial fluid culture is positive approximately 10% to 50% of the time, versus 75% to 95% of the time for nongonococcal infection [26]. However, cultures of genitourinary

sites and mucosal sites in gonococcal infection are positive approximately 80% to 90% of the time [38,39]. Therefore, when suspicion of gonococcal arthritis is high (e.g., in a young, healthy, sexually active individual with a dermatitis-arthritis syndrome), the diagnosis must often be confirmed by a positive culture from the urethra, cervix, rectum, or pharynx [37].

In addition to documenting infection and identifying a specific organism, synovial fluid culture can be useful in determining antibiotic sensitivities and subsequent treatment. Furthermore, serial synovial fluid cultures can help in assessing response to therapy. For example, a negative follow-up culture associated with a decrease in synovial fluid polymorphonuclear cell count is highly suggestive of improvement.

Other studies on synovial fluid (e.g., glucose, protein, lactate dehydrogenase, complement, immune complexes) generally are not helpful. Specifically, in a study by Shmerling et al., the investigators observed that synovial fluid glucose and protein were "highly inaccurate": The synovial fluid glucose and protein misclassified effusions as inflammatory versus noninflammatory 50% of the time [40]. In contrast, synovial fluid cell count and differential were found to be reliable and complementary: Sensitivity and specificity of cell count was 84% for both and for the differential was 75% and 92%, respectively [40]. Although synovial fluid lactate dehydrogenase was also found to be accurate, it did not offer any additional information above and beyond the cell count and differential; therefore, it is not recommended as part of the routine synovial fluid analysis [40]. Other studies such as rheumatoid factor, antinuclear antibodies, immune complexes, and complements are generally considered unnecessary and unhelpful.

Of note, there are special stains for synovial fluid that can be helpful when the clinical picture correlates; these include Congo red staining for amyloid arthropathy. Amyloid deposits display an apple-green birefringence with polarized light [41,42]. Prussian blue stain for iron deposition may reveal iron in synovial lining cells in hemochromatosis [27]. However, neither of these studies should be considered a routine component of synovial fluid analysis.

References

1. Gatter RA: *A Practical Handbook of Joint Fluid Analysis.* Philadelphia, Lea & Febiger, 1984.
2. Stein R: *Manual of Rheumatology and Outpatient Orthopedic Disorders.* Boston, Little, Brown, 1981.
3. Krey PR, Lazaro DM: *Analysis of Synovial Fluid.* Summit, NJ, CIBA-GEIGY, 1992.
4. Ropes MW, Bauer W: *Synovial Fluid Changes in Joint Disease.* Cambridge, MA, Harvard University Press, 1953.
5. Hollander JL, Jessar RA, McCarty DJ: Synovianalysis: an aid in arthritis diagnosis. *Bull Rheum Dis* 12:263, 1961.

6. Gatter RA, McCarty DJ: Synovianalysis: a rapid clinical diagnostic procedure. *Rheumatism* 20:2, 1964.

7. Coggeshell HC: *Arthritis and Allied Conditions.* 6th ed. Philadelphia, Lea & Febiger, 1960.

8. Hasselbacher P: *Primer on the Rheumatic Diseases.* 9th ed. Atlanta, Arthritis Foundation, 1988.

9. Eisenberg JM, Schumacher JM, Davidson PK, et al: Usefulness of synovial fluid analysis in the evaluation of joint effusions: use of threshold analysis and likelihood ratios to assess a diagnostic test. *Arch Intern Med* 144:715, 1984.

10. Schumacher HR: Synovial fluid analysis. *Orthop Rev* 13:85, 1984.

11. Polley HF, Hunder GG: *Rheumatologic Interviewing and Physical Examination of the Joints.* 2nd ed. Philadelphia, WB Saunders, 1978.

12. Doherty M, Hazelman BL, Hutton CW, et al: *Rheumatology Examination and Injection Techniques.* London, WB Saunders, 1992.

13. Hoppenfeld S: *Physical Examination of the Spine and Extremities.* Norwalk, CT, Appleton-Century-Crofts, 1976.

14. Ruddy S, Harris ED Jr, Sledge CB, et al. (eds): *Kelley's Textbook of Rheumatology.* 6th ed. Philadelphia, WB Saunders, 2001.

15. Greenwald RA: Oxygen radicals inflammation and arthritis: pathophysiological considerations and implications for treatment. *Semin Arthritis Rheum* 20:219, 1991.

16. Robinson DR, Tashjian AH, Levine L: Prostaglandin E2 induced bone resorption by rheumatoid synovia: a model for bone destruction in RA. *J Clin Invest* 56:1181, 1975.

17. Hollander JL, Brown EM Jr, Jessar RA, et al: Hydrocortisone and cortisone injected into arthritic joints. *JAMA* 147:1629, 1951.

18. Hollander JL: Intrasynovial corticosteroid therapy in arthritis. *Md Med J* 19:62, 1970.

19. Steinbrocker P, Neustadt DH: *Aspiration and Injection Therapy in Arthritis and Musculoskeletal Diseases.* Hagerstown, MD, Harper & Row, 1972.

20. Gray RG, Tenenbaum J, Gottlieb NL: Local corticosteroid injection treatment in rheumatic disorders. *Semin Arthritis Rheum* 10:231, 1981.

21. McCarthy DJ Jr: A basic guide to arthrocentesis. *Hosp Med* 4:77, 1968.

22. Gottlieb NL, Riskin WG: Complications of local corticosteroid injections. *JAMA* 243:1547, 1980.

23. Hollander JL: Intrasynovial corticosteroid therapy, in *Arthritis and Allied Conditions.* 8th ed. Philadelphia, Lea & Febiger, 1972.

24. Owen DS Jr: Aspiration and injection of joints and soft tissues, in Kelly WN, Harris ED, Ruddy S, et al. (eds): *Textbook of Rheumatology.* 3rd ed. Philadelphia, WB Saunders, 1989.

25. Gottlieb NL: Hypodermic needle separation during arthrocentesis. *Arthritis Rheum* 24:1593, 1981.

26. Shmerling RH: Synovial fluid analysis. A critical reappraisal. *Rheum Dis Clin North Am* 20(2):503, 1994.

27. Schumacher HR Jr: Synovial fluid analysis, in Katz WA (ed): *Diagnosis and Management of Rheumatic Diseases.* 2nd ed. Philadelphia, JB Lippincott, 1988.

28. Tanphaichitr K, Spilberg I, Hahn B: Lithium heparin crystals simulating calcium pyrophosphate dihydrate crystals in synovial fluid. *Arthritis Rheum* 9:966, 1976 [letter].

29. Kerolus G, Clayburne G, Schumacher HR Jr: Is it mandatory to examine synovial fluids promptly after arthrocentesis? *Arthritis Rheum* 32:271, 1989.

30. Krey PR, Bailen DA: Synovial fluid leukocytosis: a study of extremes. *Am J Med* 67:436, 1979.

31. Reginato AJ, Schumacher HR Jr: Crystal-associated arthropathies. *Clin Geriatr Med* 4(2):295, 1988.

32. Paul H, Reginato AJ, Schumacher HR: Alizarin red S staining as a screening test to detect calcium compounds in synovial fluid. *Arthritis Rheum* 26:191, 1983.

33. Hoffman G, Schumacher HR, Paul H, et al: Calcium oxalate microcrystalline associated arthritis in end stage renal disease. *Ann Intern Med* 97:36, 1982.

34. Reginato AJ, Feweiro JL, Barbazan AC, et al: Arthropathy and cutaneous calcinosis in hemodialysis oxalosis. *Arthritis Rheum* 29:1387, 1986.

35. Schumacher HR, Reginato AJ, Pullman S: Synovial fluid oxalate deposition complicating rheumatoid arthritis with amyloidosis and renal failure. Demonstration of intracellular oxalate crystals. *J Rheumatol* 14:361, 1987.

36. Dornan TL, Blundell JW, Morgan AG: Widespread crystallization of paraprotein in myelomatosis. *QJM* 57:659, 1985.

37. Sack K: Monoarthritis: differential diagnosis. *Am J Med* 102(1A):30S, 1997.

38. Goldenberg DL: Arthritis related to infection: bacterial arthritis, in Ruddy S, Harris ED Jr, Sledge CB, et al. (eds): *Kelley's Textbook of Rheumatology.* 6th ed. Philadelphia, WB Saunders, 2001.

39. Mahowald ML: Gonococcal arthritis, in Klippel JH, Dieppe PA, et al. (eds): *Rheumatology.* 2nd ed. London, Mosby, 1998.

40. Shmerling RH, Delbanco TL, Tosteson ANA, et al: Synovial fluid tests. What should be ordered? *JAMA* 264:1009, 1990.

41. Lakhanpal S, Li CY, Gertz MA, et al: Synovial fluid analysis for diagnosis of amyloid arthropathy. *Arthritis Rheum* 30(4):419, 1987.

42. Gordon OA, Pruzanski W, Ogryzlo MA: Synovial fluid examination for the diagnosis of amyloidosis. *Ann Rheum Dis* 32:428, 1973.

25. *Anesthesia for Bedside Procedures*

Mark Dershwitz, Laurence Landow,
and Wandana Joshi-Ryzewicz

When a patient in an intensive care unit (ICU) requires a bedside procedure, it is usually the attending intensivist, as opposed to a consultant anesthesiologist, who directs the administration of the necessary hypnotic, analgesic, or paralytic drugs. Furthermore, unlike in the operating room, the ICU usually has no equipment for the administration of gaseous (e.g., nitrous oxide) or volatile (e.g., isoflurane) anesthetics. Anesthesia for bedside procedures in the ICU is thus accomplished via a technique involving total intravenous anesthesia (TIVA).

Common Pain Management Problems in Intensive Care Unit Patients

DOSING OF AGENT. Selecting the proper dose of an analgesic to administer is problematic for several reasons, including difficulty in assessing the effectiveness of pain relief, pharmacokinetic (PK) differences between the critically ill and other patients, and normal physiologic changes associated with aging.

Assessing the Effectiveness of Pain Relief. Critically ill patients often are incapable of communicating their feelings because of delirium, obtundation, or endotracheal intubation. This makes psychological evaluation quite difficult, because surrogate markers of pain intensity (e.g., tachycardia, hypertension, and diaphoresis) are inherent in the host response to critical illness.

Pharmacokinetic Considerations. Most of the pressors and vasodilators administered in the ICU by continuous intravenous (IV) infusion have relatively straightforward PK behavior: They are water-soluble molecules that are bound very little to plasma proteins. In contrast, the hypnotics and opioids used in TIVA have high lipid solubility, and most are extensively bound to plasma proteins, causing their PK behavior to be far more complex. Figure 25-1 shows the disappearance curves of fentanyl and nitroprusside after bolus injection. The fentanyl curve has three phases: a very rapid phase (with a half-life of 0.82 minutes) lasting approximately 10 minutes, during which the plasma concentration decreases more than 90% from its peak value; an intermediate phase (with a half-life of 17 minutes) lasting from approximately 10 minutes to an hour; and, finally, a terminal, very slow phase (with a half-life of 465 minutes) beginning approximately an hour after bolus injection. After a single bolus injection of fentanyl, the terminal phase occurs at plasma concentrations below which there is no pharmacologic effect. However, after multiple bolus injections or a continuous infusion, this latter phase occurs at therapeutic plasma concentrations. Thus, fentanyl behaves as a short-acting drug after a single bolus injection but as a very long-lasting drug after a continuous infusion of more than 1 hour in duration (i.e., fentanyl accumulates). Thus, it is inappropriate to speak of *the* half-life of fentanyl.

The disappearance curve of nitroprusside has two phases: a very rapid phase (with a half-life of 0.89 minutes) lasting approximately 10 minutes, during which the plasma concentration decreases more than 85% from its peak value, and a terminal phase (with a half-life of 14 minutes). It may be slightly

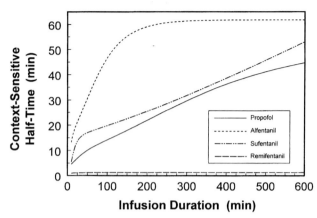

Fig. 25-2. The context-sensitive half-times for propofol, alfentanil, sufentanil, and remifentanil as a function of infusion duration. (Adapted from Shafer A, Doze VA, Shafer SL: Pharmacokinetics and pharmacodynamics of propofol infusions during general anesthesia. *Anesthesiology* 69:348, 1988; Scott JC, Stanski DR: Decreased fentanyl and alfentanil dose requirements with age. A simultaneous pharmacokinetic and pharmacodynamic evaluation. *J Pharmacol Exp Ther* 240:159, 1987; Hudson RJ, Bergstrom RG, Thomson IR, et al: Pharmacokinetics of sufentanil in patients undergoing abdominal aoritc surgery. *Anesthesiology* 70:426, 1989; and Egan TD, Lemmens HGM, Fiset P, et al: The pharmacokinetics of the new short acting opioid remifentanil [G187084B] in healthy adult male volunteers. *Anesthesiology* 79:881, 1993.)

slower in offset as compared with fentanyl during the initial 10 minutes after a bolus injection, but it does not accumulate at all even after a prolonged infusion.

The PK behavior of the lipid-soluble hypnotics and analgesics given by infusion can be described by their context-sensitive half-times (CSHT). This concept can be defined as follows: When a drug is given as an IV bolus followed by an IV infusion designed to maintain a constant plasma drug concentration, the time required for the plasma concentration to fall by 50% after termination of the infusion is the CSHT [1]. Figure 25-2 depicts the CSHT curves for the medications that are most likely to be used for TIVA in ICU patients.

PK behavior in critically ill patients is unlike that in normal subjects for several reasons. Because ICU patients frequently have renal or hepatic dysfunction, or both, drug excretion is significantly impaired. Hypoalbuminemia, common in critical illness, decreases protein binding and increases free drug concentration [2]. Because free drug is the only moiety available to tissue receptors, decreased protein binding increases the pharmacologic effect for a given plasma concentration. It is, therefore, more important in the ICU patient that the doses of medications used for TIVA are individualized for a particular patient.

Physiologic Changes Associated with Aging. Persons 65 years of age and older comprise the fastest-growing segment of the population and constitute the majority of patients in many ICUs. Aging leads to (a) a decrease in total body water and lean body mass; (b) an increase in body fat and, hence, an increase in the volume of distribution of lipid-soluble drugs; and (c) a decrease in drug clearance rates, due to reductions in liver mass, hepatic enzyme activity, liver blood flow, and renal excretory function. A progressive, age-dependent increase in pain relief and electroencephalographic suppression occurs among elderly patients who receive the same dose of opioid as younger patients. Central nervous system (CNS) depression is also increased in elderly patients after administration of identical doses of benzodiazepines.

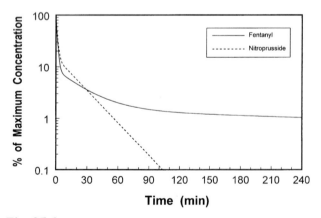

Fig. 25-1. The time courses, on a semilogarithmic scale, of the plasma concentrations of fentanyl and nitroprusside following a bolus injection. Each concentration is expressed as the percentage of the peak plasma concentration. The fentanyl curve has three phases with half-lives of 0.82, 17, and 465 minutes. The nitroprusside curve has two phases with half-lives of 0.89 and 14 minutes. (Adapted from Shafer SL, Varvel JR, Aziz N, et al: Pharmacokinetics of fentanyl administered by computer-controlled infusion pump. *Anesthesiology* 73:1091, 1990; and Vesey CJ, Sweeney B, Cole PV: Decay of nitroprusside. II: in vivo. *Br J Anaesth* 64:704, 1990.)

Table 25-1. Bedside Procedures and Associated Levels of Discomfort

Mildly to moderately uncomfortable
    Transesophageal echocardiography[a]
    Transtracheal aspiration
    Thoracentesis[a]
    Paracentesis[a]
Moderately to severely uncomfortable
    Endotracheal intubation[a]
    Flexible bronchoscopy[a]
    Thoracostomy[a]
    Bone marrow biopsy
    Colonoscopy
    Peritoneal dialysis catheter insertion[a]
    Peritoneal lavage[a]
    Percutaneous gastrostomy[a]
    Percutaneous intraaortic balloon insertion[a]
Extremely painful
    Rigid bronchoscopy
    Débridement of open wounds
    Dressing changes
    Orthopedic manipulations
    Tracheostomy[a]
    Pericardiocentesis/pericardial window[a]
    Open lung biopsy
    Ventriculostomy[a]

[a]Procedures in which the level of discomfort may be significantly mitigated by the use of local anesthesia.

SELECTION OF AGENT. Procedures performed in ICUs today (Table 25-1) span a spectrum that extends from those associated with mild discomfort (e.g., esophagogastroscopy) to those that are quite painful (e.g., orthopedic manipulations, wound débridement, tracheostomy). Depending on their technical difficulty, these procedures can last from minutes to hours. To provide a proper anesthetic, medications should be selected according to the nature of the procedure and titrated according to the patient's response to surgical stimulus. In addition, specific disease states should be considered so that safety and effectiveness are maximized.

Head Trauma. Head-injured patients require a technique that provides effective yet brief anesthesia so that the capacity to assess neurologic status is not lost for extended periods of time. In addition, the technique must not adversely affect cerebral perfusion pressure. If the effects of the anesthetics dissipate too rapidly, episodes of agitation and increased intracranial pressure (ICP) may occur that jeopardize cerebral perfusion. In contrast, if the medications last too long, there may be difficulty in making an adequate neurologic assessment following the procedure.

Coronary Artery Disease. Postoperative myocardial ischemia following cardiac and noncardiac surgery strongly predicts adverse outcome [3]. Accordingly, sufficient analgesia should be provided during and after invasive procedures to reduce plasma catecholamine and stress hormone levels.

Renal or Hepatic Failure. The association between sepsis and acute renal failure has been recognized for many years. The risk of an adverse drug reaction is at least three times higher in azotemic patients than in those with normal renal function. This risk is magnified by excessive unbound drug or drug metabolite(s) in the circulation and changes in the target tissue(s) induced by the uremic state.

    Liver failure alters many drugs' volumes of distribution by impairing synthesis of the two major plasma-binding proteins, albumin and α_1-acid glycoprotein. In addition, reductions in hepatic blood flow and hepatic enzymatic activity decrease drug clearance rates.

Table 25-2. Characteristics of Intravenous Hypnotic Agents[a]

	Propofol	Etomidate	Ketamine	Midazolam
Bolus dose (mg/kg)	1–2	0.2–0.3	1–2	0.05–0.10
Onset	Fast	Fast	Fast	**Intermediate**
Duration	Short	Short	Intermediate	Intermediate
Cardiovascular effects	↓	**None**	↑	Minimal
Respiratory effects	↓	↓	**Minimal**	↓
Analgesia	None	None	**Profound**	None
Amnesia	Mild	Mild	**Profound**	**Profound**

[a]The listed doses should be reduced 50% in elderly patients. Entries in bold type indicate noteworthy differences among the drugs.

Characteristics of Specific Agents Used for Bedside Procedures

HYPNOTICS. The characteristics of the hypnotics are listed in Table 25-2. When rapid awakening is desired, propofol or etomidate is the hypnotic agent of choice. Ketamine may be useful when a longer duration of anesthesia is needed. Midazolam is rarely used alone as a hypnotic; however, its profound anxiolytic and amnestic effects render it useful in combination with other agents.

Propofol

DESCRIPTION. Propofol is a hypnotic agent associated with pleasant emergence and little hangover. It has essentially replaced thiopental for induction of anesthesia, especially in outpatients. It is extremely popular because it is readily titratable and has more rapid onset and offset kinetics than midazolam. Thus, patients emerge from anesthesia more rapidly after propofol than after midazolam, a factor that may make propofol the preferred agent for sedation and hypnosis in general, and in particular for patients with altered level of consciousness.

    The CSHT for propofol is approximately 10 minutes following a 1-hour infusion, and the CSHT increases approximately 5 minutes for each additional hour of infusion for the first several hours, as shown in Figure 25-2. Thus, the CSHT is approximately 20 minutes after a 3-hour infusion. The CSHT plateaus for infusions longer than a day; patients sedated for weeks may be expected to wake up within a few hours after the propofol infusion is stopped [4]. This rapid recovery of neurologic status makes propofol a good sedative in ICU patients, especially those with head trauma, who may not tolerate mechanical ventilation without pharmacologic sedation.

    Even though recovery after termination of a continuous infusion is faster with propofol than with midazolam, a comparative trial showed that the two drugs were roughly equivalent in effectiveness for overnight sedation of ICU patients [5]. For long-term sedation (e.g., more than 1 day), however, recovery is significantly faster in patients given propofol.

    In spontaneously breathing patients sedated with propofol, respiratory rate appears to be a more predictable sign of adequate sedation than hemodynamic changes. The ventilatory response to rebreathing carbon dioxide during a maintenance propofol infusion is similar to that induced by other sedative drugs (i.e., propofol significantly decreases the slope of the carbon dioxide response curve). Nevertheless, spontaneously breathing patients anesthetized with propofol are able to maintain normal end-tidal carbon dioxide values during minor surgical procedures.

Bolus doses of propofol in the range of 1 to 2 mg per kg induce loss of consciousness within 30 seconds. Maintenance infusion rates of 100 to 200 μg per kg per minute are adequate in younger subjects, whereas doses should be reduced by 20% to 50% in elderly individuals.

ADVERSE EFFECTS

Cardiovascular. Propofol depresses ventricular systolic function and lowers afterload but has no effect on diastolic function [6,7]. Vasodilation results from calcium channel blockade. In patients undergoing coronary artery bypass surgery, propofol (2 mg per kg IV bolus) produced a 23% fall in mean arterial blood pressure, a 20% increase in heart rate, and a 26% decrease in stroke volume. In pigs, propofol caused a dose-related depression of sinus node and His-Purkinje system functions but had no effect on atrioventricular node function or on the conduction properties of atrial and ventricular tissues. In patients with coronary artery disease, propofol administration may be associated with a reduction in coronary perfusion pressure and increased myocardial lactate production [8].

Neurologic. Propofol may improve neurologic outcome and reduce neuronal damage by depressing cerebral metabolism. Propofol decreases cerebral oxygen consumption, cerebral blood flow, and cerebral glucose use in humans and animals to the same degree as reported for thiopental and etomidate [9].

Metabolic. The emulsion used as the vehicle for propofol contains soybean oil and lecithin and supports bacterial growth; iatrogenic contamination leading to septic shock is possible. Currently available propofol preparations contain either ethylenediaminetetraacetic acid or sulfite as a bacteriostatic agent. Because ethylenediaminetetraacetic acid chelates trace metals, particularly zinc, serum zinc levels should be measured daily during continuous propofol infusions. Hyperlipidemia may occur, particularly in infants and small children. Accordingly, triglyceride levels should be monitored daily in this population whenever propofol is administered continuously for more than 24 hours.

Etomidate

DESCRIPTION. Etomidate has onset and offset PK characteristics similar to propofol and an unrivaled cardiovascular profile, even in the setting of cardiomyopathy [10]. Not only does etomidate lack significant effects on myocardial contractility, but baseline sympathetic output and baroreflex regulation of sympathetic activity are well preserved. Etomidate depresses in a dose-related manner cerebral oxygen metabolism and blood flow without changing the intracranial volume-pressure relationship.

Etomidate is particularly useful (rather than thiopental or propofol) in certain patient subsets. These include hypovolemic patients, multiple trauma victims with closed-head injury, and those with low ejection fraction, severe aortic stenosis, left main coronary artery disease, or severe cerebrovascular disease.

ADVERSE EFFECTS: METABOLIC. Etomidate, when given by prolonged infusion, may increase mortality associated with low plasma cortisol levels [11]. Even single doses of etomidate can produce adrenocortical suppression that lasts for 24 hours or more in normal patients undergoing elective surgery [12]. These effects are more pronounced as the dose is increased or if continuous infusions are used for sedation. Etomidate-induced adrenocortical suppression occurs because the drug blocks a key step in the metabolic pathway in adrenal steroidogenesis. Because etomidate does not affect the response of tissue cortisol receptors, supplementation with exogenous steroids in physiologic doses should prevent the adverse effects of adrenocortical suppression and allow clinical use of etomidate for brain protection or anesthetic induction. It is also noteworthy that etomidate causes the highest incidence of postoperative nausea and vomiting of any of the IV anesthetic agents.

Ketamine

DESCRIPTION. Ketamine induces a state of sedation, amnesia, and marked analgesia in which the patient experiences a strong feeling of dissociation from the environment. It is unique among the hypnotics in that it reliably induces unconsciousness by the intramuscular route. Ketamine is rapidly metabolized by the liver to norketamine, which is pharmacologically active. Ketamine is slower in onset and offset as compared with propofol or etomidate following IV infusion.

Many clinicians consider ketamine to be the analgesic of choice in patients with a history of bronchospasm. In the usual dosage, it decreases airway resistance, probably by blocking norepinephrine uptake, which in turn stimulates β-adrenergic receptors in the lungs. In contrast to many β-agonist bronchodilators, ketamine is not arrhythmogenic when given to asthmatic patients who are receiving aminophylline.

Ketamine may be safer than other hypnotics or opioids in unintubated patients because it depresses airway reflexes and respiratory drive to a lesser degree. It may be particularly useful for procedures near the airway, where physical access and ability to secure an airway is limited (e.g., gunshot wounds to the face). Because ketamine increases salivary and tracheobronchial secretions, an anticholinergic (e.g., 0.2 mg glycopyrrolate) should be administered before its administration. In patients with borderline hypoxemia despite maximal therapy, ketamine may be the drug of choice, because it does not inhibit hypoxic pulmonary vasoconstriction.

Another major feature that distinguishes ketamine from most other IV anesthetics is that it stimulates the cardiovascular system (i.e., raises heart rate and blood pressure). This action appears to result from direct stimulation of the CNS, with increased sympathetic nervous system outflow and from blockade of norepinephrine reuptake in adrenergic nerves.

Because pulmonary hypertension is a characteristic feature of acute respiratory distress syndrome, drugs that increase right ventricular afterload should be avoided. In infants with either normal or elevated pulmonary vascular resistance, ketamine does not affect pulmonary vascular resistance as long as constant ventilation is maintained, a finding also confirmed in adults.

Cerebral blood flow does not change when ketamine is injected into cerebral vessels. In mechanically ventilated pigs with artificially produced intracranial hypertension in which ICP is on the shoulder of the compliance curve, 0.5 to 2.0 mg per kg IV ketamine does not raise ICP; likewise, in mechanically ventilated preterm infants, 2.0 mg per kg IV ketamine does not increase anterior fontanel pressure, an indirect monitor of ICP [13,14].

ADVERSE EFFECTS

Psychological. Emergence phenomena of ketamine have been described as floating sensations, vivid dreams (pleasant or unpleasant), hallucinations, and delirium. These effects are more common in patients older than 16 years, in female patients, after short operative procedures, after large doses (greater than 2 mg per kg IV), and after rapid administration (greater than 40 mg per minute). Pre- or concurrent treatment with benzodiazepines or propofol usually prevents these phenomena [15].

Cardiovascular. Because ketamine increases myocardial oxygen consumption, using ketamine alone risks precipitating myocardial ischemia in patients with coronary artery disease. On the other hand, combinations of ketamine plus diazepam, ketamine plus midazolam, or ketamine plus sufentanil are well tolerated for induction in patients undergoing coronary artery bypass surgery. Repeated bolus doses are often associated with tachycardia. This can be reduced by administering ketamine as a constant infusion.

Ketamine produces myocardial depression in the isolated animal heart. Hypotension has been reported following ketamine administration in hemodynamically compromised patients with chronic catecholamine depletion.

Neurologic. Ketamine does not lower the minimal electroshock seizure threshold in mice. When it is administered with aminophylline, however, a clinically apparent reduction in seizure threshold is observed.

Midazolam

DESCRIPTION. Although capable of inducing unconsciousness in high doses, midazolam is more commonly used as a sedative. Along with its sedating effects, midazolam produces anxiolysis, amnesia, and relaxation of skeletal muscle.

Anterograde amnesia following midazolam (5 mg IV) peaks 2 to 5 minutes after IV injection and lasts for 20 to 40 minutes. Because midazolam is highly (95%) protein bound (to albumin), drug effect is likely to be exaggerated in ICU patients. Recovery from midazolam is prolonged in obese and elderly patients and after continuous infusion because it accumulates to a significant degree. In patients with renal failure, active conjugated metabolites of midazolam may accumulate and delay recovery. Although flumazenil can be used to reverse excessive sedation or respiratory depression from midazolam, its duration of action is only 15 to 20 minutes. In addition, flumazenil may precipitate acute anxiety reactions or seizures, particularly in patients who are receiving chronic benzodiazepine therapy.

Midazolam causes dose-dependent reductions in cerebral metabolic rate and cerebral blood flow, suggesting that it may be beneficial in patients with cerebral ischemia. Due to its combined sedative, anxiolytic, and amnestic properties, midazolam is ideally suited for brief, relatively painless procedures (e.g., endoscopy) as well as for prolonged sedation (e.g., during mechanical ventilation).

ADVERSE EFFECTS

Respiratory. Midazolam (0.15 mg per kg IV) depresses the slope of the carbon dioxide response curve and increases the dead space–tidal volume ratio and partial arterial pressure of carbon dioxide. Respiratory depression is even more marked and prolonged in patients with chronic obstructive pulmonary disease. Midazolam also blunts the ventilatory response to hypoxia.

Cardiovascular. Small (less than 10%) increases in heart rate and small decreases in systemic vascular resistance are frequently observed after administration of midazolam. It has no significant effects on coronary vascular resistance or autoregulation.

Neurologic. Because recovery of cognitive and psychomotor function may be delayed for up to 24 hours, midazolam as the sole hypnotic may not be appropriate in situations in which rapid return of consciousness and psychomotor function is a high priority.

OPIOIDS

Morphine

DESCRIPTION. Pain relief by morphine and its surrogates is relatively selective in that other sensory modalities (touch, vibration, vision, hearing) are not obtunded. Opioids blunt pain by (a) inhibiting pain processing by the dorsal horn of the spinal cord, (b) decreasing transmission of pain by activating descending inhibitory pathways in the brain stem, and (c) altering the emotional response to pain by actions on the limbic cortex.

Various types of opioid receptors (denoted by Greek letters) have been discovered in the spinal cord, brain stem, thalamus, limbic system, and cerebral cortex. Their stimulation causes the subject to experience emotions that can be described as pleasant [analgesia (μ) and sedation (κ)] or unpleasant [hallucinations (δ)]. Morphine is an agonist at each of these receptors.

Transmission of impulses from these receptors to other centers is modulated by many substances, including substance P, neurotensin, vasoactive intestinal peptide, serotonin, cholecystokinin, gamma-aminobutyric acid, and norepinephrine.

PK data suggest that differences in lipid solubility affect the ease with which opioids cross the blood-brain barrier and reach the target-effector site. Morphine enters the brain and spinal cord with difficulty. Peak analgesic effects may not occur for more than an hour after IV injection; hence, the plasma profile of morphine does not parallel its clinical effects [16].

Morphine is unique among the opioids in causing significant histamine release after IV injection that occurs almost immediately. The beneficial effect of giving morphine to a patient with acute pulmonary edema is far more related to this hemodynamic effect than to its analgesic and sedating effects.

ADVERSE EFFECTS

Gastrointestinal. Constipation, nausea, and vomiting are well-described side effects of morphine administration. Reduced gastric emptying and bowel motility (small and large intestine), often leading to adynamic ileus, appear to be mediated peripherally (by opioid receptors located in the gut) and centrally (by the vagus nerve).

Cardiovascular. Hypotension is not unusual after morphine administration, especially if it is given rapidly (i.e., 5 to 10 mg per minute). In patients who are pretreated with H_1- and H_2-receptor antagonists, the hypotensive response following morphine administration is significantly attenuated, despite comparable increases in plasma histamine concentrations. These data strongly implicate histamine as the mediator of these changes.

Respiratory. Morphine administration is followed by a dose-dependent reduction in responsiveness of brain stem respiratory centers to carbon dioxide. Key features of this phenomenon include a reduction in the slope of the ventilatory and occlusion pressure responses to carbon dioxide, a rightward shift of the minute ventilatory response to hypercarbia, and an increase in resting end-tidal carbon dioxide and the apneic threshold (i.e., the partial pressure of carbon dioxide value below which spontaneous ventilation is not initiated without hypoxemia). The duration of these effects often exceeds the time course of analgesia. In addition to blunting the carbon dioxide response, morphine decreases hypoxic ventilatory drive. Morphine administration in patients with renal failure has been associated with prolonged respiratory depression secondary to persistence of its active metabolite, morphine 6-glucuronide [17].

The practice of administering small doses of IV naloxone (40 μg) to patients to reverse the respiratory depression of excessive morphine effects is risky and inadvisable for a number of reasons. Anecdotal reports describe the precipitation of vomiting, delirium, arrhythmias, pulmonary edema, cardiac arrest, and sudden death subsequent to naloxone administration in otherwise healthy patients after surgery. Furthermore, naloxone levels decline rapidly, whereas morphine levels may remain elevated for much longer. Recurring respiratory depression, therefore, remains a distinct possibility and, in the unintubated patient, is a source of potential morbidity.

Reversal with a mixed opioid agonist-antagonist such as nalbuphine or butorphanol appears to be safer than with naloxone. Mixed opioid agonist-antagonist agents may either increase or decrease the opioid effect, depending on the dose administered, the particular agonist already present, and the amount of agonist remaining. For bedside procedures in the ICU, many of these problems can be obviated by using a shorter-acting opioid.

Neurologic. Morphine has little effect on cerebral metabolic rate or cerebral blood flow when ventilation is controlled. It may affect cerebral perfusion pressure adversely by lowering mean arterial pressure.

Fentanyl and Its Congeners

DESCRIPTION. Fentanyl, alfentanil, sufentanil, and remifentanil enter and leave the CNS much more rapidly than morphine, thereby causing a much faster onset of effect after IV administration. These medications are also more selective opioid agonists in that they are active only at μ-opioid receptors. The only significant difference among these agents is their PK behavior.

Fentanyl may be useful when given by intermittent bolus injection (50 to 100 μg), but when given by infusion, its duration becomes prolonged [18]. Alfentanil, originally marketed as an "ultra-short"–duration medication, is not; Figure 25-2 shows that its CSHT is almost 1 hour after a 2-hour infusion. Thus, for TIVA in ICU patients in whom rapid emergence is desirable, sufentanil or remifentanil is the preferred choice for continuous infusion. When the procedure is expected to be followed by postoperative pain, sufentanil is preferred. Figure 25-2 shows that its CSHT is similar to that of propofol for infusions of up to 10 hours. When the procedure is expected to be followed by minimal postoperative pain (e.g., bronchoscopy), remifentanil is preferred. Its CSHT is approximately 4 minutes regardless of the duration of the infusion.

Remifentanil owes its extremely short duration to rapid metabolism by tissue esterases, primarily in skeletal muscle [19]. Its PK behavior is unchanged in the presence of severe hepatic [20] or renal [21] failure.

Sufentanil infusion for TIVA can be initiated with a 0.5- to 1.5-μg per kg bolus followed by an infusion at 0.01 to 0.03 μg per kg per minute. If given with a propofol infusion, the two infusions can be stopped simultaneously as governed by the curves in Figure 25-2. Remifentanil infusion for TIVA can be initiated with a 1- to 2-μg per kg bolus followed by an infusion at 0.25 to 1 μg per kg per minute. The remifentanil infusion should be continued until after the procedure is completed; if the patient is expected to have postoperative pain, another opioid must be given because the remifentanil effect dissipates within a few minutes.

ADVERSE EFFECTS

Cardiovascular. Although fentanyl, sufentanil, alfentanil, and remifentanil do not affect plasma histamine concentrations, bolus doses can be associated with hypotension, especially when they are infused rapidly (i.e., less than 1 minute). This action is related to medullary vasomotor center depression and vagal nucleus stimulation.

Neurologic. Fentanyl and sufentanil have been reported to increase ICP in ventilated patients after head trauma. Fentanyl, sufentanil, and alfentanil may adversely affect cerebral perfusion pressure by lowering mean arterial pressure. All of the fentanyl derivatives may cause chest wall rigidity when a large bolus is given rapidly. This effect may be mitigated by neuromuscular blocking (NMB) agents as well as by coadministration of a hypnotic agent.

NEUROMUSCULAR BLOCKING AGENTS. The two pharmacologic classes of NMB agents are depolarizing agents (e.g., succinylcholine) and nondepolarizing agents (e.g., vecuronium, cisatracurium). Succinylcholine is an agonist at the nicotinic acetylcholine receptor of the neuromuscular junction. Administration of succinylcholine causes an initial intense stimulation of skeletal muscle, manifested as fasciculations, followed by paralysis due to continuing depolarization. Nondepolarizing agents are competitive antagonists of acetylcholine at the neuromuscular junction; they prevent acetylcholine, released in response to motor nerve impulses, from binding to its receptor and initiating muscle contraction. Distinctions among the nondepolarizing agents are made based on PK differences as well as by their cardiovascular effects. Table 25-3 summarizes the NMB agents.

NMB agents are used to facilitate endotracheal intubation and to improve surgical conditions by decreasing skeletal muscle tone. Before intubation, the administration of an NMB agent results in paralysis of the vocal cords, increasing the ease with which the endotracheal tube can be inserted and decreasing the risk of vocal cord trauma. During surgery, the decrease in skeletal muscle tone may aid in surgical exposure (as during abdominal surgery), decrease the insufflation pressure needed during laparoscopic procedures, and make joint manipulation easier during orthopedic surgery. NMB agents should *not* be used to prevent patient movement, which is indicative of inadequate anesthesia. Dosing of NMB agents should be based on monitoring evoked twitch response; ablation of two to three twitches of the train-of-four is sufficient for the majority of surgical procedures and permits easy reversal.

Succinylcholine

DESCRIPTION. Succinylcholine has the fastest onset and shortest duration of the NMB agents. A dose of 1 mg per kg succinylcholine results in fasciculations within seconds and excellent intubating conditions in less than 1 minute. Succinylcholine is usually considered the drug of choice when the airway must be quickly secured, such as when the patient has a full stomach or has symptomatic gastroesophageal reflux.

A small dose (e.g., 0.5 mg vecuronium) of a nondepolarizing agent given before succinylcholine prevents the fasciculations caused by succinylcholine. When succinylcholine is given after

Table 25-3. Characteristics of the Neuromuscular Blocking Agents

Drug	Indication	Dose (mg/kg)	Onset (min)	Time to 25% recovery (min)
Succinylcholine	Routine intubation	1.0	0.7	10
	Rapid-sequence intubation			
Rocuronium	Rapid-sequence intubation in a patient in whom succinylcholine is contraindicated	0.6	1.5	40
		1.2	1.1	70
Cisatracurium	Intubation and/or maintenance for a case of up to several hours in duration	0.1	3	40
		0.2	2	60
Vecuronium	Intubation and/or maintenance for a case of up to several hours in duration	0.1	2	50
Pancuronium	Maintenance of long-term muscle paralysis by infusion at a rate of 0.025–0.050 mg/kg/h	0.1	3	90
Pipecuronium	Maintenance of long-term muscle paralysis by infusion at a rate of 0.02–0.04 mg/kg/h in a patient requiring strict hemodynamic stability	0.09	3	110
Doxacurium	Maintenance of long-term muscle paralysis by infusion at a rate of 0.01–0.02 mg/kg/h in a patient requiring strict hemodynamic stability	0.05	6	90

a small dose of a nondepolarizing agent, there is a delay in onset (to approximately 1.5 minutes) of its peak effect.

Succinylcholine is metabolized by plasma cholinesterase, a circulating enzyme. In most people, its duration of action is approximately 5 to 10 minutes. A number of inherited abnormalities of plasma cholinesterase may prolong the duration of succinylcholine. If a patient is deficient in plasma cholinesterase but has normal renal function, succinylcholine is eliminated unchanged with a half-life of approximately 20 to 30 minutes.

ADVERSE EFFECTS

Neurologic. Succinylcholine may trigger malignant hyperthermia in genetically susceptible persons. Its use in the pediatric population is controversial because of the possibility that a child may have a genetically determined myopathy that has not yet become symptomatic but that is associated with malignant hyperthermia.

Succinylcholine may cause a malignant rise in the extracellular potassium concentration in patients with major acute burns, upper or lower motor neuron lesions, prolonged immobility, massive crush injuries, and various myopathies. Although the usual doses of succinylcholine cause a transient increase in the plasma potassium concentration of approximately 0.5 mEq per L, preexisting hyperkalemia is generally not a contraindication to its use.

Cardiovascular. Succinylcholine often causes transient tachycardia as a result of its vagolytic effect. Interestingly, a second dose of succinylcholine, given before the complete dissipation of the first dose, may cause bradycardia or asystole. Preceding such a second dose with a dose of atropine or glycopyrrolate prevents this vagomimetic effect.

Nondepolarizing Neuromuscular Blocking Agents

DESCRIPTION. Vecuronium, rocuronium, and cisatracurium are commonly used to facilitate intubation in persons in whom succinylcholine is contraindicated. They are also used for maintenance of muscle paralysis for surgical procedures lasting up to several hours. These three agents are essentially devoid of cardiovascular effects, and the choice among them is usually made on the basis of desired PK parameters as listed in Table 25-3. Vecuronium and rocuronium are metabolized by the liver; their durations may be increased in persons with hepatic dysfunction or decreased in persons who take medications that induce hepatic cytochrome P450 (e.g., phenytoin). Cisatracurium is metabolized enzymatically (by plasma cholinesterase) and by nonenzymatic ester hydrolysis, which occurs at physiologic pH; the drug is supplied at an acidic pH and kept refrigerated before use to prevent this nonenzymatic degradation. The PK of cisatracurium are thus affected less by coexisting disease (e.g., hepatic or renal dysfunction) or by interaction with concomitantly administered medications.

Pancuronium, pipecuronium, and doxacurium are longer-lasting NMB agents. In the ICU, they are commonly used for longer-term therapy to facilitate mechanical ventilation. Pancuronium has a vagolytic effect that may cause tachycardia, which may persist throughout its administration. Pipecuronium and doxacurium are devoid of cardiovascular effects. Doses of these medications are listed in Table 25-3.

ADVERSE EFFECTS. Any patient who receives NMB agents should be properly sedated. Longer-term therapy with NMB agents may cause muscle weakness that persists for months afterward. The risk factors for developing such a myopathy are coadministration with a glucocorticoid and long duration of NMB therapy [22]. It is controversial as to whether NMB agents in the steroidal class (pancuronium, vecuronium, rocuronium, pipecuronium) have a higher propensity of causing myopathy than the NMB agents in the benzyliso-

quinoline class (atracurium, cisatracurium, mivacurium, and doxacurium).

Reversal of Muscle Paralysis. When there is no longer any need for muscle paralysis, it is reasonable to permit the agent to wear off as long as the patient remains properly sedated until muscle strength has recovered. Adequate recovery of muscle strength is indicated by the absence of fade using the double-burst mode of the evoked twitch response.

Alternatively, pharmacologic reversal of muscle paralysis can be achieved by the administration of an anticholinesterase such as neostigmine, 0.04 to 0.06 mg per kg. To counter the parasympathomimetic effects of neostigmine, glycopyrrolate, 0.008 to 0.012 mg per kg, is given concomitantly.

Practical Considerations for Total Intravenous Anesthesia

Electing to perform common procedures (e.g., tracheostomy, percutaneous gastrostomy) in the ICU instead of the operating room represents a potential cost savings of tremendous scope. Not only does this strategy eradicate costly operating room time and support resources, it eliminates misadventures that sometimes occur in hallways and on elevators. Cost analyses estimate an average overall cost reduction of 50% or more compared with traditional operative procedures [23]. TIVA represents the most cost-effective method of facilitating this.

In most patients, safe and effective TIVA can be achieved via the infusions of propofol plus sufentanil or propofol plus remifentanil. Premedication with midazolam decreases the required propofol doses and decreases the likelihood of recall for intraoperative events. Bolus doses should not be used in hemodynamically unstable patients, and lower bolus doses should be used in elderly individuals. NMB agents are also given if needed.

The opioid infusion rate is titrated to minimize signs of inadequate analgesia (e.g., tachycardia, tachypnea, hypertension, sweating, mydriasis). The propofol infusion rate is titrated to the endpoint of loss of consciousness; the new depth of anesthesia monitors (bispectral index or patient state index) facilitate locating this endpoint more accurately. Loss of consciousness should be achieved before the initiation of muscle paralysis. It is possible for patients to be completely aware of intraoperative events at times when there is no change in hemodynamics or any manifestation of increased sympathetic activity [24,25]. Hence, administering an opioid to blunt incisional pain without inducing loss of consciousness with a hypnotic is inappropriate.

The following additional points deserve consideration in this context:

1. In subhypnotic doses, propofol is less effective than midazolam in producing amnesia. In the absence of coadministration of a benzodiazepine, propofol must cause unconsciousness to reliably prevent recall. Prompt treatment of patient responses (movement, tachycardia, hypertension) is important.
2. Medications infused for TIVA should be given via a carrier IV fluid running continuously at a rate of at least 50 mL per hour. This method not only helps deliver medication into the circulation, but it also serves as another monitor of occlusion of the drug delivery system. Occlusion of the infusion line for more than a few minutes may lead to patient awareness.

3. To take advantage of the known CSHT values for the TIVA agents, communication with the surgeon during the procedure is important to anticipate the optimum time for stopping the infusions. The sufentanil and propofol infusions are stopped in advance of the end of the procedure, whereas remifentanil is infused until the procedure is complete.

4. To maintain reasonably constant propofol and sufentanil blood concentrations, the maintenance infusion rates should be decreased during the procedure because the plasma concentrations increase over time at constant infusion rates. An approximate guideline is a 10% reduction in infusion rate every 30 minutes.

5. Strict aseptic technique is especially important during the handling of propofol.

References

1. Hughes MA, Glass PSA, Jacobs JR: Context-sensitive half-time in multicompartment pharmacokinetic models for intravenous anesthetic drugs. *Anesthesiology* 76:334, 1992.
2. Koch-Weser J, Sellers EM: Binding of drugs to serum albumin. *N Engl J Med* 294:311, 1976.
3. Mangano DT, Browner WS, Hollenberg M: Association of perioperative myocardial ischemia with cardiac morbidity and mortality in men undergoing noncardiac surgery. *N Engl J Med* 323:1781, 1990.
4. Albanese J, Martin C, Lacarelle B, et al: Pharmacokinetics of long-term propofol infusion used for sedation in ICU patients. *Anesthesiology* 73:214, 1990.
5. Ronan KP, Gallagher TH, Hamby BG: Comparison of propofol and midazolam for sedation in intensive care unit patients. *Crit Care Med* 23:286, 1995.
6. Pagel PS, Warltier DC: Negative inotropic effects of propofol as evaluated by the regional preload recruitable stroke work relationship in chronically instrumented dogs. *Anesthesiology* 78:100, 1993.
7. Pagel PS, Schmeling WT, Kampine JP, et al: Alteration of canine left ventricular diastolic function by intravenous anesthetics in vivo: ketamine and propofol. *Anesthesiology* 76:419, 1992.
8. Mayer N, Legat K, Weinstabl C, et al: Effects of propofol on the function of normal, collateral-dependent, and ischemic myocardium. *Anesth Analg* 76:33, 1993.
9. Van Hemelrijck J, Fitch W, Mattheussen M, et al: Effect of propofol on cerebral circulation and autoregulation in baboons. *Anesth Analg* 71:49, 1990.
10. Goading JM, Wang JT, Smith RA, et al: Cardiovascular and pulmonary responses following etomidate induction of anesthesia in patients with demonstrated cardiac disease. *Anesth Analg* 58:40, 1979.
11. Ledingham IM, Finlay WEI, Watt I, et al: Etomidate and adrenocortical function. *Lancet* 1:1434, 1983.
12. Fragen RJ, Shanks CA, Molteni A, et al: Effects of etomidate on hormonal responses to surgical stress. *Anesthesiology* 61:652, 1984.
13. Pfenninger E, Dick W, Ahnefeld FW: The influence of ketamine on both normal and raised intracranial pressure of artificially ventilated animals. *Eur J Anaesthesiol* 2:297, 1985.
14. Friesen RH, Thieme RE, Honda AT, et al: Changes in anterior fontanel pressure in preterm neonates receiving isoflurane, halothane, fentanyl, or ketamine. *Anesth Analg* 66:431, 1987.
15. White PF: Pharmacologic interactions of midazolam and ketamine in surgical patients. *Clin Pharmacol Ther* 31:280, 1982.
16. Dershwitz M, Walsh JL, Morishige RJ, et al: Pharmacokinetics and pharmacodynamics of inhaled versus intravenous morphine in healthy volunteers. *Anesthesiology* 93:619, 2000.
17. Aitkenhead AR, Vater M, Achola K, et al: Pharmacokinetics of single-dose intravenous morphine in normal volunteers and patients with end-stage renal failure. *Br J Anaesth* 56:813, 1984.
18. Shafer SL, Varvel JR: Pharmacokinetics, pharmacodynamics, and rational opioid selection. *Anesthesiology* 74:53, 1991.
19. Dershwitz M, Rosow CE: Remifentanil: an opioid metabolized by esterases. *Exp Opin Invest Drugs* 5:1361, 1996.
20. Dershwitz M, Hoke JF, Rosow CE, et al: Pharmacokinetics and pharmacodynamics of remifentanil in volunteer subjects with severe liver disease. *Anesthesiology* 84:812, 1996.
21. Hoke JF, Shlugman D, Dershwitz M, et al: Pharmacokinetics and pharmacodynamics of remifentanil in subjects with renal failure compared to healthy volunteers. *Anesthesiology* 87:533, 1997.
22. Leatherman JW, Fluegel WL, David WS, et al: Muscle weakness in mechanically ventilated patients with severe asthma. *Am J Respir Crit Care Med* 153:1686, 1996.
23. Barba CA, Angood PB, Kauder DR, et al: Bronchoscopic guidance makes percutaneous tracheostomy a safe, cost effective, and easy to teach procedure. *Surgery* 118:879, 1995.
24. Ausems ME, Hug CC Jr, Stanski DR, et al: Plasma concentrations of alfentanil required to supplement nitrous oxide anesthesia for general surgery. *Anesthesiology* 65:362, 1986.
25. Philbin DM, Rosow CE, Schneider RC, et al: Fentanyl and sufentanil anesthesia revisited: how much is enough? *Anesthesiology* 73:5, 1990.

26. Routine Monitoring of Critically Ill Patients

Frederick J. Curley and Nicholas A. Smyrnios

When intensive care units (ICUs) came into being in the late 1950s, vital signs were monitored intermittently by a nurse, and continuous measurement either was unavailable or necessitated invasive procedures. The explosion in the use of computers and other technology over the past few decades has significantly changed critical care. In no part of the hospital is the patient more intensively and continuously monitored, with the possible exception of the operating room, than in the ICU. All vital signs can now be monitored accurately, noninvasively, and continuously.

Over the past several years, the trend in monitoring systems has been to become multipurpose. This means that one system monitors a variety of parameters. Commercial systems now have the ability to monitor multiple invasive and noninvasive blood pressures, core temperature, respiration, oxygenation, end-tidal carbon dioxide, mixed venous oxygen saturation, electrocardiographic (ECG) rhythm, and ST segments. A multipurpose system eliminates the need for multiple, freestanding devices and makes it easier to coordinate the monitoring of different parameters. It may also manage data from other sources such as a ventilator or infusion pump or work in conjunction with a bedside clinical information system that provides data management.

Monitoring systems for ICUs may be either configured or modular. Configured systems have all of their functions hardwired directly into the system. Modular systems have removable modules that interface with the monitor. These modules contain the information for each parameter to be monitored. Modular systems have gained popularity as the physiologic parameters being monitored have changed and expanded. This allows a system to be upgraded more easily. It is an axiom in critical care monitoring that systems typically become clinically obsolete before they are technically obsolete.

This chapter deals with the routine, predominantly noninvasive monitoring that should be done for most patients in critical care units. It also examines the indications for, the fundamental technology of, and the problems encountered in the routine monitoring of temperature, blood pressure, ECG rhythm and ST segments, respiratory rate and pattern, oxygenation and carbon dioxide levels, and gastric intramucosal pH (pHi).

Temperature Monitoring

Abnormal temperature is common in critically ill patients. In the surgical ICU in one study, rectal temperatures on admission were normal in only 30% of patients, were above 37.6°C in 37.6%, and were below 36.8°C in 32.3% [1]. Recognition of abnormal temperature is clinically important. Abnormal temperature is frequently the earliest clinical sign of infection, inflammation, central nervous system dysfunction, or drug toxicity. Hypothermia and hyperthermia are associated with a significant morbidity and mortality (see Chapters 65 and 66). Accurate measurement of temperature depends on the type of thermometer used and the site of temperature measurement.

TYPES OF THERMOMETERS. A mercury-in-glass thermometer has been the type in most common clinical use. Due to environmental concerns regarding mercury, however, these thermometers are gradually being phased out. Mercury remains the clinical gold standard. Falsely low measurements may result from failure to leave the thermometer in place for a minimum of 3 minutes' equilibration time. Falsely high temperatures result from failure to shake the mercury down. Because of practical limitations in length, different models of mercury thermometers are used for the hypothermic temperature range.

Liquid crystal display (LCD) thermometers usually involve liquid crystals embedded in thin adhesive strips that are directly attached to the patient's skin. The crystals may be sensitive to temperature changes as small as 0.2°C, but the displays usually limit discrimination of temperature changes to no more than 0.5°C. LCD thermometers can be applied to any area of the skin but are most commonly applied to the forehead for ease of use and steady perfusion. Like all skin temperature measurements, they poorly reflect core temperature when the skin is hypoperfused. Forehead skin temperature is typically lower than core temperatures by 2.2°C [2], and changes in LCD forehead temperature lag behind changes in core temperature by more than 12 minutes [3]. The LCD strip can be left in place for several hours without skin irritation but must be discarded after use [4]. LCD skin thermometry is probably best used in patients with stable, normal hemodynamics who are not anticipated to experience major tempera-

ture shifts and in whom the trend of temperature change is more important than the accuracy of the measurement.

Thermocouples and thermistors are frequently used as probes in electric thermometers that convert the electrical temperature signal into analog or digital displays. Thermocouples consist of a tight junction of two dissimilar metals. The voltage change across the junction can be precisely related to temperature. The measuring thermocouple must be calibrated against a second constant-temperature junction for absolute temperature measurements. The measured voltage changes are on the order of 50 µV per degree Celsius and must be amplified to generate a usable temperature display. In the range of 20° to 50°C, thermocouples may have a linearity error of less than 0.1 [4]. Thermocouples are faster and cheaper but less sensitive than thermistors and semiconductors.

Thermistors consist of semiconductor metal oxides in which the electrical resistance changes inversely with temperature. A linearity error of up to 4°C may occur over the temperature range of 20° to 50°C, but this can be substantially reduced by making mathematical adjustments or placing a fixed resistance in parallel with the thermistor, which decreases its sensitivity and usable temperature range [4]. Thermistors are more sensitive, faster responding, and less linear and costly than thermocouples or semiconductors [4,5]. Semiconductors measure temperature by taking advantage of the fact that the base-to-emitter voltage change is temperature dependent, whereas the collector current of the silicon resistor is constant. Thermocouples and thermistors can be fashioned into thin wires and embedded in flexible probes that are suitable for placing in body cavities to measure deep temperature.

Zero–heat-flow thermometry involves placing a thermistor, a heat-flow sensor, and a heater immediately adjacent to the skin. Heat loss from the skin is detected by the flow sensor and is compensated for by the heater. In this manner, the skin beneath the probe is isolated from ambient temperature changes and more directly reflects deep body temperature or core temperature [6,7]. Response time to changes in core temperature is approximately 10 minutes [7] but may be substantially longer in obese patients [5]. Inaccuracies during hypoperfusion have been reported [5]. Despite its convenience, this type of thermometer remains infrequently used in the clinical setting because of its cost, 30-minute warm-up time, and inadequate data on local variation of deep body temperature at different sites.

Radiotelemetry thermometers have been made in the form of ingestible pills. The temperature sensor in the pill is an inductor and functions in such a way that temperature-dependent changes in inductance result in changes in radiofrequency. Changes in radiofrequency can then be detected by a remote unit and translated electronically into a digital display of temperature. These thermometers have little application in the ICU because temperature differences of up to 2°C may occur simply as a result of the pill's transit in the intestine [8].

Infrared emission detection tympanic thermometers [9] are probably now most commonly used in the hospital setting. These thermometers use an infrared sensor that detects infrared energy emitted by the core-temperature tissues behind the tympanic membrane. The infrared emissions through the tympanic membrane vary linearly with core temperature. The thermometer's sensor sends a signal to a microprocessor, which converts the signal into a digitally displayed temperature. Measurements are most accurate when the measuring probe blocks the entrance of ambient air into the ear canal and when the midposterior external ear is tugged posterosuperiorly so as to direct the probe to the anterior, inferior third of the tympanic membrane. Operator error due to improper calibration, setup, or poor probe positioning can significantly alter temperatures [10]. Mathematical corrections are available so that tympanic temperature can be compared with that at other sites.

SITES OF MEASUREMENT. *Core temperature* refers to the deep body temperature that is carefully regulated by the hypothalamus so as to be independent of transient small changes in ambient temperature. Core temperature exists more as a physiologic concept than as the temperature of an anatomic location. Ideal sites of temperature measurement would be protected from heat loss, painless, and convenient to use and would not interfere with the patient's ability to move and communicate. No one location provides an accurate measurement of core temperature in all clinical circumstances. Rectal, bladder, and tympanic temperatures are in general the most reliable sites for measuring approximate core temperatures.

Sublingual temperature measurement is convenient but suffers numerous limitations. Although open- versus closed-mouth breathing [11] and use of nasogastric tubes do not alter temperature measurement [12], oral temperature is obviously altered if measured during or immediately after the patient has consumed hot or cold drinks. Falsely low oral temperatures may occur because of cooling from tachypnea [13]. Sixty percent of sublingual temperatures are more than 1°F lower than simultaneously measured rectal temperatures; 53% differ by 1° to 2°F, and 6% differ by more than 2°F. Continuous sublingual measurement interferes with the patient's ability to eat and speak, and it is difficult to maintain a good probe position. Sublingual measurement is best suited for intermittent monitoring when highly accurate measurement of core temperature is unnecessary.

Axillary temperatures have been used as an index of core temperature and can be taken with a mercury-in-glass thermometer or a flexible probe. Temperatures average 1.5° to 1.9°C lower than tympanic temperatures [14]. Positioning the sensor over the axillary artery is thought to improve accuracy. The accuracy and precision of axillary temperature measurement are less than at other sites [14], perhaps in part because of the difficulty of maintaining a good probe position.

Rectal temperature is conveniently measured with a mercury-in-glass thermometer or a flexible temperature sensor. It is clearly the most widely accepted standard of measuring core temperature in clinical use. Before a rectal thermometer is inserted, a digital rectal examination should be performed because feces can blunt temperature measurement. Readings are more accurate when the sensor is passed more than 10 cm (4 in.) into the rectum [5]. Rectal temperature correlates well in most patients with distal esophageal, bladder, and tympanic temperatures [14,15]. Because of thermal inertia in the rectum, it is typically the slowest of the central measurement sites to respond to induced changes in temperature [16,17].

Esophageal temperature is usually measured with an electric, flexible temperature sensor and varies greatly with the position of the sensor in the esophagus. In the proximal esophagus, as well as in the midportion near the trachea and bronchi, temperature is influenced by that of the ambient air [18]. During hypothermia, temperatures in different portions of the esophagus may differ by up to 6°C [18]. Stable, more accurate temperatures are reached when the sensor is 45 cm from the nose [18,19]. Esophageal temperatures on average are 0.6°C lower than rectal temperatures [20]. Because of the proximity of the distal esophagus to the great vessels and heart, distal esophageal temperature responds rapidly to changes in core temperature [5]. Changes in esophageal temperature may inaccurately reflect changes in core temperature when induced temperature change occurs because of the inspiration of heated air, warm or cold gastric lavage, or car-

diac bypass or assist [5]. Complications apart from mild discomfort and epistaxis are rare.

Tympanic temperature must be measured with a specifically designed thermometer and correlates well with rectal and distal esophageal temperature [5]. In clinical practice, tympanic measurements correlate poorly with traditional oral measurements [21]. Tympanic temperature measurement should always be preceded and followed by an otoscopic examination. Current thermometers do not permit continuous measurement, which limits their utility in the ICU. Accuracy depends on operator experience, and even when trained, experienced ICU nurses use tympanic thermometers the variability in repeated measurements is more than 0.5°F in 20% of patients [22]. Perforation of the tympanic membrane [23] and bleeding from the external canal due to trauma from the probe have been reported. One series had a 1.25% complication rate [17].

Urinary bladder temperature can be easily measured with a specially designed temperature probe embedded in a Foley catheter [14–17]. In patients undergoing induced hypothermia and rewarming, bladder temperatures correlate well with great vessel and rectal temperatures and less well with esophageal temperatures [15–17]. Bladder temperature under steady-state conditions is more reproducible than that taken at other sites [15].

Central venous temperature can be easily measured with a thermistor-equipped pulmonary artery catheter. The temperature sensor is located at the distal tip and can record accurate great vessel temperatures when the tip of the catheter is in the distal vena cava. Temperatures would differ from core temperatures when heated air was breathed or warm or cold intravenous fluids were infused.

Temperature measured on the medial aspect of the great toe varies with core temperature and toe perfusion [1]. The gradient between toe and core temperature is therefore an index of perfusion. A normal rectal-to-toe temperature difference of 3° to 7°C occurs once patient hemodynamics have been optimized. Abnormal toe-to-rectal temperature gradients occur during hypovolemia, low cardiac output, pain, and hypoxemic acidosis [1,24]. The absolute value of great toe temperature has been predictive of mortality in some populations. Great toe temperatures of less than 27°C that persist for more than 3 hours after admission are associated with death in 67% of adults [24], and temperatures less than 32°C that last for 4 hours after cardiac surgery predicted significantly increased mortality in children [25]. Toe temperature is an unreliable indicator of core temperature because it is so greatly affected by perfusion. It should be used only to assess peripheral circulatory flow in comparison with other measurements of core temperature.

The choice of site used to monitor temperature must be individualized, but certain generalizations can be made. Tympanic, bladder, and esophageal temperatures in general appear to be most accurate and reproducible [26]. In a study of 56 patients undergoing general anesthesia, esophageal, bladder, and rectal temperatures were more accurate than forehead and axillary measurements, and esophageal and bladder temperatures were more precise than rectal, axillary, and forehead temperatures when compared with tympanic temperature [15,27]. Because bladder, esophageal, tympanic, and rectal sites appear comparable, convenience may help dictate appropriate site selection. Routine measurement of esophageal temperatures would necessitate insertion of a nasal probe in all patients. In addition, accuracy varies greatly with small changes in position. Therefore, routine esophageal temperature measurement is probably of benefit only in patients undergoing treatment for hyperthermia or hypothermia. Tympanic temperature measurement requires physician involvement for otoscopy and decreases the patient's ability to hear. Placement of probes may also be traumatic. Rectal probes are frequently extruded and may be refused by patients. Reusable, electronic, sheath-covered rectal thermometers have been associated with the transmission of *Clostridium difficile* and vancomycin-resistant *Enterococcus* [28,29]. Because of the risk of infecting other patients, all rectal thermometers should be used only once. Patients with a thermistor-tipped pulmonary artery catheter already in place require no additional monitoring, but insertion of a central venous thermistor to monitor temperature is probably warranted only in hyperthermia or hypothermia. Because most critically ill patients have an indwelling Foley catheter, bladder temperature could be easily measured at a cost of less than $10 per thermistor-equipped catheter. Continuous temperature monitoring is in general probably best accomplished by measurement of bladder, great vessel, or rectal temperature [30,31]. Intermittent measurements for reasons of accuracy should probably be rectal rather than sublingual.

INDICATIONS FOR TEMPERATURE MONITORING. Temperature monitoring was identified as an essential service for critical care units by the Task Force on Guidelines of the Society of Critical Care Medicine recommendations for services and personnel for delivery of care in a critical care setting [32]. Critically ill patients are at high risk for temperature disorders because of debility, impaired voluntary control of temperature, frequent use of sedative drugs, and high predisposition to infection. All critically ill patients should have core temperature measured at least every 4 hours. Because the morbidity and mortality associated with hypothermia and hyperthermia vary with the severity and duration of the abnormality, patients with temperatures above 39°C or below 36°C should have their temperature continuously monitored. Patients who are undergoing active interventions to alter temperature, such as breathing heated air or using a cooling-warming blanket, should have continuous monitoring to prevent overtreatment or undertreatment of temperature disorders.

Arterial Pressure Monitoring

Arterial pressure has traditionally been measured with a mercury sphygmomanometer and a stethoscope. Techniques of direct blood pressure measurement by intraarterial catheter were initially developed in the 1930s and popularized in the 1950s [33,34]. These measurements were soon accepted as representing true systolic and diastolic pressures.

Since that time, a variety of alternative indirect methods have been developed that equal and even surpass auscultation in reproducibility and ease of measurement. This section examines the advantages and disadvantages of the various methods of arterial pressure monitoring and provides recommendations for their use in the ICU.

INDIRECT BLOOD PRESSURE MEASUREMENT. Several methods of indirect blood pressure monitoring can be performed [35–39], most of which describe the external pressure applied when flow is observed in an artery distal to the occlusion. Therefore, what is actually detected is blood flow, not intraarterial pressure [35]. One method describes the pressure required to maintain a distal artery with a transmural pressure of zero. These differences in what is actually measured are the major points of discrepancy between direct and indirect measurements and are discussed further later.

Indirectly measured pressures vary depending on the size of the cuff used. Cuffs of inadequate width and length can provide falsely elevated readings. Bladder width should equal 40% and bladder length at least 60% of the circumference of the extremity measured [40]. Anyone who makes indirect pressure measurements must be aware of these factors and carefully select the cuff to be used.

Manual Methods

AUSCULTATORY (RIVA-ROCCI) PRESSURES. The traditional method of blood pressure measurement involves inflating a sphygmomanometer cuff around an extremity and auscultating over an artery distal to the occlusion. Sounds from the vibrations of the artery under pressure (Korotkoff sounds) indicate systolic and diastolic pressures [38]. The level at which the sound first becomes audible is taken as the systolic pressure. The point at which there is an abrupt diminution in or disappearance of sounds is used as diastolic pressure [39]. This method continues to be used commonly in the ICU and yields an acceptable value in most situations. Its advantages include low cost, time-honored reliability, and simplicity. Disadvantages include operator variability and the absence of Korotkoff sounds when pressures are very low.

Auscultatory pressures also correlate poorly with directly measured pressures at the extremes of pressure [35,41]. The tendency is for pressures obtained by auscultation to fall increasingly below those measured directly as the pressure increases. However, the difference between these values is unpredictable, and at times the indirectly measured value can exceed its direct counterpart by as much as 20 mm Hg [35]. Therefore, auscultatory pressures must be interpreted with full knowledge of their limitations in the critically ill.

OSCILLATION METHOD. The oscillation method has served as the basis for the development of several automated blood pressure monitoring devices. The first discontinuity in the needle movement of an aneroid manometer indicates the presence of blood flow in the distal artery and is taken as systolic pressure [35]. This oscillation is caused by vibration of the walls of the artery when blood begins to flow through it. Diastolic pressure is not measured by this technique. The advantages of the oscillation method are low cost and simplicity. The disadvantages include the inability to measure diastolic pressure, poor correlation with directly measured pressures [35], and lack of utility in situations in which Riva-Rocci measurements are also unobtainable. In one study, 34% of all aneroid manometers in use in one large medical system gave inaccurate measurements, even when more lenient standards were used than those advocated by the National Bureau of Standards and the Association for the Advancement of Medical Instrumentation [42]. In the same survey, 36% of the devices were found to be mechanically defective. This points out the need for regular maintenance of these devices. Although the manometers themselves can also be used for auscultatory measurements, oscillometric readings probably provide no advantage over auscultation in the ICU.

PALPATION METHOD. Palpatory systolic pressures are obtained by detecting the pulse in the radial artery as the cuff is slowly deflated. This resembles the oscillation method because it does not measure diastolic pressure. Palpation is most useful in emergency situations in which Korotkoff sounds cannot be heard and an arterial line is not in place. The inability to measure diastolic pressure makes the palpation method less valuable for continuous monitoring. In addition, palpation obtains no better correlation with direct measurements than the previously described techniques. In one study, variation from simultaneously obtained direct pressure measurements was as high as 60 mm Hg [41]. Like other indirect methods, palpation tends to underestimate actual values to greater degrees at higher levels of arterial pressure.

Automated Methods. Automated indirect blood pressure devices provide measurements of arterial blood pressure without manual inflation and deflation of the sphygmomanometer cuff. They operate on one of seven principles: Doppler flow, infrasound, oscillometry, volume clamp, arterial tonometry, Doppler echocardiography, and pulse wave arrival time.

DOPPLER FLOW. Doppler systems operate on the Doppler principle, which takes advantage of the change in frequency of an echo signal when there is movement between two objects. These devices emit brief pulses of sound at a high frequency that are reflected back to the transducer [43]. The compressed artery exhibits a large amount of wall motion when flow first appears in the vessel distal to the inflated cuff. This causes a change in frequency of the echo signal, called a *Doppler shift*. The first appearance of flow in the distal artery represents systolic pressure. In an uncompressed artery, the small amount of motion does not cause a change in frequency of the reflected signal. Therefore, the disappearance of the Doppler shift in the echo signal represents diastolic pressure [44,45].

INFRASOUND. Infrasound devices use a microphone to detect low-frequency (20 to 30 Hz) sound waves associated with the oscillation of the arterial wall [37,46]. These sounds are processed by a minicomputer, and the processed signals are usually displayed in digital form [47].

OSCILLOMETRY. Oscillometric devices operate on the same principle as manual oscillometric measurements. The cuff senses pressure fluctuations caused by vessel wall oscillations in the presence of pulsatile blood flow [37,48]. Maximum oscillation is seen at mean pressure, whereas wall movement greatly decreases below diastolic pressure [49]. As with the other automated methods described, the signals produced by the system are processed electronically and displayed in digital form.

VOLUME CLAMP TECHNIQUE. The volume clamp method avoids the use of an arm cuff. A finger cuff is applied to the proximal or middle phalanx to keep the artery at a constant size [50]. The pressure in the cuff is changed as necessary by a servocontrol unit strapped to the wrist. The feedback in this system is provided by a light source and detector that measure absorption at a frequency specific for arterial blood. The pressure needed to keep the artery at a constant size is always equal to the intraarterial pressure, thereby creating a transmural pressure of zero [51].

ARTERIAL TONOMETRY. Arterial tonometry provides continuous noninvasive measurement of arterial pressure, including pressure waveforms. Essentially, it involves flattening a superficial artery against a bone to remove any force due to wall tension and then placing a pressure transducer on the skin over the flattened artery. The resultant force sensed by the pressure transducer is thought to measure intraarterial pressure only [52,53]. This method is being researched actively, although studies have come to differing conclusions regarding its accuracy [54,55]. It has been reported that tonometrically measured pressures can be made to describe accurately central aortic pressure waveforms by mathematically adjusting them [56]. The clinical value of this practice is unknown.

ECHOCARDIOGRAPHY. The Doppler echocardiogram has been used occasionally to estimate aortic pressures. This is primarily of value for the rare patient in whom peripheral pressures cannot be obtained. This measurement takes advantage of the Bernoulli equation, which describes the relationship between pressure gradient and flow ($\dot{V}$). In its modified form, this relationship is [57]

$$\text{Pressure gradient} = 4 \dot{V}^2$$

In patients who demonstrate regurgitation across the aortic valve, the pressure gradient measured is that seen across the valve. This can give an estimation of systolic pressure that is accurate only to within the wide range of variation of the left ventricular diastolic pressure. Therefore, this method should be used only when all other methods have failed.

PULSE WAVE ARRIVAL TIME. The time interval between the R wave of the ECG and the arrival of the pulse wave peripherally has been reported to be a measure of blood pressure change. This theory was tested in 15 critically ill infants and children. The relationship between systolic blood pressure and 1/pulse wave arrival time was not found to be close enough to be clinically useful [58].

Utility of Noninvasive Blood Pressure Measurements. Only four of the methods described previously (infrasound, oscillometry, Doppler flow, volume clamp) are associated with significant clinical experience. Of these, methods using infrasound technology correlate least well with direct measures, obtaining correlation coefficients of 0.58 to 0.84 compared with arterial lines [36,37,59]. Therefore, infrasound is rarely used in systems designed for critical care. Oscillometric methods can correlate to within 1 mm Hg of the directly measured group average values [37,60,61], but they have traditionally varied greatly from predicting intraarterial pressures in individual subjects.

Studies have shown improved correlation with simulated arterial pressures [62], although individual variation from simultaneously measured intraarterial pressures is still frequently beyond accepted standards [63]. Doppler sensing devices offer a slightly better correlation but still vary sufficiently to be clinically suspect. Correlation coefficients range from 0.83 to 0.99 for systolic pressures and 0.71 for diastolic pressures [36]. More than 30% of systolic measurements may vary from a simultaneously measured direct pressure by greater than 10 mm Hg, although only 2.7% vary by more than 20 mm Hg [62]. Volume clamp using a finger cuff has been compared with standard methods in multiple studies [39,62–67]. These devices respond rapidly to changes in blood pressure and give excellent correlation in group averages. In one study looking at a large number of measurements, 95% of all measurements using this method were within 10 mm Hg of the directly measured values [68]. Therefore, this technique may be more appropriate for use in critically ill patients.

Although they have not been consistently accurate, automated methods have the potential to yield as accurate a value as pressures derived by auscultation [68–70]. One study revealed as good a correlation with directly measured pressures as Riva-Rocci pressures have traditionally obtained [37]. Studies by Aitken et al. [64] and Hirschl et al. [39] demonstrated acceptable correlation of volume clamp technique with systolic pressures measured directly. Another study demonstrated that mean arterial pressures (MAPs) determined by auscultation were extremely close to those measured by automated devices [69].

One of the proposed advantages of automated noninvasive monitoring is patient safety [71]. The incidence of vessel occlusion and hemorrhage is thought to be reduced when arterial lines are avoided. Automated methods have complications of their own, however. Ulnar nerve palsies have been reported with frequent inflation and deflation of a cuff [72]. Decreased venous return from the limb and eventually reduced perfusion to that extremity can also be seen when the cuff is set to inflate and deflate every minute [71–73].

In summary, automated noninvasive blood pressure monitors have improved in recent years. Volume clamp devices are probably acceptable for use in critically ill patients with moderate severity of illness. Oscillometric and Doppler-based devices are adequate for frequent blood pressure checks in essentially stable patients, in patient transport situations in which arterial lines cannot be easily used, and in the severely burned patient, in whom direct arterial pressure measurement may lead to an unacceptably high risk of infection [74]. Automated noninvasive blood pressure monitors have a role in following trends of pressure change [75] and when group averages, not individual measurements, are most important. In general, they are of little value in situations in which blood pressure is likely to fluctuate rapidly. Also, they exhibit such divergence from directly obtained values that critical patient management decisions should not be made based on information derived from automated monitors unless confirmation using a more reliable method is not possible.

DIRECT INVASIVE BLOOD PRESSURE MEASUREMENT. Direct blood pressure measurement is performed with an intraarterial catheter. The techniques of insertion and care of arterial lines are covered thoroughly in Chapter 3. Here, we discuss the advantages and disadvantages of invasive monitoring compared with noninvasive means.

Arterial catheters contain a fluid column that transmits the pressure back through the tubing to a transducer. A low-compliance diaphragm in the transducer creates a reproducible volume change in response to the applied pressure change. The volume change alters the resistance of a Wheatstone bridge and is thus converted into an electrical signal [76]. In most systems, the pressure is displayed in wave and in digital forms.

Problems in Direct Pressure Monitoring

PATIENT-RELATED PROBLEMS. Several technical problems can affect the measurement of arterial pressure with the arterial line. Transducers must be calibrated to zero at the level of the heart. Improper zeroing can lead to erroneous interpretation of essentially accurate measurements. Thrombus formation at the catheter tip can cause occlusion of the catheter, making accurate measurement impossible. This problem can be largely eliminated by using a 20-gauge polyurethane catheter, rather than a smaller one, with a slow, continuous heparin flush [77,78]. Because movement of the limb may interrupt the column of fluid and prevent accurate measurement, it should be immobile during readings.

SYSTEM-RELATED PROBLEMS. Direct pressure values are also affected by several factors specific to the measurement system itself. For example, effective transducer design must take into account the natural frequency of the transducer system. The natural frequency is the frequency at which the system oscillates independent of changes in the measured variable. Signals that approach the natural frequency in wavelength become amplified and may result in an exaggerated reported pressure [79]. This phenomenon is referred to as *overshoot*. Above the natural frequency, the signal is attenuated and an erroneously low pressure can be reported. Accurate recording systems require a natural frequency at least five times greater than the fundamental frequency (i.e., the range of expected heart rates) [80,81]. This is necessary to account for the multiple harmonic frequencies produced along with the main (fundamental) frequency.

The frequency response of the system is a phenomenon not only of transducer design but of the tubing and the fluid in it. The length, width, and compliance of the tubing all affect the system's response to change. Tubing shorter than 60 cm should be used [82]. Small-bore catheters are preferable to minimize the mass of fluid that can oscillate and amplify the pressure [81]. The compliance of the system (change in volume of the tubing and the transducer for a given change in pressure) should be low [81]. In addition, bubbles in the tubing can affect measurements in two ways. Large amounts of air in the measurement system damp the system response and cause underestimation of pressure [83]. This is usually easily

detectable. Small air bubbles cause an increase in the compliance of the system and can lead to significant amplification of the reported pressure [81–83].

SITE-RELATED PROBLEMS. Other problems arise in relation to the location of catheter placement. The radial artery is the most common site of arterial cannulation for pressure measurement. This site is accessible and easily immobilized for protection of the catheter and the patient. The major alternative site is the femoral artery. Both sites are relatively safe for insertion [77,84,85]. Other available sites include the brachial, dorsalis pedis, and axillary arteries [85,86]. Site-specific problems with arterial lines center on whether pressures measured directly at one site can be compared with pressures measured at another site. Although it was thought that upper extremity pressures were different from those measured in the leg, this probably reflects the location of measurement rather than the extremity. Systolic pressure is augmented toward the periphery by reflection of the pressure from the distal vessels due to impedance discontinuity [87], the abrupt increase in resistance due to the narrowing of peripheral vessels. Changes in the pressure-pulse contour as it approaches the periphery are manifestations of this. This waveform becomes narrower and more peaked as it proceeds distally [74]. In practice, this means that systolic pressures measured in the radial artery are, on average, 6 mm Hg higher than those in the brachial artery [87]. Similarly, in the absence of a significant arterial obstruction, dorsalis pedis pressures are higher than femoral pressures. These differences are less significant in older patients and those with noncompliant vessels. The elevation of central systolic pressures in these situations eliminates the increase seen along the course of the vessels in young, healthy people. One way of avoiding these problems is to use the MAP for decision making in the ICU. The MAP varies less along the course of the arterial tree, making it a more accurate indication of the pressure in the aorta. In addition, the MAP is the driving pressure for blood flow in the periphery. Despite this, comparisons between pressures measured at different sites should be avoided.

Advantages. Despite technical problems, direct arterial pressure measurement offers several advantages. Arterial lines actually measure the end-on pressure propagated by the arterial pulse. This is in contrast to indirect methods, which report the external pressure necessary either to obstruct flow or to maintain a constant transmural vessel pressure. Arterial lines can also detect pressures at which Korotkoff sounds are either absent or inaccurate [72]. Arterial lines provide a continuous measurement. They provide an immediate report of changes in blood pressure without the need for repeated inflation and deflation of a cuff. In situations in which frequent blood drawing is necessary, indwelling arterial lines eliminate the need for multiple percutaneous punctures.

CONCLUSIONS. Indirect methods of blood pressure monitoring report the external pressure necessary to obstruct flow or to maintain a constant transmural vessel pressure. Arterial lines measure the end-on pressure propagated by the arterial pulse. Direct arterial pressure measurement offers several advantages. Arterial lines provide a continuous measurement, can detect pressures at which Korotkoff sounds are either absent or inaccurate, and provide an immediate report of changes in pressure without the need for repeated inflation and deflation of a cuff. In situations in which frequent blood drawing is necessary, arterial lines eliminate the need for multiple percutaneous punctures. Regardless of the method used, the MAP should be the basis for decision making in most critically ill patients.

Electrocardiographic Monitoring

Continuous ECG monitoring is performed routinely in almost all ICUs in the United States. It combines the principles of ECG, which have been known since 1903, with the principles of biotelemetry, first put into practical application in 1921 [88,89]. Here we review the principles of arrhythmia monitoring and the problems associated with it. We also discuss the automatic detection of arrhythmias and the role of automated ST segment analysis. Although telemetry is not usually used in ICUs, it is a useful adjunct in the advancement of recuperating patients to more routine levels of care and is briefly discussed here.

ECG monitoring in most ICUs is done over hard-wired apparatus. Skin electrodes detect cardiac impulses and transform them into an electrical signal, which is transmitted over wires directly to the signal converter and display unit. This removes the problems of interference and frequency restrictions seen in telemetry systems, at the cost of reduced mobility for the patient. Most often, mobility is not an immediate concern for this group of individuals.

Arrhythmia monitoring was shown to improve the prognosis of patients admitted to the ICU for acute myocardial infarction (AMI) many years ago [90–92]. It has been a standard of care in the United States since that time. In coronary care, arrhythmia monitoring is necessary for the following reasons: First, up to 95% of patients with AMI have some disturbance of their rate or rhythm within 48 hours of admission [93]. Ventricular premature beats are the most common arrhythmia, present in up to 100% of patients [92–94]. Monitoring allows the recognition and treatment of minor arrhythmias such as frequent ventricular premature beats, which may be entirely asymptomatic but also may predict sudden death [95]. Second, ventricular tachycardia (VT) occurs in approximately one-third of patients with AMI. Other serious arrhythmias are seen less frequently. Monitoring enables the rapid detection of ventricular fibrillation or VT, increasing the likelihood of successful resuscitation. Arrhythmia monitoring has been shown to improve prognosis in the post-myocardial infarction period when combined with an aggressive, formalized approach to the treatment of arrhythmias [92]. It also can demonstrate the response to therapy so that alternative treatments can be begun, if necessary. Thrombolytic therapy for AMI leads to a slight increase in arrhythmias within 8 to 12 hours after successful reperfusion [96–98]. This can be used as one indicator of successful reperfusion. Arrhythmia monitoring also allows the measurement of heart rate variability, which may be useful in postinfarction risk stratification [99].

The impact of monitoring in a general medical or surgical ICU is less certain. One study demonstrated a 23.9% incidence of atrial fibrillation and a 17.4% incidence of VT in a medical ICU [100]. Twenty-five percent of the episodes of VT were not detected by an experienced ICU staff. It is not known whether assigning a dedicated monitor watcher would change this finding [101]. The effect of monitoring on the prognosis of these patients is also not known. However, there is a growing body of evidence that myocardial ischemia is a barrier to weaning from mechanical ventilation [102]. If this proves to be true, ischemia monitoring may become a standard of care in medical, surgical, and respiratory ICUs.

EVOLUTION OF ARRHYTHMIA MONITORING SYSTEMS FOR CLINICAL USE. After continuous ECG monitoring in ICUs was begun, some deficiencies with the systems were recognized. Initially, the responsibility for arrhythmia detection was assigned to specially trained coronary care nurses. Despite this, several studies documented that manual methods of arrhythmia detection failed to identify arrhythmias, including salvos of VT, in

up to 77% of cases [94,103,104]. This failure was probably due to an inadequate number of staff nurses to watch the monitors, inadequate staff education, and faulty monitors [103]. Subsequently, monitors equipped with built-in rate alarms that sounded when a preset maximum or minimum rate was detected proved inadequate because some runs of VT are too brief to exceed the rate limit for a given time interval [94,104]. Ultimately, computerized arrhythmia detection systems were incorporated into the monitors. The software in these systems is capable of diagnosing arrhythmias based on recognition of heart rate, variability, rhythm, intervals, segment lengths, complex width, and morphology [105,106]. These systems have been validated in coronary care and general medical ICUs [104,107]. Computerized arrhythmia detection systems are well accepted by nursing personnel, who must work most closely with them [108].

ISCHEMIA MONITORING. Just as episodes of VT and ventricular fibrillation are missed with simple monitoring systems, significant episodes of myocardial ischemia often go undetected [109]. This is either because the episode is asymptomatic or because the patient's ability to communicate is impaired owing to intubation or altered mental status. ECG monitoring systems with automated ST segment analysis have been devised to attempt to deal with this problem.

In most ST segment monitoring systems, the computer initially creates a template of the patient's normal QRS complexes. It then recognizes the QRS complexes and the J points of subsequent beats and compares an isoelectric point just before the QRS with a portion of the ST segment 60 to 80 milliseconds after the J point [110]. It compares this relationship to that of the same points in the QRS complex template. The system must decide whether the QRS complex in question was generated and conducted in standard fashion or whether the beats are aberrant, which negates the validity of comparison. Therefore, an arrhythmia detection system must be included in all ischemia monitoring systems designed for use in the ICU. In standard systems, three leads can be monitored simultaneously. These leads are usually chosen to represent the three major axes (anteroposterior, left-right, and craniocaudal). They can be displayed individually, or the ST segment deviations can be summed up and displayed in a graph over time [110].

Automated ST segment analysis has gained widespread popularity among cardiologists. The American Heart Association Task Force has recommended since 1989 that ischemia monitoring be included in new monitoring systems developed for use in the coronary care unit [111]. Information is now available that demonstrates its value. Early detection of ischemic episodes could lead to early interventions, such as rate control or thrombolysis, to prevent further damage [112]. Continuous ST segment monitoring can lead to the treatment of an expanded group of patients with thrombolytic therapy, including patients whose initial 12-lead ECG may not have demonstrated changes characteristic of AMI [113]. The degree of ST segment resolution after thrombolytic therapy may be a marker for prognosis after AMI [114].

Newer Techniques. Some authors now advocate the use of continuous 12-lead ECG systems in the care of acute coronary syndromes [113,115]. The actual value of the broad clinical application of this is unknown. Signal-averaged ECG for the detection of heart rate variability has also been reported to predict outcomes in coronary and surgical critical care [116,117]. A great deal more study is needed before recommendations for its use can be made. Within the next several years, noninvasive central hemodynamic monitoring may be commercially available. Although this technology has the potential to revolutionize critical care, the accuracy and utility of such systems have yet to be proved.

TECHNICAL CONSIDERATIONS. As with any other biomedical measurement, technical problems can arise in the monitoring of cardiac rhythm. Standards have been devised to guide manufacturers and purchasers of ECG monitoring systems [111,118].

Whenever a patient is directly connected to an electrically operated piece of equipment by a low-resistance path, the possibility of electrical shock exists. This would most commonly occur with improper grounding of equipment when a device such as a pacemaker is in place. Precautions that are necessary to avoid this potential catastrophe include (a) periodic checks to ensure that all equipment in contact with the patient is at the same ground potential as the power ground line; (b) insulation of exposed lead connections; and (c) use of appropriately wired three-prong plugs [119,120].

The size of the ECG signal is important for accurate recognition of cardiac rate and rhythm. Several factors may affect signal size. The amplitude can be affected by mismatching between skin-electrode and preamplifier impedance. The combination of a high skin-electrode impedance, usually the result of poor contact between the skin and electrode with low-input impedance of the preamplifier can result in a decrease in the size of the ECG signal [121]. Low skin-electrode impedance can be promoted by good skin preparation, site selection, and conducting gels. A high preamplifier input impedance or the use of buffer amplifiers can also improve impedance matching and thereby improve the signal obtained.

Another factor that affects complex size is critical damping, the system's ability to respond to changes in the input signal. An underdamped system responds to changes in input with displays that exaggerate the signal, called *overshoot*. An overdamped system responds slowly to a given change and may exhibit a complex that underestimates the actual amplitude. The ECG signal can also be affected by the presence of inherent, unwanted voltages at the point of input into the ECG. These include the common mode signal, a response to surrounding electromagnetic forces; the direct current skin potential produced by contact between the skin and the electrode; and a potential caused by internal body resistance. Finally, the ECG system must have a frequency response that is accurate for the signals being monitored. Modern, commercially available systems have incorporated features to deal with each of these problems.

PERSONNEL. The staff's ability to interpret the information received is crucial to the effectiveness of ECG monitoring [111]. Primary interpretation may be by nurses or technicians under the supervision of a physician. All personnel responsible for interpreting ECG monitoring must have formal training developed cooperatively by the hospital's medical and nursing staffs. At a minimum, this training should include basic ECG interpretation skills and arrhythmia recognition. Formal protocols for responding to and verifying alarms should be established and adhered to. Finally, a physician should be available in the hospital to assist with interpretation and make decisions regarding therapy.

PRINCIPLES OF TELEMETRY. Intensive care patients frequently continue to require ECG monitoring after they are released from the ICU. At this point, increased mobility is important to allow physical and occupational therapy as well as other rehabilitation services. Telemetry systems can facilitate this.

Telemetry means measurement at a distance [122]. Biomedical telemetry consists of measuring various vital signs, including heart rhythm, and transmitting them to a distant terminal [123]. Telemetry systems in the hospital consist of four major components [123]: (a) A signal transducer detects heart activity through skin electrodes and converts it into electrical signals; (b) a radio transmitter broadcasts the electrical signal over ultrahigh frequencies or very high frequencies; (c) the radio receiver detects the transmission and converts it back into an electrical signal; and (d) the signal converter and display unit present the signal in its most familiar format.

Telemetry can be continuous or intermittent. Post-ICU patients, when monitored, are almost always followed continuously. Continuous telemetry requires an exclusive frequency so the signal can be transmitted without interruption from other signals [124], which means the hospital system must have multiple frequencies available to allow monitoring of several patients simultaneously. The telemetry signal may be received in one location or simultaneously in multiple locations, depending on staffing practices. The signal transducer and display unit should also be equipped with an automatic arrhythmia detection and alarm system to allow rapid detection and treatment of arrhythmias.

SUMMARY. Continuous ECG monitoring for the detection of arrhythmias is and should be ubiquitous in the ICU because it has been shown to improve the prognosis in post-AMI patients. Because a large percentage of arrhythmias can be missed by ICU staff when monitors without computerized arrhythmia detection systems are used, these computerized systems should be standard equipment in ICUs that care for patients with AMI. It appears that computerized monitoring devices can detect a significant number of arrhythmias not noted manually in noncardiac patients as well. A large percentage of these lead to an alteration in patient care. Therefore, it seems wise to include them as standard equipment in all medical and surgical ICUs. Automated ST segment analysis facilitates the early detection of ischemic episodes. Telemetry provides close monitoring of recuperating patients while allowing them increased mobility.

Respiratory Monitoring

The primary respiratory parameters that must be monitored in critically ill patients include respiratory rate, tidal volume or minute ventilation, and oxygenation. Routine monitoring of carbon dioxide levels and pH would be desirable, but the technology for monitoring these parameters is not yet developed enough to consider continuous monitoring mandatory. In mechanically ventilated patients, many physiologic functions can be monitored routinely and continuously by the ventilator. This section does not discuss monitoring by the mechanical ventilator (see Chapter 58) but examines devices that might be routinely used to monitor continuously and noninvasively the aforementioned parameters.

RESPIRATORY RATE, TIDAL VOLUME, AND MINUTE VENTILATION. Clinical suspicion of a new respiratory problem in a critically ill patient may lead to further evaluation with arterial blood gases (ABG), a chest radiograph, or other testing. Visual inspection of the patient frequently is inadequate to detect changes in respiratory rate or tidal volume. Physicians, nurses, and hospital staff frequently report inaccurate respiratory rates, possibly because they underestimate the importance of the measurement [125]. Two studies in which physicians and staff were asked to assess tidal volume and minute ventilation indicate that tidal volume is (a) assessed poorly, (b) frequently overestimated, and (c) not reproducible on repeat assessment [126,127]. In another study, ICU staff had a greater than 20% error more than one-third of the time when the recorded respiratory rate was compared with objective tracings [128]. Objective monitoring must be used because clinical evaluation is inaccurate.

Impedance Monitors. Impedance monitors are commonly used to measure respiratory rates and approximate tidal volume in ICUs and home apnea alarms. These devices typically use ECG leads and measure changes in impedance generated by the change in distance between leads as a result of the thoracoabdominal motions of breathing. To obtain a quality signal, leads must be placed at points of maximal change in thoracoabdominal contour, or sophisticated computerized algorithms must be used. Alarms can then be set for a high and low rate or for a percentage drop in the signal that is thought to correlate with a decrease in tidal volume.

In clinical use, impedance monitors suffer confounding problems. They have failed to detect obstructive apnea when it has occurred and falsely detected apnea when it has not [100,129,130]. Although computerized impedance monitors may falsely report bradypnea in up to 17% of patients, they detect tachypnea more accurately [100]. Detection of obstructive apnea by impedance monitors is poor because chest wall motion may persist and be counted as breaths by these monitors as the apneic patient struggles to overcome airway obstruction [129,130]. Tidal volume estimates may be artifactually affected by changes in patient position or patient movement. Impedance monitors offer the advantage of being very inexpensive when ECG is already in use but lack accuracy when precise measurements of tidal volume, change in tidal volume, or bradypnea-apnea are required.

Respiratory Inductive Plethysmography. The most commonly used respiratory inductive plethysmograph (RIP) measures changes in the cross-sectional area of the chest and abdomen that occur with respiration and processes these signals into respiratory rate and tidal volume. Two 3- to 10-cm–wide bands consisting of elastic fabric containing a wire sewn in a zigzag fashion are placed around the patient's upper chest and around the abdomen below the ribs. As the cross-sectional area of the bands changes with respiration, the self-inductance of the coils changes the frequency of attached oscillators. The signals from the oscillator pass through a demodulator, yielding a voltage signal. The voltage signals may be calibrated by numerous methods to within 10% of spirometry or may be internally calibrated so that further measurements reflect a percentage change from baseline. RIP can accurately measure respiratory rate and the percentage change in tidal volume as well as detect obstructive apnea [131–133]. These measurements are more accurate than impedance measurements [130].

In addition to displaying respiratory rate and percentage change in tidal volume, RIP can provide continuous measurement of asynchronous and paradoxical breathing and signal an alarm for predetermined changes in these values. Studies of patients during weaning have demonstrated that asynchronous and paradoxic movements are common during early weaning and may be helpful in predicting respiratory failure [134,135]. However, as a single parameter, an increase in respiratory rate is more predictive of imminent failure to wean [136]. The noninvasive nature of the tidal volume measurement may be extremely helpful in patients in whom direct measurement of expired volume is confounded because of technical problems or leaks (e.g., patients with bronchopleu-

ral fistulas, undergoing ventilation with nasal ventilators, or on nasal constant positive airway pressure). In addition, RIP can display changes in functional residual capacity, which permits rapid assessment of the effect of changing positive end-expiratory pressure (PEEP). Determinations of the presence and estimation of the amount of auto (intrinsic) PEEP can be made by observing the effect of applied (extrinsic) PEEP on functional residual capacity [137].

RIP systems are available with central station configurations designed specifically for ICU use. Routine use of RIP has resulted in decreased ICU length of stay and reduced hospital cost [138]. Compared with inductance methods, RIP is more accurate and offers a variety of other useful measurements but is slightly less convenient and more expensive. It is useful for the careful monitoring of patients with obstructive apnea.

Other Methods. Although respiratory rate can be measured accurately with a pneumotachometer, capnographs, or electromyography, none of these methods has achieved a level of popular usage in the ICU. A pneumotachometer requires complete collection of exhaled gas and, therefore, either intubation or use of a tight-fitting face mask. Because of this inconvenience and difficulties with calibration and maintenance, pneumotachometers are infrequently used routinely in the ICU. Surface electromyography of respiratory muscles can be used to calculate respiratory rate accurately [139] but cannot detect obstructive apnea or provide a measure of tidal volume. Electromyography works well in infants but presents difficulties in adults, especially in obese adults and those with edema. Capnography works exceedingly well as a respiratory rate monitor, does not require intubation or a face mask, and is a useful tool in many circumstances. Capnography is discussed in more detail later. A pneumotachometer can assess tidal volume but suffers from the same limitations as those discussed for respiratory rate.

Measurements of Gas Exchange

PULSE OXIMETRY. Medical professionals poorly estimate oxygen saturation when forced to rely on clinical criteria [140,141]. Oximeters offer a noninvasive method of determining whether oxygen supplementation is needed and, once delivered, whether supplementation is adequate. Cooximeters perform measurements on whole blood obtained from an artery or a vein. They frequently measure absorbance at multiple wavelengths and compute the percentage of oxyhemoglobin, deoxyhemoglobin, methemoglobin, and carboxyhemoglobin (COHB) in total hemoglobin. They are mostly free of the artifacts that limit the accuracy of tissue oximeters and are regarded as the gold standard by which other methods of assessing saturation are measured. Noninvasive tissue oximeters usually measure only the percentage of oxyhemoglobin of total hemoglobin. Early oximeters tended to be bulky and inconvenient, in that they required exposed vessels, heat, or histamine to induce vasodilation, arterial occlusion to render a tissue bloodless for calibration, or multistep calibration procedures [142]. Because pulse oximeters circumvent most of these problems with no significant loss of accuracy, they have supplanted virtually all older types of oximeters in clinical use. Pulse oximeters measure the saturation of hemoglobin in the tissue during the arterial and venous phases of pulsation and mathematically derive arterial saturation. However, up to 97% of physicians and nurses who use pulse oximeters do not understand the fundamental principles of use [143]. This section reviews the fundamental technology involved in pulse oximetry, practical problems that limit its use, and indications for the use of oximeters in critically ill patients.

More than 20 manufacturers now market pulse oximeters. Because of the variety of manufacturers, the numerous algorithms used, and the diverse patient populations studied, it is difficult to generalize the studies performed with one particular instrument, with its specific version of software, in one defined group of patients to critically ill patients in general. The reader should always check with an oximeter's manufacturer before generalizing the following discussion to his or her oximeter and patient population.

Technology. Oximeters distinguish between oxyhemoglobin and reduced hemoglobin on the basis of their different absorption of light. Oxyhemoglobin absorbs much less red (±660 nm) and slightly more infrared (±910 to 940 nm) light than reduced hemoglobin. Oxygen saturation thereby determines the ratio of red to infrared absorption. When red and infrared light are directed from light-emitting diodes (LEDs) to a photodetector across a pulsatile tissue bed, the absorption of each wavelength by the tissue bed varies cyclically with pulse. During diastole, absorption is due to the nonvascular tissue components (e.g., bone, muscle, and interstitium) and venous blood. During systole, absorption is determined by all of these components and arterialized blood. The pulse amplitude accounts for only 1% to 5% of the total signal [144]. Thus, the difference between absorption in systole and diastole is in theory due to the presence of arterialized blood. The change in ratio of absorption between systole and diastole can then be used to calculate an estimate of arterial oxygen saturation. Absorption is typically measured hundreds of times per second. Signals usually are averaged over several seconds and then displayed digitally. The algorithm used for each oximeter is determined by calibration on human volunteers. Most oximeters under ideal circumstances measure the saturation indicated by the pulse oximeter (SpO_2) to within 2% of arterial oxygen saturation [145].

Oximeters are typically equipped to display the measured SpO_2 and pulse and to sound alarms for high and low values of each. Most use software algorithms to send warning messages or stop display analysis when signal quality deteriorates.

Problems Encountered in Use. Any process that affects or interferes with the absorption of light between the LEDs and photodetector or alters the quality of pulsatile flow has the potential for artifactually distorting the oximeter's calculations. Pulse oximeters should be able to obtain valid readings in 98% of patients in an operating room or postanesthesia care unit [146]. Up to 9% of patients undergoing surgery may have a 10-minute or longer interruption in monitoring because of technical difficulty with oximetric measurement [147]. Table 26-1 lists the problems that must be considered in clinical use.

CALIBRATION. Because early attempts to calibrate pulse oximeters in accord with the principles of Beer's law of absorbance proved unsuccessful, manufacturers now use normal volunteers to derive calibration algorithms. This results in three problems. First, manufacturers use different calibration algorithms, which results in a difference in SpO_2 of up to 2.7% between different manufacturers' oximeters used to measure the same patient [148]. Secondly, manufacturers define SpO_2 differently for calibration purposes. Calibration may or may not account for the interference of small amounts of dyshemoglobinemia (e.g., methemoglobin or COHB). For example, if an oximeter is calibrated on the basis of a study of nonsmokers with a 2% COHB level, the measured SpO_2 percentage would differ depending on whether the value used to calibrate SpO_2 included or excluded the 2% COHB [148]. Thirdly, it is difficult, for ethical reasons, for manufacturers to obtain an adequate number of validated readings in people with an SpO_2 of less

Table 26-1. Conditions Adversely Affecting Accuracy of Oximetry

May result in poor signal detection	
Probe malposition	No pulse
Motion	Vasoconstriction
Hypothermia	Hypotension

Falsely lowers SpO_2	Falsely raises SpO_2
Nail polish	Elevated carboxyhemoglobin
Dark skin	Elevated methemoglobin
Ambient light	Ambient light
Elevated serum lipids	Hypothermia
Methylene blue	
Indigo carmine	
Indocyanine green	

SpO_2, saturation indicated by the pulse oximeter.

than 70% to develop accurate calibration algorithms in this saturation range. Most oximeters give less precise readings and underestimate saturation in this saturation range [149]. Until better calibration algorithms are available, oximeters should be considered unreliable when SpO_2 is less than 70%. The accuracy of a unit can be checked by systematically comparing the oximetry values of the oximeter with simultaneous cooximeter values measured from arterial blood. An *in vitro* system to evaluate oximeter performance has been designed but is too complex for routine validation of individual oximetry devices [150].

SITE OF MEASUREMENT. Accurate measurements can be obtained from fingers, forehead, and earlobes [151,152]. The response time from a change in the partial pressure of arterial oxygen (PaO_2) to a change in displayed SpO_2 is delayed in finger and toe probes compared with ear, cheek, or glossal probes [151,153]. Forehead edema, wetness, and head motion have resulted in inaccurate forehead SpO_2 values [154]. Motion and perfusion artifacts are the greatest problems with digital measurements. Glossal pulse oximetry has been useful in some patients in whom no other measuring site was available [155], and specific glossal probes may be developed soon. The earlobe is believed to be the site least affected by vasoconstriction artifact [156]. Sensor positioning is crucial to obtaining accurate results [157].

FINGERNAILS. Long fingernails may prevent correct positioning of the finger pulp over the LEDs used in inflexible probes and therefore produce inaccurate SpO_2 readings without affecting the pulse rate [158]. Synthetic nails have produced erroneous results [145]. Nail polish of several colors has been shown to lower SpO_2 falsely [159]. Not surprisingly, those colors with the greatest difference in absorption between 660 and 940 nm produced the greatest artifact. Although thickness of applied polish may also be a factor, adhesive tape, even when placed over both sides of a finger, did not affect measured SpO_2 [160].

SKIN COLOR. The effect of skin color on SpO_2 was assessed in a study of 655 patients [161]. Although patients with the darkest skin had significantly less accurate SpO_2 readings, the mean difference in SpO_2 between subjects with light skin and those with the darkest skin compared with control cooximeter readings was only 0.5%, a clinically insignificant difference. Pulse oximeters, however, encountered major difficulties in obtaining readings in darker-skinned patients; 18% of patients with darker skin triggered warning lights or messages versus 1% of lighter-skinned patients. Thus, dark skin may prevent a measurement from being obtained, but when the oximeter reports an error-free value, the value is accurate enough for clinical use [162].

AMBIENT LIGHT. Ambient light that affects absorption in the 660- or 910-nm wavelengths, or both, may affect calculations of saturation and pulse. Xenon arc surgical lights [163], fluorescent lights [164], and fiberoptic light sources [165] have caused falsely elevated saturation but typically obvious dramatic elevations in pulse. An infrared heating lamp [166] has produced falsely low saturations and a falsely low pulse, and a standard 15-watt fluorescent bulb resulted in falsely low saturation without a change in heart rate [167]. Interference from surrounding lights should be suspected by the presence of pulse values discordant from the palpable pulse or ECG or changes in the pulse-saturation display when the probe is transiently shielded from ambient light with an opaque object. Most manufacturers have now modified their probes to minimize this problem.

HYPERBILIRUBINEMIA. Bilirubin's absorbance peak is maximal in the 450-nm range but has tails extending in either direction [168]. Bilirubin, therefore, does not typically affect pulse oximeters that use the standard two-diode system [168,169]. However, it may greatly interfere with the measurement of saturation by cooximeters. Cooximeters typically use four to six wavelengths of light and measure absolute absorbance to quantify the percentage of all major hemoglobin variants. Serum bilirubin values as high as 44 mg per dL had no effect on the accuracy of pulse oximeters but led to falsely low levels of oxyhemoglobin measured by cooximetry [168].

DYSHEMOGLOBINEMIAS. Conventional two-diode oximeters cannot detect the presence of fetal hemoglobin, methemoglobin, or COHB. Fetal hemoglobin may confound readings in neonates but is rarely a problem in adults. Because methemoglobin absorbs more light at 660 nm than at 990 nm, oxygen saturation is falsely elevated whenever methemoglobin levels exceed 6% [170]. Moreover, higher levels of methemoglobin tend to bias the reading toward 85% to 90% [171]. COHB is typically read by a two-diode oximeter as 90% oxyhemoglobin and 10% reduced hemoglobin [172], resulting in false elevations of SpO_2. Because COHB may be 10% in smokers, pulse oximetry may fail to detect significant desaturation in this group of patients. Oxygen saturation in smokers when measured by cooximetry was on average 5% lower than pulse oximetric values [173]. Hemolytic anemia may also elevate COHB up to 2.6% [174]. Because other etiologies of COHB are rare in the hospital and the half-life of COHB is short, this problem is unusual in the critical care setting except in new admissions or patients with active hemolysis. Emergency physicians must be aware of the gap between pulse oximetric saturation and arterial saturation on patients with smoke inhalation or carbon monoxide overdose [175].

ANEMIA. Few clear data are available on the effect of anemia on pulse oximetry. In dogs, there was no significant degradation in accuracy until the hematocrit was less than 10% [176]. In one study of humans who had hemorrhagic anemia, there appeared to be little effect on pulse oximetry accuracy [177].

LIPIDS. Patients with elevated chylomicrons and those receiving lipid infusions may have falsely low SpO_2 because of interference in absorption by the lipid [178].

HYPOTHERMIA. Good-quality signals may be unobtainable in 10% of hypothermic (less than 35°C) patients [179], and signal detection fails at temperatures less than 26.5°C [180]. The decrease in signal quality probably results from hypothermia-induced vasoconstriction. When good-quality signals could be obtained, SpO_2 differed from cooximetry-measured saturation by only 0.6% [179] in one series and tended to be falsely elevated by 0.9% to 3.0% SpO_2 in another [180].

INTRAVASCULAR DYES. Methylene blue, used to treat methemoglobinemia, has a maximal absorption at 670 nm and therefore falsely lowers measured SpO_2 [181]. Indocyanine green and indigo carmine also lower SpO_2, but the changes are minor and brief [182]. Fluorescein has no effect on SpO_2 [182]. Because of the rapid vascular redistribution of injected dyes, the effect on oximetry readings typically lasts only 5 to 10 minutes [183]. Patent V dye, which is used to visualize lymphatics, confounds pulse oximetry [184].

MOTION ARTIFACT. Shivering and other motions that change the distance from diode to receiver may result in artifact. Oximeters account for motion by different algorithms. Some oximeters display a warning sign, others stop reporting data, and others display erroneous values. The display of a pulsatile waveform rather than a signal strength bar helps to indicate that artifact has distorted the pulse signal and lowered the quality of the subsequent SpO_2 analysis [185].

HYPOPERFUSION. During a blood pressure cuff inflation model of hypoperfusion, most oximeters remained within 2% of control readings [186]. Increasing systemic vascular resistance and decreasing cardiac output can also increase the difficulty in obtaining a good-quality signal. In one series, the lowest cardiac index and highest systemic vascular resistance at which a signal could be detected were 2.4 L per minute per m² and 2,930 dynes second per cm⁵ per m², respectively [180]. Warming the finger [187], sympathetic digital block [188], or applying a vasodilating cream [180] tended to extend the range of signal detection in individual patients. The oximeter's ability to display a waveform and detect perfusion degradation of the signal were crucial in determining when the readings obtained were valid [186].

PULSATILE VENOUS FLOW. In physiologic states in which venous and capillary flows become pulsatile, the systolic pulse detected by the oximeter may no longer reflect the presence only of arterial well-saturated blood. In patients with severe tricuspid regurgitation or hyperperfusion, the measured saturation may be falsely low [189,190].

Indications. Unsuspected hypoxemia is common in critically ill patients. Sixteen percent of patients not receiving supplemental oxygen in the recovery room have saturations of less than 90% [191]. In 35% of patients, saturations of less than 90% develop during transfer out of the operating room [192]. Because of the high frequency of hypoxemia in critically ill patients, the frequent need to adjust oxygen flow to avoid toxicity and insufficiency, and the unreliability of visual inspection to detect mild desaturation, oximeters should be used in most critically ill patients for routine, continuous monitoring. In one study that randomized more than 20,000 operative and perioperative patients to continuous or no oximetric monitoring, the authors concluded that oximetry permitted detection of more hypoxemic events, prompted increases in the fraction of oxygen in inspired air, and significantly decreased the incidence of myocardial ischemia but did not significantly decrease mortality or complication rates [193]. In the ICU, continuous oximetric monitoring may spare patients' oxygen toxicity by facilitating the rapid tapering of fraction of oxygen in inspired air [194].

Oximeters have been used in the ICU for reasons other than continuous monitoring. They can be useful in locating an artery that is difficult to palpate. When the oximeter is placed distal to the artery, the signal strength decreases, and the saturation may decrease when the more proximal vessel is compressed [195,196]. Oximeters may be helpful during difficult intubations. Once desaturation occurs, attempts to intubate should be postponed until manual ventilation restores saturation. Oximetry is not helpful in promptly detecting inadvertent esophageal intubation, in that desaturation may lag behind apnea by more than 30 seconds in this setting [197]. Oximeters can be useful in detecting systolic blood pressure. In one study in which the blood pressure cuff was inflated proximal to the oximeter, the point at which the pulse signal was lost was within 2 mm Hg of Doppler measurements of systolic pressure [198]. In trauma patients, an abrupt, sustained 10% drop in saturation in the presence of a stable chest radiograph and static compliance was highly predictive of pulmonary embolism [199]. Oximetry has had low sensitivity when used to evaluate potential compartment syndromes [200].

TRANSCUTANEOUS OXYGEN AND CARBON DIOXIDE MEASUREMENT.

Transcutaneous systems measure partial pressures of oxygen ($PtcO_2$) and carbon dioxide ($PtccO_2$) that diffuse out of the vasculature and through the skin. This section examines the technology most commonly used to measure transcutaneous partial pressures, the differences between the values obtained by cutaneous measurement and arterial measurement, and the indications for use of transcutaneous gas measurement.

Technology. The technology used to obtain transcutaneous gas measurements varies slightly between manufacturers but in general uses similar techniques. Typically, a unit less than 1 inch in diameter is attached to the skin with an adhesive. An electrode is used to heat the skin, which promotes arterialization of capillaries and improves diffusion of gases through the skin's lipid layers. A temperature sensor measures skin temperature at the skin surface and adjusts the heater to provide a constant temperature. In adults, temperatures of 43.5° to 44.5°C produce the most satisfactory results. Some systems do not rely on heating to improve diffusion of gas. Similar results may be produced by stripping off the stratum corneum with adhesive tape or measuring from a site with a thinner layer of skin, such as the conjunctiva.

Oxygen and carbon dioxide diffuse out of the capillaries into the interstitium and through the skin to measuring electrodes. The diffusing distance from capillary to sensor may be as small as 0.3 mm. Precalibrated Clarke- and Severinghaus-type electrodes, similar to those used in blood gas machines, then measure the partial pressure of oxygen and carbon dioxide. The temperature at which partial pressure is measured and reported can be adjusted on some units. These signals are then electronically averaged and converted into a continuous digital display. Alarms can be set for high and low values of both gases measured. Many units also display trend signals to indicate whether and in which direction a change occurs.

Because units use electrodes for partial pressure measurement, problems with calibration and electrode drift during prolonged monitoring can clearly alter measurements. Drift may alter readings by up to 12% over a 2-hour period [201].

Differences between Arterial and Transcutaneous Measurements. Numerous factors may cause $PtcO_2$ and $PtccO_2$ to differ from PaO_2 and partial pressures of arterial carbon dioxide ($PaCO_2$). Most differences can be traced to factors involving probe temperature, blood flow, local metabolism, or skin thickness.

The increased temperature of the heating probe shifts the oxygen dissociation curve to the right and promotes offloading of bound oxygen, which increases the PO_2 in the surrounding interstitium. Different temperature settings alter this effect to varying degrees and may directly influence the final value measured at the skin surface. Heat-induced artifacts may be avoided by using a measurement site that does not require heating, such as the conjunctiva [202].

Blood flow is a critical determinant of the value measured at the skin. If there is no flow to the region below the sensor, there is no delivery of oxygen and no elimination of carbon dioxide by the vasculature, resulting in lower PO_2 and higher PCO_2 than in an adjacent artery. Some units provide an index of cutaneous blood flow by displaying changes in the amount of heat necessary to keep the probe at a constant temperature. As perfusion increases, heat is carried away from the probe faster and more heat must be applied to maintain a constant temperature. As perfusion decreases, the opposite occurs. Thus, a decrease in probe heat output may reflect a fall in perfusion.

Local metabolism alters values from arterial levels, in that gases diffusing from the capillaries may be consumed or added to by local metabolism. Local oxygen consumption by the tissues between the capillary and skin surface can reduce

$PtcO_2$ by 20 to 40 mm Hg during hypoperfused states [203]. The $PtccO_2$ in hypoxemic or underperfused regions may also be dramatically increased, in some cases more than 30 mm Hg higher than in arterial samples.

Thick or edematous skin provides a diffusion barrier that amplifies all of the aforementioned effects. The longer the distance the gases must diffuse to be measured, the more important are the effects of temperature, perfusion, and local metabolism. This appears to be the fundamental reason why transcutaneous measurements are usually more accurate in neonates than in adults. Edema, burns, abrasions, or scleroderma would all alter transcutaneous values.

Clinical Correlations and Utility. In healthy adults, $PtcO_2$ and $PtccO_2$ accurately reflect PaO_2 and $PaCO_2$ [201,204]. The measured transcutaneous values of oxygen and carbon dioxide are typically 10 mm Hg lower [205] and 5 to 23 mm Hg higher [206,207] than arterial values, respectively. Fever and tissue edema alter the correlation between arterial and transcutaneous values. Systemic hypoperfusion due to low cardiac output, regional hypoperfusion due to sepsis or shock, and local hypoperfusion due to cutaneous vasoconstriction caused by medication or cold produce discrepancies. In these cases, transcutaneous measurements cease to reflect arterial values and better track oxygen delivery and tissue metabolism [203,208].

Several studies have demonstrated the value of transcutaneous oxygen measurements as indices of perfusion or oxygen delivery. When PaO_2 remains constant, a decrease in $PtcO_2$ is probably due to changes in perfusion. Changes in local perfusion and metabolism may cause $PtcO_2$ values to fall to zero and $PtccO_2$ values to climb to more than 30 mm Hg above arterial values [206]. When the cardiac index is less than 2 L per minute, $PtcO_2$ correlates best with PaO_2 [203]. In hemorrhagic shock, the ratio of $PtcO_2$ to PaO_2 decreases, even though PaO_2 may remain normal [209,210]. Values are more sensitive to changes in flow than in pressure, but flow is always compromised at a blood pressure less than 50 mm Hg. Deterioration of $PtcO_2$ values may occur up to 4 minutes before a decrease in blood pressure [210]. Improvements in flow were detected within 1 minute by a rise in $PtcO_2$ [203]. Because the measurements are very sensitive to changes in flow, they can be useful in predicting or warning of imminent change before a blood pressure response is seen. In perioperative patients, declines in the $PtcO_2$ to PaO_2 ratio to less than 0.77 were predictive of hemodynamic collapse within the next 50 minutes [211]. In cardiogenic shock, $PtcO_2$ values of 25 mm Hg or less have been predictive of death [203].

In other circumstances, transcutaneous measurements may be helpful in assessing a complex interaction between perfusion and oxygenation factors. During the titration of PEEP in critically ill patients, $PtcO_2$ correlates well and directly with PaO_2 and pulmonary artery PO_2 and correlates inversely with a shunt fraction [207]. In this setting, in which the clinical goal is to optimize oxygen delivery, the single noninvasive measurement of $PtcO_2$ might replace more invasive blood measurements.

Measurements of PCO_2 are affected in virtually all situations that alter $PtcO_2$. In most cases, the variations have been less sensitive predictors of changes in perfusion [203]. Studies in hemodynamically stable patients have shown that $PtccO_2$ reliably tracks arterial $PaCO_2$ values in patients who are being weaned from mechanical ventilation. $PtccO_2$ remained within 5.2 ± 1.5 mm Hg of $PaCO_2$ [206]. In cases in which $PaCO_2$ remains near constant, changes in $PtcO_2$ would be expected to track changes in minute ventilation or dead space.

Transcutaneous equipment also requires meticulous attention to provide good-quality readings. Probes must be firmly attached to the skin, or leaks from the surrounding atmosphere lower $PtccO_2$ and alter $PtcO_2$ values. Adhesion is a problem in diaphoretic patients. Patient motion may produce tension on the cable that connects the sensor to the processing unit, causing leaks or disconnection. Probe sites must be changed at least every 4 to 6 hours to prevent burns. Units must be recalibrated whenever the probe temperature is changed and every 4 to 6 hours to prevent artifact from electrode drift. Many units take 15 to 60 minutes to warm the skin and establish stable readings. These factors can combine in many patients to make transcutaneous measurements very inconvenient.

Indications. Transcutaneous monitors have little role in the ICU as simple tools to replace other means of measuring arterial gas. Their application in practice is not complex but is far from simple. They predictably reflect arterial values only in hemodynamically stable patients, who are least likely to demand intensive care or to benefit from ICU monitoring. As monitors of trends in P_{CO_2} and P_{O_2}, they can be regarded as effective only in the sense that they typically do not produce false-negative alarms—that is, if the arterial values change, the transcutaneous values reflect the change. So many other factors, such as changes in tissue edema and perfusion, may result in alterations in transcutaneous trends that the supervising staff can initially determine only that *something* has changed. An accurate interpretation of the clinical event usually requires reassessment of either cardiac status or arterial gases.

Therefore, transcutaneous monitors are inadequate cardiac monitors and inadequate pulmonary monitors but are good cardiopulmonary monitors. Transcutaneous monitoring is most useful in patients in whom changes in either perfusion or gas exchange are likely, but not both. When perfusion is stable, values reflect gas exchange. When gas exchange is stable, values reflect perfusion. When both are unstable, the results cannot be interpreted without additional information. In the future, transcutaneous measurements could be combined with noninvasive monitors of cardiac output or with results from indwelling arterial monitors of blood gases to provide continuous analysis of perfusion, gas exchange, and local metabolism. Until such time, this complex assessment must be provided by the supervising staff.

CAPNOGRAPHY. Capnography involves the measurement and display of expired P_{CO_2} concentrations. This section reviews the technology, the sources of difference between end-tidal P_{CO_2} and Pa_{CO_2}, and the indications for capnography in the ICU.

Technology. Expired P_{CO_2} concentration is usually determined by infrared absorbance or mass spectrometry. The infrared technique relies on the fact that carbon dioxide has a characteristic absorbance of infrared light, with maximal absorbance near a wavelength of 4.28 mm. A heated wire with optical filters is used to generate an infrared light of appropriate wavelength. When carbon dioxide passes between a focused beam of light and a semiconductor photodetector, an electronic signal can be generated that, when calibrated, accurately reflects the P_{CO_2} of the tested gas. A mass spectrometer bombards gas with an electron stream. The ion fragments that are generated can be deflected by a magnetic field to detector plates located in precise positions to detect ions that are characteristic of the molecule being evaluated. The current generated at the detector can be calibrated to be proportional to the partial pressure of the molecule being evaluated.

The two techniques have different strengths. Mass spectrometers can detect the partial pressures of several gases simultaneously and can monitor several patients at once. Infrared techniques measure only P_{CO_2} and are usually used on only one patient at a time. The calibration and analysis time required for mass spectrometry is significantly longer than with infrared techniques. Infrared systems respond to changes in approxi-

mately 100 milliseconds, whereas mass spectrometers take 45 seconds to 5 minutes to respond [212]. Although costs vary widely, mass spectrometers are in general far more expensive and are most frequently purchased to be the central component of a carbon dioxide monitoring system. In the operating room, mass spectrometry has the advantage of being able to measure the partial pressure of anesthetic gases, and the need for a technical specialist to oversee its operation can be more easily justified. For these reasons, mass spectrometry has achieved much more popularity in the operating room than in the ICU.

Gases can be sampled by mainstream or sidestream techniques. Mainstream sampling involves placing the capnometer directly in line in the patient's respiratory circuit. All air leaving the patient passes through the capnometer. The sidestream sampling techniques pump 100 to 300 mL expired air per minute through thin tubing to an adjacent analyzing chamber. The mainstream method can be used only on patients who are intubated or wearing a tight-fitting face or nose mask. Because of the size of mass spectrometer equipment, mainstream sampling is applicable only to infrared analysis. Mainstream sampling offers the advantage of almost instantaneous analysis of sampled air, but it increases the patient's dead space and adds uncomfortable weight to the endotracheal tube. Sidestream sampling removes air from the expiratory circuit, confounding measurement of tidal volume. The aspirating flow rate and tubing length significantly affect the ability to detect a rapid rise in carbon dioxide and the delay between physiologic change in the patient and display of the change at the monitor [213]. When the delay exceeds the respiratory cycle time, the generated data are inaccurate [213]. The sidestream sampling line is also prone to clogging with pulmonary secretions, saliva, or water condensation. Clogging affects accuracy and delay time. Sidestream sampling can detect cyclic changes in carbon dioxide concentration easily in the unintubated patient if the sampling tube is located near the mouth or nose. Because of all of these issues, accurate sidestream sampling requires short tubes and constant attention to the possibility of clogged sample lines.

Differences between End-Tidal and Arterial Carbon Dioxide. The P_{CO_2} in exhaled air measured at the mouth changes in a characteristic pattern in normal people that reflects the underlying physiologic changes in the lung (Fig. 26-1). During inspiration, the P_{CO_2} is negligible, but it rises abruptly with expiration. The rate of rise reflects the washout of dead-space air with air from perfused alveoli. A plateau concentration is reached after dead-space air has been exhaled. The plateau level is determined by the mean alveolar P_{CO_2}, which is in equilibrium with pulmonary artery P_{CO_2} (Pv_{CO_2}). The end alveolar plateau level of P_{CO_2} measured during the last 20% of exhalation is the end-tidal P_{CO_2} [183]. In normal people at rest, the difference between end-tidal P_{CO_2} and Pa_{CO_2} is ±1.5 mm Hg. A difference exists because of the presence of dead space (i.e., ventilation without perfusion) and a physiologic shunt (i.e., perfusion without ventilation). Any change in anatomic dead space or pulmonary perfusion alters ventilation-perfusion mismatch so as to increase the difference between end-tidal and arterial P_{CO_2} values. As dead space increases, the end-tidal P_{CO_2} represents more the P_{CO_2} of nonperfused alveoli, thereby diverging from the Pa_{CO_2} value. As perfusion decreases, fewer alveoli are perfused, creating a similar effect.

In most equipment, the end-tidal P_{CO_2} level is determined by a computerized algorithm. Because algorithms are imperfect, a waveform display is considered essential for accurate interpretation of derived values [214]. In slowly breathing patients, cardiac pulsations may cause the intermittent exhalation of small amounts of air at the end of the lungs' expiratory effort. This results in oscillations that may obscure the plateau phase. An irregular respiratory pattern or large increases in

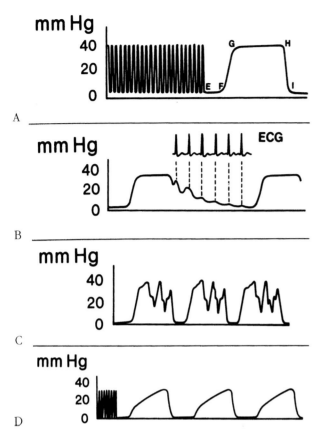

mm Hg
40
20
0

A

mm Hg
40
20
0
ECG

B

mm Hg
40
20
0

C

mm Hg
40
20
0

D

Fig. 26-1. Normal and abnormal capnograms. In the normal capnogram **(A)**, on the right of the trace, the paper speed has been increased. The *EF* segment is inspiration. The *FG* segment reflects the start of expiration with exhalation of dead space gas. The *GH* segment is the alveolar plateau. End-tidal values are taken at point *H*. *HI* is the beginning of inspiration. In the abnormal capnograms, the alveolar plateau is distorted and the end-tidal point cannot be clearly determined because of cardiac oscillations **(B)**, erratic breathing **(C)**, and obstructive airway disease **(D)**. ECG, electrocardiogram. (Modified from Stock MC: Noninvasive carbon dioxide monitoring. *Crit Care Clin* 4:511, 1988.)

dead space can also distort the plateau phase. Visual inspection of traces can detect situations in which algorithms are prone to produce errors [212].

Indications. In the ICU, capnography is most useful for determining the presence or absence of respiration. Such determinations do not require that end-tidal PCO_2 be measured accurately, only that changes be detected reliably. Apnea can be defined as an absence of variation in PCO_2 levels. Alarms for apnea and tachypnea can be set and relied on. However, capnography cannot discriminate between obstructive and central apnea because it cannot reliably detect muscular efforts of the thorax or abdomen.

For similar reasons, capnography is a useful adjunct for detecting unintentional extubation, malposition of the endotracheal tube, or absence of perfusion. Cyclic variation of end-tidal PCO_2 is absent in esophageal intubation or disconnection from the ventilator [215]. Pharyngeal intubation with adequate ventilation may, however, produce a normal capnogram. Capnography can demonstrate the return of circulation after cardiopulmonary arrest or bypass [216].

Because of changes in dead space and perfusion, end-tidal PCO_2 measurements are unreliable indicators of $PaCO_2$ in critically ill patients. In one study of anesthetized, stable, generally healthy adults, $PaCO_2$ could not be reliably determined from end-

tidal values [217]. In patients undergoing weaning from mechanical ventilation, end-tidal PCO_2 was also shown to have no predictable relationship to $PaCO_2$ [218,219]. Although end-tidal and arterial values correlated well ($r = 0.78$) and rarely differed by more than 4 mm Hg, changes in end-tidal PCO_2 correlated poorly with changes in arterial PCO_2 ($r^2 = 0.58$). Because of changes in dead space and perfusion, arterial and end-tidal measurements at times moved unpredictably in opposite directions.

If arterial PCO_2 is followed, the difference between end-tidal PCO_2 and $PaCO_2$ can be used as an index of the severity of ventilation-perfusion mismatch. The alveolar-arterial gradient of oxygen is more easily calculated and in most clinical settings provides similar information. Although theoretically attractive, use of end-tidal carbon dioxide measurements to evaluate changes in ventilation-perfusion mismatch have failed to yield clinical benefits [220].

Capnography has been helpful in the operating room in detecting air and pulmonary embolism as well as malignant hyperthermia [212,216]. In these situations, the capnograph does not provide a diagnosis; it records a change that, if limits are exceeded, signals an alarm. The responsibility for accurately interpreting the subtleties of changes in the capnogram remains the task of an experienced physician.

Conclusions. Capnography is of very limited use in the critically ill patient. It cannot reliably replace $PaCO_2$ monitoring. Although it monitors respiratory rate accurately, it is far more expensive and inconvenient than other types of respiratory rate monitors. Capnography is better suited to the operating room, where its value is increased because of its ability to help detect endotracheal tube malposition, air embolism, pulmonary embolism, and malignant hyperthermia and the immediate availability of a highly skilled anesthesiologist to interpret subtle changes in the capnogram.

CONTINUOUS INVASIVE INTRAARTERIAL OXYGEN AND CARBON DIOXIDE MONITORS. Devices specifically designed to measure intraarterial pH, PCO_2, and PO_2 continuously are now available [221]. Arterial blood may be continuously monitored by the placement of a fiberoptic sensor catheter into a 20-gauge radial artery catheter or intermittently monitored by creating a flow of blood from a radial artery catheter past an external fiberoptic sensor. Sensors are designed so that chemical indicators responsive to pH, PCO_2, and PO_2 are exposed to blood at the distal tip of the sensor. Light in the fiber may be reflected, absorbed, or otherwise altered when the indicator reacts with the analyte of interest. The change in the light is measured at the other end of the fiber and converted by a microprocessor into a digital readout. Systems that use optical detection of altered light have been named *optodes*. Fluorescence and transmission optodes are the primary technologies in use. Transmission optodes carry light to the indicator through one fiber path and measure attenuation of the light by the indicator in another fiber path. Fluorescence optodes have a dye at the tip of the sensor, which increases or decreases fluorescence as the concentration of the analyte changes in the dye. These systems require an *in vitro* calibration against known standards before use and intermittent *in vivo* calibration against arterial samples processed on a traditional ABG analyzer.

Initial studies have shown such monitoring systems to be safe, reliable, and accurate [222,223]. The optode catheters have a tremendous potential to improve quality of care by more rapidly and reliably detecting adverse events than transcutaneous, capnographic, or oximetric monitors. When coupled with these other monitors or with intramucosal monitors, they should be able to enhance our knowledge of regional organ perfusion and lung ventilation. In addition, changes in these parameters could be measured quickly in response to a therapeutic intervention. The technology has not been available long enough to assess its impact on clinical outcome or any measure of cost effectiveness. Further studies are needed to evaluate the clinical impact of these devices before they can be recommended for routine use in the ICU.

Gastric Intramucosal pH Monitoring

pHi monitoring is used to monitor trends in tissue pH in response to changes in local oxygen delivery and metabolism. The trends can be used to identify impending distress and predict survival. The technique measures P_{CO_2} and pH in fluid in a gas-permeable balloon placed in the lumen of a viscus. The pH and P_{CO_2} of the adjacent mucosa equilibrate with the fluid. The pH and P_{CO_2} of the fluid can be measured by withdrawing it from the balloon and analyzing it with a blood gas machine. Although several sites can be used to monitor intramucosal values, the stomach is most frequently monitored in the ICU setting.

BACKGROUND AND THEORY. Most authors define *shock* as a state of inadequate perfusion that leads to diffuse cellular hypoxia and organ dysfunction. Many parameters have been considered in an attempt to detect early changes in tissue oxygenation, including arterial oxygen saturation, pH, and serum lactate levels; subcutaneous and transcutaneous P_{O_2}; arterial blood pressure; cardiac output; urine output; and mixed venous oxyhemoglobin saturation. None of these can accurately and noninvasively predict the development of shock (or other common complications) in a broad range of ICU patients.

Anaerobic metabolism causes acidosis because the hydrolysis of adenosine triphosphate produces protons that cannot be used up by simultaneous oxidative phosphorylation of adenosine 5-diphosphate to adenosine triphosphate. The presence of these protons drives the carbonic anhydrase reaction to produce more carbon dioxide, which subsequently diffuses into and develops an equilibrium with any adjacent intraluminal fluid. Thus, the measurement of an intraluminal P_{CO_2} and the capillary HCO_3^- (estimated as equivalent to the arterial HCO_3^-) allows calculation of the pHi by the modified Henderson-Hasselbalch equation:

$$pH = pK - \log (HCO_3^-)/(f \times Pa_{CO_2})$$

where f is a correction factor used to account for differing periods of measurement.

Intramucosal acidosis is therefore a marker of local hypoperfusion. Several factors other than acidosis may alter cellular metabolism and intramucosal values: (a) loss of adenine nucleotides, (b) formation of oxygen free radicals, (c) increases in intracellular calcium, (d) degradation of membrane phospholipids, and (e) mechanical alterations due to cellular edema [224]. However, an accurate, noninvasive way of measuring tissue acidosis could be beneficial if it allows detection of hypoperfusion of vital organs before systemic signs can be detected.

TECHNICAL CONSIDERATIONS

Procedure. The technique of pHi monitoring has evolved steadily since the mid-1960s. Measurement of pHi in the gallbladder and urinary bladder was initially described by Bergofsky [225]. Subsequently, it was shown that the pHi of the small intestine could also be determined [226]. Early pHi monitors consisted of glass or wire electrodes that were surgically implanted in the wall of the organ being studied. These devices

were limited to research applications because an operation was required to place them and their presence in the mucosa of the organ causing tissue damage, therefore altering the conditions being measured. This prompted investigators to search for a less invasive, equally accurate way to obtain this measurement.

In 1973, an implantable catheter made of silicone impregnated with silver was described [227]. This material is extremely permeable to oxygen and carbon dioxide and allowed rapid equilibration between the tensions of these gases in the tissues and the saline that filled the catheter. Because this catheter, too, required surgical implantation and caused injury to the tissue surrounding it, it was limited to research applications. However, it was confirmed that the gases in tissue equilibrate rapidly with saline in proximity to it; it was subsequently confirmed that this principle would hold for the fluid in the lumen of a hollow viscus [228]. The current gastrointestinal tonometry catheter consists of a fluid-filled silicone balloon attached near the end of a nasogastric or sigmoid tube. Before insertion, the balloon is repeatedly infused with fluid until all air is eliminated. The upper gastrointestinal catheter is inserted with standard technique for nasogastric tube placement, and placement is confirmed radiographically. The stopcock is flushed with fluid to eliminate any trapped air, the balloon is filled to the manufacturer's specifications with fluid, and the tonometer lumen is closed to the outside environment. The fluid is allowed to equilibrate with the fluid in the lumen of the organ being monitored. It is believed that the fluid in the balloon requires approximately 90 minutes to equilibrate with the fluid in the lumen, although mathematical formulas are available to correct the values obtained with 30 to 90 minutes of equilibration [229]. After adequate time for equilibration, the dead space (usually 1.0 mL) is aspirated and discarded, and the fluid in the balloon is completely aspirated under anaerobic conditions. The tonometer lumen is closed until a decision is made to refill it for subsequent measurement. An ABG sample is taken simultaneously, and both samples are sent for analysis. The P_{CO_2} of the tonometer sample and the HCO_3^- of the arterial blood are used in the modified Henderson-Hasselbalch equation to calculate pHi.

Sites of Measurement. As already described, original descriptions of viscus tonometry used the gallbladder and urinary bladder as primary sites of monitoring [225]. Tonometry of the gastrointestinal tract was described soon thereafter and is by far the preferred site for monitoring tissue metabolism. This site is preferred because the intestine is easily accessible and can be cannulated from above or below, is sensitive to decreases in perfusion, and may be involved in initiating sepsis. The intestinal mucosa is thought to be affected early during circulatory insufficiency because blood is shunted away from it to preserve the function of the brain and heart. Ironically, because of the unique countercurrent microcirculation in the walls of the intestine, it may be particularly vulnerable to reductions in blood flow and may demonstrate conversion to anaerobic metabolism and tissue acidosis before other tissues. Finally, many have postulated that the intestine has a role in propagation of sepsis. Ischemia of the intestinal mucosa may damage the mucosal barrier and allow bacteria and toxins from the lumen to enter the bloodstream and exacerbate an early shock state.

Several sites in the gastrointestinal tract can serve as sites for pHi monitoring. The most easily accessible is the stomach. In many cases, the patient requires nasogastric tube placement independent of the placement of the tonometer, and therefore no additional procedures are necessary. Tubes that serve for nasogastric drainage as well as tonometry are commercially available. In animals, gastric pHi moves in parallel with changes in small intestinal and sigmoid pHi, although both alternative sites appear more sensitive to changes in intravascular volume and oxygen delivery induced by experimental bleeding [230]. Gastric pHi has been shown to have significant correlations with important measures of disease, although measurement in the small bowel or sigmoid may be more effective in specific situations.

INDICATIONS FOR USE. In general, the goals of monitoring in the ICU are to (a) measure key indices of underlying disease, (b) aid with diagnosis, (c) alert the health care team to changes in the patient's condition, (d) guide therapy, and (e) track trends and assess prognosis [231]. Because of its ability to detect early changes in intestinal perfusion and the potential for therapeutic actions to improve ICU survival based on this information, pHi monitoring satisfies many of these goals. In addition, because it is relatively noninvasive, it can be performed rapidly and by anyone with the ability to place a nasogastric tube. However, although proponents advocate its use in all seriously ill hospitalized patients, no clear survival or cost savings advantage has been demonstrated [232]. Therefore, an attempt should be made to identify patients who are most likely to benefit from this form of monitoring.

pHi monitoring has been better studied in postoperative ICU patients than in other critically ill patients. In particular, intraoperative and postoperative cardiac surgery patients have been well studied, and in that group gastric pHi appears to predict complications well [233,234]. Patients who have had abdominal aortic surgery and are at risk for postoperative intestinal ischemia may benefit from a tonometer placed in their sigmoid colon [235]. Some authors have gone so far as to advocate its use for all critically ill patients with a high likelihood for development of hemodynamic instability, including those with myocardial infarction and pulmonary edema or high creatine phosphokinase elevations; fever, leukocytosis, and tachycardia; positive blood cultures; APACHE II score greater than 18; overdoses of potentially vasoactive drugs; overt gastrointestinal bleeding and orthostatic hypotension; and unexplained respiratory failure, and for postoperative patients with a history of cardiac disease or intraoperative hemodynamic instability. Its efficacy in many of these situations remains unproven.

The level of gastric pHi has been correlated with survival. In a study by Gutierrez et al., gastric pHi of less than 7.32 was associated with increased mortality [236]. Gastric pHi is also useful in predicting complications after cardiac surgery [233] and has been used to predict the development of gastrointestinal bleeding and mesenteric ischemia, although small intestinal pHi appears to be a more sensitive indicator of the latter [237]. Therapeutic interventions based on gastric pHi have been reported to improve survival in critically ill patients who presented with initially normal pHi values [238]. Infusions of dobutamine and saline given in response to changes in gastric pHi improved survival in patients who presented with initial pHi levels greater than 7.35. No difference was seen in the survival rates of patients whose initial gastric pHi levels were less than 7.35. On the other hand, gastric pHi was unable to distinguish survivors from nonsurvivors in cardiac surgery patients with low cardiac output syndrome [239]. Gastric pHi (a) failed to predict outcome in a study of children with sepsis and multiple organ failure, and (b) in adults, was not as well correlated with shock as were the blood lactate levels [240,241].

Evolving Issues

1. *Timing of measurements.* The fluid in the tonometer balloon requires 90 minutes to equilibrate with the fluid in the stomach. Although correction equations are available to normalize values obtained at less than 90 minutes, in general the full time period should be used.
2. *Tonometer fluid.* Saline has been the fluid used in the balloon most often. However, evidence suggests that phosphate-buffered solution provides more consistent results [242]. This is currently the preferred material.
3. *Acid secretion.* Tonometrically derived gastric pHi can be affected by the acid-secretory status of the stomach. In one study, mean gastric pHi was 7.30 in untreated normal volunteers but 7.39 in a similar group treated with ranitidine [243]. This was because the PCO_2 in the gastric fluid of the treated patients was 42 ± 4 mm Hg, compared with 52 ± 14 mm Hg in the untreated group. The difference in carbon dioxide content of the fluid is thought to be due to production of carbon dioxide by the conversion of secreted H^+ and HCO_3^- into water and carbon dioxide. This is particularly important because some have suggested that inhibition of gastric acid secretion predisposes to nosocomial pneumonia [244]. At present, treating patients with H_2-receptor antagonists is considered standard [245].
4. *Tube feedings.* Enteral feeding may also affect pHi reading. Tube feedings may lead to increased production of carbon dioxide through the interaction of secreted hydrogen ions and HCO_3^-. One study has suggested temporarily discontinuing tube feeds before doing pHi measurements [246]. No clear consensus has been established on this matter.
5. *Analysis equipment.* Measurements of gastric PCO_2 for determination of pHi have been validated on a limited number of blood gas analyzers. Machines other than those previously validated may show errors in the measurement of gastric PCO_2 despite the ability to measure systemic arterial PCO_2 accurately. To our knowledge, all such errors identified to date have been systematic in nature and therefore could be adjusted with appropriate correction factors. Before making clinical decisions based on the information derived, the clinician should determine whether the blood gas analyzer in use has been validated and, if a systematic error has been found, that correction factors are available.

CONCLUSIONS. Conventional methods of determining the adequacy of tissue oxygenation may be insensitive to the localized changes that may precede systemic hemodynamic collapse. Inadequate tissue oxygenation causes tissue acidosis because of the shift to anaerobic metabolism. Because the carbon dioxide present in the tissue is in equilibrium with that in the intraluminal fluid of a viscus, the pHi of that organ can be determined by measuring intraluminal PCO_2 and arterial HCO_3^-. The stomach, small intestine, or sigmoid colon can be used, with the stomach being most popular because of the ease of cannulation. The results of these tests may be helpful in determining prognosis in critically ill patients, and therapy based on these findings may improve survival.

Definite indications for use have not been clearly established, but the procedure may be beneficial to any critically ill patient at risk of local ischemia or the systemic hypoperfusion state of shock.

References

1. Kholoussi AM, Sufian S, Pavlides C, et al: Central peripheral temperature gradient: its value and limitations in the management of critically ill surgical patients. *Am J Surg* 140:609, 1980.
2. Burgess GE III, Cooper JR, Marino RJ: Continuous monitoring of skin temperature using a liquid-crystal thermometer during anesthesia. *South Med J* 71:516, 1978.
3. Roberts NH: The comparison of surface and core temperature devices. *J Am Assoc Nurse Anesth* 48:53, 1980.
4. Silverman RW, Lomax P: The measurement of temperature for thermoregulatory studies. *Pharmacol Ther* 27:233, 1985.

5. Vale RJ: Monitoring of temperature during anesthesia. *Int Anesthesiol Clin* 19:61, 1981.

6. Fukuoka M, Yamori Y, Toyoshima T: Twenty-four hour monitoring of deep body temperature with a novel flexible probe. *J Biomed Eng* 9:173, 1987.

7. Lees DE, Kim YD, MacNamara TE: Noninvasive determination of core temperature during anesthesia. *South Med J* 73:1322, 1980.

8. Watson BW: Clinical uses of radio pills. *Br J Hosp Med* 25:618, 1981.

9. Terndrup TE: An appraisal of temperature assessment by infrared emission detection tympanic thermometry. *Ann Emerg Med* 21:1483, 1992.

10. Terndrup TE, Rajk J: Impact of operator technique and device on infrared emission detection tympanic thermometry. *J Emerg Med* 10:683, 1992.

11. Erickson R: Thermometer placement for oral temperature measurement in febrile adults. *Int J Nurs Stud* 13:199, 1976.

12. Heinz J: Validation of sublingual temperatures in patients with nasogastric tubes. *Heart Lung* 14:128, 1985.

13. Tandberg D, Sklar D: Effect of tachypnea on the estimation of body temperature by an oral thermometer. *N Engl J Med* 313:945, 1985.

14. Cork RC, Vaughan RW, Humphrey LS: Precision and accuracy of intraoperative temperature monitoring. *Anesth Analg* 62:211, 1983.

15. Bone ME, Feneck RO: Bladder temperature as an estimate of body temperature during cardiopulmonary bypass. *Anaesthesia* 43:181, 1988.

16. Ramsay JG, Ralley FE, Whalley DG, et al: Site of temperature monitoring and prediction of afterdrop after open heart surgery. *Can Anaesth Soc J* 32:607, 1985.

17. Moorthy SS, Winn BA, Jallard MS, et al: Monitoring urinary bladder temperature. *Heart Lung* 14:90, 1985.

18. Severinghaus JW: Temperature gradients during hypothermia. *Ann N Y Acad Sci* 80:515, 1962.

19. Webb GE: Comparison of esophageal and tympanic temperature monitoring during cardiopulmonary bypass. *Anesth Analg* 52:729, 1973.

20. Crocker BD, Okumura F, McCuaig DI, et al: Temperature monitoring during general anaesthesia. *Br J Anaesth* 52:1223, 1980.

21. Manian FA, Griesenauer S: Lack of agreement between tympanic and oral temperature measurements in adult hospitalized patients. *Am J Infect Control* 26(4):428, 1998.

22. Amoateng-Adjepong Y, Del Mundo J, Manthous CA: Accuracy of infrared tympanic thermometer. *Chest* 115(4):1002, 1999.

23. Wallace CT, Marks WE, Adkins WY, et al: Perforation of the tympanic membrane: a complication of tympanic thermometry during anesthesia. *Anesthesiology* 41:290, 1974.

24. Joly HR, Weil MH: Temperature of the great toe as an indication of the severity of shock. *Circulation* 39:131, 1969.

25. Knight RW, Opie JC: The big toe in the recovery room: peripheral warm-up patterns in children after open-heart surgery. *Can J Surg* 24:239, 1981.

26. Nierman DM: Core temperature measurement in the intensive care unit. *Crit Care Med* 19:818, 1991.

27. Heidenreich T, Giuffre M, Doorley J: Temperature and temperature measurement after induced hypothermia. *Nurs Res* 41:296, 1992.

28. Brooks SE, Veal RO, Kramer M, et al: Reduction in the incidence of *Clostridium difficile* associated diarrhea in an acute care hospital and a skilled nursing facility following replacement of electronic thermometers with single-use disposables. *Infect Control Hosp Epidemiol* 13:98, 1992.

29. Livnorese LL, Dias S, Samel C, et al: Hospital-acquired infection with vancomycin-resistant *Enterococcus faecium* transmitted by electronic thermometers. *Ann Intern Med* 117:112, 1992.

30. Rotello LC, Crawford L, Terndrup TE: Comparison of infrared ear thermometer derived and equilibrated rectal temperatures in estimating pulmonary artery temperatures. *Crit Care Med* 24:1501, 1996.

31. Schmitz T, Bair N, Falk M, et al: A comparison of 5 methods of temperature measurement in febrile intensive care unit patients. *Am J Crit Care* 4:286, 1995.

32. Task Force on Guidelines: Recommendations for services and personnel for delivery of care in a critical care setting. *Crit Care Med* 16:809, 1988.

33. Pierce EC: Percutaneous arterial catheterization in man with special reference to aortography. *Surg Gynecol Obstet* 93:56, 1951.

34. Donald DC Jr, Kesmodel KF Jr, Rollins SL Jr, et al: An improved technique for percutaneous cerebral angiography. *Arch Neurol Psychiatry* 65:500, 1951.

35. Bruner JMR, Krenis LJ, Kunsman JM, et al: Comparison of direct and indirect methods of measuring arterial blood pressure: Pt III. *Med Instrum* 15:182, 1981.

36. Reder RF, Dimich I, Cohen ML, et al: Evaluating indirect blood pressure measurement techniques: a comparison of three systems in infants and children. *Pediatrics* 62:326, 1978.

37. Nystrom E, Reid KH, Bennett R, et al: A comparison of two automated indirect arterial blood pressure meters: with recordings from a radial arterial catheter in anesthetized surgical patients. *Anesthesiology* 62:526, 1985.

38. DeGowin EL, DeGowin RL: The thorax and cardiovascular system, in DeGowin EL, DeGowin RL (eds): *Bedside Diagnostic Examination*. New York, Macmillan, 1981, p 229.

39. Hirschl MM, Binder M, Herkner H, et al: Accuracy and reliability of noninvasive continuous finger blood pressure measurement in critically ill patients. *Crit Care Med* 24:1684, 1996.

40. Carrol GC: Blood pressure monitoring. *Crit Care Clin* 4:411, 1988.

41. Van Bergen FH, Weatherhead S, Treloar AE, et al: Comparison of direct and indirect methods of measuring arterial blood pressure. *Circulation* 10:481, 1954.

42. Bailey RH, Knaus VL, Bauer JH: Aneroid sphygmomanometers: an assessment of accuracy at a university hospital and clinics. *Arch Intern Med* 151:1409, 1991.

43. Zagzebski JA: Physics and instrumentation in Doppler and B-mode ultrasonography, in Zwiebel WJ (ed): *Introduction to Vascular Ultrasonography*. Orlando, FL, Grune & Stratton, 1986, p 21.

44. Kirby RR, Kemmerer WT, Morgan JL: Transcutaneous Doppler measurement of blood pressure. *Anesthesiology* 31:86, 1969.

45. Hochberg HM, Salomon H: Accuracy of automated ultrasound blood pressure monitor. *Curr Ther Res* 13:129, 1971.

46. Chastonay P, Morel D, Forster A, et al: Evaluation of a new monitoring device for arterial blood pressure and heart rate measurement by automatic sphygmomanometry. *Anaesth Intensivther Notfallmed* 17:348, 1982.

47. Puritan Bennett Corporation: *Infrasonde Model D4000 Electronic Blood Pressure Monitor Operating Manual*. Los Angeles, Puritan Bennett Corporation.

48. Cullen PM, Dye J, Hughes DG: Clinical assessment of the neonatal Dinamap 847 during anesthesia in neonates and infants. *J Clin Monit* 3:229, 1987.

49. Borow KM, Newberger JW: Non-invasive estimation of central aortic pressure using the oscillometric method for analyzing systemic artery pulsatile blood flow: comparative study of indirect systolic, diastolic, and mean brachial artery pressure with simultaneous direct ascending aortic pressure measurements. *Am Heart J* 103:879, 1982.

50. Van Egmond J, Hasenbros M, Crul JF: Invasive v. non-invasive measurement of arterial pressure. *Br J Anaesth* 57:434, 1985.

51. Boehmer RD: Continuous, real-time, noninvasive monitor of blood pressure: Penaz methodology applied to the finger. *J Clin Monit* 3:282, 1987.

52. Kemmotsu O, Ueda M, Otsuka H, et al: Arterial tonometry for non-invasive, continuous blood pressure monitoring during anesthesia. *Anesthesiology* 75:333, 1991.

53. Kemmotsu O, Ueda M, Otsuka H, et al: Blood pressure measurement by arterial tonometry in controlled hypotension. *Anesth Analg* 73:54, 1991.

54. Siegel LC, Brock-Utne JG, Brodsky JB: Comparison of arterial tonometry with radial artery catheter measurements of blood pressure in anesthetized patients. *Anesthesiology* 81:578, 1994.

55. Kemmotsu O, Ohno M, Takita K, et al: Noninvasive, continuous blood pressure measurement by arterial tonometry during anesthesia in children. *Anesthesiology* 81:1162, 1994.

56. Chen CH, Nevp E, Fetics B, et al: Estimation of central aortic pressure waveform by mathematical transformation of radial tonometry pressure: validation of generalized transfer function. *Circulation* 95:1827, 1997.

57. Jawad IA: Quantitative applications of Doppler ultrasonography, in Jawad IA (ed): *A Practical Guide to Echocardiography and Cardiac Doppler Ultrasound*. Boston, Little, Brown, 1993.

58. Wipperman CF, Schranz D, Huth RG: Evaluation of the pulse wave arrival time as a marker for pressure changes in critically ill infants and children. *J Clin Monit* 11:324, 1995.

59. Edwards RC, Goldberg AD, Bannister R, et al: The infrasound blood pressure monitor: a clinical evaluation. *Lancet* 2:398, 1976.

60. Baker LK: Dinamap monitor versus direct blood pressure measurements. *Dimensions of Critical Care Nursing* 5:228, 1986.

61. Amoore JN, Geake WB, Scott DHT: Oscillometric non-invasive blood pressure measurements: the influence of the make of instrument on readings. *Med Biol Eng Comput* 35:131, 1997.
62. Derrico DJ: Comparison of blood pressure measurement methods in critically ill children. *Dimensions of Critical Care Nursing* 12:31, 1993.
63. Latman NS: Evaluation of finger blood pressure monitoring instruments. *Biomed Instrum Technol* 26:52, 1992.
64. Aitken HA, Todd JG, Kenny GNC: Comparison of the Finapres and direct arterial pressure monitoring during profound hypotensive anesthesia. *Br J Anaesth* 67:36, 1991.
65. Kermode JL, Davis NJ, Thompson WR: Comparison of the Finapres blood pressure monitor with intra-arterial manometry during induction of anaesthesia. *Anaesth Intensive Care* 17:470, 1989.
66. Farquhar IK: Continuous direct and indirect blood pressure measurement (Finapres) in the critically ill. *Anaesthesia* 46:1050, 1991.
67. Bos WJW, Imholz BPM, van Goudoever J, et al: The reliability of non-invasive continuous finger blood pressure measurement in patients with both hypertension and vascular disease. *Am J Hypertens* 5:529, 1992.
68. Rutten AJ, Isley AH, Skowronski GA, et al: A comparative study of the measurement of mean arterial blood pressure using automatic oscillometers, arterial cannulation and auscultation. *Anaesth Intensive Care* 14:58, 1986.
69. Yelderman M, Ream AK: Indirect measurement of mean blood pressure in the anesthetized patient. *Anesthesiology* 50:253, 1979.
70. Modesti PA, Gensini GF, Conti C, et al: Clinical evaluation of an automatic blood-pressure monitoring device. *J Clin Hyper* 3:631, 1987.
71. Paulus DA: Noninvasive blood pressure measurement. *Med Instrum* 15:91, 1981.
72. Sy WP: Ulnar nerve palsy possibly related to use of automatically cycled blood pressure cuff. *Anesth Analg* 60:687, 1981.
73. Betts EK: Hazard of automated noninvasive blood pressure monitoring. *Anesthesiology* 55:717, 1981.
74. Bainbridge LC, Simmons HM, Elliot D: The use of automatic blood pressure monitors in the burned patient. *Br J Plast Surg* 43:322, 1990.
75. Hutton P, Prys-Roberts C: An assessment of the Dinamap 845. *Anaesthesia* 39:261, 1984.
76. Sladen A: Complications of invasive hemodynamic monitoring in the intensive care unit. *Curr Probl Surg* 25:69, 1988.
77. Davis FM, Stewart JM: Radial artery cannulation. *Br J Anaesth* 52:41, 1980.
78. Gardner RM, Schwarz R, Wong HC, et al: Percutaneous indwelling radial-artery catheters for monitoring cardiovascular function. *N Engl J Med* 290:1227, 1974.
79. Schwid HA: Frequency response evaluation of radial artery catheter-manometer systems: sinusoidal frequency analysis versus flush method. *J Clin Monit* 4:181, 1988.
80. Bruner JMR, Krenis LJ, Kunsman JM, et al: Comparison of direct and indirect methods of measuring arterial blood pressure: Pt II. *Med Instrum* 15:97, 1981.
81. Rothe CF, Kim KC: Measuring systolic arterial blood pressure: possible errors from extension tubes or disposable transducer domes. *Crit Care Med* 8:683, 1980.
82. Hughes VG, Prys-Roberts C: Intra-arterial pressure measurements: a review and analysis of methods relevant to anaesthesia and intensive care. *Anaesthesia* 26:511, 1971.
83. Shinozaki T, Deane RS, Mazuzan JE: The dynamic responses of liquid filled catheter systems for direct measurements of blood pressure. *Anesthesiology* 53:498, 1980.
84. Russell JA, Joel M, Hudson RJ, et al: Prospective evaluation of radial and femoral artery catheterization sites in critically ill adults. *Crit Care Med* 11:936, 1983.
85. Colvin MP, Curran JP, Jarvis D, et al: Femoral artery pressure monitoring. *Anaesthesia* 32:451, 1977.
86. Bryan-Brown CW, Kwun KB, Lumb PD, et al: The axillary artery catheter. *Heart Lung* 12:492, 1983.
87. Bruner JMR, Krenis LJ, Kunsman JM, et al: Comparison of direct and indirect methods of measuring arterial blood pressure: Pt I. *Med Instrum* 15:11, 1981.
88. Thys DM: The normal ECG, in Thys DM, Kaplan JA (eds): *The ECG in Anesthesia and Critical Care*. New York, Churchill Livingstone, 1987, p 1.
89. Winters SR: Diagnosis by wireless. *Sci Am* 124:465, 1921.
90. Lown B, Klein MD: Coronary and precoronary care. *Am J Med* 46:705, 1969.
91. Yu PN, Fox SM, Imboden CA, et al: A specialized intensive care unit for acute myocardial infarction. *Mod Concepts Cardiovasc Dis* 34:23, 1965.
92. Kimball JT, Killip T: Aggressive treatment of arrhythmias in acute myocardial infarction: procedures and results. *Prog Cardiovasc Dis* 10:483, 1968.
93. Julian DG, Valentine PA, Miller GG: Disturbances of rate, rhythm, and conduction in acute myocardial infarction. *Am J Med* 37:915, 1964.
94. Romhilt DW, Bloomfield SS, Chou T, et al: Unreliability of conventional electrocardiographic monitoring for arrhythmia detection in coronary care units. *Am J Cardiol* 31:457, 1973.
95. American Heart Association: Myocardial infarction, in *Textbook of Advanced Cardiac Life Support*. Dallas, American Heart Association, 1987, p 11.
96. Cercek B, Lew AS, Laramee P, et al: Time course and characteristics of ventricular arrhythmias after reperfusion in acute myocardial infarction. *Am J Cardiol* 60:214, 1987.
97. Buckingham TA, Devine JE, Redd RM, et al: Reperfusion arrhythmias during coronary reperfusion therapy in man: clinical and angiographic correlations. *Chest* 90:346, 1986.
98. Linnik W, Tintinalli JE, Ramos R: Associated reactions during and immediately after rtPA infusion. *Ann Emerg Med* 18:234, 1989.
99. Singh N, Mironov D, Armstrong PW, et al: Heart rate variability assessment early after acute myocardial infarction: pathophysiological and prognostic correlates. GUSTO ECG Substudy Investigators. Global Utilization of Streptokinase and TPA for Occluded Arteries. *Circulation* 93:1388, 1996.
100. Bartter T, Curley FJ, Larrivee G, et al: The value of arrhythmia monitoring in medical intensive care units. *Am Rev Respir Dis* 139:A152, 1989.
101. Funk M, Parkosewich JA, Johnson CR, Stukshis I: Effect of dedicated monitor watchers on patients' outcomes. *Am J Crit Care* 6:318, 1997.
102. Chatila W, Ani S, Guaglianone D, et al: Cardiac ischemia during weaning from mechanical ventilation. *Chest* 109:1577, 1996.
103. Holmberg S, Ryden L, Waldenstrom A: Efficiency of arrhythmia detection by nurses in a coronary care unit using a decentralized monitoring system. *Br Heart J* 39:1019, 1977.
104. Vetter NJ, Julian DG: Comparison of arrhythmia computer and conventional monitoring in coronary-care unit. *Lancet* 1:1151, 1975.
105. Pierpoint GL: Pitfalls of computer use in acute care medicine. *Heart Lung* 16:207, 1987.
106. Watkinson WP, Brice MA, Robinson KS: A computer-assisted electrocardiographic analysis system: methodology and potential application to cardiovascular toxicology. *J Toxicol Environ Health* 15:713, 1985.
107. Alcover IA, Henning RJ, Jackson DL: A computer-assisted monitoring system for arrhythmia detection in a medical intensive care unit. *Crit Care Med* 12:888, 1984.
108. Badura FK: Nurse acceptance of a computerized arrhythmia monitoring system. *Heart Lung* 9:1044, 1980.
109. Cecchi AC, Dovellini EV, Marchi F, et al: Silent myocardial ischemia during ambulatory electrocardiographic monitoring in patients with effort angina. *J Am Coll Cardiol* 1:934, 1983.
110. Clements FM, Bruijn NP: Noninvasive cardiac monitoring. *Crit Care Clin* 4:435, 1988.
111. Mirvis DM, Berson AS, Goldberger AL, et al: Instrumentation and practice standards for electrocardiographic monitoring in special care units. *Circulation* 79:464, 1989.
112. Patel DJ, Holdright DR, Knight CJ, et al: Early continuous ST segment monitoring in unstable angina: prognostic value additional to the clinical characteristics and the admission electrocardiogram. *Heart* 75:222, 1996.
113. Fesmire FM, Wharton DR, Calhoun FB: Instability of ST segments in the early stages of acute myocardial infarction in patients undergoing continuous 12-lead ECG monitoring. *Am J Emerg Med* 13:158, 1995.
114. Pepine CJ: Prognostic markers in thrombolytic therapy: looking beyond mortality. *Am J Cardiol* 78[Suppl 12A]:24, 1996.
115. Drew BJ, Adams MG, Pelter MM, Wung SF: ST segment monitoring with a derived 12-lead electrocardiogram is superior to routine cardiac care unit monitoring. *Am J Crit Care* 5:198, 1996.
116. Winchell RJ, Hoyt DB: Spectral analysis of heart rate variability in the ICU: a measure of autonomic function. *J Surg Res* 63:11, 1996.
117. Singh N, Mironov D, Armstrong PW, et al: Heart rate variability assessment early after acute myocardial infarction: pathophysiologic and prognostic correlates. GUSTO Substudy Investigators. *Circulation* 93:1388, 1996.

118. Association for the Advancement of Medical Instrumentation: *American National Standard for Cardiac Monitors, Heart Rate Meters, and Alarms (EC 13-1983)*. Arlington, VA, ANSI/AAMI, 1984.

119. Starmer CF, Whalen RE, McIntosh HD: Hazards of electric shock in cardiology. *Am J Cardiol* 14:537, 1964.

120. Bruner JMR: Hazards of electrical apparatus. *Anesthesiology* 28:396, 1967.

121. Hewlett-Packard Corporation: *ECG Measurement—Application Note AN711*. Waltham, MA, Hewlett Packard.

122. Hanley J: Telemetry in health care. *Biomed Eng* 11:269, 1976.

123. Pittman JV, Blum MS, Leonard MS: *Telemetry Utilization for Emergency Medical Services Systems*. Atlanta, Health Systems Research Center, Georgia Institute of Technology, 1974.

124. Anderson GJ, Knoebel SB, Fisch C: Continuous prehospitalization monitoring of cardiac rhythm. *Am Heart J* 82:642, 1971.

125. McFadden JP, Price RC, Eastwood HD, et al: Raised respiratory rate in elderly patients: a valuable physical sign. *Br J Med* 284:626, 1982.

126. Mithoefer JC, Bossman OG, Thibeault DW, et al: The clinical estimation of alveolar ventilation. *Am Rev Respir Dis* 98:868, 1968.

127. Semmes BJ, Tobin MJ, Snyder JV, et al: Subjective and objective measurement of tidal volume in critically ill patients. *Chest* 87:577, 1985.

128. Krieger B, Feinerman D, Zaron A, et al: Continuous noninvasive monitoring of respiratory rate in critically ill patients. *Chest* 90:632, 1986.

129. Shelly MP, Park GR: Failure of a respiratory monitor to detect obstructive apnea. *Crit Care Med* 14:836, 1986.

130. Sackner MA, Bizousky F, Krieger BP: Performance of impedance pneumograph and respiratory inductive plethysmograph as monitors of respiratory frequency and apnea. *Am Rev Respir Dis* 135:A41, 1987.

131. Chadha TS, Watson H, Birch S, et al: Validation of respiratory inductive plethysmography using different calibration procedures. *Am Rev Respir Dis* 125:644, 1982.

132. Sackner MA, Watson H, Belsito AS, et al: Calibration of respiratory inductive plethysmograph during natural breathing. *J Appl Physiol* 66:410, 1989.

133. Tobin MJ, Jenouri G, Lind B, et al: Validation of respiratory inductive plethysmography in patients with pulmonary disease. *Chest* 83:615, 1983.

134. Tobin MJ, Jenouri G, Birch S, et al: Effect of positive end-expiratory pressure on breathing patterns of normal subjects and intubated patients with respiratory failure. *Crit Care Med* 11:859, 1983.

135. Tobin MJ, Guenther SM, Perez W, et al: Konno-Mead analysis of ribcage-abdominal motion during successful and unsuccessful trials of weaning from mechanical ventilation. *Am Rev Respir Dis* 135:1320, 1987.

136. Krieger BP, Chediak A, Gazeroglu HB, et al: Variability of breathing pattern before and after extubation. *Chest* 93:767, 1988.

137. Hoffman RA, Ershowsky P, Krieger BP: Determination of auto-PEEP during spontaneous and controlled ventilation by monitoring changes in end-expiratory thoracic gas volume. *Chest* 96:613, 1989.

138. Krieger BP, Ershowsky P, Spivack D, et al: Initial experience with a central respiratory monitoring unit as a cost-saving alternative to the intensive care unit for Medicare patients who require long-term ventilator support. *Chest* 93:395, 1988.

139. O'Brien MJ, Van Eykern LA, Oetomo SB, et al: Transcutaneous respiratory electromyographic monitoring. *Crit Care Med* 15:394, 1987.

140. Mower WR, Sachs C, Nicklin EL, et al: A comparison of pulse oximetry and respiratory rate in patient screening. *Respir Med* 90:593, 1996.

141. Brown LH, Manring EA, Korengay HB, et al: Can prehospital personnel detect hypoxemia without the aid of pulse oximetry? *Am J Emerg Med* 14:43, 1996.

142. Chapman KR, Rebuck AS: Oximetry, in Nochomovitz ML, Cherniak NS (eds): *Noninvasive Respiratory Monitoring*. New York, Churchill Livingstone, 1986, p 803.

143. Stoneham MD, Saville GM, Wilson IH: Knowledge about pulse oximetry among medical and nursing staff. *Lancet* 344:1339, 1994.

144. Huch A, Huch R, Konig V, et al: Limitations of pulse oximetry. *Lancet* 2:357, 1988.

145. New W: Pulse oximetry. *J Clin Monit* 1:126, 1985.

146. Moller JT, Pederen T, Rasmussen LS, et al: Randomized evaluation of pulse oximetry in 20,802 patients: I. Design, demography,

147. Reich DL, Timcenko A, Bodian CA, et al: Predictors of pulse oximetry data failure. *Anesthesiology* 84:859, 1996.

148. Choe H, Tashiro C, Fukumitsu K, et al: Comparison of recorded values from six pulse oximeters. *Crit Care Med* 17:678, 1989.

149. Severinghaus JW, Naifeh KH, Koh SO: Errors in 14 pulse oximeters during profound hypoxia. *J Clin Monit* 5:72, 1989.

150. Reynolds KJ, Moyle JTB, Gale LB, et al: In vitro performance test system for pulse oximeters. *Med Biol Eng Comput* 30:629, 1992.

151. Severinghaus JW, Naifeh KH: Accuracy of responses of six pulse oximeters to profound hypoxia. *Anesthesiology* 67:551, 1987.

152. Cheng EY, Stommel KA: Quantitative evaluation of a combined pulse oximetry and end-tidal CO_2 monitor. *Biomed Instrum Technol* 23:216, 1989.

153. Reynolds LM, Nicolson SC, Steven JM, et al: Influence of sensor site location on pulse oximetry kinetics in children. *Anesth Analg* 76:751, 1993.

154. Cheng EY, Hopwood MB, Kay J: Forehead pulse oximetry compared with finger pulse oximetry and arterial blood gas measurement. *J Clin Monit* 4:223, 1988.

155. Hickerson W, Morrell M, Cicala RS: Glossal pulse oximetry. *Anesth Analg* 69:72, 1989.

156. Evans ML, Geddes LA: An assessment of blood vessel vasoactivity using photoplethysmography. *Med Instrum* 22:29, 1988.

157. Barker SJ, Hyatt J, Shah NK, et al: The effect of sensor malpositioning on pulse oximetry accuracy during hypoxemia. *Anesthesiology* 79:248, 1993.

158. Tweedie IE: Pulse oximeters and finger nails. *Anaesthesia* 44:268, 1989.

159. Cote CJ, Goldstein EA, Fuchsman WH, et al: The effect of nail polish on pulse oximetry. *Anesth Analg* 67:683, 1988.

160. Read MS: Effect of transparent adhesive tape on pulse oximetry. *Anesth Analg* 68:701, 1989.

161. Ries AL, Prewitt LM, Johnson JJ: Skin color and ear oximetry. *Chest* 96:287, 1989.

162. Bothma PA, Joynt GM, Lipman J, et al: Accuracy of pulse oximetry in pigmented patients. *S Afr Med J* 86:594, 1996.

163. Costarino AT, Davis DA, Keon TP: Falsely normal saturation reading with the pulse oximeter. *Anesthesiology* 67:830, 1987.

164. Hanowell L, Eisele JH Jr, Downs D: Ambient light affects pulse oximeters. *Anesthesiology* 67:864, 1987.

165. Block FE Jr: Interference in a pulse oximeter from a fiberoptic light source. *J Clin Monit* 3:210, 1987.

166. Brooks TD, Paulus DA, Winkle WE: Infrared heat lamps interfere with pulse oximeters. *Anesthesiology* 61:630, 1984.

167. Amar D, Neidzwski J, Wald A, et al: Fluorescent light interferes with pulse oximetry. *J Clin Monit* 5:135, 1989.

168. Beall SN, Moorthy SS: Jaundice, oximetry, and spurious hemoglobin desaturation. *Anesth Analg* 68:806, 1989.

169. Veyckemans F, Baele P, Guillaume JE, et al: Hyperbilirubinemia does not interfere with hemoglobin saturation measured by pulse oximetry. *Anesthesiology* 70:118, 1989.

170. Watcha MF, Connor MT, Hing AV: Pulse oximetry in methemoglobinemia. *Am J Dis Child* 143:845, 1989.

171. Reynolds KJ, Palayiwa E, Moyle JTB, et al: The effect of dyshemoglobins on pulse oximetry: I. Theoretical approach. II. Experimental results using an in vitro system. *J Clin Monit* 9:81, 1993.

172. Barker SJ, Tremper KK: The effect of carbon monoxide inhalation on pulse oximetry and transcutaneous PO_2. *Anesthesiology* 66:677, 1987.

173. Glass KL, Dillard TA, Phillips YY, et al: Pulse oximetry correction for smoking exposure. *Mil Med* 16:273, 1996.

174. Coburn RF, Williams WJ, Kahn SB: Endogenous carbon monoxide production in patients with hemolytic anemia. *J Clin Invest* 45:460, 1966.

175. Buckley RG, Aks SE, Eshom JL, et al: The pulse oximetry gap in carbon monoxide intoxication. *Ann Emerg Med* 24:252, 1994.

176. Lee SE, Tremper KK, Barker SJ: Effects of anemia on pulse oximetry and continuous mixed venous oxygen saturation monitoring in dogs. *Anesth Analg* 67:S130, 1988.

177. Jay GD, Hughes L, Renzi FP: Pulse oximetry is accurate in acute anemia from hemorrhage. *Ann Emerg Med* 24:32, 1994.

178. Cane RD, Harrison RA, Shapiro BA, et al: The spectrophotometric absorbance of intralipid. *Anesthesiology* 53:53, 1980.

179. Gabrielczyk MR, Buist RJ: Pulse oximetry and postoperative hypothermia: an evaluation of the Nellcor N-100 in a cardiac surgical intensive care unit. *Anaesthesia* 43:402, 1988.

180. Palve H, Vuori A: Pulse oximetry during low cardiac output and hypothermia states immediately after open heart surgery. *Crit Care Med* 17:66, 1989.

181. Rieder HU, Frei FJ, Zbinden AM, et al: Pulse oximetry in methemoglobinemia: failure to detect low oxygen saturation. *Anaesthesia* 44:326, 1989.

182. Scheller MS, Unger RJ, Kelner MJ: Effects of intravenously administered dyes on pulse oximetry readings. *Anesthesiology* 65:550, 1986.

183. Unger R, Scheller MS: More on dyes and pulse oximeters. *Anesthesiology* 67:148, 1987.

184. Larsen VH, Freudendal-Pedersen A, Fogh-Andersen N: The influence of patent blue V on pulse oximetry and haemoximetry. *Acta Anaesthesiol Scand Suppl* 107:53, 1995.

185. Taylor MB: Erroneous actuation of the pulse oximeter. *Anaesthesia* 42:1116, 1987.

186. Morris RW, Nairn M, Torda TA: A comparison of fifteen pulse oximeters: I: a clinical comparison. II: a test of performance under conditions of poor perfusion. *Anaesth Intensive Care* 17:62, 1989.

187. Paulus DA: Cool fingers and pulse oximetry. *Anesthesiology* 71:168, 1989.

188. Mineo R, Sharrock NE: Pulse oximeter waveforms from the finger and the toe during lumbar epidural anesthesia. *Reg Anesth* 18:106, 1993.

189. Broome IJ, Mills GH, Spiers P, et al: An evaluation of the effect of vasodilatation on oxygen saturations measured by pulse oximetry and venous blood gas analysis. *Anaesthesia* 48:415, 1993.

190. Stewart KG, Rowbottam SJ: Inaccuracy of pulse oximetry in patients with severe tricuspid regurgitation. *Anaesthesia* 46:668, 1991.

191. Smith DC, Canning JJ, Crul JF: Pulse oximetry in the recovery room. *Anaesthesia* 44:345, 1989.

192. Tyler IL, Tantisera B, Winter PM: Continuous monitoring of arterial oxygen saturation with pulse oximetry during transfer to the recovery room. *Anesth Analg* 64:1108, 1985.

193. Moller JT, Johannenssen NW, Espersen K, et al: Randomized evaluation of pulse oximetry in 20,802 patients: II. Perioperative events and postoperative complications. *Anesthesiology* 78:423, 1993.

194. Rotello LC, Warren J, Jastremski MS, et al: A nurse directed protocol using pulse oximetry to wean mechanically ventilated patients from toxic oxygen concentrations. *Chest* 102:1833, 1992.

195. Introna RPS, Silverstein PI: A new use for the pulse oximeter. *Anesthesiology* 65:342, 1986.

196. Katz Y, Lee ME: Pulse oximetry for localization of the dorsalis pedis artery. *Anaesth Intensive Care* 17:114, 1989.

197. Guggenberger H, Lenz G, Federle R: Early detection of inadvertent esophageal intubation: pulse oximetry vs. capnography. *Acta Anaesthesiol Scand* 33:112, 1989.

198. Korbon GA, Wills MH, D'Lauro F, et al: Systolic blood pressure measurement: Doppler vs. pulse oximeter. *Anesthesiology* 67:A188, 1987.

199. Brathwaite CEM, O'Malley KF, Ross SE, et al: Continuous pulse oximetry and the diagnosis of pulmonary embolism in critically ill trauma patients. *J Trauma* 33:528, 1992.

200. Mars M, Maesjo S, Thompson S, et al: Can pulse oximetry detect raised intracompartmental pressure? *S Afr J Surg* 32:48, 1994.

201. Wimberley PD, Pedersen KG, Thode J, et al: Transcutaneous and capillary pCO_2 and pO_2 measurements in healthy adults. *Clin Chem* 29:1471, 1983.

202. Abraham E, Smith M, Silver L: Continuous monitoring of critically ill patients with transcutaneous oxygen and carbon dioxide and conjunctival oxygen sensors. *Ann Emerg Med* 13:1021, 1984.

203. Tremper KK, Keenan B, Applebaum R, et al: Clinical and experimental monitoring with transcutaneous PO_2 during hypoxia, shock, cardiac arrest, and CPR. *J Clin Eng* 6:149, 1981.

204. Rooth G, Hedstrand U, Tyden H, et al: The validity of the transcutaneous oxygen tension method in adults. *Crit Care Med* 4:162, 1976.

205. Gothgen I, Jacobsen E: Transcutaneous oxygen tension measurement: I. Age variation and reproducibility. *Acta Anaesthesiol Scand* 67:66, 1978.

206. Eletr S, Jimison H, Ream AK, et al: Cutaneous monitoring of systemic PCO_2 on patients in the respiratory intensive care unit being weaned from the ventilator. *Acta Anaesthesiol Scand* 68:123, 1978.

207. Tremper KK, Waxman K, Shoemaker WC: Use of transcutaneous oxygen sensors to titrate PEEP. *Ann Surg* 193:206, 1981.

208. Tremper KK, Shoemaker WC: Transcutaneous oxygen monitoring of critically ill adults, with and without low flow shock. *Crit Care Med* 9:706, 1981.

209. Shoemaker WC, Fink S, Ray CW, et al: Effect of hemorrhagic shock on conjunctival and transcutaneous oxygen tensions in relation to hemodynamic and oxygen transport changes. *Crit Care Med* 12:949, 1984.

210. Abraham E, Oye R, Smith M: Detection of blood volume deficits through conjunctival oxygen tension monitoring. *Crit Care Med* 12:931, 1984.

211. Nolan LS, Shoemaker WC: Transcutaneous O_2 and CO_2 monitoring of high risk surgical patients during the perioperative period. *Crit Care Med* 10:762, 1982.

212. Stock MC: Noninvasive carbon dioxide monitoring. *Crit Care Clin* 4:511, 1988.

213. Schena J, Thompson J, Crone R: Mechanical influences on the capnogram. *Crit Care Med* 12:672, 1984.

214. Paulus DA: Capnography. *Int Anesthesiol Clin* 27:167, 1989.

215. Murray IP, Modell JM: Early detection of endotracheal tube accidents by monitoring of carbon dioxide concentration in respiratory gas. *Anesthesiology* 59:344, 1983.

216. Falk JL, Rackow EC, Weil MH: End tidal carbon dioxide concentration during cardiopulmonary resuscitation. *N Engl J Med* 318:607, 1988.

217. Raemer DB, Francis D, Philip JH, et al: Variation in PCO_2 between arterial blood and peak expired gas during anesthesia. *Anesth Analg* 62:1065, 1983.

218. Hoffman RA, Krieger BP, Kramer MR, et al: End-tidal carbon dioxide in critically ill patients during changes in mechanical ventilation. *Am Rev Respir Dis* 140:1265, 1989.

219. Morley TF, Giaimo J, Maroszan E, et al: Use of capnography for assessment of the adequacy of alveolar ventilation during weaning from mechanical ventilation. *Am Rev Respir Dis* 148:339, 1993.

220. Jardin F, Genevray B, Pazin M, et al: Inability to titrate PEEP in patients with acute respiratory failure using end tidal carbon dioxide measurements. *Anesthesiology* 62:530, 1985.

221. Shapiro BA: In-vivo monitoring of arterial blood gases and pH. *Respir Care* 37:165, 1992.

222. Shapiro BA, Mahutte CK, Cane RD, et al: Clinical performance of a blood gas monitor: a prospective, multicenter trial. *Crit Care Med* 21:487, 1993.

223. Zimmerman JI, Dellinger RP: Initial evaluation of a new intraarterial blood gas system in humans. *Crit Care Med* 4:495, 1993.

224. Gutierrez G: Cellular energy metabolism during hypoxia. *Crit Care Med* 19:619, 1991.

225. Bergofsky EM: Determination of tissue O_2 tensions by hollow visceral tonometers: effects of breathing enriched O_2 mixtures. *J Clin Invest* 43:193, 1964.

226. Dawson AM, Trenchard D, Guz A: Small bowel tonometry: assessment of small gut mucosal oxygen tension in dog and man. *Nature* 206:943, 1965.

227. Kivisaari J, Niinikoski J: Use of Silastic tube and capillary sampling technic in the measurement of tissue pO_2 and pCO_2. *Am J Surg* 125:623, 1973.

228. Fiddian-Green RG, Pittenger G, Whitehouse WM: Back-diffusion of CO_2 and its influence on the intramural pH in gastric mucosa. *J Surg Res* 33:39, 1982.

229. Fiddian-Green RG: Tonometry: theory and applications. *Intensive Care World* 9:1, 1992.

230. Hartmann M, Montgomery A, Jonsson K, et al: Tissue oxygenation in hemorrhagic shock measured as transcutaneous oxygen tension, subcutaneous oxygen tension, and gastric intramucosal pH in pigs. *Crit Care Med* 19:205, 1991.

231. Gutierrez G: Advances in ICU monitoring. Presented at the Annual Meeting of the American College of Chest Physicians, Chicago, October, 1992.

232. Fiddian-Green RG: Should the measurements of tissue pH and pO_2 be included in the routine monitoring of intensive care unit patients? *Crit Care Med* 19:141, 1991.

233. Fiddian-Green RG, Baker S: Predictive value of the stomach wall pH for complications after cardiac operations: comparison with other monitoring. *Crit Care Med* 15:153, 1987.

234. Landow L, Phillips DA, Heard SO, et al: Gastric tonometry and venous oximetry in cardiac surgery patients. *Crit Care Med* 19:1226, 1991.

235. Shiedler MG, Cutler BS, Fiddian-Green RG: Sigmoid intramural pH for prediction of ischemic colitis during aortic surgery. *Arch Surg* 122:881, 1987.
236. Gutierrez G, Bismar H, Dantzker DR, et al: Comparison of gastric intramucosal pH with measures of oxygen transport and consumption in critically ill patients. *Crit Care Med* 20:451, 1992.
237. Fiddian-Green RG, McGough E, Pittenger G: Predictive value of intramural pH and other risk factors for massive bleeding from stress ulceration. *Gastroenterology* 85:613, 1983.
238. Gutierrez G, Palizas F, Doglio G, et al: Gastric intramucosal pH as a therapeutic index of tissue oxygenation in critically ill patients. *Lancet* 1339:195, 1992.
239. Bohrer H, Schmidt H, Motsch J, et al: Gastric intramucosal pH: a predictor of survival in cardiac surgery patients with low cardiac output? *J Cardiothorac Vasc Anesth* 11:184, 1997.
240. Duke TD, Butt W, South M: Predictors of mortality and multiple organ failure in children with sepsis. *Intensive Care Med* 23:684, 1997.
241. Joynt GM, Lipman J, Gomersall CD, et al: Gastric intramucosal pH and blood lactate in severe sepsis. *Anaesthesia* 52:726, 1997.
242. Knichwitz G, Kuhmann M, Brodner G, et al: Gastric tonometry: precision and reliability are improved by a phosphate buffered solution. *Crit Care Med* 24:512, 1996.
243. Heard SO, Helsmoortel CM, Kent JC, et al: Gastric tonometry in healthy volunteers: effect of ranitidine on calculated intramural pH. *Crit Care Med* 19:271, 1991.
244. Eddleston JM, Vohra A, Scott P, et al: A comparison of stress ulceration and secondary pneumonia in sucralfate or ranitidine treated intensive care unit patients. *Crit Care Med* 19:1491, 1991.
245. Taylor DE, Gutierrez G: Tonometry: a review of clinical studies. *Crit Care Clin* 12:1007, 1996.
246. Marik PE, Lorenzana A: Effect of tube feedings on the measurement of gastric intramucosal pH. *Crit Care Med* 24:1498, 1996.

27. Indirect Calorimetry

Nicholas A. Smyrnios and
Frederick J. Curley

Indirect calorimetry is a technique that uses measurements of inspired and expired gas flows, volumes, and concentrations to calculate oxygen consumption and carbon dioxide production. Oxygen consumption and caloric expenditure are determined by directly measuring inhaled and exhaled gases and analyzing them with a computerized metabolic cart. Energy expenditure, respiratory quotient (RQ), and other values can be derived from the measured values. By contrast, *direct calorimetry* measures energy by quantitating the person's heat production. Because it requires placing the person in a thermally isolated whole-body enclosure for more than 1 hour [1], it is virtually impossible to use in a critical care setting. Therefore, the indirect method is much more suitable to the intensive care environment. Indirect calorimetry provides a noninvasive, accurate method of measuring caloric requirements and oxygen consumption. It should be the preferred technique when measurements of oxygen consumption and energy expenditure are needed in the intensive care unit (ICU). This chapter focuses on the technique of performing indirect calorimetry in the ICU setting. Chapters 197, 198, and 199 more fully discuss the use of energy expenditure estimates to determine caloric requirements in the critically ill.

Theoretical Basis of Indirect Calorimetry

Indirect calorimetry systems rely on measures of inhaled and exhaled air flow, volume, and concentrations of oxygen and carbon dioxide. Indirect calorimetry systems can be classified as *open-circuit systems*, which measure the difference between inspired and expired gas concentrations, or *closed-circuit systems*, which measure changes in the amount of gases in a fixed reservoir over time [2]. This chapter reviews only open-circuit systems because most ICUs use this technique.

DEFINITIONS. Chemical energy used to fuel the human body is directly provided by adenosine triphosphate, which is formed by the oxidation of carbohydrate, protein, and lipid. The stores of adenosine triphosphate in the body are small, but they are in a constant, high-volume, well-balanced state of formation and utilization. Indirect calorimetry measures the oxygen used and carbon dioxide produced when carbohydrate, protein, and lipid are oxidized to produce adenosine triphosphate. Therefore, it is the production of chemical energy that is indirectly measured by the gas exchange parameters. Despite this, it is the convention to describe this quantity as energy expended. Therefore, we use the term *energy expenditure* to describe the amount of energy measured by indirect calorimetry.

In any discussion of energy expenditure, it is important to define what level of energy expenditure is being considered. Basal metabolic rate or basal energy expenditure (BEE) is the energy used by the body at complete rest and in the postabsorptive state (absence of active nutritional intake for at least 4 to 6 hours). This measurement can be obtained reliably only in deep sleep. If such a measurement is made, BEE takes into account the effects of illness and stress. However, BEE often is taken to be a value calculated from a standardized equation that does not account for stress, such as the Harris-Benedict equation. Resting energy expenditure (REE) is obtained from an awake person at rest and includes the energy used at rest in the awake state plus the energy used to metabolize foodstuffs, also called *diet-induced thermogenesis*. It is expected to be approximately 10% greater than BEE [3–5]. Total energy expenditure (TEE) is REE plus the energy used during activity. For most ICU patients, we wish to know the 24-hour REE or TEE rather than the BEE.

CALCULATION OF ENERGY EXPENDITURE. Most indirect calorimetry systems use the modified Weir equation to calculate energy expenditure. In its more complete form, this equation uses oxygen consumption ($\dot{V}O_2$), carbon dioxide production ($\dot{V}CO_2$), and nonprotein urinary nitrogen (UN):

Energy expenditure = $3.9(\dot{V}O_2) - 1.1(\dot{V}CO_2) - 2.17(UN \ g/day)$

The Weir equation is not experimentally derived from measurements on humans but is mathematically derived based on physiologic facts. The derivation relies on the knowledge that (a) TEE is equal to the sum of the energy expended from the combustion of carbohydrate, fat, and protein; (b) the caloric equivalents of glucose (3.7 kcal per g), fat (9.5 kcal per g), and protein (4.1 kcal per g) are known; (c) the oxygen consumed and carbon dioxide produced in metabolizing each of these fuels is known; and (d) therefore, the equation for energy expenditure can be expressed in terms of oxygen consumption and carbon dioxide production by solving the system of equations that describes the stoichiometry of fuel combustion. The reader is referred to other sources for a complete derivation of the equation [6]. In practice, the amount of urea nitrogen in the urine is sometimes not measured because of the inconvenience of measurement and the fact that its contribution to TEE is considered minimal.

CALCULATION OF OXYGEN CONSUMPTION. The essential measurements of indirect calorimetry are the inspired and expired oxygen fractions (FIO_2 and FEO_2, respectively), carbon dioxide fractions ($FICO_2$ and $FECO_2$, respectively), and minute ventilation. Oxygen consumption and carbon dioxide production can be calculated using similar equations, which compute the difference between inspired (I) and expired (E) volumes:

Oxygen consumption = $\dot{V}O_2 = \dot{V}I(FIO_2) - \dot{V}E(FEO_2)$

Carbon dioxide production = $\dot{V}CO_2 = \dot{V}E(FECO_2) - \dot{V}I(FICO_2)$

To avoid the need to measure the concentrations and volumes of expiratory and inspiratory gases, techniques that preferentially measure only the expiratory gases have been developed. Most systems measure only exhaled volumes and mathematically derive the inhaled volume. Any assumption that the volume exhaled is equal to the volume inhaled is erroneous whenever $\dot{V}CO_2$ and $\dot{V}O_2$ are not equal (i.e., RQ is not equal to 1) and becomes more erroneous as FIO_2 increases. A mathematic relationship of $\dot{V}E$ to $\dot{V}I$ called the *Haldane transformation* can be used to explain this phenomenon. It takes advantage of the fact that nitrogen is an essentially inert gas. Therefore,

Volume inspired ($\dot{V}I$) × FIN_2 = volume expired ($\dot{V}E$) × FEN_2

Rearranged, this reads

$\dot{V}I = \dot{V}E \times FEN_2 / FIN_2$

Because $FIO_2 + FIN_2 = 1$ and $FEO_2 + FECO_2 + FEN_2 = 1$,

$FIN_2 = 1 - FIO_2$

and

$FEN_2 = 1 - FECO_2 - FEO_2$

If we substitute back into the previous equation,

$$\dot{V}I = \dot{V}E \times \frac{(1 - FECO_2 - FEO_2)}{1 - FIO_2}$$

As the inspired oxygen concentration increases, the denominator decreases and the difference between inspired and expired gas volume becomes greater. The Haldane equation can therefore be used to determine the value of $\dot{V}I$ without measuring inspired volume. The accuracy of the Haldane equation in estimating inspired volume, and thereby oxygen consumption and energy expenditure, therefore depends greatly on the accuracy of measurement of FIO_2 and $\dot{V}E$. Any error in measuring exhaled volumes or gas concentrations directly produces an error of a greater magnitude in the calculation of oxygen consumption, carbon dioxide production, or energy expenditure. At a minute ventilation of 10 L per minute and an inspired-to-expired oxygen concentration difference of 0.03, the oxygen consumption would be 300 mL per minute. If the FIO_2 was measured to be 0.46 instead or 0.45 and the FEO_2 remained at 0.42, the oxygen consumption would be 400 mL per minute, a 33% change. If the measured minute ventilation was 10.1 L per minute and the actual value was 10 L per minute, there would be an error in the oxygen consumption of 30 mL per minute, or 10%. The analysis system must be free of leaks, and extremely accurate sensors must be used. Most oxygen sensors are less accurate at higher FIO_2. Because of the difficulty in obtaining accurate measures at higher FIO_2, most indirect calorimetry studies are usually limited to patients on 60% oxygen or less. Although some systems have provided accurate results *in vitro* with higher levels of oxygen, no system has proved its accuracy at higher levels in clinical trials on critically ill adults [7,8].

CALCULATION OF SUBSTRATE USE. Indirect calorimetry can be used to determine what percentage of energy expenditure comes from each of the major foodstuffs. Once carbon dioxide production and oxygen consumption have been measured, their relationship and a measure of protein metabolism can be used to solve mathematically for the percentage of calories burned derived from fat or carbohydrate (CHO) [9]. The equations used for these calculations are [10]

CHO (g) = $4.113 \ \dot{V}CO_2 - 2.907 \ \dot{V}O_2 - 2.544 \ UN$ (g/day)

FAT (g) = $1.689 \ (\dot{V}CO_2 - \dot{V}O_2) - 1.943 \ UN$ (g/day)

Protein (g) = $6.25 \ (UN + 4)$ (g/day)

These calculations yield only an estimate of substrate use. Important items to be remembered from this exercise include

1. The amount of protein catabolized in a day can be estimated to be the sum of UN and daily losses from skin and stool, assumed to be approximately 4 g per day, multiplied by 6.25.
2. The RQ is the ratio of carbon dioxide produced to oxygen consumed, or $\dot{V}O_2$ to $\dot{V}CO_2$.
3. The primary foodstuffs have established RQs: fat, 0.7; protein, 0.8; and carbohydrate, 1.0. Because a combination of processes is almost always occurring, the normal range of RQ is from 0.7 to 1.0. RQs greater than 1.0 indicate that the net outcome of all the reactions occurring is the synthesis of fat (lipogenesis). Values less than 0.7 may be encountered when ketones are the primary fuel.

Equipment and Technique

Open-circuit indirect calorimetry systems all involve certain basic components, typically an oxygen analyzer, a carbon dioxide analyzer, and a flowmeter (usually a pneumotach). Various systems include masks, canopies, mixing chambers, tubing, desiccants, and pumps, and most have a personal computer with a monitor for graphic displays. We describe only the equipment necessary for the techniques discussed in this chapter.

METHODS OF MEASUREMENT. Oxygen sensors in commercially available systems are either zirconium or differential paramagnetic sensors. The zirconium oxide sensor is coated with an oxygen-permeable substance. At temperatures of approximately 800°C, oxygen diffuses across this outer layer and an electrical signal that is proportional to the partial pressure of oxygen is created [2,11]. Differential paramagnetic analyzers measure the difference in concentration of the gas between the inspiratory and expiratory lines. These analyzers typically have an accuracy of ±0.02% and a response time of 130 milliseconds or less. Essentially all available carbon dioxide analyzers are nondispersed infrared devices. A gas sample in the path of infrared energy creates an alteration in an electrical signal that is proportional to the concentration of carbon dioxide. These analyzers have an accuracy of ±0.02% with a response time of 110 milliseconds. Some systems measure inspired and expired carbon dioxide, and some measure only expired, assuming the inspired value to be negligible. Volume is measured by measuring flow and integrating the result over time to obtain volume. Flow is usually either measured with a pneumotach or a mass flow sensor or generated by the device and kept constant in response to changes in ventilation.

Gas concentrations are measured using one of three techniques: mixing chamber, breath by breath, and dilution. All devices must have well-validated calibration procedures for essential components. Newer machines have automated much of this process.

Mixing Chamber Method. The mixing chamber is the best-established method and has been considered the gold standard. A mixing chamber is an automated Douglas bag that mixes expired gases over a predetermined interval and provides the material to be sampled [11]. Expired gas is passed from a mouthpiece or the ventilator exhalation port into a collection chamber, which is in series with the flowmeter and gas analyzers. Inside the chamber, flow is interrupted by baffles to allow more even mixing of gases. A sample of mixed gas is withdrawn from the chamber, the gas concentrations analyzed, and the sample returned to the chamber. Depending on the design, the gas is either vented or passed through the flowmeter. The concentrations of inspiratory gas are sampled from the inspiratory side of a mouthpiece or a ventilator circuit. Inspiratory volumes are calculated from expiratory volumes as explained previously. A computer compares mixed expired versus inspired concentrations and multiplies by volume to yield a measure of consumption or production. The results reflect the values of gases mixed over time and are reported as values per time interval of measurement (e.g., milliliters of oxygen consumed per minute).

Breath-by-Breath Method. The collection and analysis of gases in the breath-by-breath method are similar to those in the mixing chamber technique, but each breath is analyzed. A sample of gases is taken for analysis from each inspiration and expiration. These samples are coupled with flow measurements for each breath to calculate $\dot{V}O_2$, $\dot{V}CO_2$, and REE. The concentrations of expiratory gases are measured directly from samples drawn from the expiratory side of the mouthpiece or ventilator circuit. Inspired concentrations are measured from samples drawn from the inspiratory side of a mouthpiece or ventilator circuit. Oxygen consumption and carbon dioxide production values are usually expressed as milliliters per minute and energy expenditure as kilocalories per day for each breath and can be averaged or summed over varying periods, depending on the clinician's needs. The crucial component in these measurements is the alignment of various signals. If the time needed for the gases to reach the analyzer and the expiratory flow to reach the flowmeter is known, the $\dot{V}O_2$, $\dot{V}CO_2$, and $\dot{V}E$ signals can be precisely aligned and accurate measurements made.

Instruments that use breath-by-breath analysis align the signals automatically by computer. Improper alignment can render the measurements useless. Oxygen and carbon dioxide sensors must have a very rapid response time. The placement of the gas analysis line just distal to the endotracheal tube can standardize transit time and eliminate artifact, which assists in this process.

Dilution Method. The dilution method is the only technique that can be used in intubated patients as well as nonintubated patients who cannot use a mouthpiece. A predetermined flow of gas of known oxygen and carbon dioxide concentration passes through a face shield mask or a hood-like canopy. The exhaled gases are diluted into the passing stream of known gas. The amount of gas the machine puts into the stream is adjusted to keep the flow constant as the patient alters his or her own ventilation. Samples of the diluted gases are removed for analysis and the values obtained multiplied by the flow rate to yield a measure of volume. Oxygen consumption and carbon dioxide production are calculated by comparing concentrations in and out of the system.

FACTORS AFFECTING ACCURACY. Accurate measurements require close attention to technique. Several problems are frequently encountered in the ICU setting. In the mixing chamber or breath-by-breath method, even a small error in measuring volume can produce a large error in calculated values. All connections to the metabolic cart and in the ventilator circuit must be checked for leaks. In intubated patients, it may be necessary to eliminate the small leak at the endotracheal tube cuff by overdistending the cuff for the brief duration of the study. It may be impossible to eliminate this leak in patients with high peak pressures. In dilution method systems, leaks in the mixing chamber and in the sampling lines may produce discrepancies between the programmed flow and the actual flow, leading to overestimation of $\dot{V}O_2$ and $\dot{V}CO_2$ [12]. In all techniques, an error in measuring oxygen or carbon dioxide concentrations leads to larger errors in the subsequently calculated values. If the patient's oxygen source produces any variation in FIO_2, inspiratory concentrations of oxygen must be continuously measured. If the equipment is not capable of this, a high-quality blender or tank of oxygen of known concentration can be used for the testing period. Any change in inspired oxygen concentration during the study renders the measurements invalid until the inspired oxygen concentration is remeasured.

Inspired and expired gas concentrations are typically sampled with long, narrow tubes leading from taps into the respiratory circuit. Tubing can easily clog with patient secretions and invalidate collected data. Most systems also somehow condition the gas from these sample tubings to standardize for temperature and water vapor. Failure to follow the manufacturer's advice on desiccant change or timing of tubing change alters the accuracy of the data.

Care must also be taken to interface the metabolic cart with the ventilator and associated equipment carefully. Disruption of the normal ventilator circuit with inappropriately placed sampling devices may lead to ventilator malfunction or trigger alarms. All connections to ventilators must be according to manufacturer's specifications. Inappropriate location of sampling tubes may also lead to artifacts in flow or concentration measurements. The use of positive end-expiratory pressure may variably alter the ventilator circuit compressible volume, leading to errors in volume and concentration measurements. Techniques to isolate sensors from the effects of positive end-expiratory pressure have been incorporated into the latest generation of equipment.

Traditionally, children have not been monitored with indirect calorimetry because of leaks due to uncuffed endotracheal tubes, frequent use of high-frequency ventilation, and the common use of high FIO_2 and low ventilator flows. Studies indicate that certain dilution method devices may be accurate in children at moderate levels of FIO_2 [13]. No equipment has yet been validated with high-frequency or oscillator ventilation.

Very few measures can be used to determine whether the data obtained are reliable. The RQ can act as a quality control when the values obtained are outside the physiologic range (approximately 0.65 to 1.30 in the ICU) [2]. Data averaged over 30 to 60 seconds can be used to determine whether the degree of variability is physiologic. Inspiratory values, which should be stable, should be frequently measured and displayed during the test. When inspiratory values are not monitored frequently, leaks in the inspiratory circuit lower FIO_2 values, falsely lower oxygen consumption and energy expenditure measurements, and falsely elevate RQ. Leaks in the expiratory circuit falsely decrease volume measurements. Leaks in the breath-by-breath sampling line produce marked variability in the derived values.

Uses of Indirect Calorimetry in the Intensive Care Unit

The primary role of indirect calorimetry in the ICU is to assess energy expenditure and nutritional requirements. Indirect calorimetry can also be used to measure oxygen consumption in shock states. The value of that is unproved. Indirect calorimetry is also useful for research into the pathophysiology of critical illness.

NUTRITIONAL ASSESSMENT. Inappropriate nutrition support causes problems in the critically ill. Malnutrition is associated with an increased mortality [14,15]. Inadequate caloric intake can cause muscle weakness, impaired immunity, and delayed wound healing [16,17]. Excess alimentation can lead to hyperglycemia, hepatic dysfunction, increased carbon dioxide production [18,19], increased minute ventilation ($\dot{V}E$), respiratory distress, and respiratory failure [20]. In most ICUs, the patient's caloric intake is determined by estimating a daily TEE. BEE is calculated from a standard equation and adjusted for level of illness, diet-induced thermogenesis, and amount of activity. Studies comparing this practice with measurement of energy expenditure by indirect calorimetry have inconsistent results. Some conclude that estimates of energy expenditure routinely overestimate caloric need [21–24]; others conclude that estimates of energy expenditure are inaccurate but in no consistent direction [25–27], and still others conclude that clinical estimates are as accurate as measured values [28–31]. The results may differ because of the different techniques and patient populations in each study.

Indirect calorimetry studies have no standard length and frequency. Studies from 5 minutes to 24 hours in duration have been used [24,32,33]. It has been shown that a 30-minute study can predict 24-hour energy expenditure well in medical ICU patients [34]. However, even if the test accurately determines that day's energy expenditure, it is unclear whether it can predict caloric need for subsequent days. Weissman et al. [35] found day-to-day changes of 12% to 46%, depending on the patient's clinical condition.

If energy expenditure can be measured more accurately than it can be estimated, does it alter clinical outcome? Some investigators believe providing an average energy requirement suffices for most patients and that indirect calorimetry can be reserved for the 10% to 20% with more complex nutritional problems [36]. Others believe that accurate determination of energy requirements is crucial [37]. This question could be answered by a randomized study comparing outcomes of large numbers of patients who have their caloric intake determined by traditional or indirect calorimetric methods.

SUBSTRATE USE. An elevated RQ may indicate excessive levels of carbohydrate metabolism or net lipogenesis due to excess calorie intake [19,20,38–40]. Although the impact of altering substrate composition has not been shown in most diseases, in complicated cases of hepatic or renal failure an analysis of substrate use can be used quickly to assess the efficacy of a change in diet.

OXYGEN CONSUMPTION. Indirect calorimetry was instrumental in demonstrating that the implied correlation of oxygen delivery (DO_2) and $\dot{V}O_2$ was due to mathematic coupling [41–45]. Similarly, reports that the use of $\dot{V}O_2$ is useful for mortality prediction or for description of lung metabolic activity have failed to demonstrate clinical utility [46].

Research and Future Applications

Although this discussion has focused primarily on the indirect calorimeter as a monitor of oxygen consumption and energy expenditure, other values measured by the calorimeter have potential value in the ICU. Many computerized indirect calorimetry systems permit inputs from other monitoring equipment into the system's computer. Values derived from the combination of device inputs have not been adequately studied to recommend routine clinical use. For example, the value of oxygen pulse, measured as oxygen consumption divided by heart rate, correlates well as an index of left ventricular stroke volume. The ventilatory equivalents of oxygen and carbon dioxide, calculated by dividing minute ventilation by oxygen consumption or carbon dioxide production, respectively, can serve as indices of ventilation-perfusion mismatch. As technology improves and high-quality equipment becomes more available, the use of indirect calorimeters as short-term monitors of complex physiologic changes resulting from disease and treatment may markedly increase.

References

1. McManus C, Newhouse H, Seitz S, et al: Human gradient-layer calorimeter: development of an accurate and practical instrument for clinical studies. *JPEN J Parenter Enteral Nutr* 8:317, 1984.
2. Branson RD: The measurement of energy expenditure: instrumentation, practical considerations, and clinical application. *Respir Care* 35:640, 1990.
3. Feurer ID, Crosby LO, Mullen JL: Measured and predicted resting energy expenditure in clinically stable patients. *Clin Nutr* 3:27, 1984.
4. Kinney J: Indirect calorimetry: the search for clinical relevance. *Nutr Clin Prac* 7:203, 1992.

5. Weissman C, Kemper M: Metabolic measurements in the critically ill. *Crit Care Clin* 11:169, 1995.
6. Ferrannini E: The theoretical bases of indirect calorimetry: a review. *Metabolism* 37:287, 1988.
7. Takala J, Keinanen O, Vaisanen P, et al: Measurement of gas exchange in intensive care: laboratory and clinical validation of a new device. *Crit Care Med* 17:1041, 1989.
8. Weissman C, Sardar A, Kemper M: An in vitro evaluation of an instrument designed to measure oxygen consumption and carbon dioxide production during mechanical ventilation. *Crit Care Med* 22:1995, 1994.
9. Bursztein S, Elwyn DH, Askanazi J, et al: *Energy Metabolism, Indirect Calorimetry, and Nutrition.* Baltimore, Williams & Wilkins, 1989.
10. Molina P, Burzstein S, Abumarad NN: Theories and assumptions on energy expenditure. *Crit Care Clin* 11:587,1995.
11. Teirlinck HC: Sensormedics 2900 metabolic measurement cart: technical and fundamental considerations in gas exchange measurements. *Cardiopulmonary Review* 1991 (Sensormedics Corporation publication, Yorba Linda, CA).
12. Bracco D, Chiolero R, Pasche O, et al: Failure in measuring gas exchange in the ICU. *Chest* 107:1406, 1995.
13. Joosten KF, Jacobs FI, van Klaarwater E, et al: Accuracy of an indirect calorimeter for mechanically ventilated infants and children: the influence of low rates of gas exchange and varying FIO_2. *Crit Care Med* 28:3014, 2000.
14. Apelgren KN, Rombeau JL, Twomey P, et al: Comparison of nutritional indices and outcome in critically ill patients. *Crit Care Med* 10:305, 1982.
15. Murray MJ, Marsh HM, Wochos DN, et al: Nutritional assessment of intensive care unit patients. *Mayo Clin Proc* 63:1106, 1988.
16. Arora NS, Rochester DF: Respiratory muscle strength and maximal voluntary ventilation in undernourished patients. *Am Rev Respir Dis* 126:5, 1982.
17. Kahan BD: Nutrition and host defense mechanisms. *Surg Clin North Am* 61:557, 1981.
18. Askanazi J, Rosenbaum SH, Hyman AI, et al: Respiratory changes induced by the large glucose loads of total parenteral nutrition. *JAMA* 243:1444, 1980.
19. Gieske T, Gurushanthaiah G, Glauser FL: Effects of carbohydrates on carbon dioxide excretion in patients with airway disease. *Chest* 71:55, 1977.
20. Covelli HD, Black JW, Olsen MS, et al: Respiratory failure precipitated by high carbohydrate loads. *Ann Intern Med* 95:579, 1981.
21. Daly JM, Heymsfield SB, Head CA, et al: Human energy requirements: overestimation by widely used prediction equation. *Am J Clin Nutr* 42:1170, 1985.
22. Cortes V, Nelson LD: Errors in estimating energy expenditure in critically ill surgical patients. *Arch Surg* 124:287, 1989.
23. Mann S, Westenkow DR, Houtchens BA: Measured and predicted caloric expenditure in the acutely ill. *Crit Care Med* 13:173, 1985.
24. Makk LJK, McClave SA, Creech PW, et al: Clinical application of the metabolic cart to the delivery of total parenteral nutrition. *Crit Care Med* 18:1320, 1990.
25. Saffle JR, Medina E, Raymond J, et al: Use of indirect calorimetry in the nutritional management of burned patients. *J Trauma* 25:32, 1985.
26. Weissman C, Kemper M, Askanazi J, et al: Resting metabolic rate of the critically ill patient: measured versus predicted. *Anesthesiology* 64:673, 1986.
27. Smyrnios NA, Curley FJ, Jederlinic PJ, et al: Indirect calorimetry in the medical ICU: comparison with traditional practice and effect on cost of care. *Am Rev Respir Dis* 141:A581, 1990.
28. Hunter DC, Jaksic T, Lewis D, et al: Resting energy expenditure in the critically ill: estimations versus measurement. *Br J Surg* 75:875, 1988.
29. Van Lanschot JB, Feenstra BWA, Vermeij CG, et al: Calculation versus measurement of total energy expenditure. *Crit Care Med* 14:981, 1986.
30. Saffle JR, Larson CM, Sullivan J: A randomized trial of indirect calorimetry-based feedings in thermal injury. *J Trauma* 30:776, 1990.
31. Liggett SB, Renfro AD: Energy expenditures of mechanically ventilated nonsurgical patients. *Chest* 98:682, 1990.
32. Vermeij CG, Feenstra BW, Van Lanschot JB, et al: Day-to-day variability of energy expenditure in critically ill surgical patients. *Crit Care Med* 17:623, 1989.
33. Rumpler WV, Seale JL, Conway JM, et al: Repeatability of 24-h energy expenditure measurements in humans by indirect calorimetry. *Am J Clin Nutr* 51:147, 1990.
34. Smyrnios NA, Curley FJ, Shaker KG: Accuracy of 30 minute indirect calorimetry studies in predicting 24-hour energy expenditure in mechanically ventilated, critically ill patients. *JPEN J Parenter Enteral Nutr* 21:168, 1997.
35. Weissman C, Kemper M, Hyman AI: Variation in the resting metabolic rate of mechanically ventilated critically ill patients. *Anesth Analg* 68:457, 1989.
36. Bursztein S, Elwyn DH: Measured and predicted energy expenditure in critically ill patients. *Crit Care Med* 21:312, 1993.
37. Mullen JL: Indirect calorimetry in critical care. *Proc Nutr Soc* 50:239, 1991.
38. Herve P, Simmonneau G, Girard P, et al: Hypercapneic acidosis induced by nutrition in mechanically ventilated patients: glucose versus fat. *Crit Care Med* 13:537, 1985.
39. Sherman BW, Hamilton C, Panacek EA: Adequacy of early enteral nutrition support by the enteral route in patients with acute respiratory failure. *Chest* 98:104S, 1990.
40. Guenst JM, Nelson LD: Predictors of total parenteral nutrition induced lipogenesis. *Chest* 105:553, 1997.
41. Archie JP Jr: Mathematic coupling of data: a common source of error. *Ann Surg* 193:296, 1981.
42. Stratton HH, Feustel PJ, Newell JC: Regression of calculated variables in the presence of shared measurement error. *J Appl Physiol* 62:2083, 1987.
43. Ronco JJ, Fenwick JC, Wiggs BR, et al: Oxygen consumption is independent of increases in oxygen delivery by dobutamine in septic patients who have normal or increased plasma lactate. *Am Rev Respir Dis* 147:25, 1993.
44. Phang PT, Cunningham KF, Ronco JJ, et al: Mathematical coupling explains dependence of oxygen consumption on oxygen delivery in ARDS. *Am J Respir Crit Care Med* 150:308, 1994.
45. Yu M, Burchell S, Takiguchi SA, et al: The relationship of oxygen consumption measured by indirect calorimetry to oxygen delivery in critically ill patients. *J Trauma* 41:41, 1996.
46. deBoisblanc BP, McClarity E, Lord K: Oxygen consumption in the intensive care unit: indirect calorimetry is the way to go, but where? *Crit Care Med* 26:1153, 1998.

28. Interventional Radiology: Drainage Techniques

Ashley Davidoff

The intensive care unit (ICU) patient has unique clinical problems and most commonly presents to the radiologist with problems of sepsis. Often, the role of the radiologist is to identify the source of sepsis and to characterize and drain problematic collections. Once the source of sepsis is identified, imaging modalities can assist in further diagnostic evaluation as well as in therapy. Plain film, ultrasound, computed tomography (CT), and nuclear medicine are the tools at hand.

General Aims

Abnormal fluid collections may be a result of physiologic stasis (e.g., cholestasis) or pathologic accumulation (e.g., hematoma, urinoma, lymphocele, seroma), each of which may be complicated by secondary infection and abscess formation. The aim, therefore, is to characterize the abnormal fluid collection and drain infected collections safely.

Indications

The indications for imaging and intervention may be diagnostic or therapeutic. Accumulation of fluid may occur in normal (e.g., pleural space, peritoneal space) or abnormal [e.g., interloop collections (Fig. 28-1), dissecting pseudocysts (Fig. 28-2), anastomotic leakages] spaces. Normal fluid may accumulate in abnormal places (e.g., biloma, hematoma, urinoma). These collections are all within the capability of percutaneous drainage. Detection of these accumulations usually requires imaging, because clinical examination lacks sensitivity. Characterization of the fluid usually requires needle aspiration, because imaging modalities lack specificity. The presence of infection in any fluid accumulation in the abdomen is almost always an absolute indication for drainage. The most common indications for bedside imaging, aspiration, and drainage are presented in Table 28-1.

Contraindications

The contraindications to intervention mostly reflect risks that may supersede the advantages of the procedure. Contraindications that relate to patient safety include perforation of organs and bleeding, specifically of lung (with resultant pneumothorax), blood vessels, large bowel, pancreas, spleen, and small bowel (Fig. 28-1). Perforations by small-gauge needles (except of the lung) commonly have a benign course, but morbidity increases significantly when these organs are traversed with a drainage catheter. An important consideration when draining fluid accumulations in the abdominal cavity is the position of the pleural space, situated at the twelfth rib anteriorly and posteriorly and at the tenth rib along the midaxillary line. The pleural space is normally not visualized. Subacute or chronic secondary infection of the pleural space is usual when this space is traversed during catheter passage to the abdomen; therefore, drainage of an abdominal collection through the pleural space is contraindicated.

Attention to clotting factors is important before embarking on an invasive procedure. When the prothrombin time is 3 seconds longer than control, the partial thromboplastin time measures 50 seconds or more, the platelet count is less than 70,000, or the bleeding time is greater than 8 minutes, a procedure is relatively contraindicated [1,2]. Each case is weighed on its own merit, however, and more liberal allowance is often made for small-gauge needle procedures and superficial collections.

A second set of relative contraindications stems from limitations of the drainage procedure related to features of the disease process. Collections surrounded by bowel or bone cannot be safely accessed (Fig. 28-1). In the past, multilocular collections were considered a contraindication because of inability to drain all but the first abscess entered. It has been suggested that drainage of multilocular collections should be attempted because the loculations may communicate, may be mechanically broken by the catheter [3], or may be lysed chemically with urokinase [4,5].

The presence of more than three abscess cavities, fistulous tracts, and fungi was previously considered a contraindication to drainage, but some of these have become only relative contraindications. Many patients with these conditions are given a trial of percutaneous therapy if they can tolerate the time necessary to show a therapeutic response.

Under many circumstances, patients are not candidates for curative surgery or curative percutaneous drainage. Temporary drainage may allow partial recovery and make subsequent surgical treatment more feasible [6].

Risks

The risk of complication is low, with minor complications reported in 9.8% [7] and serious complications in 5.0% [8] of procedures. Risks include bleeding, perforation, and secondary infection. Death as a result of the procedure is rare, but mortality after the maneuver can be as high as 14.2%, with the cause of death attributed to sepsis and underlying multisystem disease rather than the procedure itself [7].

Benefits

The benefits of drainage include avoidance of surgery and anesthesia and the ability to mobilize immediately after the procedure. Drainage has a cure rate of 60% to 85% [1,7,9–11].

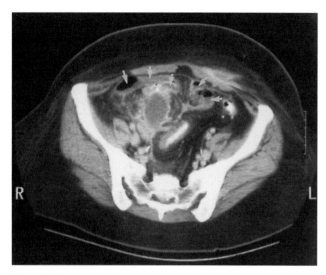

Fig. 28-1. Computed tomography scan demonstrating an interloop collection characterized by an enhancing rim and low-density center. Access to the collection through a drainage catheter is prohibited anteriorly by surrounding bowel loops (*arrows*) and posteriorly and laterally by the bony pelvis.

Method

PATIENT PREPARATION. Informed consent is imperative. Although most procedures are relatively safe, it is important that the patient and family understand the risks.

Prothrombin time, partial thromboplastin time, and the international normalized ratio are essential tests; platelet count and bleeding time are requested only if there are clinical concerns. For ultrasound, enteric nutrition should be discontinued 4 hours before the procedure because the introduction of air into the gastrointestinal tract or added peristalsis limits visualization. For CT, oral contrast is given 4 to 8 hours before the procedure. The contrast is a 2% solution, close to water. Unless there are contraindications to drinking water, the use of oral contrast is not contraindicated. Water-soluble contrast media (as opposed to barium-based solutions) are used in patients with suspected gastrointestinal leakage. Broad-spectrum antibiotic coverage is essential before procedures that involve infected collections and should be continued as dictated by the sensitivities of the bacteria.

EQUIPMENT AND SPECIAL NEEDS. Portable ultrasound is now well established as the workhorse for diagnostic and interventional procedures at the bedside. The overall strength of ultrasound in this setting is its portability and ability to identify and characterize fluid collections. It can provide very

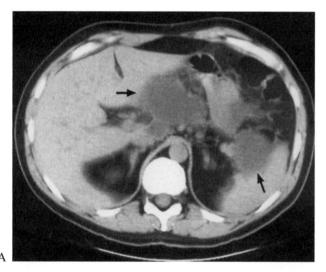

A

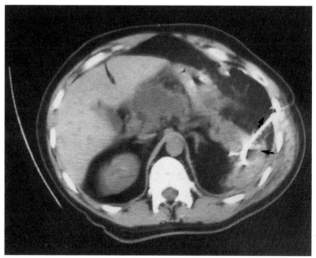

B

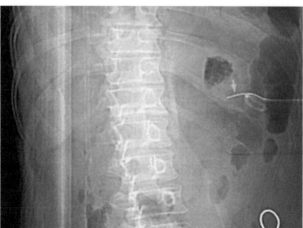

C

Fig. 28-2. A: Two pseudocysts superior to the pancreas (*arrows*), the first in the lesser sac and the second near the hilum of the spleen. **B:** Drainage of the latter was accomplished using an angled approach to avoid the spleen (*arrow*) and colon (*curved arrow*). Access to the first was accomplished using an unimpeded inferior approach. **C:** The scout film, performed after the first drainage, shows the catheter coiled and fixed in shape. The arrow indicates the safety guidewire that is left in place until the position of the catheter is deemed satisfactory.

Table 28-1. Indications for Imaging, Aspiration, and Drainage

Imaging
    Evaluation of the gallbladder for cholecystitis
    Evaluation of the pleural space for pleural fluid
    Evaluation of the peritoneal cavity for peritoneal fluid
Aspiration
    Thoracentesis for characterization of pleural fluid
    Paracentesis for characterization of peritoneal fluid
    Characterization of an intraabdominal fluid collection
Drainage
    Abscess drainage
    Cholecystostomy for acalculous cholecystitis

specific information in the ICU setting. Ultrasound is best used when the collection is superficial [pleural, peritoneal, or gallbladder (Fig. 28-3)]; CT is best used when the fluid is thought to be deeper in the peritoneal cavity or in the retroperitoneum (Fig. 28-2).

When the questions are of a global nature, such as ruling out abdominal abscess; when they relate to the retroperitoneum; or if the disease lies beyond bowel (Fig. 28-1), CT is the diagnostic and therapeutic tool of choice. Although ultrasound can portray needles and catheters as they pass through the tissues to the final target, CT is far more consistent in this regard. When a treacherous path has to be taken and bowel, spleen, and pleural space have to be avoided, CT is preferred (Fig. 28-2).

Procedures done in the ICU require the assistance of an ultrasound technologist and ICU nursing staff. Because sterile method is used, the ultrasound technologist is needed to operate the equipment. The nursing staff assists in monitoring the patient during the procedure, administers required analgesic and anxiolytic medication (see Chapter 25), maintains optimal patient positioning, and provides additional equipment as needed.

Kits for aspiration and drainage containing lidocaine, needles, syringes, test tubes, gloves, and vacutainers should be readily available. Needles, catheters, and guidewires should be selected in the radiology department because they are not usually available in the ICU.

Standard sterile precautions are used, including hand-washing and patient skin preparation using 10% povidone-iodine, sterile drapes, and sterile surgical gloves. If the Seldinger technique, in which guidewire exchange is usually cumbersome, is contemplated, gown, mask, and cap should be worn to prevent unintentional contamination.

A spinal needle is used for the initial aspiration. A conventional 22-gauge spinal needle with a 0.7-mm outside diameter does not accept the skinny guidewire (0.018 in.). Thus, if the Seldinger technique is used, the small-gauge needle used initially is of the manufacture that accepts the skinny wire. If the collection cannot be aspirated, a 20- or 18-gauge needle is used.

Appropriate tests are ordered on the aspirated fluid, depending on the indications for the procedure. A vacuum-protected culture medium is used for culture of fungi and aerobic and anaerobic bacteria.

A wide selection of guidewires is available. We routinely use the 15-cm Bentson guidewire (Cook, Bloomington, IN) with a flexible straight tip. When the Seldinger technique is used, a small-gauge stainless steel wire is used initially. A series of dilators should be available so that the Seldinger tract can be progressively dilated to 1 French (Fr) larger than the catheter to be inserted.

Many types of catheters are available. In general, we use 5- to 10-Fr catheters, depending on the character of the fluid aspirated. When the fluid is thin and not obviously infected, the 5-Fr catheter is adequate; the thicker the fluid, the larger the catheter used. The Luer lock at the end of the catheter is usually only 5- or 6-Fr, thus limiting the ability of even a 14-Fr

catheter. The tendency is to think that the largest catheter with a sump yields the best results, but we have not found this to be the case. We tend to place 7- to 9-Fr catheters without a sump, with comparable success.

TECHNIQUES

Diagnostic Aspirates. The key to successful diagnostic aspiration is a well-planned needle path. The site of insertion, angle of introduction, and depth of the needle are the three important factors to consider. A right-angle entry (needle to skin) and the shortest path to the collection are optimal but not always possible (Fig. 28-2). Real-time guided ultrasonography allows the path of the needle to be traced as it passes along the planned course. If aspiration is unsuccessful after the needle has been introduced, either the needle is placed incorrectly or the fluid is too thick to be aspirated through a small-gauge needle. The collection is imaged to identify the needle position; a larger-bore needle is usually substituted if the fluid is too thick for the small-gauge needle.

Drainage
INTRODUCTION OF THE CATHETER. The catheter is introduced by using either the trocar or the Seldinger technique. When the fluid collection appears to be easily accessible, the trocar technique is preferred. This technique is easier to perform but carries the risk of more severe complications if a viscus is perforated, because the hole produced by a catheter is larger than that from the first step in the Seldinger technique. Usually, a guiding small-gauge needle is used to sound out the direction and course of the final catheter path. Once the needle is placed, it is imaged and its placement revised until an optimal course has been accomplished. An attempt is made to aspirate the fluid to confirm appropriate placement and to evaluate the character and thickness. The aspirated fluid is evaluated to determine whether drainage is needed. Often, the referring physician's instructions are to drain if infected, leave if not. In practice, waiting 10 minutes for this decision is impractical, and late growth on a previously negative Gram's stain is common. We have adopted a policy of liberal placement of catheters, particularly if clinical suspicion is high and the fluid appears complex. If, on subsequent culture, no growth of organisms occurs, the catheter is removed. Secondary infection of a previously sterile collection is possible, but we have found that cautious and judicious use of this policy has been effective and uncomplicated, particularly when decisions are made in conjunction with the referring clinician.

The catheter is inserted alongside the guiding needle. Attention to depth of the collection, position of the sideholes in relation to this depth, and the final position and shape of the catheter are considerations at this stage.

In the Seldinger technique, needle, guidewire, and dilators are progressively introduced until an appropriate tract has been formed to allow for the final introduction of the catheter. In theory, it is the safer of the two procedures. However, when the procedure is performed under CT or ultrasound guidance, the needles, guidewires, dilators, and catheter cannot be optimally visualized in real time and the technique loses some of its advantage. It is the better method when the path to the collection is hazardous, the catheter size required is large, or fluoroscopic guidance is needed.

The considerations of catheter choice are similar to those outlined for the trocar technique. Once the collection has been entered and there is free drainage of fluid, careful manipulation is suggested. At this point, with free drainage of fluid from the catheter, it is useful to document the satisfactory position of the catheter (Figs. 28-2C and 28-3C). Distention of the abscess cavity by contrast, air, or aggressive manipulation

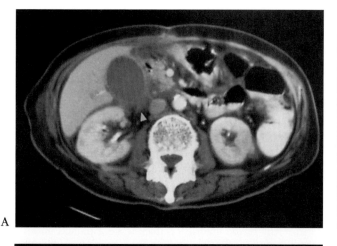

A

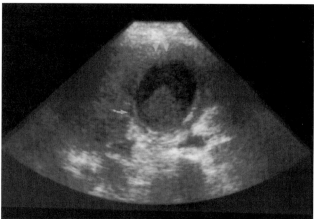

B

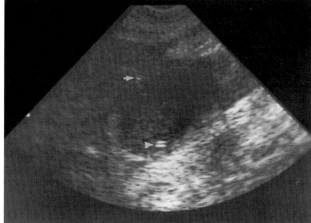

C

Fig. 28-3. **A:** Computed tomography scan demonstrating a distended gallbladder with a small amount of pericholecystic fluid (*arrow*) and induration of the surrounding fat (*arrowhead*), suggesting cholecystitis with extension of the inflammatory process or early perforation. **B:** Transverse ultrasound image of the gallbladder, confirming the presence of pericholecystic fluid (*arrow*), the rounded and distended shape of the gallbladder, and tumefactive bile in the lumen. A small amount of liver tissue anterior to the gallbladder (*arrowheads*) is the planned path to the gallbladder. **C:** Transverse ultrasound image of the gallbladder showing two echogenic foci. The first reflects the path of the catheter through the liver (*arrow*) and bare area of the gallbladder; the second (*arrowhead*) reflects the satisfactory intracystic position of the catheter.

is discouraged, to prevent bacteremia or septicemia that may originate from the inflamed and bleeding surface of the cavity. It is reasonable, however, to aspirate obviously purulent material, with the aim of evacuating the contents as completely as possible. The sudden appearance of blood-tinged material is usually an indication to discontinue aspiration and to rely on gravity drainage.

FIXING THE CATHETER. Anchoring the catheter with self-retaining locks is essential to prevent it from being accidentally pulled out. These locks consist of a string that threads through the catheter to its tip. When the string is pulled and fixed in position, the tension retains the pigtail in a fixed, rounded, more stable position. In addition, the catheter is fixed to the skin using a disk or belt. It is important to anchor the bag to the patient's clothing so that it does not put tension on the catheter.

Aftercare and Follow-Up. Frequent flushing of the catheter is necessary starting a few hours after insertion. Normal saline is injected initially in small amounts (5 to 10 mL) every 4 hours to flush the catheter and prevent clogging of the sideholes. After 24 hours, the aim of flushing is to agitate the dependent debris of the collection so that the sediment can eventually work its way into the catheter. Larger volumes, approximating the size of the cavity, are used to prevent the development of adhesions and loculation. We recommend 4-hourly flushing until the drainage fluid clears. When the fluid is too viscous to permit drainage, it can be liquefied with *N*-acetylcysteine [12]; loculations can be loosened by mechanical [3] or chemical means with urokinase [4,5].

Follow-up study of the abscess should be performed using CT or fluoroscopy 3 to 4 days after catheter insertion to eval-

uate the extent of the abscess and identify undrained collections and fistulous tracts. This is an important and often-ignored procedure. Frequently, the findings drastically alter management when unsuspected fistulous tracts are revealed, indicating the need for surgery.

Kinking, blockage by debris, and dislodgment of the catheter are common causes of failed drainage. The interventional team should evaluate daily for these problems.

When to Remove the Catheter. Once the patient has defervesced (usually within 24 hours), the cavity has decompressed (5 to 10 days), antibiotics are discontinued, and drainage has ceased or is minimal, it is recommended that the three-way stopcock of the catheter be turned off to the patient and a trial of 24 hours with the patient off antibiotics be performed. If fever, leukocytosis, or reaccumulation of fluid occurs, the catheter should be left in. Otherwise, it can be withdrawn.

Expected Results

Defervescence usually occurs within 24 hours but may take up to 4 to 5 days. Successful drainage may take 2 weeks or even longer. Successful drainage and cure are usually accomplished in 60% to 85% of patients [1,7,9,13,14], with partial success attained in 7% to 18% [10,11]. The procedure fails in 8% to 20% of patients [7,8,10,11] and must be repeated in 2.1% [7].

Minor complications occur in 9.8% [7] and serious complications in 5.0% [8]. Mortality after the procedure ranges from

1.4% to 14.2% [3,8,13], although most groups who report mortality after the procedure suggest that death was due not to the technique but to the patient's severely compromised condition.

Special Circumstances

CHOLECYSTOSTOMY. A cholestatic situation exists in most ICU patients, and distention of the gallbladder is common. Cholecystostomy is indicated in the patient with a distended gallbladder and sepsis of unknown origin (Fig. 28-3). This relatively simple procedure is safe when performed by an experienced physician, and can be performed at the bedside. The trocar technique, using the liver as a window to the gallbladder fossa, is our method of choice. Special attention should be paid to the exact depth of the gallbladder because there is little room for error. If the catheter is advanced too far, it may perforate the wall, with resultant bile peritonitis. The bile in acalculous cholecystitis is black (like crank-case oil) and does not appear grossly purulent. Frequently, neither organisms nor white cells are present, and the real test of successful drainage is the patient's subsequent clinical course.

EMPYEMA. The percutaneous insertion of large chest tubes by a thoracic surgeon is the procedure of choice for empyemas in our institution (see Chapter 11). Occasionally, small, inaccessible empyemas require imaging guidance. Special considerations for this procedure include the use of a large-bore catheter and underwater seal and care to prevent introduction of air through the needles and catheters into the pleural space, because inspiratory effort by the patient causes a negative intrathoracic pressure. Urokinase has been used in the pleural space to lyse loculated collections [4,5].

PSEUDOCYSTS. Percutaneous drainage has an 80% cure rate and is an effective front-line treatment for most pancreatic pseudocysts, whether the collection is sterile or infected. It is particularly suitable for the ICU patient. Cure is likely if sufficient time is allowed for closure of fistulas from the pancreatic duct [6]. Because low-output fistulas are present in 44% of patients [2], it is recommended that the catheter be maintained for an average of 7 weeks, sometimes longer. Paradoxically, infected pseudocysts require a shorter period. Duvnjak et al.

[14] suggest that the amylase concentration in the pseudocyst correlates to some degree with the potential for cure and recommend that this level be evaluated during the course of drainage.

References

1. Ferrucci JT, Wittenberg J, Mueller PR, et al. (eds): *Interventional Radiology of the Abdomen*. 2nd ed. Baltimore, Williams & Wilkins, 1985.
2. Kandarpa K: *Handbook of Cardiovascular and Interventional Radiologic Procedures*. Boston, Little, Brown, 1989.
3. Lang EK, Springer RM, Glorioso LW, et al: Abdominal abscess drainage under radiologic guidance: causes of failure. *Radiology* 159:329, 1986.
4. Couser JI Jr, Berley J, Timm EG: Intrapleural urokinase for loculated effusion. *Chest* 101:1467, 1992.
5. Lieberman RP, Hahn FJ, Imray TJ, et al: Loculated abscesses: management by percutaneous fracture of septations. *Radiology* 161:827, 1986.
6. van Sonnenberg E, Mueller PR, Ferrucci JT Jr: Percutaneous drainage of 250 abdominal abscesses and fluid collections: I. Results, failures, and complications. *Radiology* 151:337, 1984.
7. Kerlan RK Jr, Jeffrey RB Jr, Pogany AC, et al: Abdominal abscess with low-output fistula: successful percutaneous drainage. *Radiology* 155:73 1985.
8. Lambiase RE, Deyoe L, Cronan JJ, et al: Percutaneous drainage of 335 consecutive abscesses: results of primary drainage with 1-year follow-up. *Radiology* 184:167, 1992.
9. Brolin RE, Flancbaum L, Ercoli FR, et al: Limitations of percutaneous catheter drainage of abdominal abscesses. *Surg Gynecol Obstet* 173:203, 1991.
10. Gerzof SG, Johnson WC: Radiographic aspects of diagnosis and treatment of abdominal abscesses. *Surg Clin North Am* 64:53, 1984.
11. Moulton JS, Moore PT, Mencini RA: Treatment of loculated pleural effusions with transcatheter intracavitary urokinase. *AJR Am J Roentgenol* 153:941, 1989.
12. van Sonnenberg E, Wittich GR, Casola G, et al: Percutaneous drainage of infected and noninfected pancreatic pseudocysts: experience in 101 cases. *Radiology* 170:757, 1989.
13. Dahnert W, Gunther R, Klose K, et al: Results of percutaneous abscess drainage. *ROFO. Fortschr Geb Röntgenstrahlen Nuklearmed Erganzungsbd* 139:400, 1983.
14. Duvnjak M, Vucelic B, Rotkvic I, et al: Assessment of value of pancreatic pseudocyst amylase concentration in the treatment of pancreatic pseudocysts by percutaneous evacuation. *J Clin Ultrasound* 20:183, 1992.

29. Lung Biopsy

Scott E. Kopec, A. Alan Conlan, and Richard S. Irwin

Overview

Lung biopsy is indicated whenever it is necessary to obtain a definitive diagnosis of a localized or diffuse pulmonary dis-

ease, usually after noninvasive diagnostic modalities have been used unsuccessfully.

Multiple lung biopsy techniques are available that have been well characterized with regard to tissue yield, diagnostic yield, complications, contraindications, and mortality rate. The relative usefulness of a particular biopsy technique depends not only on the availability of local expertise, but also on the clinical situation. Each of the commonly used biopsy procedures is briefly described, and an approach to the lung biopsy procedure in the critically ill patient that focuses on the following questions is outlined: (a) When should a lung biopsy be considered in the critically ill patient? (b) Which biopsy technique should be chosen? (c) How should the specimens be handled?

Biopsy Procedures

GENERAL CONSIDERATIONS. Lung biopsy procedures can be grouped into two broad categories: open (i.e., surgical) and closed (i.e., nonsurgical). The major distinction between the two is that closed procedures avoid major surgical intervention and general anesthesia at the expense of a lower likelihood of obtaining a definitive diagnosis. Contraindications and relative contraindications for open and closed lung biopsy procedures are listed in Table 29-1 [1–8].

OPEN THORACOTOMY LUNG BIOPSY. Because thoracotomy allows the surgeon to obtain relatively large specimens of lung tissue under direct observation, open lung biopsy is a consistently accurate lung biopsy technique. The procedure requires endotracheal intubation, general anesthesia, and pleural catheter drainage for at least 24 hours after the biopsy. A "conventional" open thoracotomy, using a posterolateral incision, is used when hilar adenopathy is present or uneven parenchymal infiltrates exist [9]. A more limited or "modified" open thoracotomy is preferred in other situations [9]. Although

Table 29-1. Contraindications and Relative Contraindications to Lung Biopsy

Open thoracotomy biopsy
   Contraindication: too ill to undergo general anesthesia
Thoracoscopic lung biopsy [1]
   Contraindications
     Too ill to undergo general anesthesia
     Extensive pleural adhesions
     Uncorrectable coagulopathy
     Patients with a single lung
   Relative contraindication: inability to place a double-lumen endotracheal tube
Closed biopsy [2–8]
   Contraindications
     Uncorrectable coagulopathy[a] (including uremia)
     Unstable cardiovascular status
     Severe hypoxia likely to worsen during bronchoscopy
     Inadequately trained bronchoscopist
     Poor patient cooperation
   Relative contraindications
     Recent myocardial infarction or unstable angina
     Nearby vascular abnormalities
     Positive-pressure ventilation
     Cavitating lesions (especially with air-fluid levels or >10 cm diameter)
     Severe pulmonary hypertension
     Emphysematous lung disease surrounding area to be biopsied
     Suspected echinococcal disease
     Uncontrollable cough

[a]Bronchoalveolar lavage can be performed safely in patients with severe thrombocytopenia.

the modified procedure limits the area from which the biopsy can be obtained, it does not require rib resection and uses a small anterior incision. The following interventions maximize diagnostic yield [10]. First, average, rather than normal or markedly abnormal, lung tissue should be preferentially sampled. Second, in cases of diffuse pulmonary disease, more than one site should be sampled, if possible. Third, areas corresponding to ground-glass appearance on high-resolution chest tomography should be biopsied, as they are more likely to reveal the inflammatory process [11]. Although some authors believe that biopsies of the tip of the lingula or right middle lobe should be avoided because prior scarring, inflammation, and passive congestion of a nonspecific nature are likely to occur in these sites [12], a recent study refutes this [10].

THORACOSCOPIC LUNG BIOPSY. Thoracoscopy is a percutaneous procedure that involves the endoscopic exploration and sampling of the contents of the thoracic cavity [1,10,13,14]. Unlike the other percutaneous procedures, thoracoscopic lung biopsy is considered a surgical procedure. Although there are a variety of potential uses for thoracoscopy, only lung biopsy is highlighted here. Thoracoscopic lung biopsy involves multiple small chest wall incisions and a controlled pneumothorax to collapse the lung. One incision allows the insertion of a sterile fiberoptic endoscope to visualize the lung and pleural surfaces. A biopsy device is inserted through another incision and guided by direct endoscopic vision/video monitoring. Multiple points of entry may be necessary to determine the ideal endoscopic approach.

An advantage of thoracoscopy is that it can obtain a larger piece of lung tissue than bronchoscopy techniques, equal in size to that obtained at open lung biopsy. Where available, it is the open procedure of choice for patients in stable condition who are not requiring mechanical ventilation. Some authors caution that ventilator-dependent patients should not routinely undergo biopsy procedures by thoracoscopy because they typically cannot tolerate the change to a double-lumen endotracheal tube or the single-lung ventilation technique (Table 29-1). The authors individualize the decision.

Although several studies of non–critically ill patients with interstitial lung disease demonstrated that thoracoscopy and open lung biopsy were identical in providing the diagnosis and complications [15–18], the authors are unaware of any study that compares open lung biopsy with thoracoscopic biopsy in critically ill patients. Due to the absolute and relative contraindications of thoracoscopic lung biopsy, critically ill patients on mechanical ventilation should preferentially undergo an open procedure.

CLOSED BIOPSY PROCEDURES

Percutaneous Transthoracic Needle Aspiration Biopsy. This procedure involves the insertion, under guidance of fluoroscopy or computed tomography, of a sterile needle through the chest wall into the area of the lung to be sampled [19]. Needles of varying sizes (18-, 20-, 22-, and 24- to 25-gauge) can be used. In general, the thinner the needle, the fewer the complications [20]. A specimen is obtained by aspiration; it usually consists of cells (e.g., neoplastic, parenchymal, inflammatory), tissue fluids, or small tissue fragments. The major advantage of this procedure is that it can be easily performed with local anesthesia. The major disadvantage is that lung architectural integrity is usually not maintained in the specimen.

Bronchoscopic Procedures. A variety of techniques, including bronchial and transbronchial biopsy, bronchial brushing, transbronchial needle aspiration, and bronchoalveolar lavage (BAL), can be easily and safely performed with the flexible bronchoscope. A detailed discussion of flexible bronchoscopy is presented in Chapter 12.

TRANSBRONCHIAL LUNG BIOPSY. Transbronchial lung biopsy is performed by passing the bronchoscope to the segmental level, instilling a dilute solution of epinephrine, and then advancing flexible biopsy forceps into the radiographically abnormal area [7]. The forceps usually are advanced under fluoroscopic guidance. They are passed in the closed position until resistance is met or the patient signals that he or she has chest (pleural) pain. If pain is felt, the forceps are withdrawn in 1-cm increments until pain is no longer perceived. If no pain is felt, the forceps are opened, pressure is gently applied, and the forceps are closed. If no chest pain is felt, the forceps are then removed. As soon as the biopsy is taken, the endoscope is wedged into the airway from which the biopsy was taken to tamponade any potential bleeding and to prevent any blood from spilling out into other airways. Synchronization of the biopsy to the respiratory phase has affected neither the amount of alveolar tissue obtained nor the integrity of the specimen [21]. Because specimens are small (not greater than 3.9 mm² on average [21]), multiple specimens should be obtained to maximize the yield of this technique.

BRONCHIAL BRUSH BIOPSY. Using a flexible wire brush, the operator performs a bronchial brush biopsy in a manner similar to forceps biopsy [22–23]. Usually under fluoroscopic guidance, the brush is passed as far as possible into the radiographically abnormal area. The usefulness of this method is limited by the fact that only cellular material can be obtained and, in general, only endobronchial processes are sampled. A nodule not in communication with the bronchial tree cannot be entered with the brush, even though the nodule can be sampled with a needle passed transthoracically.

TRANSBRONCHIAL NEEDLE ASPIRATION. Transbronchial needle aspiration technique allows the clinician to pierce the walls of airways and aspirate cellular contents and tissue fluid or processes not in communication with the tracheobronchial tree. Specially designed catheters with attached needles are passed through the suction channel of the bronchoscope to the abnormal area [8,24,25]. As long as the vascularity of the area to be aspirated is appreciated or has been defined, transbronchial puncture with aspiration can be safely performed [26]. This procedure has a role in the diagnosis and staging of lung cancer and in the diagnosis of some benign mediastinal diseases, such as bronchogenic cysts. When appropriately applied and with good cytopathologic support, this procedure can eliminate the need for surgical staging in a substantial number of patients with inoperable lung cancer [27,28].

BRONCHOALVEOLAR LAVAGE. BAL is a quick, safe diagnostic extension of routine flexible bronchoscopy [29]. The tip of the bronchoscope is wedged into a segmental or smaller airway, and physiologic saline is instilled and withdrawn through the suction channel. Using this technique, it is possible to sample cellular and soluble components from the distal airways and alveoli. It can be useful in diagnosing some infectious or other diffuse parenchymal diseases (e.g., *Pneumocystis carinii* pneumonitis [30], intraalveolar hemorrhage [31], bronchogenic carcinoma [32], exogenous lipoid pneumonia [33], alveolar proteinosis [34], and eosinophilic granuloma [35]). A detailed discussion of the use of BAL analysis in a variety of lung diseases can be found elsewhere [29]. The usefulness of BAL and bronchoscopy-protected brush-catheter cultures in diagnosing lung infections is reviewed in Chapters 12 and 68. Because BAL is not really a biopsy procedure and little or no associated bleeding occurs, it may be performed in patients with bleeding abnormalities and pulmonary hypertension.

Expected Results from Lung Biopsy

GENERAL CONSIDERATIONS. To determine what type of lung biopsy procedure should be performed, and when, it is important to appreciate the expected results. The yield of positive diagnoses and the complications incurred depend on the procedure performed, the disease process, and the clinical stability of the patient.

DIFFUSE PARENCHYMAL DISEASE IN CLINICALLY STABLE PATIENTS. To maximize the diagnostic yield, the ideal biopsy procedure is one that maintains the architectural lung integrity in the specimen. The procedures that best meet this requirement are (a) open lung biopsy, (b) thoracoscopic biopsy, and (c) transbronchoscopic lung biopsy. A number of reports on stable patients with diffuse lung have documented average rates of mortality, complications, and diagnostic yield for these procedures (Table 29-2) [1,36–39]. The highest tissue and diagnostic yields with low morbidity and very low mortality rates are obtained with open and thoracoscopic lung biopsies. Transbronchoscopic lung biopsy has lower diagnostic yields, but carries the lowest morbidity and mortality rates of any of these biopsy procedures.

Although open and thoracoscopic lung biopsies more consistently yield adequate tissue and an increased likelihood of definitive diagnosis than transbronchoscopic forceps lung biopsy, the latter may be preferred as an initial procedure to avoid the morbidity of general anesthesia, postoperative chest tube drainage, residual parenchymal and pleural scarring, postoperative pain, and increased length of hospital stay. The potential morbidity of empyema that may complicate an open or thoracoscopic lung biopsy procedure is also avoided with transbronchoscopic lung biopsy. This closed procedure is much less expensive and less painful, and carries less mortality than open lung biopsy.

The overall complication rate for transbronchoscopic lung biopsy is less than 10%. The most common complication is pneumothorax, which may require chest tube drainage in up to 50% of cases [38]. Although the definitive diagnostic accuracy of transbronchoscopic lung biopsy is less than that of open and thoracoscopic lung biopsy (the tissue is smaller in quantity, often crushed, usually only peribronchiolar in origin, and not obtained under direct vision), its diagnostic yield is sufficiently high under certain conditions to justify its use as the initial biopsy procedure. For instance, in diffuse diseases such as carcinomatosis, sarcoidosis, and *P. carinii* infection, transbronchoscopic forceps lung biopsy yields a specific diagnosis in 80% to 90% of cases [30,40,41].

Percutaneous needle aspiration (lung tap) also has a role in patients with diffuse parenchymal disease due to infection. The diagnostic yield in this setting varies from 40% to 82% [42–

Table 29-2. Representative Results of Lung Biopsy Procedures in Diffuse Lung Disease

Procedure	Mortality (%)	Complications (%)	Diagnostic yield (%)
Open	0.0–4.7	5–7[a]	94–95
Thoracoscopy	0–8	0–15[b]	96–100
Transbronchial forceps	≤0.12	≤10[c]	84

[a]Pneumothorax, empyema, and bleeding into pleural space.
[b]Subcutaneous emphysema, infection, persistent air leak, and hemorrhage with conversion to open thoracotomy.
[c]Pneumothorax, hemorrhage in uremic or thrombocytopenic patients.

45]. Although percutaneous needle aspiration rarely causes mortality or air embolism, pneumothorax is common, occurring in approximately 25% of cases [42,44]. Hemoptysis occurs in 1% to 11% of patients [42,44]. Complication rates can be reduced by using an ultrathin needle (24- or 25-gauge) [43].

LUNG MASS IN CLINICALLY STABLE PATIENTS. Because solid or cavitary masses are most often due to malignant or infectious causes, and because these diagnoses can often be readily confirmed by analyzing cellular material and fluid, open lung biopsy is usually not the preferred initial procedure. When open or thoracoscopic biopsy is performed, however, tissue and diagnostic yields should consistently approach 100%. Because nodules are usually resected in their entirety, surgical mortality depends on the severity of illness and extent of the resection [46]. The operative mortality associated with wedge resections by open thoracotomy of benign nodules in otherwise healthy, young patients is less than 1%, whereas it may vary from 2% to 12% in older patients with bronchogenic carcinomas who undergo pneumonectomy [47]. Complications of thoracotomy for lung masses in clinically stable patients are similar to those in such patients with diffuse lung disease. In a report of 242 solitary pulmonary nodules excised by video-assisted thoracoscopic surgery, there was a complication rate of 3.6% and no mortality [12] in patients undergoing thoracoscopy alone.

Percutaneous needle aspiration is extremely useful in evaluating lung masses. It carries the highest diagnostic yield. A definite diagnosis is obtained in 80% to 97% of all masses, and adequate samples are obtained in 82% to 98% of cases [48–52]. If the lesion is less than 2 cm in diameter, the likelihood of obtaining adequate material is significantly decreased [48,52]. The diagnostic yield in solid malignant nodules can approach 96% [49]; in malignant and infectious cavitary lesions, 90% to 100% [48]; and in "benign" inflammatory disease, such as granulomatous nodules, only 19% [53]. Although percutaneous needle aspiration is rarely associated with fatalities, complications such as pneumothorax, hemoptysis, and intraparenchymal hemorrhage or hemothorax are not uncommon [48,49,52,53]. The risk of pneumothorax increases with smaller-size lesions and the presence of surrounding emphysema [54]. Hemorrhage and pneumothorax occur much more frequently in cavitary lesions. It has been demonstrated that aspiration biopsy using smaller, ultrathin 24- to 25-gauge needles results in a significant decrease in complications without loss of excellent diagnostic yield [55]. Although some authors feel the risk of needle-track implantation of cancer is remote and it should not be considered a contraindication to the procedure [56], a recent study suggests that the risk of spread of malignant cells may be as high as 60% [57]. In this study, 12 of 20 lung resections had evidence of malignant cells on the visceral pleura after a needle aspirate was performed.

Peripheral lung nodules and masses can also be sampled using the transbronchoscopic brush and forceps techniques. Complication rates are less than those for percutaneous needle aspiration biopsy. Although the diagnostic yield is also diminished and the procedures are more difficult and time consuming than percutaneous needle biopsy, transbronchial biopsies more frequently yield tissue with architectural integrity. This may allow the pathologist a better opportunity to diagnose benign conditions. In peripheral malignant lesions, the diagnostic yield of transbronchial biopsy relates directly to the number of biopsies obtained under fluoroscopic guidance. With brushing alone, the diagnostic yield is approximately 40%; with brushing plus one transbronchoscopic forceps lung biopsy, diagnostic accuracy improves to 55%; with brushing plus four transbronchoscopic forceps lung

biopsies, accuracy reaches 60%; and with brushing plus five transbronchoscopic forceps lung biopsies, diagnostic accuracy improves to 75% [58].

DIFFUSE AND LOCALIZED DISEASE IN CLINICALLY UNSTABLE PATIENTS. Lung biopsy in critically ill, clinically unstable patients is most commonly considered in those who are immunocompromised hosts or who have the acute respiratory distress syndrome.

Numerous studies have considered the merits of various lung biopsy procedures in the non–acquired immunodeficiency syndrome (AIDS)-immunocompromised host. The choice of which biopsy procedure to perform depends on a number of factors, including the severity and rate of progression of the illness, differential diagnosis, underlying medical conditions, radiographic findings, and level of experience and expertise of the physician performing the procedure. The diagnostic yields of the different biopsy procedures also depend on a number of factors, including differential diagnosis, underlying medical conditions, and radiographic findings.

For critically ill patients with rapidly progressing hypoxemia and radiographic infiltrates, open lung biopsy is the procedure of first choice as it is associated with the highest yield and can be surprisingly well tolerated in critically ill patients [59]. However, mortality rates of 8.6% to 13.6% have been reported [60,61]. For less severely ill patients in whom progressive hypoxemia is not an immediate problem, less invasive procedures can be attempted first.

In solid-organ transplant patients with diffuse infiltrates, bronchoscopy with BAL can result in the correct diagnosis up to 85% of the time (range, 27% to 85%), and is associated with little to no morbidity [62]. In neutropenic leukemic patients with diffuse infiltrates, however, BAL is of little value as it is associated with a very low yield for invasive aspergillosis, has a very high false-positive rate for bacterial pathogens, and does not aid in diagnosing drug-induced pulmonary processes [59]. In addition, in neutropenic patients, the bronchoscopic procedure itself can result in the development of pneumonia, bacteremia, and sepsis [63,64]. In patients with AIDS, the sensitivity of lavage alone for diagnosing *P. carinii* can be as high as 97% [65]. In nonneutropenic patients, BAL does not increase the already low complication rate of routine diagnostic flexible bronchoscopy (see Chapter 12).

Transbronchial biopsy in patients with diffuse pulmonary infiltrates and solid-organ transplants is associated with yields of 46% to 78% [59,66], and in patients with hematologic malignancies, a yield of 55% [66]. Transbronchial biopsy has the highest frequency in diagnosing tuberculosis, fungal pneumonia, and pulmonary involvement of hematological malignancies [66]. In non-AIDS patients, BAL in combination with transbronchial biopsy has a higher yield for identifying *P. carinii*, *Legionella* sp., and cytomegalovirus infections than BAL or transbronchial biopsy alone [62,67]. In this setting, the combination of BAL and transbronchial biopsy can increase yield by 33% [62].

Transthoracic needle aspiration biopsy has the highest yield in immunocompromised hosts with focal pulmonary processes, especially peripheral lung lesions. In these clinical settings, sensitivities of a transthoracic needle biopsy can be greater than 80% for infectious processes and greater than 90% for malignant processes [59]. Yields for fungi, tuberculosis, and *Nocardia* can be greater than 90% [59,68].

In critically ill patients requiring mechanical ventilation, lung biopsy may be considered to assist in diagnosis and management, and to ensure that no treatable disease process is overlooked. Specific diagnosis may be made in up to 80% of the cases [59]. Other studies report lower yields, however, and suggest that the results of the biopsy may not alter management. One retrospective study of 24 patients requiring mechanical ventilation demonstrated that open lung biopsy provided a specific diagnosis 46% of the time and provided information that altered therapy in 47% of the cases [60]. The overall mortality rate was 8.4%, and this rate increased with a higher multiple organ dysfunction score. Another study of 49 patients demonstrated that open lung biopsy led to a specific diagnosis in 88% but resulted in a change in management in only 45% [69]. Open lung biopsy may be more helpful in the critically ill pediatric population. A study of 26 children demonstrated that open lung biopsy was diagnostic in 96% and associated with no mortalities [70].

There is no consensus about which biopsy technique is best and under which clinical circumstances. A wide range of expected diagnostic yields exists for all procedures, and the etiology of lung disease in these patients may remain unknown in 19% to 45%, even when adequate tissue is obtained by open lung biopsy. Deciding who, when, and how to sample is further complicated by the occasionally excessive mortality rates associated with lung biopsy procedures, and by the knowledge that even with adequate biopsy material and appropriate therapy, the high mortality rates seen in this group of patients may not be altered [71]. Consequently, the clinician must adopt a practical approach to management that combines empiric therapy with available biopsy procedures.

In patients with AIDS, open lung biopsy is the most sensitive and specific procedure. However, open or thoracoscopic lung biopsy should not be the first procedure contemplated or attempted because diffuse infiltrates are most likely due to opportunistic infection, and bronchoscopic procedures accurately diagnose infection in 90% or more of the cases [72]. Open lung biopsy or thoracoscopic biopsy is appropriate when at least one bronchoscopic examination with BAL and transbronchial biopsy (unless contraindicated) has been nondiagnostic [59]. It is rarely useful in patients who worsen after treatment for a diagnosis established by bronchoscopy [72], and it should not be repeated often.

Indications for Lung Biopsy in Critically Ill Patients

GENERAL CONSIDERATIONS. A lung biopsy is indicated in critically ill patients when (a) the pulmonary disease process progresses and its etiology remains unknown, (b) an initial evaluation short of lung biopsy has failed to reveal the etiology and logical empiric therapy has failed to reverse the process, (c) no contraindications exist to performing the procedures, (d) the prognosis of the patient's underlying disease is good, and (e) the potential benefit from performing the procedure outweighs associated morbidity and mortality [71].

MANAGEMENT OF CRITICALLY ILL PATIENTS WITH PULMONARY DISEASE. The lung biopsy is part of an extensive evaluation of a pulmonary abnormality, yet in critically ill patients it is never the initial step. Any critically ill patient is, for clinical purposes, a compromised host and should be managed as such (Table 29-3).

Because of their altered defense mechanisms, critically ill patients are particularly susceptible to infection by opportunistic as well as pathogenic organisms. Nonimmunologic defenses (e.g., altered physical barriers, altered indigenous microbiologic flora) as well as immunologic defenses (e.g., altered humoral or

Table 29-3. Management of the Compromised Host with Pulmonary Disease

Identify the patient as a compromised host.
Construct a list of differential possibilities that remains constant from patient to patient.
Integrate the history, physical examination, and laboratory data with the chest radiographic pattern to narrow the diagnostic possibilities.
Assess the urgency of the situation and the need for invasive diagnostic studies, including lung biopsy.

cellular immunity) may be impaired. These impairments may be partial or transient (e.g., alcoholism, diabetes mellitus, sickle cell anemia, uremia, malnutrition), as well as prolonged or permanent (e.g., Hodgkin's disease, chronic lymphatic leukemia, acute myelogenous leukemia, multiple myeloma, inherited immune deficiency diseases, cytotoxic chemotherapy, corticosteroids, irradiation).

Four major differential diagnostic possibilities should be considered in every critically ill (compromised) patient with pulmonary disease (Table 29-4). After general diagnostic considerations, the diagnostic possibilities are narrowed by integrating the history, physical examination, and laboratory data (i.e., routine blood work; serologic studies; and smears and cultures of blood, urine, sputum, cerebrospinal fluid, ascites, and pleural effusion) with the chest radiographic pattern. A previous recent or remote chest radiograph may confirm or rule out the presence of another stable process. Although unilateral or focal infiltrates suggest bacterial infection, the presence of bilateral disease does not rule out infectious processes [70]. Unusual and opportunistic organisms, such as *P. carinii*, often present as bilateral infiltrates after administration of immunosuppressive drugs or chemotherapy [73].

The final step involves assessing clinical urgency to evaluate the need for invasive diagnostic studies such as lung biopsy. In some clinical cases, empiric therapy should be considered and invasive biopsy avoided. These cases include patients with underlying diseases that limit life expectancy, such as advanced AIDS or advanced cancer; leukemia before treatment, as the risk for opportunistic infection is low, and there is a high probability of successful treatment with antibacterial therapy; uncontrolled coagulopathies; severely impaired pulmonary function such that an invasive procedure would not be tolerated; and patient refusal to undergo an invasive procedure [59].

In other clinical settings, other less invasive treatment options should be attempted first. For example, in an intubated, elderly patient with diffuse pulmonary infiltrates associated with pancreatitis, the first diagnostic procedure might be pulmonary artery catheterization. If the pulmonary artery occlusion pres-

Table 29-4. Differential Diagnosis of Pulmonary Disease in the Compromised Host

Manifestations of basic disease
Complications of management
  Lipid embolization
  Pulmonary edema
  Pulmonary hemorrhage
  Leukoagglutinin reaction
  Radiation pneumonitis
  Drug-induced pneumonitis
Presence of another, unrelated basic disease
Infection
  Bacterial
  Viral
  Fungal
  Parasitic

sure is normal, acute respiratory distress syndrome is likely to have developed. In this case, a biopsy is unlikely to add additional information that may alter the management. In the thrombocytopenic, immunocompromised host who has diffuse pulmonary infiltrates and who is clinically stable with supplemental oxygen, platelet transfusions and observation may be adequate therapy. As many as 70% of infiltrates in these patients may be due to intrapulmonary bleeding [31].

Finally, in other clinical settings, lung biopsy (especially open lung biopsy) should be considered early on in the management plan. Solid-organ transplant patients and patients with other immunocompromised states (with life expectancies measured in years) who develop hypoxemia with fever and diffuse infiltrates are more likely to benefit from a biopsy [59].

Selection of Lung Biopsy Procedure

Three factors should be considered in choosing a particular lung biopsy procedure: (a) local expertise, (b) the patient's condition, and (c) the potential yield of the procedure.

LOCAL EXPERTISE. This factor includes the availability of personnel skilled in performing the procedure and laboratory personnel skilled in specimen processing and analysis. If local expertise is limited (e.g., a skilled cytopathologist is not available to read bronchial brush or percutaneous needle aspiration specimens, or the microbiology laboratory is not equipped to process reliably specimens for the variety of organisms seen in immunocompromised hosts), the patient should be transferred to another institution with expanded resources.

PATIENT CONDITION. Once it has been decided that the patient's prognosis is potentially good enough to justify a lung biopsy technique, the next decision is the choice of biopsy procedure. If it is determined that the patient's condition allows time for only one diagnostic procedure (i.e., the patient is rapidly deteriorating), then an open or thoracoscopic lung biopsy should be performed. If there are no contraindications to a closed procedure and the patient's condition is such that there will be time for another diagnostic procedure if necessary, then one of the closed procedures may be preferable. Mechanical ventilation should not be considered an absolute contraindication to transbronchial biopsy [74,75]. Useful information has been obtained with transbronchial lung biopsy with acceptable morbidity (e.g., pneumothorax, hemorrhage) in a limited number of hemodynamically stable, mechanically ventilated patients.

POTENTIAL YIELD. The potential yield of a particular biopsy procedure depends on local expertise and the individual clinical setting. For example, in the elderly patient with a solitary pulmonary nodule and clinically obvious disseminated carcinomatosis, percutaneous needle aspiration biopsy, which has a high diagnostic yield and relatively low complication rate, should be the initial procedure of choice to document whether the nodule is malignant. When a patient with a solitary pulmonary nodule has a clinical picture of vasculitis, however, open lung biopsy (or thoracoscopy biopsy if the lesion is peripheral) might be considered first or performed after bronchial brushing and forceps biopsies and percutaneous needle aspirations yield nonspecific findings without evidence of malignancy or infection.

In patients with diffuse pulmonary disease, the clinical setting influences the choice of procedure. When a biopsy is performed to document the presence and type of inorganic pneumoconiosis, open lung biopsy and thoracoscopic biopsy [76] are the only procedures that yield a sufficient amount of tissue for all the requisite analyses (chemical analysis must be included). When diffuse pulmonary infiltrates suggesting sarcoidosis or carcinomatosis occur in the appropriate clinical setting, transbronchoscopic forceps lung biopsy should be initially considered because it has an extremely high yield in these situations [40,41]. In the non–AIDS-immunocompromised host with diffuse pulmonary infiltrates, transbronchoscopic lung biopsy may yield a diagnosis overall up to 78% of the time [66]. In chronic interstitial pneumonias (e.g., idiopathic pulmonary fibrosis), open or thoracoscopic lung biopsy is diagnostically superior to transbronchoscopic lung biopsy [40]. If chronic eosinophilic pneumonia, desquamative interstitial pneumonitis, or bronchiolitis obliterans organizing pneumonia can be ruled in by transbronchoscopic forceps lung biopsy, however, open or thoracoscopic lung biopsy may not be necessary. If infection and malignancy can be ruled out by transbronchoscopic forceps lung biopsy and other nonbiopsy laboratory techniques, it also may be unnecessary to perform an open procedure. If the diffuse process worsens, corticosteroids can be empirically initiated, and the response to therapy can be assessed by noninvasive means (e.g., chest radiograph, gallium scan, pulmonary function studies).

Handling of Specimens

To maximize the diagnostic yield from any lung biopsy procedure, specimens must be rapidly transported to the appropriate laboratories by a person directly involved in the patient's management. All analyses should be planned in advance by the team involved in the case (e.g., pathologist, microbiologist, pulmonologist, infectious disease specialist).

Because large samples of tissue are obtained from open lung and thoracoscopy biopsies, multiple pieces should be processed for a variety of analyses. First, under sterile conditions, a piece of fresh tissue should be kept moist with physiologic saline and transported immediately to the microbiology laboratory to be minced, ground, and cultured for aerobic and anaerobic bacteria, fungi, and *Mycobacterium* and *Legionella* sp. A second piece should be snap-frozen and stored at –60°C to ensure that immunofluorescent studies (e.g., immunoglobulin deposition as well as T- and B-lymphocyte markers, direct fluorescent antibody staining for *Legionella* sp.), Oil-Red-O staining, and viral cultures can be performed if necessary. If pneumoconiosis is suspected, special studies can be performed on formalin-fixed, paraffin-embedded tissue. At this juncture, touch preparations of a freshly cut surface of the tissue can be made for cytologic analysis, and special stains can be used for rapid diagnosis of microorganisms. The pathologist should perform a frozen-section analysis to (a) advise the surgeon whether an adequate biopsy has been obtained (i.e., the tissue does or does not exhibit a pathologic lesion), (b) obtain information that could focus the work-up of the specimen (e.g., order a lymphoma work-up or specific viral culture), and (c) attempt to obtain a rapid definitive diagnosis. The remainder of the tissue should be placed in 10% formalin for routine histologic study and special stains.

Unlimited analysis on specimens from transbronchoscopic forceps lung biopsies cannot be performed because of the relatively small amount of tissue obtained. To maximize the diagnostic yield, four to six pieces should be obtained [58,77].

In immunocompromised patients, touch preparations of transbronchial biopsies should be obtained and stained for microorganisms. If an exogenous lipoid pneumonia, immunologic disease, or *Legionella* infection is suspected, one piece should be snap-frozen for fat stains and immunofluorescent studies. One piece can be submitted to microbiology and the remaining pieces processed for routine and special pathologic stains. Once the slides have been made from bronchial brush biopsies, they can be stained in a manner similar to needle aspiration specimens.

A specimen obtained by percutaneous transthoracic needle aspiration should be sent for microbiologic as well as cytologic analyses unless infection is not even a remote possibility. For cytologic analysis, a few drops of the aspirate can first be smeared onto frosted glass slides that are immediately placed in 95% alcohol. Then, a portion can be injected into a test tube with physiologic saline so that it can be processed using the Millipore filter or cytocentrifuge, or into a vial containing a fluid preservative for use in one of the instruments capable of preparing cell monolayers [78]. Filters and slides can be stained routinely by the Papanicolaou technique and specifically by Gomori-methenamine silver (for fungi and *P. carinii*), periodic acid-Schiff (for fungi), and Ziehl-Neelsen stains (for acid-fast organisms). When evaluating for the possibility of *P. carinii* pneumonia, immunofluorescent staining with monoclonal antibodies can increase the yield. Sensitivity and specificity of this test have been reported to be greater than 90% [79]. The portion for microbiology should be immediately injected into prereduced anaerobic transport medium and transported to the microbiology laboratory. In the laboratory, drops of the specimen are placed on several sterile slides and allowed to air dry for Gram's, Ziehl-Neelsen, and direct fluorescent antibody stains for *Legionella* organisms. The remaining specimen can be cultured for anaerobic and aerobic bacteria, fungi, and *Mycobacterium* and *Legionella* sp.

After submitting an aliquot of BAL fluid for microbiologic analysis, the specimen should be handled in the cytology laboratory in a manner similar to that of percutaneous aspiration specimens.

References

1. Fountain SW: Pulmonary wedge biopsy: technique and application in interstitial lung disease, in Walker WS (ed): *Video-Assisted Thoracic Surgery*. Oxford, Isis Medical Media, 1995, p 115.
2. Utz JP, Prakash UB: Indications for and contraindications to bronchoscopy, in Praskash UB (ed): *Bronchoscopy*. New York, Raven Press, 1994, p 81.
3. Baughman RP, Golden JA, Keith FM: Bronchoscopy, lung biopsy, and other diagnostic procedures, in Murrary JF, Nadel JA, Mason RJ, et al. (eds): *Textbook of Respiratory Medicine*. 3rd ed. New York, WB Saunders, 2000, p 728.
4. Raoof S, Mehrishi S, Prakash UB: Role of bronchoscopy in modern medical intensive care unit. *Clin Chest Med* 22:241, 2001.
5. Sokolowski JW, Burgher LW, Jones FL, et al: Guidelines for fiberoptic bronchoscopy in adults. *Am Rev Respir Dis* 136:1066, 1987.
6. Rai NS, Arroliga AC: Indications, contraindications, and medications, in Wang KP, Mehta AC (eds): *Flexible Bronchoscopy*. Cambridge, MA, Blackwell Science, 1995, p 34.
7. McDougall JC, Cortese DA: Bronchoscopic lung biopsy, in Praskash UB (ed): *Bronchoscopy*. New York, Raven Press, 1994, p 141.
8. Midthun DE, Cortese DA: Bronchoscopy needle aspiration and biopsy, in Praskash UB (ed): *Bronchoscopy*. New York, Raven Press, 1994, p 147.
9. Gaensler EA, Carrington CB: Open lung biopsy for chronic diffuse infiltrative lung disease: clinical, roentgenographic, and physiologic correlations in 502 patients. *Ann Thorac Surg* 30:411, 1980.
10. Ponn RB, Knight H: Diffuse lung disease, in Shields TW (ed): *General Thoracic Surgery*. 5th ed. Philadelphia, Lippincott Williams & Wilkins, 2000, p 1151.
11. Chechani V, Landrenau RJ, Shaikh SS: Open lung biopsy for diffuse interstitial lung disease. *Ann Thorac Surg* 54:296, 1992.
12. Gaensler EA: Open and closed lung biopsy, in Sackner MA (ed): *The Human Lung in Biology: Techniques in Pulmonary Disease, Part 2*. New York, Marcel Dekker Inc, 1980, p 579.
13. Harris RJ, Kavuru MS, Rice TW, et al: The diagnostic and therapeutic utility of thoracoscopy: a review. *Chest* 108:828, 1995.
14. Kaiser LR: Video-assisted thoracic surgery: current state of the art. *Ann Surg* 220:720, 1994.
15. Miller JD, Urschel JD, Cox G, et al: A randomized, controlled trial comparing thoracoscopy and limited thoracotomy for lung biopsy in interstitial lung disease. *Ann Thorac Surg* 70:1674, 2000.
16. Trivedi UH, Millner RW, Griffiths EM, et al: Three-year review of video-assisted thoracoscopic lung biopsy. *Thorax* 49:1060, 1994.
17. Carnochen FM, Walker WS, Cameron EW: Efficiency of video-assisted thoracoscopic lung biopsy: an historical comparison with open lung biopsy. *Thorax* 49:361, 1994.
18. Ferson PF, Landreneau RJ, Dowling RD, et al: Comparison of open vs. thoracoscopic lung biopsy for diffuse infiltrative pulmonary disease. *J Thorac Cardiovasc Surg* 106:194, 1993.
19. Sinner WN: Technique of needle aspiration biopsy, in Sinner WN (ed): *Needle Biopsy and Transbronchial Biopsy*. New York, Thieme-Stratton, 1982, p 35.
20. Zavala DC, Schoell JE: Ultrathin needle aspiration of the lung in infections and malignant diseases. *Am Rev Respir Dis* 123:125, 1981.
21. Schure D, Abraham JL, Konopka R: How should transbronchial biopsies be performed and processed? *Am Rev Respir Dis* 126:342, 1982.
22. Cortese DA, McDougall JC: Biopsy and brushing of peripheral lung cancer with fluoroscopic guidance. *Chest* 75:141, 1979.
23. Cortese DA, McDougall JC: Bronchoscopy in peripheral and central lesions, in Praskash UB (ed): *Bronchoscopy*. New York, Raven Press, 1994, p 135.
24. Wang KP: Transbronchial needle aspiration for cytology specimens, in Wang KP, Mehta AC (eds): *Flexible Bronchoscopy*. Cambridge, MA, Blackwell Science, 1995, p 195.
25. Mehta AC, Meeker DP: Transbronchial needle aspiration for histology specimens, in Wang KP, Mehta AC (eds): *Flexible Bronchoscopy*. Cambridge, MA, Blackwell Science, 1995, p 199.
26. Wang KP, Terry PB: Transbronchial needle aspiration in the diagnosis and staging of bronchogenic carcinoma. *Am Rev Respir Dis* 127:344, 1983.
27. Haponik EF, Cappellari JO, Chin R, et al: Education and experience improve transbronchial needle aspiration procedure. *Am J Respir Crit Care Med* 151:1998, 1995.
28. Shannon JJ, Bude RO, Orens JB, et al: Endobronchial ultrasound-guided needle aspiration of mediastinal adenopathy. *Am J Respir Crit Care Med* 153:1424, 1996.
29. Helmers RA, Pisani RJ: Bronchoalveolar lavage, in Praskash UB (ed): *Bronchoscopy*. New York, Raven Press, 1994, p 155.
30. Weldon-Linne CM, Rhone DP, Bourassa R: Bronchoscopy specimens in adults with AIDS: comparative yields of cytology, histology, and cultures for diagnosis of infectious agents. *Chest* 98:24, 1990.
31. Drew WL, Finley TH, Golde DW: Diagnostic lavage and occult pulmonary hemorrhage in thrombocytopenic immunocompromised patients. *Am Rev Respir Dis* 116:215, 1977.
32. Linder J, Radio SR, Robbins RA, et al: Bronchoalveolar lavage in the cytologic diagnosis of carcinoma of the lung. *Acta Cytol* 31:796, 1987.
33. Corwin RW, Irwin RS: Sensitivity and specificity of the lipid-laden macrophage in diagnosing exogenous lipoid pneumonia. *Am Rev Respir Dis* 127[Suppl]:94, 1983.
34. Prakash UB, Barham SS, Carpenter HA, et al: Pulmonary alveolar phospholipoproteinosis: experience with 34 cases and a review. *Mayo Clin Proc* 62:499, 1987.
35. Basset F, Soler P, Jaurand ML, et al: Ultrastructural examination of bronchoalveolar lavage for diagnosis of pulmonary histiocytosis X: preliminary report of 4 cases. *Thorax* 32:303, 1977.
36. Shah SS, Tsang V, Goldstraw P: Open lung biopsy: a safe, reliable, and accurate method for diagnosing diffuse lung disease. *Respiration* 59:243, 1992.
37. Neuhaus SJ, Matar KS: The efficacy of open lung biopsy. *Aust N Z J Surg* 67:181, 1997.

38. Anderson HA: Transbronchoscopic lung biopsy for diffuse pulmonary disease: results in 939 patients. *Chest* 73:734, 1978.
39. Simpson FG, Arnold AG, Purvis A, et al: Postal survey of bronchoscopic practice by physicians in the United Kingdom. *Thorax* 41:311, 1986.
40. Schwarz MI: Approach to the understanding, diagnosis, and management of interstitial lung disease, in Schwarz MI, King TE (ed): *Interstitial Lung Disease*. 3rd ed. London, BC Decker, 1998, p 3.
41. Gilman MJ, Wang KP: Transbronchial lung biopsy in sarcoidosis. *Am Rev Respir Dis* 122:721, 1980.
42. Palmer DL, Davidson M, Lusk R: Needle aspiration of the lung in complex pneumonias. *Chest* 78:16, 1980.
43. Zalacain R, Llorente JL, Gaztelurrutia L, et al: Influence of three factors on the diagnostic effectiveness of transthoracic needle aspiration in pneumonia. *Chest* 107:96, 1995.
44. Busk MF, Rosenow EC, Wilson WR: Invasive procedures in the diagnosis of pneumonia. *Semin Respir Infect* 3:113, 1988.
45. Matthay RA, Mortiz ED: Invasive procedures for diagnosing pulmonary infections. A critical review. *Clin Chest Med* 2:3, 1981.
46. Lillington GA: The solitary pulmonary nodule—1974. *Am Rev Respir Dis* 110:699, 1974.
47. Kopec SE, Irwin RS, Umali-Torres CB, et al: The postpneumonectomy state. *Chest* 144:1158; 1998.
48. Berquist TH, Bailey PB, Cortese DA, et al: Transthoracic needle biopsy. *Mayo Clin Proc* 55:475, 1980.
49. Lopez Hanninen E, Vogl TJ, Ricke J, et al: CT-guided percutaneous core biopsies of pulmonary lesions. Diagnostic accuracy, complications, and therapeutic impact. *Acta Radiologica* 42:151, 2001.
50. Conces DJ, Schwenk GR, Doering PR, et al: Thoracic needle biopsy. Improved results utilizing a team approach. *Chest* 91:813, 1987.
51. Wallace JM, Deutsch L: Flexible fiberoptic bronchoscopy and percutaneous needle lung aspiration for evaluating the solitary pulmonary nodule. *Chest* 81:665, 1982.
52. Poe RH, Robin RE: Sensitivity and specificity of needle biopsy in lung malignancy. *Am Rev Respir Dis* 122:755, 1980.
53. Sinner WN: Material and results, in Sinner WN (ed): *Needle Biopsy and Transbronchial Biopsy*. New York, Thieme-Stratton, 1982, p 18.
54. Cox JE, Chiles C, McManus CM, et al: Transthoracic needle aspirate biopsy: variables that affect risk of pneumothorax. *Radiology* 212:165, 1999.
55. Zavala DC, Schoell JU: Ultrathin needle aspiration of the lung in infectious and malignant diseases. *Am Rev Respir Dis* 123:125, 1981.
56. Sinner WN: Complications, in Sinner WN (ed): *Needle Biopsy and Transbronchial Biopsy*. New York, Thieme-Stratton, 1982, p 44.
57. Sawabata N, Ohta M, Maeda H: Fine-needle aspiration cytologic technique for lung cancer has a high potential of malignant cell spread through the tract. *Chest* 118:936, 2000.
58. Popovich J, Koace PA, Eichenhorn MS, et al: Diagnostic accuracy of multiple biopsies from flexible fiberoptic bronchoscopy. *Am Rev Respir Dis* 125:521, 1982.
59. Rubin RH, Greene R: Clinical approach to the compromised host with fever and pulmonary infiltrates, in Rubin RH, Young LS (eds): *Clinical Approach to Infections in the Compromised Host*. 3rd ed. New York, Plenum Publishing, 1994, p 121.
60. Flabouris A, Myburgh J: The utility of open lung biopsy in patients requiring mechanical ventilation. *Chest* 115:811, 1999.
61. Potter D, Pass HI, Brower S, et al: Prospective randomized study of open lung biopsy versus empirical antibiotic therapy for acute pneumonitis in non-neutropenic cancer patients. *Ann Thorac Surg* 40:422, 1985.
62. Nusair S, Kramer MR: The role of fiber-optic bronchoscopy in solid organ, transplant patients with pulmonary infections. *Respir Med* 93:621, 1999.
63. Robbins H, Goldman AL: Failure of a prophylactic antimicrobial drug to prevent sepsis after fiberoptic bronchoscopy. *Am Rev Respir Dis* 116:325, 1977.
64. Beyt BE, King DK, Glew RH: Fatal pneumonitis and septicemia after fiberoptic bronchoscopy. *Chest* 72:105, 1977.
65. Hopewell PC: *Pneumocystis carinii* pneumonia: diagnosis. *J Infect Dis* 157:1115, 1988.
66. Cazzadori A, DiPerri G, Todeschini G, et al: Transbronchial biopsy in the diagnosis of pulmonary infiltrates in immunocompromised patients. *Chest* 107:101, 1995.
67. Springmeyer SC, Silvestri RC, Sale GE, et al: The role of transbronchial biopsy for the diagnosis of diffuse pneumonias in immunocompromised marrow transplant recipients. *Am Rev Respir Dis* 126:763, 1982.
68. Scott WW, Kuhlman JE: Focal pulmonary lesions in patients with AIDS: percutaneous transthoracic needle biopsy. *Radiology* 180:419, 1991.
69. Wong P, Downey R, White D: Open lung biopsy in the ICH: analysis of 49 cases. *Am J Respir Crit Care Med* 149:A560, 1999.
70. Steinberg R, Freud E, Ben-Ari J, et al: Open lung biopsy—successful diagnostic tool with therapeutic implications in the critically ill paediatric population. *Acta Peadiat* 87:945, 1998.
71. Hiatt JR, Gong H, Mulder DG, et al: The value of open lung biopsy in the immunosuppressed patient. *Surgery* 92:285, 1982.
72. Fitzgerald W, Bevelaqua FA, Garay SM, et al: The role of open lung biopsy in patients with the acquired immunodeficiency syndrome. *Chest* 91:659, 1987.
73. Tenholder MF, Hooper RG: Pulmonary infiltrates in leukemia. *Chest* 78:468, 1980.
74. Pincus PS, Kallenbach JM, Hurwitz MD, et al: Transbronchial biopsy during mechanical ventilation. *Crit Care Med* 15:1136, 1987.
75. Olopade CO, Prakash UB: Bronchoscopy in the intensive care critical care unit. *Mayo Clinic Proc* 64:1255, 1989.
76. Bensard DD, McIntyre RC Jr, Waring BJ, et al: Comparison of video thoracoscopic lung biopsy to open lung biopsy in the diagnosis of interstitial lung disease. *Chest* 103:765, 1993.
77. Roethe RA, Fuller PD, Byrd RB, et al: Transbronchoscopic lung biopsy in sarcoidosis. Optimal number and site for diagnosis. *Chest* 77:400, 1980.
78. Hutchinson ML, Cassin CM, Ball HG: The efficacy of an automated preparation device for cervical cytology. *Am J Clin Pathol* 96:300, 1991.
79. Kovacs JA, Ng JL, Masur H, et al: Diagnosis of *Pneumocystis carinii* pneumonia: improved detection in sputum with use of monoclonal antibodies. *N Engl J Med* 318:589, 1988.

30. Dialysis Therapy in the Intensive Care Setting

Joseph A. Coladonato, Todd F. Griffith, and William F. Owen, Jr.

Overview of Dialysis Modalities

Bones can break, muscles can atrophy, glands can loaf, even the brains can go to sleep, without immediately endangering our survival; but should the kidneys fail neither bone, muscle, gland, nor brain could carry on.

Homer W. Smith (1895–1962)

In 1839, Addison [1] reported that stupor, coma, and convulsions were consequences of diseased kidneys, referred to for much of that century as Bright's disease [2]. Almost 50 years later, Tyson [3] noted that

Uremic symptoms are dependent on retention of urea and allied substances in the blood, which when they have accumulated to a sufficient quantity, act on the nervous system producing delirium and convulsions or coma.

These rudimentary observations relevant to the pathobiology of symptomatic renal failure suggested that therapy should be directed at the reversal or attenuation of the retention of nitrogenous products of metabolism. In September 1945, Kolff [4] dialyzed a 67-year-old woman with acute oliguric renal failure. Although this was a successful effort, dialysis remained an experimental tool until Teschan [5] described its use in treating Korean war casualties with posttraumatic renal failure in 1955. In 1960, Scribner et al. [6] devised an exteriorized arteriovenous access for long-term hemodialysis and initiated a 39-year-old man with end-stage renal disease (ESRD) on regular dialysis treatments. By the mid-1960s, hemodialysis was becoming conventional therapy for acute renal failure (ARF) and its application was expanding to patients with ESRD.

Conceptually, peritoneal dialysis is an older technique than hemodialysis, but its practical application was delayed by numerous unsuccessful attempts to treat both acute and end-stage renal disease patients [7]. Results were poor because of technical problems with catheters, peritonitis, and dialysate fluid composition. The subsequent development of commercially prepared dialysate and the introduction of the silicon cuffed catheter by Tenckhoff and Schechter [8] in 1968 heralded the modern era of peritoneal dialysis. Despite those improvements, peritoneal dialysis was still a somewhat unsatisfactory technique until 1976, when Popovich et al. [9] advocated "portable equilibration" from which continuous ambulatory peritoneal dialysis is modeled.

Because ARF is potentially reversible, an aggressive pursuit should be undertaken to identify and correct the cause. Within the intensive care unit (ICU) setting, although elements of chronicity may or may not be present, most cases of renal failure that require dialytic support are acute in nature. Therefore, most of the subsequent discussion focuses on dialysis for ARF within the ICU. Except where specifically denoted, all subsequent discussions are applicable to both patients with ARF and those with advanced chronic renal failure. A full discussion of the clinical pathophysiology, epidemiology, and treatment of ARF is found in Chapter 74.

Dialysis fulfills two biophysical goals: the addition or removal ("clearance") of solute and the elimination of excess fluid from the patient ("ultrafiltration"). These two processes can be performed simultaneously or at different times. The dialysis procedures in common use are hemodialysis, hemofiltration, a combination of these, and peritoneal dialysis (Table 30-1).

Hemodialysis

Hemodialysis is a diffusion-driven and size-discriminatory process for the clearance of relatively small solutes such as electrolytes and urea [less than 300 daltons (Da)]. Larger solutes are typically cleared far less readily. During hemodialysis, ultrafiltration is engendered by the generation of negative hydraulic pressure on the dialysate side of the dialyzer. The major components of the hemodialytic system are the artificial kidney or dialyzer; the respective mechanical devices that pump the patient's blood and the dialysate through the dialyzer; and the dialysate, which is the fluid having a specified chemical composition used for solute clearance. During the performance of "conventional" intermittent hemodialysis, the patient's blood and dialysate are pumped continuously through the dialyzer in opposite (countercurrent) directions at flow rates averaging 300 and 500 mL per minute, respectively. The dialysate passes through the dialyzer only once (single-pass system) and is discarded after interaction with the blood across the semipermeable membrane of the dialyzer. The efficiency of hemodialysis can be augmented by the use of dialyzers that are more porous to water and solutes. Those kidneys with enhanced performance characteristics are described as high-efficiency or high-flux dialyzers, depending on their ability to ultrafilter and remove larger molecular weight solutes like β_2-microglobulin. High-efficiency hemodialysis uses a high-porosity dialyzer that has an ultrafiltration coefficient greater than 10 and less than 20 mL per mm Hg per hour. High-flux hemodialysis uses an even more porous dialyzer with an ultrafiltration coefficient greater than 20 mL per mm Hg per hour and greater clearances of solutes greater than 300 Da.

Variables of the hemodialysis procedure that may be manipulated by the dialysis care team are the type of dialyzer (determines the solute clearance and ultrafiltration capacity of the dialysis treatment), the dialysate composition (influences solute clearance and loading), the blood and dialysate flow (influences solute clearance), the hydraulic pressure that drives ultrafiltration, and the duration of dialysis.

These dialytic parameters should be prescribed, so patients may derive the optimal "dose" of dialysis. Although numerous patient outcome studies have demonstrated a strong statistical relationship between the measured dose of hemodialysis and ESRD patient survival, dialysis dose has not yet been established in ARF. Nonetheless, due to the strong concordant rela-

Table 30-1. Dialysis Modalities

Technique	Dialyzer	Physical principle
Hemodialysis		
Conventional	Hemodialyzer	Concurrent diffusive clearance and UF
Sequential UF/ clearance	Hemodialyzer	UF followed by diffusive clearance
UF	Hemodialyzer	UF alone
Hemofiltration		
SCUF	Hemofilter	Arteriovenous UF without a blood pump
CAVH	Hemofilter	Arteriovenous convective transport without a blood pump
CAVHD	Hemofilter	Arteriovenous hemodialysis without a blood pump
CAVHDF	Hemofilter	Arteriovenous hemofiltration and hemodialysis without a blood pump
CVVH	Hemofilter	Venovenous convective transport with a blood pump
CVVHD	Hemofilter	Venovenous hemodialysis with a blood pump
CVVHDF	Hemofilter	Venovenous hemofiltration and hemodialysis with a blood pump
Peritoneal dialysis		
Intermittent	None	Exchanges performed for 10–12 h every 2–3 d
CAPD	None	Manual exchanges performed daily during waking hours
CCPD	None	Automated cycling device performs exchanges nightly

CAPD, continuous ambulatory peritoneal dialysis; CAVH, continuous arteriovenous hemofiltration; CAVHD, continuous arteriovenous hemodialysis; CAVHDF, continuous arteriovenous hemodiafiltration; CCPD, continuous cycling peritoneal dialysis; CVVH, continuous venovenous hemofiltration; CVVHD, continuous venovenous hemodialysis; CVVHDF, continuous venovenous hemodiafiltration; SCUF, slow continuous ultrafiltration; UF, ultrafiltration.

tionship between dose of dialysis and ESRD patient survival, consideration should be given to measuring the dose of dialysis in the setting of ARF [10]. The currently preferred measurement of hemodialysis dose is the volume-adjusted fractional clearance of urea, Kt/V_{urea}, where K is the dialyzer's urea clearance, t is the time on dialysis, and V is the volume of distribution of urea. Alternatively, the dose of hemodialysis may be expressed as the percentage reduction in urea during a single hemodialysis treatment, the urea reduction ratio (URR) [11], which is defined mathematically as

$$[1 - (\text{postdialysis blood urea nitrogen concentration} \div \text{preblood urea nitrogen concentration})] \times 100$$

HEMOFILTRATION AND HEMODIAFILTRATION.

In contrast to the diffusion-driven solute clearance of hemodialysis, hemofiltration also depends substantially on convective transport. In its simplest form, the patient's blood is conveyed through an extremely high-porosity dialyzer (hemofilter). The result is the formation of a protein-free hemofiltrate that resembles plasma water in composition. In the case of arteriovenous hemofiltration, the major determinant of perfusion of the hemofilter is the patient's mean arterial pressure, whereas the hydrostatic pressure in the hemofiltrate compartment provides the driving force for the formation of the filtrate. For effective hemofiltration, the mean arterial pressure should be maintained at more than 70 mm Hg. Blood is usually conveyed into the hemofilter from an arterial cannula and is returned into a large-caliber vein.

If a hemofiltrate is formed but is not replaced by a replacement fluid, the process is called slow continuous ultrafiltration. Little solute clearance occurs during slow continuous ultrafiltration. An alternative technique that enhances solute clearance is to continually replace the lost volume with a physiologic solution lacking the solute to be removed. If an arteriovenous blood path is used, the process is called continuous arteriovenous hemofiltration (CAVH). A venovenous circuit may be used with blood flow driven by a blood pump, and this procedure is referred to as *continuous venovenous hemofiltration* (CVVH). Optimal solute clearance is achieved by combining diffusive clearance and convective transport. This is accomplished by circulating dialysate through the hemofilter with or without high ultrafiltration rates [continuous arteriovenous hemodiafiltration (CAVHDF) and continuous arteriovenous hemodialysis (CAVHD), respectively]. Alternatively, these procedures may be performed using venovenous access with a blood pump to generate adequate flow rates [continuous venovenous hemodiafiltration (CVVHDF) and continuous venovenous hemodialysis (CVVHD), respectively]. Hemodiafiltration combines high ultrafiltration rate (requiring replacement fluid) and dialysate flow for clearance. Collectively, all these modalities are termed *continuous renal replacement therapies* (CRRT). Due to the availability of reliable blood pumps, precise ultrafiltration controllers, and the desire to avoid the morbidity of arterial cannulation, venovenous therapies have greatly diminished the use of arteriovenous modes of CRRT.

PERITONEAL DIALYSIS. Solute clearance in peritoneal dialysis is gradient driven, whereas ultrafiltration during peritoneal dialysis depends on the osmolality of the dialysis solution. In stable ESRD patients, maintenance peritoneal dialysis is performed daily, either by manual instillation and drainage of the dialysate during waking hours [continuous ambulatory peritoneal dialysis (CAPD)] or while sleeping using an automated dialysate cycling device [continuous cycling peritoneal dialysis (CCPD)]. The dialysate is allowed to dwell in the peritoneal cavity for variable intervals depending on the clearance and ultrafiltration goals (described as an "exchange"). The dialysate volume is usually 1.5 to 2.0 L per instillation, but can be as great as 3 L for the overnight dwell while the patient is recumbent.

In the acute setting, after the placement of a peritoneal dialysis catheter, peritoneal dialysis is easily initiated and discontinued with limited personnel and equipment. As in ambulatory ESRD patients, peritoneal dialysis for ARF may be performed manually, as in CAPD or using an automated cycler, as in CCPD. If it is performed acutely using an uncuffed dialysis catheter, rather than the conventional Dacron-cuffed catheters used for ESRD patients, 60 to 80 L of dialysate are exchanged over 48 to 72 hours, and the catheter is removed. The risk of peritonitis increases significantly thereafter without a cuffed catheter. A soft Dacron-cuff catheter is preferred if extended periods of peritoneal dialysis are expected.

A major disadvantage of peritoneal dialysis is its relative inefficiency for solute clearance, which may be problematic for patients in the ICU, who are often hypercatabolic and require high clearance of nitrogenous wastes. The advantages of peritoneal dialysis are that it obviates the use of anticoagulation, uses a biologic membrane (the peritoneum) for dialysis, and demands much less nursing time if automated cycling is used. Careful attention has to be paid to the patient's nitrogen balance because substantial losses of protein and amino acid may occur through the peritoneum [12].

Indications for Dialysis in Renal Failure

In patients with ARF, the goal of dialytic therapy is to support the patient while awaiting the recovery of adequate renal function to sustain life, whereas in chronic renal failure and ESRD, the objective is for dialysis to substitute for absent renal function indefinitely. In patients with ARF, who have had insufficient time to establish compensatory or adaptive physiologic alterations, it is mandatory that dialysis be initiated promptly. Absolute indications for the initiation of dialysis are uremic serositis, uremic encephalopathy, hyperkalemia resistant to conservative therapy, hypervolemia unresponsive to high doses of diuretics, and acidosis that is not adequately corrected with alkali. In addition, there are selected conditions that typically are not life-threatening and that can be managed by more conservative means. These conditions are relative indications for the initiation of dialysis. Examples include azotemia in the absence of uremia, hypercalcemia, hyperuricemia, hypermagnesemia, and bleeding exacerbated by uremia.

ABSOLUTE DIALYSIS INDICATIONS

Uremic Encephalopathy and Serositis. Historically, uremic encephalopathy and hyperkalemia were the principal absolute indications for the initiation of dialysis [13]. Of the complications of uremia, few are corrected as dramatically with dialysis as those involving the central nervous system (CNS). Tremor, asterixis, diminished cognitive function, neuromuscular irritability, seizures, somnolence, and coma are all reversible manifestations of uremia that merit the provision of dialysis [14].

Reversible cardiopulmonary complications of uremia, such as uremic pericarditis and uremic lung, respond to the initiation of an adequate dialysis regimen, but clinical resolution is more protracted than for the CNS manifestations of uremia [15,16]. Uremic pericarditis is characterized by the presence of noninfectious inflammation of both layers of the pericardium. It is accompanied by pericardial neovascularization and the development of a serofibrinous exudative effusion. Injudicious use of systemic anticoagulation for hemodialysis or other indications may induce intrapericardial hemorrhage and cardiac tamponade, although these complications may also occur spontaneously. Uremic pericarditis may also be associated with systolic dysfunction of the left ventricle and serosal inflammation with pleural hemorrhage. Uremic lung is a poorly understood late pulmonary complication of uremia demonstrating a roentgenographic pattern of atypical pulmonary edema that is not necessarily associated with elevated pulmonary capillary wedge pressures. It is also treated by the initiation of dialysis.

There is a poor correlation between the blood urea nitrogen (BUN) and the development of uremic signs and symptoms. The BUN is determined not just by the degree of renal insufficiency but also by dietary protein intake, hepatocellular function, and protein catabolic rate. Therefore, it is not surprising that uremic manifestations may arise with a BUN less than 100 mg per dL. In addition to the absolute level, the temporal rate of increase of the BUN seems to influence the development of uremia. Patients with a sudden and rapid decline in renal function, such as those with ARF, typically manifest uremic symptoms at lesser degrees of azotemia than do patients with more gradual declines in renal function, such as those with chronic progressive kidney disease. This is especially true for uremic encephalopathy. Finally, selected patient populations, such as children, the elderly, and individuals with diabetes mellitus, appear to have a lower threshold for manifesting uremic symptoms.

Hyperkalemia. During the course of progressive renal insufficiency, the capacity to excrete potassium is compromised and the adaptive cellular uptake declines [17]. Although hyperkalemia is a frequent complication of renal failure, its severity and timing are influenced by the cause of the renal failure, comorbid conditions, medications administered (e.g., angiotensin-converting enzyme inhibitors, nonsteroidal antiinflammatory drugs, potassium-sparing diuretics, and nonselective beta-blockers), and exogenous and endogenous potassium loads (see Chapter 73).

The need for emergent treatment is based on the degree of hyperkalemia, rate of rise, symptoms, and presence of electrocardiographic changes. It should be noted that patients with chronic renal failure develop adaptive mechanisms to excrete potassium [18]. In contrast, hyperkalemia in the setting of ARF is usually poorly tolerated. In the absence of indications for urgent treatment, conservative measures will suffice. These interventions include limiting daily intake of potassium (oral or parenteral), discontinuing incriminating medications, augmenting potassium excretion in the urine or stool (if oliguric), and implementing strategies to minimize cardiotoxicity [17,19,20]. Although hemodialysis is perhaps the quickest means for removing potassium, its efficiency may not be that achievable with polystyrene sulfonate resin (Kayexalate). Depending on the venue, presence or absence of dialysis access, and time of day, it may take up to 4 hours to set up for hemodialysis; in the interim, nondialytic measures can be applied that are life-saving.

Hypervolemia. Hypervolemia is a common complication of renal insufficiency, both in and out of hospital settings. For an outpatient with established ESRD, overzealous fluid intake and dietary indiscretion are major causes of hypervolemia. For hospitalized patients, the obligatory volume of fluids, medications, and food administered in caring for patients often exceed their excretory capacity, even in nonoliguric renal failure. There are also many ways in which clinicians caring for acutely ill patients may inadvertently overload them with fluids.

Integral to the prevention and treatment of hypervolemia is the administration of diuretics. Even patients with advanced renal insufficiency [glomerular filtration rate (GFR) less than 15 mL per minute] may respond to aggressive doses of loop diuretics.

The absence of an adequate diuretic response (diuresis that is inadequate to meet the volume challenge from obligatory fluids) is an absolute indication for dialysis. Fluid removal can be accomplished by hemodialysis, hemofiltration, or peritoneal dialysis (ultrafiltration). Ultrafiltration rates of more than 3 L per hour can be achieved during hemodialysis, 1 to 3 L per hour during hemofiltration, and usually less than 1 L per hour during peritoneal dialysis.

Acidosis. As renal function declines, endogenously generated organic acids and exogenously ingested acids are retained, and the capacity to generate and reclaim bicarbonate becomes increasingly compromised [21]. In patients who are not hypercatabolic or receiving an acid load, acid generation occurs at a rate of approximately 1 mEq per kg per day, resulting in an uncorrected decline in serum bicarbonate concentration to approximately 12 mEq per L [22]. Therefore, in patients with renal failure, metabolic acidosis is the typical acid-base disturbance. The severity of the acidosis in ICU patients with ARF is influenced by comorbid occurrences that may further contribute to the acidemia such as sepsis, uncontrolled diabetes mellitus, and poor cardiac output.

Severe acidosis in the context of ARF can result in changes in mental state leading to coma and can provoke hypotension by depressing myocardial contractility and causing vasodilation. The correction of acidosis is thus a major concern, especially in the intensive care setting. Less severe acidosis may be corrected by administration of exogenous oral alkali therapy. Sodium bicarbonate is the treatment of choice.

The use of alkali agents should be judicious in patients with renal failure. Both bicarbonate and citrate are administered as sodium salts. Therefore, volume overload is a risk. Excessive correction of severe metabolic acidosis (plasma bicarbonate less than 10 mEq per L) may have adverse consequences, including paradoxical acidification of the cerebrospinal fluid (CSF) and increased tissue lactic acid production. An initial partial correction to 15 to 20 mEq per L is quite appropriate. As with acidemia, patients with kidney failure do not tolerate alkalemia well. The diseased kidney cannot increase bicarbonate excretion, and severe alkalemia (from excessive alkaline therapy) may have grave consequences [23].

With these concerns in mind, if progressively larger doses of alkali therapy are required to control acidosis in renal failure, dialysis is indicated. Hemodialysis is especially useful in treating acidosis accompanying salicylate [24], methanol [25], and ethylene glycol poisonings [26]. An added benefit is the ability of hemodialysis to remove the parent compounds and their toxic metabolites [methanol (formic acid) and ethylene glycol (glycolic acid, oxalate)].

RELATIVE DIALYSIS INDICATIONS. Non–life-threatening indications for dialysis can typically be managed with more conservative interventions. Multiple relatively mild manifestations of ARF may provoke consideration of dialysis when present simultaneously. For example, a hypercatabolic trauma patient with ARF manifested by a gradually increasing serum potassium concentration, declining serum bicarbonate concentration, falling urine output, and a mildly diminished sensorium does not fulfill any of the absolute criteria for the initiation of dialysis. However, in such a case, the need for dialysis is almost inevitable, and the patient's care is not improved by withholding dialysis until a life-threatening complication of renal failure develops.

Hypercalcemia and hyperuricemia associated with ARF are common in patients with malignancies and tumor lysis syndrome, respectively [27,28]. Hypermagnesemia in renal failure is usually the result of the injudicious use of magnesium containing cathartics or antacids [29]. These metabolic disorders are readily corrected by deletion of the excessive electrolyte from the dialysate. For example, hypercalcemia that is unresponsive to conventional conservative interventions may be corrected by hemodialysis with a reduced calcium dialysate (less than 2.5 mEq per L).

Bleeding from the skin and gastrointestinal tract are common manifestations of platelet dysfunction in renal insufficiency. The hemostatic defect of renal insufficiency, an impairment of platelet aggregation and adherence, is reflected in the typical threefold prolongation of the bleeding time [30–33]. Although either peritoneal or hemodialysis can correct the platelet defect [34,35], more conservative therapies are available. Platelet dysfunction can be rapidly corrected by erythrocyte transfusion to a hematocrit level above 35% [31]; infusion of 10 U of cryoprecipitate, which is rich in von Willebrand factor, every 12 to 24 hours [36]; or intravenous (0.3 µg per kg) or subcutaneous (0.3 µg per kg) administration of deamino-8-D-arginine vasopressin, which induces the endothelial release of factor VIII–von Willebrand multimers [37]. Although not uniformly effective and of diminishing benefit after repeated administration, deamino-8-D-arginine vasopressin is the safest and most rapid way to correct the platelet defect of renal insufficiency. Interventions that produce a more protracted response that have a delayed onset of action are the administration of erythropoietin [38], conjugated estrogens (0.6 mg per kg for 5 days), or Premarin (25 mg per day for 7 days) [39,40].

Prophylactic Dialysis and Residual Renal Function

The presence of definitive indications such as severe hyperkalemia and overt uremia prompts the decision to initiate dialysis without further delay. However, in the absence of such emergent indications, the timing of the initiation of dialysis is more a matter of judgment. Prevailing opinion dictates that dialysis should be initiated prophylactically in ARF when life-threatening events appear imminent, understanding that it may be difficult to predict imminent events in a condition that is highly volatile in nature.

An additional consideration in the timing of dialysis is its influence on residual renal function and the length of recovery from ARF. Numerous observations suggested an important and possibly deleterious effect of dialysis on residual renal function. Several investigators have observed that in posttraumatic ARF treated with hemodialysis, there were pathologically demonstrable fresh, focal areas of tubular necrosis 3 to 4 weeks after the initial renal injury [41,42]. The only culpable hemodynamic insults experienced during this period were short-lived episodes of intradialytic hypotension. Furthermore, the initiation of dialysis is frequently associated with an acute decline in urine output [43]. It has been observed that in patients with advanced renal failure, the institution of hemodialysis results in progressive deterioration in GFR over several months [44]. The fact that peritoneal dialysis does not provoke a similar relentless decline in residual renal function [45] suggests this may be a consequence of combined hemodialysis-induced hypotension with abnormal vascular compensation and complement-mediated injury resulting from immunogenic dialyzer membrane materials [46,47]. Preserving residual renal function must be a high priority in managing patients with severe renal insufficiency [48]. Even modest preservation of GFR may ease fluid management in patients with ARF. A residual GFR of approximately 15 mL per minute is equivalent to 5 hours of hemodialysis with a dialyzer, having a urea clearance of 160 mL per minute. The clearance of middle-molecular-weight solutes is especially enhanced with endogenous function compared with hemodialysis.

Relatively few studies have examined the issue of the timing of dialysis initiation, and most are reports from the early days of dialytic therapy. In 1960, Teschan et al. [49] described their success with the initiation of hemodialysis before the onset of frank uremia. Using this protocol, dialysis was continued on a daily basis to maintain the BUN less than 150 mg per dL until recovery occurred. Compared with historical control subjects, who were dialyzed for severe uremia alone, patient survival was greatly improved. Another study reported similar favorable outcome of early dialysis based on a retrospective analysis of 500 patients [50]. In later years, two relevant randomized prospective studies were performed. In one study, 18 posttraumatic ARF patients were randomized to initiate hemodialysis at low (predialysis BUN and creatinine levels less than 70 mg per dL and 5 mg per dL, respectively) or high BUN threshold treatment groups (predialysis BUN approximately 150 mg per dL or overt uremia as an indication for dialysis). Continued hemodialysis was performed only when these thresholds were reached. The study reported 64% survival in the low BUN group compared with 20% in the high BUN group [51]. Sepsis and hemorrhage were frequent complications in the high BUN group. As intriguing as these observations are, none of these studies was sufficiently optimally designed as to allow definitive conclusions.

To address these inadequacies, Gillum et al. [52] performed a larger intervention study involving 34 patients and segregated them into medical and surgical causes of ARF. In this investigation, the low-BUN group was dialyzed as needed to maintain the BUN and creatinine at levels less than 60 and 5 mg per dL, respectively, and the high-BUN group to BUN and creatinine concentrations of 100 and 9 mg per dL, respectively. Neither group began dialysis until the creatinine was at least 8 mg per dL. The investigators observed no statistically significant difference in patient mortality between the two groups (41% for the low-BUN group vs. 53% for the high-BUN group). It must be appreciated that this study design evaluated the impact of the intensity of dialysis and not the timing of its initiation.

In summary, although dialytic therapy is an essential tool in the management of ARF, its use or abuse may have detrimental effects on patient outcome. The physician must avoid the temptation to intervene in the course of ARF based on the achievement of a threshold BUN value alone. Proper consideration of the patient's overall condition, expected course of the type of renal failure experienced, fluid and nutritional requirements, and the presence of comorbid conditions is a more reasoned approach.

Practical Application of Engineering Principles

HEMODIALYSIS AND HEMOFILTRATION

Clearance. The most fundamental biophysical principle of dialysis is solute movement across a semipermeable membrane by diffusion. Diffusional movement of a solute from a region of higher concentration to that of a lower concentration is governed by Fick's law:

$$J = -DA \times (dc/dx)$$

where J is the solute flux, D its diffusivity, A is the area available for diffusion, and dc is the change in the concentration of the solute over the intercompartmental distance, dx. For a particular model of dialyzers, dx and A are constant, and for an individual solute, D is constant. It is clear that solute flux is influenced by the surface area and the physical structure of the membrane, the variables that define the clearance characteristic of a given dialyzer.

In clinical practice, the clearance of a solute is not only dependent on the dialyzer but also the blood and dialysate flow rates, expressed by the following equation:

$$K = [Q_{Bi} \times (C_{Bi} - C_{B0})] \div C_{Bi}$$

In this expression, K is the diffusive clearance of the solute from the blood, Q_{Bi} is the rate at which blood containing the solute flows into the dialyzer, C_{Bi} is the concentration of the solute in the blood entering the dialyzer (arterial end), and C_{B0} is the remaining concentration of the solute in the egress side of the blood compartment (venous end) [53]. This mathematical description is accurate for the situation in which the solute is not initially present in the dialysate ($C_{Di} = 0$). Usually, the dialysate passes through the dialyzer only once (single-pass dialysis system), and there is minimal convective transport of the solute during its clearance. Thus, the clearance of a solute during dialysis may be functionally defined as the volumetric removal of the solute from the patient's blood. Within the practical application of this formulation, the clearance of a solute can be modified by altering the patient's blood flow into the dialyzer (Q_{Bi}).

A similar relationship exists for the dialysate and the diffusive clearance of a solute from the blood:

$$K = [Q_{Di} \times (C_{D0} - C_{Di})] \div C_{Bi}$$

where Q_{Di} is the flow rate of the dialysate into the dialyzer, and C_{D0} and C_{Di} are the concentrations of solute at the dialysate outlet and inlet ends of the hemodialyzer, respectively [53]. Thus, an additional means of augmenting the diffusive clearance of a solute from the blood into the dialysate, or vice versa, is to increase the dialysate flow rate. Increases in blood, dialysate flow, or both do not improve the clearance proportionally. As blood and dialysate flow rates are increased, resistance and turbulence within the dialyzer occur, resulting in a decline in clearance per unit flow of blood or dialysate. For conventional dialyzers, this limitation occurs above 300 and 500 mL per minute, respectively, for blood and dialysate flows. Limitations for high-flux dialyzers are observed at above 400 and 800 mL per minute for blood and dialysate flow rates.

The clearance characteristics of dialyzers provided by their manufacturers are determined *in vitro*; the influence of plasma proteins on solute clearance is not accounted for, and the actual *in vivo* diffusivity is usually lower [54]. The clearance of a solute by a given dialyzer is a unique property of that solute. Molecules larger than 300 Da, such as vitamin B_{12} or β_2-microglobulin, typically have lower K values compared with smaller solutes, such as urea and potassium. The clearance of these larger solutes from blood depends to a greater extent on ultrafiltration and the passive movement of solute (convective transport). The summary interaction between the diffusive clearance and convective transport of a solute is expressed as

$$J = (K \times [1 - Q_f/Q_B] + Q_f) \times C_{Bi} = KC_{Bi}$$

where Q_f is the ultrafiltration rate, and K is the sum of the convective and diffuse clearances [53,55]. If the diffusive clearance (K) is large, as is true for urea, the influence of the ultrafiltration rate is not great. As the diffusive clearance for a solute declines because of increasing molecular weight (value of K approaches Q_f), the proportionate contribution of convective transport to solute movement increases greatly [56]. The practical application of convective transport of solutes alone is observed during pure hemofiltration (CAVH, CVVH), because no dialysate is passed through the hemofilter (preventing diffusive clearance).

Ultrafiltration. An equally important operational variable in the dialysis procedure is the ultrafiltration coefficient (K_f), defined by

$$K_f = Q_f \div (P_B - P_D)$$

where Q_f is the ultrafiltration rate, and P_B and P_D are the mean pressures in the blood and dialysate compartments, respectively [53,55]. Analogous to the information derived for the clearance of a particular solute for a specific dialyzer, each dialyzer also has an ultrafiltration coefficient. Because these values are typically derived *in vitro*, similar limitations exist for their application to the *in vivo* situation. It is not unusual for an individual dialyzer's *in vitro* and *in vivo* ultrafiltration coefficients to vary by 10% to 20% in either direction.

The ultrafiltration coefficient for a dialyzer operationally defines the volume of ultrafiltrate formed for a given pressure across the dialysis membrane per unit time (mL per mm Hg per hour), which is P_B minus P_D. Therefore, it is possible to use the ultrafiltration coefficient to calculate the quantity of pressure that must be exerted across the dialysis membrane [transmembrane pressure (TMP)] to achieve a given volume of ultrafiltration during a dialysis session. To make this calculation, it is first necessary to quantitate the pressure that is exerted across the dialysis membrane from the blood to the dialysate compartment. During ultrafiltration, the serum oncotic pressure increases in the dialyzer's blood compartment from the arterial to the venous end, but this is usually a relatively negligible biophysical factor. Therefore, the net pressure across the dialysis membrane that arises from the flow of blood and dialysate is calculated by

$$P_{net} = [(P_{Bi} - P_{B0}) \div 2] - [(P_{Di} + P_{D0}) \div 2]$$

where P_{Bi}, P_{B0}, P_{D0}, and P_{Di} are the pressures measured at the inflow and outflow ports of the blood and dialysate compartments, respectively. If the P_{net} is too low to provide for adequate ultrafiltration during a dialysis session ($P_{net} \times$ ultrafiltration coefficient × dialysis time < target ultrafiltrate volume), additional pressure can be generated across the dialysis membrane by creating negative pressure in the dialysate compartment. The effective pressure, or TMP, required can be derived from TMP = desired weight loss ÷ (ultrafiltration coefficient × dialysis time).

The performance of ultrafiltration during hemodialysis has been greatly simplified by the development of dialysis machines that possess volumetric control systems ("ultrafiltration controllers"). Ultrafiltration with these devices is remarkably precise, and weight loss can be effected in a linear manner per unit of time. Such exact volumetric control is a prerequisite for high flux hemodialysis in which high porosity dialyzers are used.

During most hemodialysis treatments, ultrafiltration and solute clearance are performed simultaneously. However, it is possible to segregate the two procedures temporally by a modification of the hemodialysis procedure described as *sequential ultrafiltration clearance* [57,58]. This modification of the conventional hemodialysis procedure is accomplished by first ultrafiltering to the desired volume and then conducting diffusive clearance without ultrafiltration. During the initial ultrafiltration phase, diffusive clearance is prevented by not pumping dialysate through the dialyzer. During the second phase, no negative pressure is instituted, and the small fluid losses secondary to P_{net} are balanced by the infusion of saline. Sequential ultrafiltration clearance has distinct hemodynamic advantages over conventional hemodialysis, making it a particularly useful technique for aggressive fluid removal within a short interval. When ultrafiltration is performed concurrently with diffusive solute clearance, intravascular volume losses may exceed the rate of translocation of fluid from the interstitium. If these losses are not counterbalanced by an appropriate increase in the peripheral vascular resistance and venous refilling, hypotension occurs [57–61]. With sequential ultrafiltration clearance, these hemodynamic abnormalities are attenuated, and up to 4 L per hour may be removed without causing hypotension. However, unless the total time allotted to dialysis is increased during sequential ultrafiltration clearance, solute clearance is compromised and inadequate dialysis may occur.

During CRRT, ultrafiltration is governed by different physical principles than those for hemodialysis. Because the driving force for blood flow during CAVH is the mean arterial pressure, and the resistance in the blood path that arises from the hemofilter and the lines is low, the hydraulic pressure in the blood compartment of the hemofilter is also low. Therefore, during CAVH, the driving force for the formation of an ultrafiltrate is the negative hydrostatic pressure within the ultrafiltrate compartment of the hemofilter. This effective negative pressure (P_h) is generated by the weight of the column within the ultrafiltration collection line and is calculated by P_h = height difference (cm) between the hemofilter and collection bag × 0.74. Therefore, to increase or decrease the rate of fluid formation during hemofiltration, the collection bag is either lowered below or raised to the level of the hemofilter. In contrast to hemodialysis, the increase in oncotic pressure at the venous end of the hemo-

filter is of sufficient magnitude that little ultrafiltration occurs at this end. Because significant convective solute clearance occurs with hemofiltration, little clearance occurs at the venous end of the hemofilter. This situation is most likely to occur when the amount of ultrafiltrate formed is maximal and when the blood flow rate through the hemofilter is low. It is therefore undesirable to have the net ultrafiltration rate greater than 25% of the blood flow rate [62]. Excessively large amounts of ultrafiltrate can result from a kinked or thrombosed venous return line, as increased back pressure will translate into significant hydraulic pressure on the blood side compartment.

The ultrafiltrate that is formed during hemofiltration is free of protein with a solute composition that closely resembles plasma water [55]. The quantity of a selected solute that is cleared is determined by the volume of ultrafiltrate formed, by its concentration in the blood (and therefore in the ultrafiltrate), and by the composition of the replacement solution. For example, if hemofiltration results in the formation of 0.5 L ultrafiltrate per hour and the ultrafiltrate and the replacement solution contain 5 mEq per L and 0 mEq per L of potassium, respectively, 30 mEq of potassium will be cleared in 12 hours.

As mentioned earlier, hemofiltration usually necessitates replacement fluid, because of the inherently high rate of ultrafiltration associated. The replacement solution can be administered immediately before (predilutional hemofiltration) or after the hemofilter (postdilutional hemofiltration), simultaneously into both locations (pre-postdilution hemofiltration), or into the peripheral venous circulation [63,64]. Predilution hemofiltration offers the advantage of diluting plasma proteins, effectively lowering the thrombogenicity of the hemofilter and increasing the ultrafiltration rate for a given hydrostatic pressure. However, this technique also reduces the concentration of solutes in the blood entering the hemofilter and therefore may compromise their clearance. Alternatively, the replacement solution can be administered incompletely before the hemofilter, with the balance being infused immediately after the hemofilter. This offers the advantages of predilutional hemofiltration and avoids the clearance disadvantages.

PERITONEAL DIALYSIS

Clearance. The simplest kinetic model of solute transport in peritoneal dialysis is that of two compartments separated by a membrane, with the two pools representing blood in the mesenteric vasculature and dialysate in the peritoneal cavity [65]. Solutes passing from the blood into the dialysate compartment encounter three structures of resistance: the capillary endothelium, the interstitial tissues, and the mesothelial cell layer of the peritoneum. Diffusion and convective transport are involved in clearance during peritoneal dialysis. As within the context of hemodialysis, diffusion (according to Fick's law) can be expressed as $J = -DA \times dc/dx$, where J is the solute flux, D is the diffusion coefficient of that solute, A is the functional surface area of the membrane, dx is the diffusion distance, and dc is the concentration gradient. DA/dx is known as the *mass transfer area coefficient* (MTAC), and the *concentration gradient* is the difference between the plasma (CP) and dialysate (CD) concentrations. Hence,

$$J = \text{MTAC} \times (\text{CP} - \text{CD})$$

As is evident from these principles of solute transfer, the diffusive clearance can clearly be influenced by the concentration gradient; the diffusion coefficient, which is solute size dependent; and the characteristics of the peritoneal membrane. As the concentrations approximate each other (CP – CD nears zero), diffusive clearance declines. Thus, to increase clearance, the concentration gradient must be maintained with frequent change of dialysate (increase the number of exchanges with shorter dwell times). The benefit of increasing dialysate exchange rate (above 3.5 L per hour) is limited by the fact that this decreases the effective time available for contact between the dialysate and the peritoneum [66]. A successful alternative to aid clearance is to increase the volume of dialysate per exchange from 2.0 to 3.0 L. These volumes are usually well tolerated by adults, especially when recumbent. The larger volume of dialysate allows more contact with the peritoneum, facilitating clearance. Increments in the dialysate volume have been shown to augment MTAC [67,68].

Because ultrafiltration and clearance occur concurrently during peritoneal dialysis, the use of hyperosmolal dialysates augments the clearance of solutes. In this situation, convective transport is added to diffusive clearance. The use of the most osmotically active dialysate (4.25% dextrose) can increase urea clearance by approximately 50% [69]. If the peritoneal vascular surface area is adequate, urea clearance and ultrafiltration are not limited by peritoneal blood flow [70–73]. For example, in patients in shock, the clearance of urea is depressed only by approximately 30%; intraperitoneal vasodilators augment small solute clearance by only 20%.

Considering that a 24 L per day exchange of 1.5% dextrose-containing dialysate typically results in a urea clearance of approximately 17 mL per minute, peritoneal dialysis is a low-efficiency procedure. Therefore, it is not surprising that this technique may be inappropriate for management of hypercatabolic patients with ARF. Likewise, an acutely ill, maintenance peritoneal dialysis patient, who has been on an adequate and stable dialysis regimen when healthy, may not achieve adequate clearance for his or her increased needs with continued peritoneal dialysis. For many adults on maintenance peritoneal dialysis, the contribution of residual renal function to solute clearance is critical for achieving adequate peritoneal dialysis. In a peritoneal dialysis patient, the loss of residual renal function due to a severe comorbid illness or nephrotoxic medication such as an aminoglycoside may render inadequate a previously satisfactory dialysis regimen. Such patients should have their daily number of exchanges increased empirically or be transferred to hemodialysis.

Ultrafiltration. In peritoneal dialysis, the net pressure generated favors movement of water from the dialysate into the capillaries. Therefore, an active osmotic solute (typically dextrose) is used to facilitate ultrafiltration. As is the situation for solute clearance, ultrafiltration is maximal at the beginning of an exchange and declines as the osmolality gradient declines during equilibration. Hyperglycemia, by decreasing the osmolality gradient, also impairs ultrafiltration. Even with optimal exchange frequency and volume, ultrafiltration rates during peritoneal dialysis are usually at least 700 mL per hour. The ultrafiltrate formed is hypoosmolal to serum, so hypernatremia is a common complication of excessive ultrafiltration.

Components of the Dialysis Process

HEMODIALYSIS AND HEMOFILTRATION

Dialyzers and Hemofilters. Virtually all commercial dialyzers available for hemodialysis in the United States are configured as large cylinders packed with hollow fibers through which the blood flows (hollow-fiber dialyzer). The dialysate flows through the dialyzer and around these fibers usually in a countercurrent direction. The membrane for these dialyzers is composed of a variety of modified biologic or synthetic materials such as regenerated cellulose, cuprophan, hemophan, cellu-

lose acetate, polysulfone, polymethylmethacrylate, and polyacrylonitrile. The surface area available for solute transport and the filling volume of the blood and dialysate compartments vary significantly among different dialyzers and are a function of the membrane material. These materials vary in their characteristics for solute transport and ultrafiltration, the degree to which they are tolerated by the patient's immune system ("biocompatibility"), costs, and capacity to be reused. The choices of dialyzer for the management of either acute or chronic renal failure are usually dictated by these three variables in this same rank order.

The impetus to develop more efficient dialyzers stems from the desire to decrease time on hemodialysis through faster solute clearance. A secondary goal is to improve clearance of larger solutes that may be toxic, such as β_2-microglobulin. The relative inability of dialyzers to clear these larger solutes may contribute to the development of neuropathy and dialysis-associated amyloidosis [74,75]. A putative disadvantage of these efficient larger pore dialyzers is that they may permit more readily the transmembrane back flux of bacterial-derived lipopolysaccharides from the dialysate into the dialyzer blood compartment (backfiltration) [76]. The resultant patient exposure to the pyrogen results in an acute nonbacteremic, febrile illness described as a pyrogen reaction. The use of bicarbonate-buffered dialysates, which permit the growth of gram-negative bacteria, and ultrafiltration controllers that limit the rate of ultrafiltration may also contribute to the occurrence of pyrogen reactions [77,78].

The characteristic requirements of a dialyzer or hemofilter used in CRRT must be considered from a different perspective. Because the driving force for hemofiltration is the mean arterial pressure of a low-speed venous pump and clearance is disproportionately dependent on convection of low resistance, a high K_{uf} hemofilter is required. Hemofilters are usually composed of polysulfone, polymethylmethacrylate, or polyacrylonitrile, because cuprophan does not have sufficient hydraulic permeability at TMP of 30 to 70 mm Hg. Hemofilters are available in two geometric configurations: the hollow-fiber or the parallel-plate configuration (blood and dialysate separated by a flat semipermeable membrane). The parallel-plate filter may be advantageous in arteriovenous systems (where arterial pressure is the driving force) because the Poiseuille resistance to flow is less and, therefore, less pressure decline occurs during blood transit through the hemofilter [79]. The flat-plate geometry is also less susceptible to clotting, and hemofilter changes are not needed as often.

In continuous hemodialysis techniques (CAVHD, CVVHD), solute transport is limited by the dialysate flow rate, unlike conventional intermittent hemodialysis. The blood flow rate is usually 100 to 150 mL per minute, and dialysate flow rate is generally 16 to 30 mL per minute. The rapidity of solute equilibration across the dialysis membrane, which is a function of the hemofilter, determines the type of hemofilter that can be used.

Dialysates for Hemodialysis. The composition of the dialysate is the other major component of the dialysis process that determines the outcome of this procedure (Table 30-2). Although sodium and potassium are typically the only components of the dialysate that are adjusted to meet the demands of specific clinical situations, the other constituents are equally critical. The dialysate is stored as a liquid or powdered concentrate that is diluted in a fixed ratio to yield the final solute concentration. The safe and appropriate proportioning of dialysate concentrates and water is monitored using online measurements of the conductivity of the dialysate before its entry into the hemodialyzer.

GLUCOSE. Before hydraulic-driven ultrafiltration became available, the dialysate glucose concentration was maintained at

Table 30-2. Dialysate Formulation for Peritoneal Dialysis and Conventional Hemodialysis

Solute	Range (usual concentration)
Peritoneal dialysis	
Na^+	132 mEq/L
K^+	0
Cl^-	96 mEq/L
Lactate	35 mEq/L
Ca^+	2.5 or 3.5 mEq/L
Mg^+	0.5 or 1.5 mEq/L
Glucose	1.5%, 2.5%, or 4.25% g/dL
Conventional hemodialysis	
Na^+	138–145 mEq/L (140)
K^+	0–4 mEq/L (2)
Cl^-	100–110 mEq/L (106)
HCO_3^-	35–45 mEq/L (38)
Ca^+	1.0–3.5 mEq/L (2.5)
Mg^+	1.5 mEq/L (1.5)
Dextrose	1.0–2.5 mEq/L (2)

above 1.8 g per day to generate an osmotic gradient between the blood and the dialysate [80]. Although this was effective for inducing ultrafiltration, some patients developed morbid symptoms and signs of hyperosmolality. Currently, dialysates are glucose free, normoglycemic (0.00% to 0.25%), or modestly hyperglycemic (more than 0.25%). Hemodialysis with a glucose-free dialysate results in a net glucose loss of approximately 30 g and stimulates ketogenesis and gluconeogenesis [81]. Such alterations in intermediary metabolism may be particularly deleterious in chronically or acutely ill hemodialysis patients who are malnourished or on a medication such as propranolol that may induce hypoglycemia [82,83]. These effects are ameliorated by the use of a normoglycemic dialysate. Additional metabolic consequences occurring from the use of a glucose-free dialysate include an accelerated loss of free amino acids into the dialysate [84], a decline in serum amino acids [85], and enhanced potassium clearance stemming from relative hypoinsulinemia [81]. Therefore, the dialysate glucose concentration should be maintained at normoglycemic concentrations.

SODIUM. Historically, the dialysate sodium concentration was maintained on the low side (more than 135 mEq per L) to prevent interdialytic hypertension, exaggerated thirst, and excessive weight gains. However, hyponatremic dialysates increase the likelihood of intradialytic hypotension, cramps, headaches, nausea, and vomiting and are provocative of the dialysis dysequilibrium syndrome [86–90]. During hemodialysis, the volume ultrafiltered may exceed intravascular volume. As solute molecules are cleared from the extracellular compartment, an osmotic gradient arises favoring movement of water into the intracellular space, which drives transcellular volume movement [91]. CNS symptoms are prominent in the dialysis dysequilibrium syndrome, reflecting the brain swelling caused by this water shift. These hemodynamic alterations are minimized in the setting of equal dialysate and serum sodium concentrations. Thus, there has been an appropriate increase in the dialysate sodium to 140 to 145 mEq per L.

Although an increase in dialysate sodium could result in polydipsia and increased interdialytic weight gains [88], it permits enhanced ability to ultrafilter these patients, offsetting this problem. The pressor response to an increased dialysate sodium varies. In patients who are hypertensive because of hyperreninemia during ultrafiltration, a higher dialysate sodium may be associated with a reduction in blood pressure. However, most patients exhibit no increment in blood pressure with physiologic dialysate sodium concentrations [88]. Some patients who typically are hypertensive at baseline have worsened vasopressor control with a higher sodium dialysate [86,89].

The newer dialysate delivery systems permit active alteration of dialysate sodium concentrations during hemodialysis by the use of variable-dilution proportioning systems. The technique of sodium "profiling" to fit a patient's hemodynamic needs has been espoused as a means of accomplishing optimal blood pressure support without increased thirst at the completion of the treatment. The modulation of dialysate sodium concentration can be executed in several patterns. Sodium profiling may reduce the frequency of hypotension during ultrafiltration without decreasing the dialysis time committed to diffusive clearance, as is the case with sequential ultrafiltration clearance [91]. However, it is unclear if this technique offers any advantage over a fixed dialysate sodium of 140 to 145 mEq per L [92–94]. Furthermore, interdialytic weight gains appear unaffected by sodium modeling [93]. For most hemodialysis patients, the dialysate sodium concentration can be maintained at 140 to 145 mEq per L.

POTASSIUM. Unlike urea, which usually behaves as a solute distributed in a single pool with a variable volume of distribution, only 1% to 2% of the total body store of 3,000 to 3,500 mEq of potassium are present in the extracellular space [95]. The flux of potassium from the intracellular compartment to the extracellular space, and subsequently across the dialysis membrane to the dialysate compartment, is unequal. Therefore, the efficacy of potassium removal in hemodialysis is highly variable, difficult to predict, and influenced by dialysis-specific and patient-specific factors [96]. In a study that controlled for dialyzer-specific components of the dialysis procedure (blood and dialysate flow, dialyzer type and surface area, duration of dialysis, dialysate composition), potassium removal varied by approximately 70%. Even for the same patient, approximately 20% variability in potassium removal was noted using identical hemodialysis conditions [97].

During hemodialysis, approximately 70% of the potassium removed is derived from the intracellular compartment [81]. Because 50 to 80 mEq of potassium are removed in a single dialysis session and only 15 to 20 mEq of potassium are present in the plasma, life-threatening hypokalemia would be the consequence of hemodialysis if this was not the case [96]. However, the volume of distribution of potassium is not constant; the greater the total body potassium, the lower its volume of distribution [98]. As a result, the fractional decline in plasma potassium during a single dialysis session is greater if the prehemodialysis level is higher. Optimal potassium elimination by hemodialysis is accomplished by daily short hemodialysis treatments instead of protracted sessions every other day. The transfer of potassium from the intracellular compartment to the extracellular compartment usually occurs more slowly than the transfer from the plasma across the dialysis membrane [98,99]. This discrepancy further complicates predicting the quantity of potassium removed during hemodialysis. A practical consequence of the discordant transfer rates is that the plasma potassium measured immediately after the completion of hemodialysis is approximately 30% less than the steady-state value measured after 5 hours. Therefore, hypokalemia based on blood measurements obtained immediately after the completion of hemodialysis should not be treated with potassium supplements.

The transcellular distribution of potassium is influenced by several variables, including the relative degree of hyperinsulinemia (promotes potassium uptake into cells, lowering its intradialytic clearance) [81], catecholamine tone (β agonists promote cellular uptake of potassium and α agonists stimulate the cellular egress of potassium, attenuating and increasing the intradialytic clearance of potassium, respectively) [95,100], sodium-potassium adenosine triphosphatase activity (pharmacologic inhibition diminishes potassium uptake into cells, which may enhance intradialytic clearance) [101], and systemic pH (alkalemia augments transcellular potassium uptake, which may diminish dialytic clearance of potassium) [95]. Although the degree of systemic alkalization is greater and more rapid in onset with bicarbonate-buffered dialysates than with acetate-buffered dialysates, the choice of buffer does not appear to be critical in determining potassium removal during hemodialysis [81,102]. Paradoxically, it has been observed that as the gradient for potassium clearance from blood into the dialysate is increased by decreasing the dialysate potassium concentration, the uptake of bicarbonate from the dialysate declines [102]. This interaction between alkali and potassium in the dialysate is significant: a 1-mEq increase in the potassium gradient results in a decline in bicarbonate loading of 50 mEq. This interaction should not be overlooked in planning the dialysate prescription for patients being dialyzed for severe acidosis [103].

Because the selection of the dialysate potassium is empirical, most patients are dialyzed against a potassium concentration of 1 to 3 mEq per L. For patients who have excessive potassium loads from their diet, medications, hemolysis, trauma, or gastrointestinal bleeding, the dialysate potassium concentration should be 0 to 1 mEq per L. For stable patients who do not have significant cardiac disease or who are not taking cardiac glycosides, a dialysate potassium concentration of 2 to 3 mEq per L is appropriate. In a patient with a history of cardiac disease, especially with arrhythmias and cardiac glycoside usage, the dialysate potassium should be increased to 3 to 4 mEq per L [104]. Such patients are at the greatest risk for the development of dysrhythmias associated with the intradialytic potassium flux. They may be best managed by tolerating a greater degree of interdialytic hyperkalemia possibly with the concomitant administration of sodium polystyrene sulfonate resin (Kayexalate), so that they may tolerate the higher dialysate potassium concentrations.

Most cardiac morbidity attributable to the dialysate potassium concentration occurs during the first half of the dialysis session. The rapidity of the fall in the plasma potassium concentration, rather than the absolute plasma concentration, appears to determine the risk of cardiac arrhythmias [99,104]. For this reason, hyperkalemic patients should be managed with an incremental decline in the dialysate potassium concentration of approximately 1.0 mEq per L per hour [105]. If the patient has a significant deficit in total body potassium, postdialysis hypokalemia can occur, even if the dialysate potassium concentration is greater than the serum potassium concentration [106]. This seemingly contradictory situation arises because of the potential for a delayed conductance of potassium from the dialysate into the patient, compared with its movement from the extracellular space into the intracellular compartment.

BASES. Initially, bicarbonate was used as the base in the dialysate. In the early 1960s, it was superseded by acetate, which is more stable in aqueous solution at neutral pH in the presence of divalent cations. Acetate is metabolized in skeletal muscle, and to a lesser extent in the liver, to acetyl coenzyme A, which is subsequently metabolized further via Krebs cycle to carbon dioxide and water. In the latter process, one proton is consumed and one molecule of bicarbonate is liberated [107]. During conventional hemodialysis with large-surface-area dialyzers, acetate flux above 300 mmoL per hour can occur, resulting in acetate accumulation as the amount translocated exceeds the capacity to metabolize the base. This complication occurs most often in women, elderly patients, and patients who are malnourished [108]. The resultant clinical consequences of acetate accumulation include variable degrees of nausea, vomiting, headache, fatigue, peripheral vasodilatation, decreased myocardial contractility, metabolic acidosis, and arterial hypoxemia [109–112]. Hence, vascular instability is much more problematic with predominantly acetate-containing dialysates than bicarbonate-containing

dialysates. The hemodynamic instability associated with acetate is worsened by hyponatremic dialysates and is lessened with a normonatremic dialysate [110,113,114].

Hemodialysis using a bicarbonate-buffered dialysate prevents these complications. The transient anion gap metabolic acidosis associated with acetate dialysis is not seen with bicarbonate based dialysis. A raised bicarbonate concentration in the dialysate not only attenuates the diffusive gradient from blood to dialysate but generally allows the patient to achieve a net positive bicarbonate balance. Additionally, dialysis-induced hypoxemia is attenuated by a bicarbonate dialysate. During hemodialysis with acetate, there is a large diffusive loss of carbon dioxide into the dialysate such that the minute ventilation falls by approximately 25%. Therefore, despite the loss of carbon dioxide across the dialytic circuit, there is little decline in the arterial carbon dioxide tension (normocapneic hypoventilation). During hemodialysis with acetate, hypoxemia is most prominent during the first 60 minutes of hemodialysis and may be associated with an approximately 35-mm Hg decline in arterial oxygen tension [115,116].

Because of the amelioration of many intradialytic symptoms with bicarbonate-containing dialysates, and the increased use of high-efficiency and high-flux hemodialysis, acetate is used for hemodialysis in less than 20% of the dialysis facilities in the United States. Bicarbonate dialysis is now feasible because of the widespread availability of proportioning systems that permit mixing of the separate concentrates containing bicarbonate and divalent cations close to the final entry point of the dialysate into the dialyzer. Unlike the more acidic and hyperosmolal acetate-based dialysate, liquid bicarbonate concentrates and reconstituted bicarbonate dialysates support the growth of Gram-negative bacteria such as *Pseudomonas, Acinetobacter, Flavobacterium,* and *Achromobacter*; filamentous fungi; and yeast [78]. Because of the propensity of the dialysate to support bacterial growth, and the morbidity associated with the presence of such growth in the dialysate, strict guidelines exist for the acceptable limit of bacterial growth, the presence of lipopolysaccharide in the dialysate, and dialyzer reuse [117].

A bicarbonate-based dialysate of 30 to 35 mEq per L is typically used. Bicarbonate concentrations above 35 mEq per L may result in the development of a metabolic alkalosis with secondary hypoventilation, hypercapnia, and hypoxemia. If a bicarbonate dialysate is unavailable, acetate at an equivalent concentration is suitable, but large-surface-area dialyzers or dialyzers with high-efficiency or high-flux transport characteristics cannot be used.

CALCIUM. Patients with renal failure are prone to develop hypocalcemia, hyperphosphatemia, hypovitaminosis D, and hyperparathyroidism. Positive calcium balance is thus useful as an adjunct during hemodialysis for controlling metabolic bone disease [118–120]. In patients with renal failure requiring dialysis, over 60% of the calcium is not bound to plasma proteins and is in a diffusible equilibrium during hemodialysis [121]. Assuming free conductance of calcium across the dialysis membrane secondary to diffusive clearance and an additional contribution secondary to convective losses, a dialysate calcium concentration of roughly 3.5 mEq per L (7.0 mg per dL) is necessary to prevent intradialytic calcium losses [122]. Because such elevated calcium dialysates transiently induce hypercalcemia, which temporarily reduces parathyroid hormone secretion [123], they had been the standard dialysate calcium concentration.

Over the last decade, increasing and appropriate concerns arose for the development of aluminum intoxication syndromes secondary to the protracted use of oral aluminum hydroxide as a phosphate binder. The three aluminum intoxication disorders, which arise because of the intestinal absorption and retention of ingested aluminum, are progressive osteomalacia, iron-resistant microcytic anemia, and progressive encephalopathy [124–126]. Instead of using aluminum salts alone, calcium carbonate, calcium acetate, or sevelamer have been increasingly used alone or with small quantities of aluminum hydroxide as oral phosphate binders [127–129]. However, because variable amounts of calcium are absorbed from the ingested calcium salt, persistent hypercalcemia is a frequent complication of a dialysate calcium of greater than 3.0 mEq per L, especially if a vitamin D supplement is also used. To minimize the likelihood of hypercalcemia and consequently soft tissue calcification [130], there is a trend toward lower dialysate calcium concentrations [118]. In most dialysis facilities, a dialysate calcium concentration of 2.5 to 3.0 mEq per L is used.

A reduction in the dialysate calcium may increase vascular instability during hemodialysis [130–132]. Dialysis-induced changes in the serum calcium concentration correlate with the intradialytic systolic and diastolic blood pressures. Intradialytic increases in serum ionized calcium concentration augment left ventricular performance without an accompanying alteration in the peripheral vascular resistance [133].

MAGNESIUM. The serum magnesium concentration, like that of potassium, is a poor determinant of total body magnesium stores. Only approximately 1% of the total body magnesium is present in the extracellular fluid and only 60% of this amount (approximately 25 mEq) is free and diffusible [134]. Because of scant extrarenal clearance, removal during hemodialysis is the primary route of elimination for magnesium in renal failure. The magnesium flux that occurs during a dialysis session is difficult to predict despite knowledge of the serum and dialysate magnesium concentrations. When using a low-magnesium dialysate, the postdialytic decline in serum magnesium concentration is virtually corrected after 24 hours [135].

Because the ideal serum magnesium concentration in patients with ESRD is debatable, the appropriate dialysate magnesium concentration is unresolved. Many centers use a 1.0-mEq per L dialysate magnesium concentration, and mild interdialytic hypermagnesemia is often observed.

CHLORIDE. Chloride is the major anion in the dialysate. Because its concentration is defined by the constraints of maintaining electrical neutrality in the dialysate, chloride concentration varies depending on the concentration of cations.

Dialysates for Continuous Hemodialysis and Hemodiafiltration.
Typical dialysate flow rates for continuous hemodialysis or hemodiafiltration are 800 to 1,000 mL per hour (vs. 500 to 800 mL per minute for conventional hemodialysis), and the dialysate is usually delivered into the dialyzer by a continuous infusion pump. Because it is impractical to mix and store conventional hemodialysis fluid for continuous hemodialysis and hemodiafiltration, and the formation of a custom dialysate in the volumes required for these techniques is cumbersome and costly, most hospitals use conventional peritoneal dialysate for CAVHD, CVVHD, CAVHDF, and CVVHDF. Despite the use of commercially prepared dialysate formulations, which typically are less costly than custom preparations, the dialysate costs associated with CAVHD and CVVHD render these techniques more expensive than CAVH or CVVH. Although peritoneal dialysate presents the most conveniently available fluid for use, its glucose concentration is higher than optimally desired. A further drawback is that it is relatively hyponatremic (sodium concentration of 132 mEq per L), although this may be beneficial for patients with hypernatremia. Peritoneal dialysate formulations are discussed in greater detail below.

The need for a custom dialysate for hemofiltration most often arises in situations in which the calcium concentration requires modification or the patient cannot tolerate a lactate-buffered dialysate. Commercial dialysates for peritoneal dialysis are usually available in three calcium concentrations: 3.5, 3.0, and 2.5 mEq per L. Such a limited selection of dialysates compromises

the treatment of hypercalcemic patients by these modalities. When such circumstances arise, the dialysate formula should be tailored to the individual using an appropriately reduced calcium concentration. The standard lactate buffering of peritoneal dialysates may become problematic for patients with an impaired capacity to metabolize lactate, such as those with reduced hepatic and renal function or hypotension with ongoing tissue ischemia. Hyperlactatemia has been shown to occur in hemodiafiltration using lactate-buffered dialysate [136]. In these circumstances, a custom dialysate should be formulated with bicarbonate as the buffer. Successful experiences have been reported with a custom bicarbonate dialysate containing sodium 144 mEq per L, bicarbonate 37 mEq per L, potassium 3 or 4 mEq per L, calcium 3 mEq per L, and magnesium 1.4 mg per dL. No solute precipitation was observed, and bacterial contamination was not a problem [137].

Replacement Solutions for Continuous Hemofiltration. The principal mechanism for solute clearance in techniques using hemofiltration is by convection. To achieve adequate solute clearance, the ultrafiltered volume is large (12 to 24 L per day), which makes fluid replacement obligatory for CAVH, CVVH, CAVHDF, and CVVHDF. Because the composition of the ultrafiltrate is similar to plasma water, the ideal replacement solution should approximate the normal plasma composition minus the solutes that need removal. Numerous replacement solutions have been used. Lactated Ringer's solution [138] and peritoneal dialysate [139] are two commonly used commercial replacement solutions. Although convenient, they do not offer the same flexibility in composition as on-site preparations. Both lactated Ringer's solution and peritoneal dialysate have lactate as buffer and may not be suitable in association with liver failure and lactic acidosis. Lactated Ringer's solution also provides an obligate potassium load, and peritoneal dialysate has a high glucose content. A specially formulated hemodiafiltration fluid is being marketed currently (Table 30-3). Although it contains lactate, it is normoglycemic and has a higher sodium concentration than peritoneal dialysis fluid or Ringer's solution (see Table 30-2 for comparison). This preparation can also be used as a dialysate for CRRT.

In situations in which lactate buffer is less than ideal and a bicarbonate solution is preferred, the latter can be prepared on

Table 30-3. Infusion Fluids for Replacement in Continuous Renal Replacement Therapies

Hyperalimentation solutions	
Lactated Ringer's solution	
Na^+	130 mEq/L
Cl^-	110 mEq/L
Lactate	28 mEq/L
K^+	4 mEq/L
Ca^+	3 mEq/L
Alternative solutions	
1 L IV D10 0.9% normal saline with 5 mEq calcium gluconate and 0–4 mEq magnesium sulfate, followed by	
1 L IV D10 0.45% normal saline with 44 mEq (1 amp) $NaHCO_3$, followed by	
1 L IV D10 0.9% normal saline with 5 mEq calcium gluconate and 0–4 mEq magnesium sulfate, followed by	
1 L IV D10 W with 132 mEq (3 amp) $NaHCO_3$	
Cycle can then be repeated	
Net: Na^+	140 mEq/L
Cl^-	96 mEq/L
HCO_3^-	44 mEq/L
K^+	0 mEq/L
Ca^+	2.5 mEq/L
Mg^+	0–2 mEq/L

D10 W, dextrose 10% in water.

site, but must be used soon after preparation because of its inherent instability. On-site replacement solutions can be made by the addition of various solutes to standard intravenous dextrose 5% water or saline. The single-bag approach is easiest, in which bicarbonate is mixed with calcium and magnesium. Because of the potential for solute precipitation, single bags have limited use. Alternately, bicarbonate can be prepared separately from the calcium- and magnesium-containing solutions, and the two bags of replacement solutions can be infused sequentially or concurrently through different infusion ports. Because these fluids are prepared when needed, they can be custom formulated to the requirements of the patient.

Anticoagulation for Intermittent Hemodialysis. Despite the impaired capacity of platelets to aggregate and adhere in most patients with advanced renal failure, the interaction of plasma with the dialysis membrane results in activation of the clotting cascade, thrombosis in the extracorporeal circuit, and the resultant dysfunction of the dialyzer [140]. Dialyzer thrombogenicity is determined by its composition, surface charge, surface area, and configuration [141]. In addition, the propensity for intradialytic clotting is influenced by the blood flow through the dialyzer; the extent of blood recirculation in the extracorporeal circuit (newly dialyzed blood reentering the dialyzer); the amount of ultrafiltration; and the length, diameter, and composition of the lines between the patient and the dialyzer. Patient-specific variables that influence thrombogenicity and determine the requirements for anticoagulants include the presence of congestive heart failure, malnutrition, neoplasia, blood transfusions, and comorbid coagulopathies such as disseminated intravascular coagulation, warfarin therapy, or hepatic synthetic dysfunction [142].

Because of its low cost, ready availability, ease of administration, simplicity of monitoring, and relatively short biologic half-life, the anionic mucopolysaccharide heparin is the most widely used anticoagulant for dialysis. The time constraints of hemodialysis are such that the partial thromboplastin time cannot be used to monitor the effectiveness of anticoagulation. Instead, an activated clotting time (ACT) is often used. In this assay, whole blood is mixed with an activator of the extrinsic clotting cascade, such as kaolin, diatomaceous earth, or ground glass, and the time necessary for the blood to first congeal is monitored. The normal range is 90 to 140 seconds.

The precise method of heparin administration is influenced by the patient's comorbid illness and varies among dialysis providers. The simplest method of heparin administration is systemic administration, in which 2,000 to 5,000 U of heparin are administered at the initiation of dialysis followed by a constant infusion of 1,000 U per hour. The target ACT is approximately 50% above baseline. Another method of systemic anticoagulation is to administer repeated boluses of heparin (100 U per kg of dry weight at the start) when the ACT falls below target. Because the degree of anticoagulation during systemic anticoagulation is relatively intensive, it is appropriate only for stable patients who are at no risk for bleeding. Therefore, in the ICU, systemic anticoagulation is rarely used. Less intensive anticoagulation is achieved with fractional heparinization, in which the target ACT is maintained at 15% ("tight fractional") or 25% ("fractional") greater than the baseline value. Five hundred to 3,000 U of heparin are administered at the initiation of dialysis, followed by a continuous heparin infusion at an initial rate of 500 to 1,000 U per hour.

Minimal heparinization occurs with "regional" heparinization. By this method, the extracorporeal circuit alone is anticoagulated with heparin and the effect reversed before the extracorporeal blood is returned to the patient [143]. Five hundred units of heparin are given at the beginning of dialysis, and 500 to 750 U per hour are infused into the arterial line. Simultaneously, 3.75 mg per hour of protamine are infused into the venous line. Using fre-

quent checks of the ACT from the arterial and venous lines as a guide, the heparin and protamine infusion rates are adjusted to maintain the ACT for the patient at baseline and for the dialytic circuit at approximately 10 seconds. Because heparin has a longer half-life than protamine, an additional 50 mg of protamine should be given at the end of dialysis [144]. Problems associated with this method of anticoagulation include complexity in balancing the infusion rate, bleeding from rebound anticoagulation because of the dissociation of the heparin–protamine complex [145], and side effects of protamine (flushing, bradycardia, dyspnea, and hypotension). Alternatively, regional anticoagulation may be achieved with sodium citrate as the anticoagulant [146]. Citrate binds to calcium and forms a dialyzable salt, thereby depleting the extrinsic and intrinsic clotting cascades of the obligatory cofactor, calcium. A 4% solution of trisodium citrate is initially infused into the arterial line at 200 mL per hour, and the infusion rate is adjusted after 20 minutes to maintain the ACT of the machine at 25% over baseline. This process is reversed on the venous side distal to the filter by infusion of 10% calcium chloride at 30 mL per hour. Although very effective [146], the principal disadvantages of this technique are the requirements for additional infusions and close monitoring of the patient's calcium and acid-base status (as citrate is metabolized to generate bicarbonate, thus increasing the risk of alkalemia). The dialysate used in citrate regional anticoagulation must be calcium free with lower sodium and bicarbonate concentration.

Regional anticoagulation can be associated with significant and relatively frequent side effects [145]. In high-risk situations in which regional anticoagulation may be contraindicated (e.g., heparin-induced thrombocytopenia, allergy to protamine, personnel unfamiliar with technique), dialysis may be performed without heparin [146–148]. In this technique, the hemodialyzer is first rinsed with 1 L of 0.45% saline containing 3,000 to 5,000 U of heparin. Hemodialysis is immediately initiated using the maximum blood flow tolerated, and the dialyzer is flushed every 15 to 30 minutes with 50 mL of saline. Although not feasible with large-volume ultrafiltration, compromised blood flow, or the intradialytic administration of blood products, heparin-free dialysis may be the safest choice for any ICU patient at risk of bleeding.

Anticoagulation must be individualized based on the patient's risk of hemorrhage. Clearly, the risk of thrombosis of the dialytic circuit is a secondary consideration. Guidelines for anticoagulation based on comorbid conditions are as follows:

1. Patients who are bleeding or are at significant risk of bleeding, have a baseline major thrombostatic defect, or are within 7 days of a major operative procedure or within 14 days of intracranial surgery should be dialyzed without heparin or by regional anticoagulation.
2. Patients who are within 72 hours of a needle or forceps biopsy of a visceral organ should be dialyzed without heparin or by regional anticoagulation.
3. Patients who are beyond the temporal limits established for items 1 and 2 can be dialyzed by fractional heparinization. If they have previously received fractional heparinization, they can now be considered for systemic anticoagulation.
4. Patients with pericarditis should be dialyzed without heparin or by regional anticoagulation.
5. Patients who have undergone minor surgical procedures within the previous 72 hours should be dialyzed under fractional anticoagulation.
6. Patients anticipated to receive a major surgical procedure within 8 hours of hemodialysis should be dialyzed without heparin or by regional anticoagulation. If they are within 8 hours of a minor procedure, fractional anticoagulation is appropriate.

Anticoagulation for Continuous Renal Replacement Therapy. The need for anticoagulation in CRRT is driven by its relatively low blood flow rate (100 to 150 mL per minute) and prolonged continuous exposure of blood to the dialyzer membrane. Thus, even by modifying the procedure to minimize thrombogenicity (using relatively short arterial and venous lines, changing to a parallel plate configuration for the hemofilter, performing predilutional hemofiltration), heparin is usually required [149]. Predictably, the use of aggressive ultrafiltration that results in hemoconcentration, reduced blood flows, and blood passage through long venous lines, is very thrombogenic. In CRRT, the required intensity of anticoagulation usually is similar to that associated with systemic heparinization for hemodialysis. After a systemic loading dose of heparin, an initial maintenance infusion of approximately 10 U per kg per hour is administered and titrated to maintain the partial thromboplastin time in the arterial line 50% greater than control. Obviously, such concentrated heparinization compromises the use of this technique for patients at risk for bleeding.

Alternatives to the standard systemic heparinization technique described above have been proposed for patients with high risk of bleeding. These include citrate regional anticoagulation [150,151] and use of heparin with protamine [152].

CRRT modalities can be performed without anticoagulation, although this usually compromises the performance of the hemofilter unless it is changed frequently. This technique involves rinsing the kidney and lines with heparinized saline in the method described for heparin-free hemodialysis [153].

Thrombosis within the hemofilter is easy to recognize by the characteristic striped clotting of the usually white fibers within the hollow-fiber dialyzer. However, the parallel-plate configuration is assembled in such a manner that the interior of the hemofilter cannot be visualized. In this circumstance, clotting of the hemofilter can be defined inferentially by the decline in the ultrafiltration rate, decrease in dialysate urea nitrogen to BUN ratio (less than 0.6 is significant), or both [154].

Hemodialysis Angioaccess. An adequately functioning angioaccess is a prerequisite for any blood-based dialytic techniques. There are two categories of access-related issues in the intensive care setting: ESRD patients with established permanent access and patients with ARF requiring temporary angioaccess for hemodialysis or CRRT. The care and maintenance of these permanent or temporary accesses are of crucial importance for the support of patients needing dialysis treatments.

The vascular access of choice for maintenance hemodialysis patients is the endogenous arteriovenous native vein fistula. This is because of its ease of construction, long-term survival, and lower incidence of infection compared with other modalities of vascular access [155]. Many older patients and diabetics with ESRD do not have adequate arterial or venous anatomy to allow the creation of an endogenous fistula. In these patients, a prosthetic arteriovenous fistula is generated. The most frequently used material for such a graft fistula is polytetrafluoroethylene. Relevant to care within the ICU, it should be appreciated that acute thrombosis of either a native vein or graft fistula may occur from intravascular volume depletion secondary to overzealous ultrafiltration, systemic hypotension from a comorbid condition like sepsis, or excessive local pressure for hemostasis after removal of the hemodialysis needles. Judicious care must be given to preserve patency of these fistulas. This includes their exclusion from use for routine cannulation or phlebotomy and prohibition of blood pressure measurements or application of constricting dressings on the fistula-side limb. An early sign of thrombotic graft failure is the observation of an increase in the pressure of the venous limb during dialysis. Although hemodialysis may still be performed at this stage, the efficiency of the treatment is compromised because turbulent nonlaminar blood flow occurs together with regurgitation of venous side blood back to the arterial side (access recirculation).

The type of angioaccess needed for dialysis in the setting of ARF in the ICU is determined by the chosen modality of dialytic therapy. If hemodialysis is adopted, a venous catheter will suffice. If CRRT is preferred, there is the option of using arteriovenous or venovenous methods. The latter is currently favored, because it allows direct regulation of blood flow and, consequently, higher blood flows can be achieved relatively independent of the mean arterial pressure [156]. Higher blood flows also permit less intense anticoagulation, because they minimize clotting of the extracorporeal circuit. Acute angioaccess for hemodialysis or venovenous CRRT may be achieved with vascular catheters. Vascular complications such as aneurysm, bleeding, and limb ischemia are less likely to occur with a venous access [157,158]. The oldest and safest means of establishing angioaccess for hemodialysis is to place a single- or double-lumen coaxial catheter in the femoral vein by the Seldinger technique [159]. The incidence of serious complication from femoral vein dialysis catheters is only 0.2% [160]. Under ideal situations, catheters should be removed within 7 days to minimize the risk of infection and thrombosis [160]. Femoral vein catheters are available in a number of lengths and diameters. The 24-cm length is preferable because it permits less blood recirculation.

Alternative sites for catheter-based angioaccess are the subclavian or internal jugular veins. Compared with the femoral vein, these sites have the advantages of fewer local infections, longer local positioning, and enhanced patient mobility [161]. Early-occurring complications such as local bleeding, hemothorax, pneumothorax, hemopericardium [162], arrhythmia [163], and hemomediastinum are usually related to catheter placement. Catheter placement under ultrasound guidance may make this procedure safer [164]. Late-occurring complications such as arteriovenous fistula formation, local catheter infection or sepsis, central vein thrombosis or stenosis [165], and catheter malfunction are particularly vexing. Infectious complications are a function of the duration of catheter usage. If the catheter is left in place for less than 2 weeks, the incidence of infections is less than 5%. Longer periods of catheter placement *in situ* are associated with an increased incidence of infections (as great as 25%) [166]. The typical pathogenesis for catheter infections is from bacteria colonizing the skin adjacent to the catheter entry site that migrate down the catheter sheath [167], which may be minimized by the use of topical antibiotics like mupirocin [168]. When an infection occurs, the usual therapy is 10 to 14 days of systemic antibiotics and removal of the dialysis catheter. Suppurative thrombophlebitis or endocarditis requires prompt discontinuation of the catheter and 4 to 6 weeks of bacteriocidal antibiotics. Central venous thrombosis (which occurs more commonly with subclavian vein positioning) necessitates immediate removal of the catheter [169].

Catheter malfunction with inadequate or absent blood flow is most often secondary to intraluminal thrombosis or catheter malposition [161]. Forced irrigation is usually of no benefit and may be detrimental. Instead, inadequate blood flow should be treated by the instillation of tissue plasminogen activator in a volume sufficiently large to fill the catheter. The solution should be aspirated out of the catheter, and dialysis reattempted. If unsuccessful, the procedure may be repeated. If thrombolytic therapy is of no benefit, catheter malposition should be considered. The catheter can be threaded with a guidewire, removed, and a replacement catheter repositioned.

Site-specific instructions for placing venous catheters via the Seldinger technique can be found in Chapter 2. Although easiest and least risky to place, the femoral vein dialysis catheter confines a patient to the supine position. For this reason, and the higher likelihood of infection in the femoral location, internal jugular and subclavian catheters are a better choice if a long course of dialysis is anticipated or if the patient is to be allowed to move. The newer tunneled, cuffed, soft catheters, such as the Tessio catheter, are preferred for this purpose.

Hemofiltration Angioaccess. The techniques used to establish venous access for CVVH or CVVHD are exactly as described above. The principal advantage of an arteriovenous access for CRRT (CAVH) is that it allows the use of a very simple extracorporeal circuit without a blood pump or an air embolus monitor. On the other hand, arteriovenous circuits require the placement of an additional catheter for arterial access. There are only two forms of arteriovenous access: wide-bore single-lumen femoral artery and vein catheters and, much less commonly, the Scribner shunt (an external plastic arteriovenous fistula). Scribner shunts should not be placed in patients with peripheral vascular disease who may develop digital ischemia.

Because patients on CRRT are, by definition, bed confined, vascular access is usually achieved by percutaneous cannulation of the common femoral vessels. Alternative sites, including the axillary artery and vein, and external shunts have been attempted but do not provide adequate blood flow for effective hemofiltration. Patients with femoral artery bypass grafts or those with severe atherosclerotic vascular disease may be extremely poor candidates for arteriovenous techniques. Before femoral artery cannulation, dorsalis pedis pulses should be examined by Doppler ultrasonography. If pulses are inaudible or if a bruit is present over the femoral artery, an alternative dialytic modality (e.g., conventional hemodialysis or CVVH or hemodialysis via the femoral, subclavian, or internal jugular vein) should be considered. The proper technique for femoral artery cannulation is described in Chapter 3.

PERITONEAL DIALYSIS

Dialysates. Compared with the dialysates used for hemodialysis or hemofiltration, the composition of the dialysates used for peritoneal dialysis is relatively constant (Table 30-2). The conventional dialysate sodium concentration is 132 mEq per L, potassium concentration 0 mEq per L, and lactate concentration 35 mEq per L. Hypokalemia in peritoneal dialysis patients is usually managed by increasing the dietary potassium intake. If oral therapy is ineffective or unfeasible, potassium can be added to the dialysate to attenuate the diffusive gradient. A typical potassium concentration in the dialysate is 1 to 4 mEq per L. The dialysate calcium concentration varies from 2.5 to 3.5 mEq per L; the choice of dialysate calcium depends on the patient's propensity to develop hypercalcemia. Many peritoneal dialysis patients, who ingest calcium salts as phosphate binders, become hypercalcemic using the traditional 3.5 mEq per L containing calcium dialysate. Therefore, as in hemodialysis, the trend has been to lower the calcium concentration in peritoneal dialysates. Magnesium is provided in the dialysate at 0.5 mEq per L. The other electrolyte present in the dialysate is chloride, the concentration of which is determined solely by the requirements to achieve electrical neutrality.

Ultrafiltration during peritoneal dialysis is achieved by the infusion of a hyperosmolal dialysate. Dextrose in concentrations of 1.5%, 2.5%, or 4.25% is used to induce ultrafiltration. Because the osmotic gradient is less with a 1.5% dextrose-containing dialysate than with a 4.25% dialysate, the fall-off in ultrafiltration develops relatively sooner using the 1.5% dextrose solution. Likewise, if the osmotic gradient is attenuated by the development of hyperglycemia, ultrafiltration will decline. Therefore, in peritoneal dialysis patients with glucose intolerance, ultrafiltration with dialysates containing high levels of glucose may be compromised if glycemic control is not maintained.

Access to the Peritoneal Cavity. Immediate access for peritoneal dialysis may be provided in the acute setting by the percutaneous placement of a stylet-guided catheter connected to a closed-gravity, manual instillation drainage system or to an automated dialysate cycler.

The procedure for placement of a temporary peritoneal dialysis catheter is as follows:

1. The urinary bladder is emptied to prevent inadvertent perforation.
2. The abdomen is prepared with povidone-iodine solution and draped, as it would be for an abdominal paracentesis. A point one-third of the distance between the umbilicus and symphysis pubis is infiltrated with local anesthetic to the peritoneum.
3. To distend the peritoneum, 1 to 2 L of 1.5% dextrose peritoneal dialysate is introduced into the peritoneal cavity via a 16-gauge spinal needle or Angiocath (Becton, Dickinson and Company, Franklin Lakes, NJ).
4. A small puncture is made at the same site with a scalpel blade.
5. The stylet-guided catheter is inserted into the skin puncture site and passed through the skin, underlying fascia, and linea alba. Entrance of the catheter tip into the peritoneum is evident by a sudden reduction in resistance and by appearance of dialysis fluid in the transparent catheter. If cloudy or feculent fluid is withdrawn, the bowel has been punctured [170], and the dialysis catheter should be left in place until a decision is made regarding the need for a diagnostic procedure (e.g., contrast computed tomography). Intravenous antibiotics to cover bowel bacteria (e.g., gentamicin and metronidazole or ampicillin-sulbactam) should be started. If peritoneal dialysis is to be continued, another access site should be chosen, and the above process repeated.
6. If the peritoneal drainage is clear, the stylet is withdrawn until the obturator point meets the catheter tip. The catheter is then advanced into the posteroinferior area of the peritoneal cavity and connected to a closed-gravity manual instillation drainage system or to an automatic cycler. The catheter can then be secured to the skin by a superficial pursestring suture.

Although simple to install and position in the peritoneal cavity, patients must remain supine, and the risk of infection is so great that the catheters must be removed after 48 hours. If dialysis is required for more than 48 to 72 hours, a new site should be selected and the original catheter removed.

An alternative means of establishing access into the peritoneal cavity with much greater permanency and one that permits patient ambulation is to install a flexible Silastic catheter with one or two Dacron cuffs. The most frequently used dual-cuffed catheter is the Tenckhoff catheter, which has an open end and multiple holes in the distal 15 cm [8]. These cuffed catheters minimize bacterial migration down the catheter tract. Such catheters are not only highly desirable for ESRD patients on continuous peritoneal dialysis but also in the ARF population, if the expected duration of dialytic support by peritoneal dialysis is more than 2 weeks. Although the placement of a chronic dialysis catheter can be performed in the ICU by experienced skilled personnel using a percutaneous technique, the method used in most hospitals is surgical placement under sterile conditions in the operating suite.

Placement of stylet-guided temporary catheters can be difficult and dangerous in patients who have intraabdominal adhesions, which usually result from prior major abdominal surgery. The most common catastrophes are vascular and visceral organ puncture. Even if successfully positioned, the resultant compartmentalization of the dialysate in the peritoneal cavity greatly decreases the surface area available for solute clearance and ultrafiltration. Similar limitations exist for the placement of surgically implanted Tenckhoff catheters. For this reason, peritoneal dialysis is not generally offered to renal failure patients with previous major abdominal surgery and likely intraabdominal adhesions.

Catheter malfunction, manifested by slow dialysate instillation, drainage, or both, may be caused by catheter malpositioning (catheter tip migration, entrapment in adhesions, or kinking) or luminal obstruction (blood clot, fibrin, or incarcerated omentum). An initial approach to this problem is to obtain an abdominal plain radiograph to determine the position of the catheter tip. If appropriately positioned, a thrombolytic may be instilled into the catheter [171]. After the liquid is aspirated, an exchange may be attempted. If catheter dysfunction continues, it should be replaced. Catheter exit site infection, as evident by local redness and drainage, needs to have antibiotic treatment and usually does not mandate a change of catheter to a new exit location. More extensive infections, such as tunnel infection with or without peritonitis, obligates removal of the catheter and transient substitution of peritoneal dialysis with another dialytic modality.

Selected Issues in Dialytic Therapy for Acute Renal Failure

MEMBRANE BIOCOMPATIBILITY IN HEMODIALYSIS. The development of a wide array of dialyzers allows an easier selection to fulfill the dialytic solute and ultrafiltration needs of the patient. However, with the advent of these newer membranes, an added criterion for selection of membranes in the management of ARF and the ESRD population is its biocompatibility [172]. The interaction of both soluble and cellular components of the blood with the dialysis membrane may be important in the pathobiology of such varied issues as duration of recovery from acute ischemic renal failure [173]; adverse intradialytic symptoms and signs such as fever, hypotension, and hypoxemia [115,174–177]; immunologic dysfunction and infectious susceptibility [178–180]; maintenance of an anabolic state [181]; development of β_2-microglobulin amyloidosis [74,182]; and the severity of hyperlipidemia [183].

A plethora of alterations in cellular functions and physiologic responses has been described in association with hemodialysis using cellulosic-based membranes, including the intradialytic generation of complement-derived anaphylatoxins, such as C3a and C5a, via the alternate complement pathway *in vivo* [184]; induction of enhanced membrane expression of selected granulocyte adhesion molecules such as membrane attack complex and leukocyte adhesion molecule *in vivo* [185,186]; inappropriate production of reactive oxygen species such as superoxide by granulocytes *in vivo* [187]; activation of the coagulation pathway *in vitro* [188]; formation of kallikrein and bradykinin [189]; enhanced monocyte elaboration of cytokines such as interleukin (IL)-1, IL-6, and tumor necrosis factor *in vitro* and perhaps *in vivo* [175,190–192]; altered IL-2 receptor expression *in vivo* [193]; altered monocyte phagocytosis *in vitro* [179]; and defective natural killer cell function [194]. Membranes without these proinflammatory effects are described as biocompatible. Another aspect of biocompatibility is the ability of the membrane to adsorb activated proinflammatory substances from the blood. Highly adsorptive membranes can efficiently reduce levels of factor D (an essential enzyme of the alternative pathway acti-

vation) [195], bradykinin, and pyrogenic cytokines such as IL-1 and tumor necrosis factor. It has been suggested that removal of these substances may offer some benefit to critically ill patients, although this remains unproven [240].

Dialyzer membranes composed of bioincompatible materials are typically derived from cellulose, whereas biocompatible membrane dialyzers are usually synthetic materials, such as polysulfone, polymethylmethacrylate, polyamide, or polyacrylonitrile. Many adverse pathobiologic consequences of hemodialysis that arise from membrane interactions are thought to be attenuated by using biocompatible membranes. This has led to an increased preference for these membrane materials for dialyzers in maintenance hemodialysis. Because of the high ultrafiltration requirement for CRRT, and the inability of cellulosic dialyzers to fulfill this requirement, CRRT is always performed with highly porous biocompatible dialyzers.

Several reviews examined the impact of dialysis membrane type on outcome in patients with ARF [196–199]. Based on *in vitro* models of ischemic ARF [200] and several *in vivo* interventional trials [173,201], the use of biocompatible membranes has been espoused to enhance patient survival, expedite recovery from ARF, and diminish the need for dialytic support [202]. However, those reports are not uniform [203–205]. Studies addressing patient symptoms such as hypotensive episodes, angina, and bronchospasm during hemodialysis have not demonstrated any difference between membrane types [206]. Although catabolic effects were demonstrated in experimental single hemodialysis sessions with bioincompatible membranes [181], a long-term study found an increase in serum albumin in both groups of patients treated with biocompatible and bioincompatible membranes [207]. In the same study, flux characteristics of the membranes were not found to have a significant effect on nutritional parameters. Because of the inconsistent nature of the available evidence, it is not justifiable to recommend the routine exclusion of bioincompatible membrane dialyzers to treat patients with ARF [208,209]. A limitation of biocompatible membrane dialyzers is their increased cost compared with cellulosic membrane dialyzers. Although the benefits of biocompatible membrane materials are not conclusive, the two well-controlled, prospective studies supporting their use demonstrated no detrimental effect when compared with cuprophan [173,201].

Comparing the results across trials is difficult because of the varying definitions of membrane biocompatibility, dialyzer flux, achieved hemodialysis adequacy, and disparity in the patients' demographics, comorbid conditions, cause of ARF, presence of oliguria, follow-up duration, and sample size. In conclusion, choosing a biocompatible membrane means paying more for uncertain but potentially improved patient outcomes in selected patients [210].

DOSE OF DIALYSIS. As is true for maintenance peritoneal and hemodialysis, the amount of solute clearance provided during ARF likely affects outcomes [211]. Using urea as a surrogate uremic toxin, the amount of urea removed can be quantitated by its fractional clearance during a dialysis session. For hemodialysis, a commonly used measure is the URR. For maintenance hemodialysis patients, a URR of less than 60% to 65% is associated with an increased odds risk of death [212,213]. An alternative measurement is the Kt/V, which is the fractional reduction of urea adjusted for the urea distribution volume. A Kt/V less than 1.2 is associated with increased death risk for maintenance hemodialysis patients [213]. Arguably, a similar dose-response relationship may exist for patients with ARF.

In an outcome analysis of patient survival with ARF, the mean delivered Kt/V was significantly higher among survivors

(0.90 ± 0.04 vs. 0.76 ± 0.05) [214]. However, it was observed that the quantity of hemodialysis exerted no influence for the highest and lowest patient disease severity quartiles but did have an impact on the survival of patients with moderate severity scores. It is not surprising that the amount of dialysis would have no discernible influence when the disease severity and comorbidity are extreme as competing risks. There is inadequate information to recommend a minimum or optimal delivered dose of hemodialysis in ARF. However, there is no reason to anticipate that the delivered hemodialysis dose should be less than a Kt/V of 1.2 or URR of 65% as recommended for maintenance hemodialysis patients [213].

CONTINUOUS VERSUS INTERMITTENT DIALYTIC THERAPY. Advocates of CRRT espouse several putative advantages of CRRT over intermittent hemodialysis. Fluid removal is a common reason for initiating dialysis in ARF, and this can easily be achieved by either CRRT or hemodialysis. However, because of its intermittent nature, significant volume expansion can occur between hemodialysis treatments, especially if the patient is receiving parenteral nutrition. In contrast, CRRT allows precise hourly adjustments of the ultrafiltration rate that readily permits the removal of more than 10 L per day. Because ultrafiltration with CRRT is gradual, hemodynamic stability may be more readily maintained. Therefore, a principal advantage of CRRT is that it permits the allocation of nutrition with less concern for volume overload [215]. Similarly, the continuous dynamic nature of CRRT may allow better correction of azotemia and acidemia [216]. Seven hours of daily intermittent hemodialysis are necessary to achieve similar levels of urea clearance as CRRT [217]. In a comparison of CVVH and hemodialysis in patients with ARF, CRRT provided better control of azotemia for equal amounts of therapy [218].

Sepsis syndrome and multiorgan failure in association with ARF [203] predict a poor outcome, perhaps related to the activity of proinflammatory substances such as activated complement fragments, platelet-activating factor, arachidonic acid metabolites, kinins, selected cytokines, and proteases [219,220]. It has been speculated that CRRT may improve patient outcomes by removing these inflammatory mediators in sepsis and multiorgan failure syndrome with renal failure. Several human studies demonstrated that hemofiltration removes inflammatory mediators like tumor necrosis factor, IL-1β, IL-6, platelet-activating factor, and complement fragments from circulation [221,222]. The mechanism of removal is through convective clearance or by the adsorption to the hemofilter membrane.

Despite these theoretical advantages, CRRT has not been demonstrated to be of added benefit over conventional dialysis to enhance patients' outcomes. Based on an analysis of data from 15 studies performed between 1986 and 1993, CRRT was not observed to improve patient outcomes when compared with the intermittent hemodialysis [223]. In a randomized crossover intervention trial comparing the hemodynamic response to intermittent hemodialysis versus CAVH in ICU patients with ARF, no difference in the hemodynamic parameters (mean arterial pressure, use of adrenergic drugs, change in body weight) occurred between the two methods [224]. In a multicenter, randomized, controlled trial of 166 patients with ARF, treatment by intermittent hemodialysis resulted in lower mortality (41.5%) compared with CRRT (59.5%) [225]. However, patients randomized to CRRT had more severe disease. After statistical adjustment for this difference, both groups had similar mortality. In a prospective study, 79 ICU patients with ARF were stratified by severity of illness and then randomized to CVVHD or intermittent hemodialysis [226]. Clinical and demographic variables, and the types of hemofilter and dialysates, were consistent

across modalities. Although a trend towards more renal recoveries was observed in the CVVHD group, their length of stay in the ICU and mortality were higher. Historically, CRRT has preferentially been used in patients who were believed to be too hemodynamically unstable for conventional hemodialysis. Therefore, the inability to demonstrate a favorable effect on mortality for CRRT may be a consequence of patient selection bias (i.e., treatment by indication), which biases towards the null. The possibility also exists that CRRT may have deleterious consequences and so contribute to competing risks. For example, by eliminating beneficial cytokines, IL-1 receptor antagonist and IL-10, peptides with antagonistic effects against IL-1, and tumor necrosis factor, respectively, adverse effects may be produced [227].

There are operational drawbacks in the use of CRRT. These include the greater need for anticoagulation, increased frequency of access-related problems due to its continuous use, intensive nursing support requirements, lack of mobility for the patient (not a consideration if the patient is ventilated), slower onset of removal of electrolytes in emergent cases, and cost, which is estimated to be 2.5 times that of conventional hemodialysis.

NUTRITION. The importance of adequate nutrition in patients with ESRD and chronic kidney disease has been strongly suggested [228–230]. Critically ill patients with ARF are at high risk for malnutrition, in part because of reduced nutritional intake and also hypercatabolic processes, such as sepsis, glucocorticoid therapy, surgical trauma, and especially multiple organ failure [231]. Dialysis itself may adversely affect nutritional status; amino acids and water-soluble vitamins are readily removed with dialysis. Peritoneal dialysis can contribute to substantial protein losses, far more so than conventional hemodialysis or CRRT. Moreover, hemodialysis with bioincompatible membranes may worsen catabolism. Inadequate nutrition in ARF can lead to endogenous protein breakdown and worsening catabolism, along with delayed postoperative healing and impaired host defenses. In turn, nutritional support may improve patients' outcomes [240].

In past years, protein intake was severely restricted in patients with ARF in an effort to reduce uremic symptoms. However, institution of adequate nutritional support has appropriately become standard practice. As stated earlier, dialysis should be initiated relatively early for ARF to permit adequate nutritional support, especially in catabolic patients. Once begun, dialysis may need to be more intensive, so that resultant nitrogenous waste products can be sufficiently cleared and adequate volume removed. Dialysis should be prescribed as needed to control azotemia without compromising nutrition, even if treatments are prolonged (5 to 6 hours) or more frequent (four to six per week). CRRT may offer especially practical and effective modalities for critically ill patients who require large volumes of hyperalimentation with their other obligate intake.

Current recommendations for nutrition in patients with ARF include enteral or parenteral administration of 25 to 35 kcal per kg per day of energy and 1.2 to 1.4 g of protein per kg per day [240].

DISCONTINUING DIALYSIS. Recovery from ARF usually occurs within 4 weeks, but may take 6 to 8 weeks if a severe insult has occurred or if preexisting renal insufficiency was present. It is imperative to periodically examine factors that may be associated with functional recovery. Generally, a urine output of less than 0.75 L per day is insufficient to provide clearance of obligate solute. However, the urine output alone cannot be used to gauge the safety of discontinuing dialysis, particularly in critically ill patients. This aspect of care must be individualized, balancing the risks of holding renal replacement therapy against the benefit and risks of continued dialysis, which includes the reduced chance for recovery of renal function with continued therapy.

Several laboratory parameters may provide clues that renal function is returning. A urine osmolality dissimilar to that of plasma or a specific gravity of greater than 1.020 or less than 1.010 indicates the ability of the kidney to concentrate or dilute the urine, a capacity lost when renal tubular function is severely impaired. Paradoxically, the BUN concentration may increase during recovery because of improved tubular reabsorptive capacity. As renal function improves, the serum creatinine concentration typically plateaus or slowly decreases. If the interdialytic rate of rise of the serum creatinine concentration is progressively less, renal function may be improving. If the serum creatinine concentration decreases between dialysis treatments and the patient is not threatened by volume overload or metabolic complications, dialysis should be withheld and the patient followed carefully.

Discontinuing dialysis based on a relentlessly declining clinical condition is far more challenging because of the frequent uncertainty in defining the patient's prognosis [232]. In most critically ill patients who develop ARF, the extent of comorbid disease (e.g., sepsis, cardiac failure, surgical trauma, etc.) determines the clinical outcome. Withdrawing dialysis may be appropriate when further aggressive care is ineffective but will almost certainly hasten death. Like most ethical dilemmas encountered by ICU staff, the care of the dying patient must be individualized to reflect the wishes of the patient or his or her designated advocate [232]. It is mandatory to fully inform the patient or his or her health care proxy, or both, of the potential risks and benefits of dialysis before it is begun. In cases in which the patient, his or her health proxy, and the proximate caregivers are ambivalent because of an uncertain outcome, it may be helpful to recommend dialysis for a defined period. After this time, the patient's clinical condition can be reassessed and the decision to proceed with additional dialysis treatments readdressed. The institution of dialysis does not mandate that this intervention is continued indefinitely. Many patients agree to short-term dialysis therapy but elect *a priori* to decline chronic dialysis if it is deemed necessary, based on quality of life considerations. A thoughtful, realistic, and compassionate approach to the patient with ARF should allow the patient, his or her family, and physicians to share in decision making [232].

MATCHING THE DIALYSIS MODALITY TO THE PATIENT. There is no consensus as to the definitive dialysis modality for a particular clinical situation [233,234]. We offer these guidelines based on our experiences and our assessment of the available evidence (Table 30-4):

1. If a large volume of fluid removal is required, hemodialysis or CRRT is the preferred treatment. In situations in which the expected ultrafiltration volume is more than 10% of the body weight, CRRT should take precedence.
2. If solute clearance is the main consideration, hemodialysis or CRRT is the choice. Note that CAVHDF and CVVHDF achieve the greatest solute clearance with time.
3. If rapid fluid or solute correction is needed (such as for hyperkalemia), hemodialysis is the most efficient in the shortest amount of time.
4. If anticoagulation is contraindicated, heparin-free hemodialysis (for those with high demands for clearance) or peritoneal dialysis (for those with lower demands for clearance) would be appropriate.

Table 30-4. Considerations Relevant to the Selection of a Dialysis Modality

Patient specific	Dialysis specific
Residual renal function	Membrane composition
Cardiovascular status	Membrane surface area
Pulmonary status	Ultrafiltration coefficient
Volume status	Dialysate composition
Volume load	Sodium
Medications	Potassium
Comorbid conditions	Base
Surgery	Calcium
Myocardial or coronary	Dextrose
disease	Magnesium
Coagulopathy	Blood and dialysate flow
Hemorrhage	Dialysis duration and frequency
Sepsis	Dialysate volume[a]
Arrhythmias	Angioaccess
Malnutrition	Peritoneal access[a]
Diabetes mellitus	Anticoagulation
Burns	
Vasculopathy	

[a]Applicable to peritoneal dialysis only.

5. If the patient is hemodynamically unstable, peritoneal dialysis is the safest option. CRRT may be considered as an alternative.
6. If vascular access cannot be established, peritoneal dialysis is the only option.
7. Because of its restrictions on mobility, CRRT may present more of a problem for conscious patients.
8. In neurosurgical patients or patients with hepatic coma and cerebral edema, CRRT and peritoneal dialysis are less likely to increase intracerebral pressure further by inducing osmotic dysequilibrium [235,236].
9. In hypercatabolic patients who require large fluid volumes for nutritional support, CRRT is advantageous.
10. If dialysis nursing support is not available, peritoneal dialysis is the simplest to manage.
11. Hemodialysis is most efficient for rapid drug or toxin removal.

Regardless of the dialysis modality selected, it is vital that the full range of dialysis techniques is available. The selection of one form of therapy does not preclude change to another when the dynamics of the clinical condition alter.

Selected Complications of Dialysis

CONVENTIONAL HEMODIALYSIS. The complications of hemodialysis are best managed conceptually as those arising from ultrafiltration, solute clearance, and from technical variances (Table 30-5).

Cardiovascular Complications. Hypotension during hemodialysis is a common complication. There are many factors that may play a role in the pathophysiology of intradialytic hypotension [237–240]. These are listed in Table 30-6. Intradialytic hypotension is typically ascribed to excessive ultrafiltration (frank intravascular volume depletion resulting in diminished left ventricular filling pressure) or to an excessive rate of ultrafiltration (volume removal from the intravascular space at a rate that exceeds the capacity of interstitial fluid to migrate into this compartment). Common additional contributory factors include left ventricular dysfunction (systolic or diastolic secondary to

Table 30-5. Dialysis Complications

Hemodialysis
  Hypotension
  Cramps
  Bleeding
  Leukopenia
  Arrhythmias
  Infections
  Hypoxemia
  Pyrogen reactions
  Dialysis dysequilibrium syndrome
  Angioaccess dysfunction
  Technical mishaps
    Incorrect dialysate mixture, contaminated dialysate, air embolism, spallation
Hemofiltration
  Bleeding
  Thrombosis of hemofilter
  Technical mishaps
    Incorrect dialysate mixture, incorrect replacement solution, contaminated dialysate, air embolism
  Hemolysis
  Angioaccess dysfunction
  Hypotension
  Congestive heart failure
Peritoneal dialysis
  Peritonitis
  Catheter infections
  Catheter dysfunction
  Abdominal pain
  Visceral perforation
  Pleural effusion
  Respiratory failure
  Technical mishaps
    Inappropriate dialysate composition, contaminated dialysate

comorbid illness or medications), autonomic dysfunction (secondary to disease processes or medications), lack of pressor hormone stimulation, inappropriate vasodilatation (secondary to sepsis, medications), disease of the pericardium or the pericardial space, and bleeding. It is important to appreciate that other critical components of the dialysis procedure may contribute to the development of hypotension. These include the choice of dialysate (buffer, sodium, and calcium concentration), dialyzer membrane composition, and porosity. Specific provocative issues are the (a) vasodilatory and cardiodepressant effects of acetate; (b) impairment of vasoconstriction, exacerbation of autonomic dysfunction, and declining serum osmolality with a hyponatremic dialysate; (c) vasodilatory and cardiodepressant

Table 30-6. Pathophysiology of Hypotension during Hemodialysis

Contributing factors	Probable mechanism(s)
Hypovolemia	Excessive fluid removal or ultrafiltration at a rate exceeding that at which interstitial fluid moves to intravascular space; hemorrhage
Reduced cardiac output	Systolic or diastolic left ventricular dysfunction due to drugs or comorbid conditions; pericardial disease
Autonomic dysfunction	Associated with uremia, comorbid states (e.g., diabetes mellitus), certain medications (e.g., beta-blockers)
Reduced vascular tone	Associated with certain medications (e.g., narcotic analgesics) and with comorbid states such as sepsis
Response to dialysis system	Acetate, low calcium, low sodium in dialysate; bioincompatible dialyzer membranes

effects of a lowered calcium dialysate; (d) cellulosic membrane-induced complement activation; (e) cellulosic membrane-induced or acetate-induced hypoxemia; (f) complement or pyrogen-induced production of proinflammatory cytokines; and (g) dialysis membrane immediate hypersensitivity mediated by kallikrein/bradykinin activation [139–145,160,161,218,228].

Preemptive strategies should be taken to prevent hypotension in the setting of hemodialysis [213,241]. The dialysate solution should have higher concentrations of sodium (140 to 145 mEq per L), calcium (3.5 mEq per L), and bicarbonate, if not otherwise contraindicated. In some cases, the temperature of the dialysate can be lowered to 34° to 36°C. Cooler dialysate results in increased myocardial contractility [242] and peripheral vasoconstriction [243]. The ultrafiltration rate (as determined to achieve the estimated dry weight) should be closely regulated, and a volumetric-controlled machine is preferable. The time on dialysis can be increased if large-volume ultrafiltration is desired (decreased rate of ultrafiltration) and sequential ultrafiltration clearance can be instituted to give better cardiovascular tolerance. The use of a biocompatible dialyzer membrane may provide additional benefit as discussed earlier. Antihypertensive medications should be withheld before each treatment in patients prone to hypotension during dialysis. Hypotension is managed acutely by intravenous infusion of saline, hypertonic saline, dextran [244], or albumin. Ultrafiltration rate should be transiently reduced with continuation of hemodialysis. In hemodynamically unstable patients, inotropic agents and supplemental oxygen may be required. Other potential causes of low blood pressure during hemodialysis should be considered, such as myocardial ischemia with left ventricular dysfunction, arrhythmias, and pericardial tamponade from hemorrhage and bleeding.

Dialysis-associated arrhythmias occur most often in patients with comorbid cardiovascular disease, cardiac glycoside administration, a concurrent rapid decline in plasma potassium concentration, or a combination of these factors [245]. In high-risk patients, the dialysate potassium concentration should be increased to 3 to 4 mEq per L. Interdialytic hyperkalemia can be managed by more frequent dialysis treatments or the supplemental administration of Kayexalate, if not contraindicated because of gastrointestinal dysfunction. Myocardial ischemia and hypoxemia must be ruled out and treated if present.

Dialysis Dysequilibrium. The dialysis dysequilibrium syndrome is an admixture of neurologic symptoms and signs associated with the excessive removal of solute that occurs with the initiation of hemodialysis or in the setting of a dramatic increase in the amount of hemodialysis delivered to a chronically poorly dialyzed patient. The precise pathobiology of this disorder is undefined but seems associated with increases in intracerebral pressure [246]. Although not uniformly supported experimentally [247,248], most evidence suggests that during rapid solute clearance with hemodialysis, urea departure from the CSF is delayed. The brain becomes relatively hyperosmolal, and water shifts into the brain [249]. Because bicarbonate entry into the CSF is also relatively delayed, an additional contributor to the increase in intracerebral pressure is the transient paradoxical development of CSF acidosis with hemodialysis. CSF acidosis increases intracerebral osmotic activity. The intracerebral accumulation of organic osmolytes, such as inositol, glutamine, and glutamate in the brain [250], is an adaptation to the hyperosmolality in chronic azotemia. These osmolytes further contribute to the discrepancy in osmolality during rapid hemodialysis. These alterations result in paradoxical intracerebral swelling. Because such adaptation occurs less in ARF, dialysis dysequilibrium is uncommon in this setting. The clinical manifestations may range from mere headache and nausea to disorientation, seizures, coma, and even death when especially severe [251].

The simplest way to prevent dialysis dysequilibrium is to slow solute clearance during hemodialysis by using a smaller surface area dialyzer, decreasing blood and dialysate flows, circulating the blood and dialysate in a concurrent direction, and decreasing the duration of dialysis. Typically, a urea clearance of 1 to 2 mL per minute per kg is well tolerated. However, such a low urea clearance may delay resolution of uremia. This limitation can be overcome by performing hemodialysis with low solute clearance for 3 consecutive days [142]. Alternatively, dialysis can also be initiated using peritoneal dialysis, with its lesser solute clearance. Additional preventive strategies include the intradialytic administration of mannitol or dextrose or the use of a hypernatremic dialysate. The use of a high-sodium dialysate appears to be the most effective strategy [90]. The intent is to minimize the decline in serum osmolality by substituting another osmolyte for urea. Finally, in high-risk patients who require aggressive solute clearance, the patient should receive a loading dose of phenytoin before the initiation of hemodialysis, and a maintenance dose should be continued over the subsequent 72 hours as a full dialysis schedule is achieved. Once dialysis dysequilibrium has developed, therapy consists of administration of antiepileptics and reducing cerebral edema by inducing hyperventilation and administering mannitol. Neurosurgical patients with stable ESRD treated by hemodialysis may exhibit a similar propensity to develop cerebral edema. Even in the setting of solute clearances that are not a consequence of major changes in the hemodialysis prescription, caution should be undertaken in performing hemodialysis in this group of patients [235,236].

Hypoxemia. In some hemodialysis patients, a 5- to 35-mm Hg decline in arterial oxygen tension is observed. For most patients, this decline in arterial oxygen tension is usually of no clinical significance. However, in critically ill, nonventilated patients with preexisting respiratory and cardiac compromise, this decline in O_2 tension can result in overt respiratory failure, CNS hypoxemia, cardiac arrhythmias, hypotension, or a combination of these. Dialysis-associated hypoxemia appears to result from the interaction of the dialysate, dialysis membrane, lungs, and respiratory control center. As discussed earlier in this chapter, with acetate-based dialysates, CO_2 is cleared from the blood into the dialysate. The dialysance of CO_2 results in hypocapnia, which causes compensatory hypoventilation and hypoxemia (normocapnic hypoventilation) [252]. Less contributory to the development of dialysis-associated hypoxemia is the interaction between blood complement and selected dialysis membrane materials. Cellulosic membrane materials activate complement by the alternate pathway, giving rise to anaphylatoxins that alter pulmonary regional ventilatory and perfusion patterns [253]. In addition, leukocyte interactions with the dialysis membrane enhance cell membrane expression of selected leukocyte adhesion molecules, causing leukocyte pulmonary sequestration [115,254]. Modifications of the hemodialysis procedure that minimize this complication include the use of a bicarbonate-based dialysate containing 30 to 35 mEq per L and use of a biocompatible dialysis membrane material. Patients at high risk should have their inspired oxygen concentration empirically increased during the hemodialysis treatment.

Technical Errors. Because the monitoring techniques for the performance of hemodialysis have improved, technical errors that compromise patient safety, such as air emboli, incorrect dialysates, and hemolysis, are now remarkably uncommon. As discussed earlier, pyrogen reactions are a persistent and vexing problem that result from the development of high-porosity dialysis membranes [76] and ultrafiltration controllers, combined with the greatly increased utility of bicarbonate-based dialysates [77]. Arguably, strict adherence to prescribed guidelines for water and dialysate purity can minimize this occurrence [255]. In the case of a suspected pyrogen reaction, blood cultures should be performed, and the patient should be treated with systemic antibiotics until the possibility of septicemia has been eliminated.

CONTINUOUS RENAL REPLACEMENT THERAPY. Technical evolution and increased experience have made CRRT a well-tolerated therapy with low complication rates. The most frequent complications are those related to the access and the need for intensive anticoagulation. Less frequently, problems arise from balancing ultrafiltration and clearance needs. Complications from establishing and maintaining angioaccess are discussed in an earlier section.

Bleeding is the most vexing problem encountered in CRRT techniques. Its risk is increased by the continuous need for anticoagulation during CRRT. Bleeding may be internal (gastrointestinal, intracerebral, or both) or localized to the catheter insertion site. Although not typically life-threatening, infection of a hematoma or distortion and compression of vascular anatomy can be problematic if protracted dialysis is needed. An infected hematoma may lead to sepsis in a critically ill patient.

Because automated safeguards are fewer with CRRT and replacement solutions are often needed, errors are more common. Hence, vigilant and experienced staff is mandatory. A host of metabolic abnormalities may develop as a consequence of variances in the replacement solution or the dialysate. For example, if CAVH is performed in the absence of a bicarbonate-containing replacement solution, severe hyperchloremic metabolic acidosis develops [21]. Excessive solute replacement can result in hypernatremia, metabolic alkalosis, hyperkalemia, hypercalcemia, and hypermagnesemia. Inadequate solute replacement may cause hyponatremia, hyperchloremic metabolic acidosis, hypokalemia, hypocalcemia, and hypomagnesemia. The removal of phospate is usually high in CRRT and may necessitate replacement.

Techniques like CRRT, that depend on convective clearance, obligate the formation of large volumes of ultrafiltrate and require the administration of a replacement fluid. This must be done with precision because errors can result in gross fluid imbalances of both extremes. Changes in key parameters (central venous pressure, mean arterial pressure, pulmonary artery wedge pressure) should prompt reassessment and changes to the prescriptions. Adequate patient and technical surveillance can prevent this problem. A meticulously maintained flow chart, recording the progress of the procedure and displaying an ongoing ledger of the patient's fluid balance, is absolutely essential.

PERITONEAL DIALYSIS. The most common complication of peritoneal dialysis is peritonitis, which is reviewed in detail elsewhere [256]. Although peritonitis may occur as a consequence of bacteremia, it usually results from introduction of bacteria through the catheter during an exchange or from bacterial migration along the catheter tunnel. The incidence of peritonitis has declined, predominantly because of improvements in apparatus [257]. The diagnosis of bacterial peritonitis is not difficult. Symptoms and signs of fever, abdominal pain and tenderness, and cloudy dialysate effluent are noted within 6 to 24 hours of the provocative event. It must be recognized that dialysate turbidity may be less apparent because of the rapid cycling and short dwell times typical of acute peritoneal dialysis. The diagnosis of peritonitis is made if the leukocyte count is more than 500 cells per µL (or 250 polymorphonuclear leukocytes per µL). Routine sentinel cell counts and cultures of dialysate fluid may help detect early infections. Antibiotics should be initiated while awaiting definitive culture results. *Staphylococcus aureus* and *epidermidis* account for more than 50% of the cases of bacterial peritonitis, although polymicrobial [258] and fungal infections should not be discounted in the ICU. Appropriate antibiotics may be administered intraperitoneally [259]. In some severe cases of peritonitis, discontinuation of peritoneal dialysis should be considered.

Common metabolic abnormalities associated with peritoneal dialysis are hyperglycemia, hyper- and hyponatremia, hypokalemia, and hypercalcemia. Insulin may be required for adequate glycemic control, and hypokalemia can be corrected with addition of potassium into the dialysate.

Less common, but with devastating ramifications, is the occurrence of a hydrothorax, which is present in approximately 5% of patients [260] and is due to tracking of dialysate into the pleural space through a defect in the diaphragm. The diagnosis is straightforward from thoracocentesis; the pleural fluid has a high glucose and urea content. At the very least, hydrothorax should prompt a reduction in dwell volume. Placing the patient in reverse Trendelenburg position may reduce the tendency of dialysate to leak into the chest cavity. If these measures fail to control the problem, changing to another dialytic modality is recommended.

Finally, dialysate in the peritoneum can also contribute to respiratory compromise by limiting lung expansion. This may pose a serious problem in patients with marginal pulmonary reserve. As with hydrothorax, if reduction in dialysate dwell volume is not possible or fails to correct the issue, alternative treatment options should be explored.

References

1. Addison T: On the disorders of the brain connected with diseased kidneys. *Guys Hosp Rep* 4:1, 1839.
2. Bright R: Cases and observations illustrative of renal disease 77 accompanied with the secretion of albuminous urine. *Guys Hosp Rep* 1:338, 1836.
3. Tyson J: Acute parenchymatous nephritis. *Boston Med Surg J* 111:193, 1884.
4. Kolff WJ: *The Artificial Kidney.* MD thesis, University of Groningen, The Netherlands, 1946.
5. Teschan PE: Hemodialysis in military casualties. *Trans Am Soc Artif Int Organs* 2:52, 1955.
6. Scribner BH, Buri R, Caner JEZ, et al: The treatment of chronic uremia by means of intermittent dialysis: a preliminary report. *Trans Am Soc Artif Int Organs* 6:114, 1960.
7. Odel HM, Ferns DO, Power H: Peritoneal lavage is an effective means of extra renal excretion. *Am J Med* 9:63, 1950.
8. Tenckhoff H, Schechter H: A bacteriologically safe peritoneal access device. *Trans Am Soc Artif Intern Organs* 14:181, 1968.
9. Popovich RP, Moncrief JW, et al: The definition of a novel portable/wearable equilibrium dialysis technique. *Trans Am Soc Artif Intern Organs* 5:64, 1976.
10. Evanson JA, Himmelfarb J, Wingard R, et al: Prescribed versus delivered dialysis in acute renal failure patients. *Am J Kindey Dis* 32:832, 1998.
11. Lowrie E, Lew N: The urea reduction ratio (URR): a simple method for evaluating hemodialysis treatment. *Contemp Dial Nephrol* 12:11, 1991.
12. Dulaney JT, Hatch FE: Peritoneal dialysis and loss of proteins: a review. *Kidney Int* 26:253, 1984.
13. Merrill JP: Medical progress: the artificial kidney. *N Engl J Med* 246:17, 1952.
14. Locke S, Merrill JP, Tyler HR: Neurologic complications of acute uremia. *N Engl J Med* 108:75, 1961.
15. Drueke T, Le Pailleur C, Zingraff J, Jungers P: Uremic cardiomyopathy and pericarditis. *Adv Nephrol* 9:33, 1980.
16. De Broe M, Lins R, De Backer W: Pulmonary aspects of dialysis patients, in Jacobs C, Kjellstrand C, Koch K, Winchester J (eds): *Replacement of Renal Function by Dialysis.* Dordrecht, The Netherlands, Kluwer Academic Publishers, 1996, p 1034.
17. Allon M: Hyperkalemia in end stage renal disease: mechanisms and management. *J Am Soc Nephrol* 6:1134, 1995.
18. Bastl C, Hayslett JP, Binder HJ: Increased large intestinal secretion of potassium in renal insufficiency. *Kidney Int* 12:9, 1977.
19. Kunis CL, Lowenstein J: The emergency treatment of hyperkalemia. *Med Clin North Am* 65:165, 1981.
20. Allon M, Shanklin N: Effect of bicarbonate administration on plasma potassium in dialysis patients: interactions with insulin and albuterol. *Am J Kidney Dis* 28:508, 1996.
21. Gennari FJ, Rimmer JM: Acid-base disorders in end stage renal disease. Part I. *Semin Dial* 3:81, 1990.
22. Van Ypersele de Strihou C, Frans A: The pattern of respiratory compensation in chronic uremic acidosis. *Nephron* 7:37, 1970.
23. Levin T: What this patient didn't need: a dose of salts. *Hosp Pract* 18:95, 1983.
24. Garella S: Extracorporeal techniques in the treatment of exogenous intoxication. *Kidney Int* 33:735, 1988.
25. Gonda A, Gault H, Churchill D, Hollomby D: Hemodialysis for methanol intoxication. *Am J Med* 64:749, 1978.
26. Peterson CD, Collins AJ, Himes JM, et al: Ethylene glycol poisoning: pharmacokinetics during therapy with ethanol and hemodialysis. *N Engl J Med* 304:21, 1981.
27. Benabe JE, Martinez-Maldonado M: Hypercalcemic nephropathy. *Arch Intern Med* 138:777, 1978.
28. Kjellstrand CM, Campbell DC, von Hartitzch B, Buselmeier TJ: Hyperuricemic acute renal failure. *Arch Intern Med* 133:349, 1974.
29. Randall RE, Cohen MD, Spray CC: Hypermagnesemia in renal failure. *Ann Intern Med* 61:73, 1964.
30. Remuzzi G: Bleeding in renal failure. *Lancet* 1:1205, 1988.
31. Livio M, Gotti E, Marchesi D, et al: Uremic bleeding: role of anemia and beneficial effect of red cell transfusion. *Lancet* 2:1013, 1982.
32. Escolar G, Cases A, Bastida E, et al: Uremic platelets have a functional defect affecting the interaction of von Willebrand factor with glycoprotein IIb–IIIa. *Blood* 76:1336, 1990.
33. Remuzzi G, Perico N, Zoja C, et al: Role of endothelium-derived nitric oxide in the bleeding tendency of uremia. *J Clin Invest* 86:1768, 1990.
34. Lindsay RM, Friesen M, Koens F, et al: Platelet function in patients on long term peritoneal dialysis. *Clin Nephrol* 6:335, 1976.
35. Nenci G, Berrittini M, Agnelli G, et al: The effect of peritoneal dialysis, hemodialysis, and kidney transplantation on blood platelet function. Platelet aggregation to ADP and epinephrine. *Nephron* 23:287, 1979.
36. Janson PA, Jubeliere SJ, Weinstein MJ, Deykin D: Treatment of the bleeding tendency in uremia with cryoprecipitate. *N Engl J Med* 308:8, 1980.
37. Mannucci PM, Remuzzi G, Pusineri F, et al: Deamino-8-D-arginine vasopressin shortens the bleeding time in uremia. *N Engl J Med* 308:8, 1983.
38. Moia M, Vizzotto L, Cattaneo M, et al: Improvement of the hemostatic defect of uraemia after treatment with recombinant human erythropoietin. *Lancet* 2:1227, 1987.
39. Livio M, Mannucchi PM, Bignano G, et al: Conjugated estrogens for the management of bleeding associated with renal failure. *N Engl J Med* 315:731, 1986.
40. Lohr JW, Schwab SJ: Minimizing hemorrhagic complications in dialysis patients. *J Am Soc Nephrol* 2:961, 1991.
41. Conger JD: Does hemodialysis delay recovery from acute renal failure? *Semin Dial* 3:146, 1990.
42. Solez L, Morel-Maroger L, Sraer J: The morphology of acute tubular necrosis in man: analysis of 57 renal biopsies and comparison with the glycerol model. *Medicine* 58:362, 1979.
43. Yeh BPY, Tomki DJ, Stacy WK, et al: Factors influencing sodium and water excretion in uremic man. *Kidney Int* 7:103, 1975.
44. Ogata K: Clinicopathological study of kidneys from patients on chronic dialysis. *Kidney Int* 37:1333, 1990.
45. Rottermbourg J: Residual renal function and recovery of renal function in patients treated by CAPD. *Kidney Int* 43(suppl 40):S-106, 1993.

46. Conger JD, Robinette JB, Schrier RW: Smooth muscle calcium and endothelial-derived relaxing factor in abnormal vascular responses of acute renal failure. *J Clin Invest* 82:532, 1988.

47. Hakim RM: Clinical implications of hemodialysis membrane biocompatibility. *Kidney Int* 44:484, 1993.

48. Lynn RI, Feinfeld DA: Importance of residual renal function in end-stage renal disease. *Semin Dial* 2:1, 1989.

49. Teschan PE, Baxter CR, O Brien TF, et al: Prophylactic hemodialysis in the treatment of acute renal failure. *Ann Intern Med* 53:992, 1960.

50. Kleinknecht D, Jungers P, Chanard J, et al: Uremic and non-uremic complications in acute renal failure: evaluation of early and frequent dialysis on prognosis. *Kidney Int* 1:190, 1972.

51. Conger JD: A controlled evaluation of prophylactic dialysis in post-traumatic acute renal failure. *J Trauma* 15:1056, 1975.

52. Gillum DM, Dixon BS, Yanover MJ, et al: The role of intensive dialysis in acute renal failure. *Clin Nephrol* 25:249:1986.

53. Sargent JA, Gotch FA: Principles and biophysics of dialysis, in Jacobs C, Kjellstrand C, Koch K, Winchester J (eds): *Replacement of Renal Function by Dialysis*. Dordrecht, The Netherlands, Kluwer Academic Publishers, 1996, p 34.

54. Babb AL, Farrell P, Uvelli DA, Scribner BH: Hemodialyzer evaluation by examination of solute molecular spectra. *Trans Am Soc Artif Int Organs* 18:98, 1972.

55. Henderson LW: Biophysics of ultrafiltration and hemofiltration, in Jacobs C, Kjellstrand C, Koch K, Winchester J (eds): *Replacement of Renal Function by Dialysis*. Dordrecht, The Netherlands, Kluwer Academic Publishers, 1996, p 114.

56. Nolph KD, Nothum RJ, Maher JF: Ultrafiltration: a mechanism for removal of intermediate molecular weight substances in coil dialyzers. *Kidney Int* 6:55, 1974.

57. Asaba H, Bergstrom J, Furst P, et al: Sequential ultrafiltration and diffusion as alternatives to conventional hemodialysis. *Proc Clin Dial Transplant Forum* 6:29, 1976.

58. Shaldon S: Sequential ultrafiltration and dialysis. *Proc Eur Dial Transplant Assoc* 13:300, 1976.

59. Wehle B, Asaba H, Castenfores J, et al: Hemodynamic changes during sequential ultrafiltration and dialysis. *Kidney Int* 15:411, 1979.

60. Fleming SJ, Wilkinson JS, Aldridge C, et al: Blood volume change during isolated ultrafiltration and combined ultrafiltration-dialysis. *Nephrol Dial Transplant* 3:272, 1988.

61. Bradley JR, Evans DB, Cowley AJ: Comparison of vascular tone during haemodialysis with ultrafiltration and during ultrafiltration followed by haemodialysis: a possible mechanism for dialysis hypotension. *BMJ* 19:300, 1990.

62. Forni LG, Hilton PJ: Continuous hemofiltration in the treatment of acute renal failure. *N Engl J Med* 336:1303, 1997.

63. Geronemus R, von Albertini B, Glabman S, et al: Enhanced molecular clearance in hemofiltration. *Proc Clin Dial Transplant Forum* 8:47, 1985.

64. Kaplan AA: Predilution vs postdilution for continuous arteriovenous hemofiltration. *Trans Am Soc Artif Int Organs* 3:28, 1985.

65. Popovich RP, Moncrief JW, Nolph KD, et al: Physiological transport parameters in peritoneal and hemodialysis. 3rd Annual Report No. N01-AM-3-2205, AK-CUP, Bethesda, MD, NIAMDD, National Institutes of Health, 1977.

66. Penzotti SC, Mattocks AM: Effects of dwell time, volume of dialysis fluid, and added accelerators on peritoneal dialysis of urea. *J Pharm Sci* 60:1520, 1971.

67. Brandes J, Emerson P, Campbell D, Keshaviah P: The relationship between body size, fill volume and mass transfer area coefficient in PD (abstract). *Am Soc Nephrol* 3:407, 1992.

68. Schonfeld P, Diaz-Buxo JA, Keen M, Gotch FA: The effect of body position, surface area (BSA), and intraperitoneal exchange volume (Vip) on the peritoneal transport constant (abstract). *Am Soc Nephrol* 4:416, 1993.

69. Henderson LW: Peritoneal ultrafiltration dialysis. Enhanced urea transfer using hypertonic peritoneal dialysis fluid. *J Clin Invest* 45:950, 1966.

70. Nolph KD, Ghods AJ, Van Stone JC: The effects of intraperitoneal vasodilators on peritoneal clearances. *Trans Am Soc Artif Int Organs* 22:586, 1976.

71. Nolph KD, Ghods AJ, Brown PA: Effects of intraperitoneal nitroprusside on peritoneal clearances with variations in dose, frequency of administration, and dwell times. *Nephron* 24:4, 1979.

72. Miller FN, Nolph KD, Harris PD: Microvascular and clinical effects of altered peritoneal solutions. *Kidney Int* 15:630, 1979.

73. Grzegorzewska AE, Moore HL, Nolph KD, Chen TW: Ultrafiltration and effective peritoneal blood flow during peritoneal dialysis in the rat. *Kidney Int* 39:608, 1991.

74. Vanholder R: Middle molecules as uremic toxins—still a viable hypothesis? *Semin Dial* 7:65, 1994.

75. Davidson AM: β_2-Microglobulin and amyloidosis: who is at risk? *Nephrol Dial Transplant* 10(suppl 10):50, 1995.

76. Urena P, Herbelin A, Zingraff J, et al: Permeability of cellulosic and non-cellulosic membranes to endotoxins subunits and cytokines production during in vitro hemodialysis. *Nephrol Dial Transplant* 7:16, 1992.

77. Mion CM, Canaud B, Francesqui MP, et al: Bicarbonate concentrate: a hidden source of microbial contamination of dialysis fluid. *Blood Purif* 7:32, 1987.

78. Klein E, Pass T, Harding GB, et al: Microbial and endotoxin contamination in water and dialysate in the central United States. *Artif Organs* 14:85, 1990.

79. Yohay DA, Butterly DW, Schwab SJ, Quarles LD: Continuous arteriovenous hemodialysis: effect of dialyzer geometry. *Kidney Int* 42:448, 1992.

80. Mendelssohn S, Swartz CD, Yudis M, et al: High glucose concentration dialysate in chronic hemodialysis. *Trans Am Soc Artif Int Organs* 13:249, 1967.

81. Ward RA, Walthen RL, Williams TE, Harding GB: Hemodialysate composition and intradialytic metabolic, acid-base, and potassium changes. *Kidney Int* 32:129, 1987.

82. Arem R: Hypoglycemia. *Endocrinol Metab Clin North Am* 18:103, 1989.

83. Grajower MM, Walter L, Albin J: Hypoglycemia in chronic hemodialysis patients: association with propranolol use. *Nephron* 26:126, 1980.

84. Kopple JD, Swendseid ME, Shinaberger JH, Umezawa CY: The free and bound amino acids removed by hemodialysis. *Trans Am Soc Artif Int Organs* 19:309, 1973.

85. Ganda OP, Aoki TT, Soeldner JS, et al: Hormone-fuel concentrations in anephric subjects: effects of hemodialysis (with special references to amino acids). *J Clin Invest* 57:1403, 1976.

86. Wilkinson R, Barber SG, Robson V: Cramps, thirst, and hypertension in hemodialysis patients. The influence of dialysate sodium concentration. *Clin Nephrol* 7:101, 1977.

87. Ogden D: A double-blind crossover comparison of high and low sodium dialysate. *Proc Clin Dial Transplant Forum* 88:157, 1978.

88. Henrich WL, Woodard TD, McPhaul JJ: The chronic efficacy and safety of high sodium dialysate: double-blind crossover study. *Am J Kidney Dis* 2:349, 1982.

89. Cybulsky AVE, Materi A, Hollomby DJ: Effects of high sodium dialysate during maintenance hemodialysis. *Nephron* 41:57, 1985.

90. Port FK, Johnson WJ, Klass DW: Prevention of dialysis disequilibrium syndrome by use of high sodium concentration in the dialysate. *Kidney Int* 3:327, 1973.

91. Raja RM: Sodium profiling in the elderly hemodialysis patients. *Nephrol Dial Transplant* 11(suppl 8):42, 1996.

92. Palmer BF: The effect of dialysate composition on systemic hemodynamics. *Semin Dial* 5:54, 1992.

93. Raja R, Kramer M, Barber K, Chin S: Sequential changes in dialysate sodium during hemodialysis. *Trans Am Soc Artif Int Organs* 29:649, 1983.

94. Paganini EP, Sandy D, Moreno L, et al: The effect of sodium and ultrafiltration modelling on plasma volume changes and hemodynamic stability in intensive care patients receiving hemodialysis for acute renal failure: a prospective, stratified, randomized, cross-over study. *Nephrol Dial Transplant* 11(suppl 8):32, 1996.

95. Williams M, Epstein FH: Internal exchanges of potassium, in Seldin DW, Giebisch G (eds): *The Regulation of Potassium Balance*. New York, Raven Press, 1989, p 3.

96. Ketchersid TL, Van Stone JC: Dialysate potassium. *Semin Dial* 4:46, 1991.

97. Sherman RA, Hwang ER, Bernholc AS, Eisinger RP: Variability in potassium removal by hemodialysis. *Am J Nephrol* 6:284, 1986.

98. Feig PU, Shook A, Sterns RH: Effect of potassium removal during hemodialysis on the plasma potassium concentration. *Nephron* 27:25, 1981.

99. Hou S, McElroy PA, Nootes S, Beach M: Safety and efficacy of low potassium dialysate. *Am J Kidney Dis* 13:137, 1989.

100. Ozuer M, Aksoy, Dortlemez O, Dortlemez H: Effects of cardioselective (β1) and nonselective (both β1 and β2) adrenergic blockade on serum potassium in patients with chronic renal failure undergoing hemodialysis. *Kidney Int* 26:584, 1984.

101. Papadakis MA, Wexman MP, Fraser C, Sedlacek SM: Hyperkalemia complicating digoxin toxicity in a patient with renal failure. *Am J Kidney Dis* 5:64, 1985.

102. Williams AJ, Barnes JN, Cunningham J, et al: Effect of dialysate buffer on potassium removal during haemodialysis. *Proc EDTA-ERA* 21:209, 1985.

103. Redaelli B, Sforzini B, Bonoldi L, et al: Potassium removal as a factor limiting the correction of acidosis during dialysis. *Proc EDTA-ERA* 19:366, 1982.

104. Morrison G, Michelson EL, Brown S, Morganroth J: Mechanism and prevention of cardiac arrhythmias in chronic hemodialysis patients. *Kidney Int* 17:811, 1980.

105. Lazarus JM: Complications in hemodialysis. An overview. *Kidney Int* 18:783, 1980.

106. Wiegand CF, Davin TD, Raij L, Kjellstrand CM: Severe hypokalemia induced by hemodialysis. *Arch Intern Med* 141:167, 1981.

107. Kveim M, Nesbakken R: Utilization of exogenous acetate during hemodialysis. *Proc Dial Transplant Forum* 5:138, 1975.

108. Vinay P, Prudhomme M, Vinet B, et al: Acetate metabolism and bicarbonate generation during hemodialysis: 10 years of observation. *Kidney Int* 31:1194, 1987.

109. Mastrangelo F, Rizzelli S, Corliano C: Benefits of bicarbonate dialysis. *Kidney Int* 28(suppl 17):S-188, 1985.

110. Henrich WL: Hemodynamic instability during hemodialysis. *Kidney Int* 30:605, 1986.

111. Wolff J, Pendersen T, Rossen M, Cleeman-Rasmussen K: Effects of acetate and bicarbonate dialysis on cardiac performance, transmural myocardial perfusion and acid-base balance. *Int J Artif Organs* 9:105, 1986.

112. Daugirdas JT: Dialysis hypotension: a hemodynamic analysis. *Kidney Int* 39:233, 1991.

113. Wehle B, Asaba H, Castenfors J, et al: The influence of dialysis fluid composition on the blood pressure response during dialysis. *Clin Nephrol* 10:62, 1978.

114. Borges HF, Fryd DS, Rosa AA, et al: Hypotension during acetate and bicarbonate dialysis in patients with acute renal failure. *Am J Nephrol* 1:24, 1981.

115. Ross EA, Nissenson AR: Dialysis associated hypoxemia: insights into pathophysiology and prevention. *Semin Dial* 1:33, 1988.

116. Garella S, Chang BS: Hemodialysis associated hypoxemia. *Am J Nephrol* 4:272, 1984.

117. Ward RA, Luehmann DA, Klein E: Are current standards for the microbiological purity of hemodialysate adequate? *Semin Dial* 2:69, 1989.

118. Sherman RA: On lowering dialysate calcium. *Semin Dial* 1:78, 1988.

119. Goodman WG, Coburn JW: The use of 1,25-dihydroxyvitamin D3 in early renal failure. *Annu Rev Med* 43:27, 1992.

120. Sutton RA, Cameron EC: Renal osteodystrophy: pathophysiology. *Semin Nephrol* 12:91, 1992.

121. Wing AJ: Optimum calcium concentration of dialysis fluid for hemodialysis. *BMJ* 4:145, 1968.

122. Raman A, Chong YK, Sreenevasan GA: Effects of varying dialysate calcium concentrations on the plasma calcium fractions in patients on dialysis. *Nephron* 16:181, 1976.

123. Bouillon R, Verberckmoes R, Moor PD: Influence of dialysate calcium concentration and vitamin D on serum parathyroid hormone during repetitive dialysis. *Kidney Int* 7:422, 1975.

124. Salusky IB, Foley J, Nelson P, Goodman WG: Aluminum accumulation during treatment with aluminum hydroxide and dialysis in children and young adults with chronic renal failure. *N Engl J Med* 324:527, 1991.

125. Touam M, Martinez F, Lacour B, et al: Aluminum-induced, reversible microcytic anemia in chronic renal failure: clinical and experimental studies. *Clin Nephrol* 19:295, 1983.

126. Alfrey AC, Le Gendre GR, Kaehny WD: The dialysis encephalopathy syndrome. Possible aluminum intoxication. *N Engl J Med* 294:184, 1976.

127. Slatopolsky E, Weerts C, Lopez-Hilker S, et al: Calcium carbonate as a phosphate binder in patients with chronic renal failure undergoing dialysis. *N Engl J Med* 315:157, 1986.

128. Mai ML, Emmett M, Sheikh MS, et al: Calcium acetate, an effective phosphorus binder in patients with renal failure. *Kidney Int* 36:690, 1989.

129. Slatopolsky EA, Burke SK, Dillon MA, et al. RenaGel, a nonabsorbed calcium- and aluminum-free phosphate binder, lowers serum phosphorus and parathyroid hormone. *Kidney Int* 55:299, 1999.

130. Fernandez E, Montoliu J: Successful treatment of massive uremic tumoral calcinosis with daily hemodialysis and very low calcium dialysate. *Nephrol Dial Transplant* 9:1207, 1994.

131. Sherman RA, Bialy GB, Gazinski B, et al: The effect of dialysate calcium levels on blood pressure during hemodialysis. *Am J Kidney Dis* 8:244, 1986.

132. Maynard JC, Cruz C, Kleerekoper M, Levin NW: Blood pressure response to changes in serum ionized calcium during hemodialysis. *Ann Intern Med* 104:358, 1986.

133. Fellner SK, Lang RM, Neumann A, et al: Physiological mechanisms for calcium-induced changes in systemic arterial pressure in stable dialysis patients. *Hypertension* 13:213, 1989.

134. Vaporean ML, Van Stone JC: Dialysate magnesium. *Semin Dial* 6:46, 1993.

135. Breuer J, Moniz C, Baldwin D, Parsons V: The effects of zero magnesium dialysate and magnesium supplements on ionized calcium concentration in patients on regular dialysis treatment. *Nephrol Dial Transplant* 2:347, 1987.

136. Davenport A, Will EJ, Davison AM: Hyperlactatemia and metabolic acidosis during hemofiltration using lactate-buffered fluids. *Nephron* 59:461, 1991.

137. Leblanc M, Moreno L, Paganini E, et al: Bicarbonate dialysate for CRRT in intensive care unit patients with acute renal failure. *Am J Kidney Dis* 26:910, 1995.

138. Kaplan AA, Longnecker RE, Folkert VW: Continuous arteriovenous hemofiltration. *Ann Intern Med* 100:358, 1984.

139. Monaghan R, Watters JM, Clancey SM, et al: Uptake of glucose during CAVH. *Crit Care Med* 21:1159, 1993.

140. Cazenave JP, Mulvihill J: Interaction of blood with surfaces: Hemocompatibility and thromboresistance of biomaterials. *Contrib Nephrol* 62:188, 1988.

141. Grant ME, Lovell HB, Wiegmann TB: Current use of anticoagulation in hemodialysis. *Semin Dial* 4:168, 1991.

142. Owen WF, Lazarus JM: Dialytic management of acute renal failure, in Lazarus JM, Brenner BM (eds): *Acute Renal Failure.* New York, Churchill Livingstone, 1993, p 487.

143. Gordon LA, Simon ER, Richards JM: Studies in regional heparinization. II. Artificial kidney hemodialysis without systemic heparinization—preliminary report of a method using simultaneous infusion of heparin and protamine. *N Engl J Med* 255:1063, 1956.

144. Hampers CL, Blaufox MD, Merrill JP: Anticoagulation rebound after hemodialysis. *N Engl J Med* 255:1063, 1966.

145. Swartz R, Port F: Preventing hemorrhage in high risk hemodialysis: regional versus low-dose heparin. *Kidney Int* 16:513, 1979.

146. Flanigan MJ, Pillsbury L, Sadewasser G, Lim VS: Regional hemodialysis anticoagulation: hypertonic tri-sodium citrate or anticoagulant citrate dextrose-A. *Am J Kidney Dis* 27:519, 1996.

147. Schwab S, Onorato J, Shara L, Dennis P: Hemodialysis without anticoagulation: 1 year prospective trial in hospitalized patients at risk for bleeding. *Am J Med* 83:405, 1987.

148. Caruna R, Raiai R, Bush J, et al: Heparin free dialysis: comparative data and results in high risk patients. *Kidney Int* 31:35, 1987.

149. Ronco C, Brendolan A, Gragantini L, et al: Continuous arteriovenous hemofiltration. *Contrib Nephrol* 48:70, 1985.

150. Palsson R, Niles JL: Regional citrate anticoagulation in continuous venovenous hemofiltration in critically ill patients with high risk of bleeding. *Kidney Int* 55:1991, 1999.

151. Tolwani AJ, Campbell RC, Schenk MB, et al: Simplified citrate anticoagulation of continuous renal replacement therapy. *Kidney Int* 60:370, 2001.

152. Kaplan AA, Petrillo R: Regional heparinization for continuous arteriovenous hemofiltration. *Trans Am Soc Artif Int Organs* 33:312, 1987.

153. Smith D, Paganini EP, Suhoza K, et al: Non-heparin continuous renal replacement therapy is possible, in Nose J, Kjellstrand CM,

Ivanovich P (eds): *Progress in Artificial Internal Organs.* Cleveland, OH, ISAO Press, 1985, p 32.
154. Mehta R: Anticoagulation strategies for continuous renal replacement therapies: what works? *Am J Kidney Dis* 28(suppl 3):S-8, 1996.
155. Fan PY, Schwab SJ: Vascular access: concepts for the 1990s. *J Am Soc Nephrol* 3:1, 1992.
156. Storck M, Hartl WH, Zimmerer E, Inthorn D: Comparison of pump-driven and spontaneous continuous hemofiltration in postoperative ARF. *Lancet* 337:452, 1991.
157. Bellomo R, Parkin G, Love J, Boyce N: A prospective comparative study of CAVHDF and CVVHDF in critically ill patients. *Am J Kidney Dis* 21:400, 1993.
158. Tominaga G, Ingegno M, Ceraldi C, Waxman K: Vascular complications of CAVH in trauma patients. *J Trauma* 35:285, 1993.
159. Nidus B, Matalon R, Katz C: Hemodialysis using femoral vein cannulation. *Nephron* 13:416, 1974.
160. Kjellstrand CN, Merino GE, Mauer SM, et al: Complications of percutaneous femoral vein catheterization for hemodialysis. *Clin Nephrol* 4:37, 1975.
161. Besarab A, Al-Ejel F: Creating and maintaining acute access for hemodialysis. *Semin Dial* 9(suppl 1):S-2, 1996.
162. Edwards H, King TC: Cardiac tamponade from central venous catheters. *Arch Surg* 117:965, 1982.
163. Fiaccadori E, Gonzi G, Zambrelli P, Tortorella G: Cardiac arrhythmias during central venous catheter procedure in ARF: a prospective study. *J Am Soc Nephrol* 7:1079, 1996.
164. Troianos C, Jobes D, Ellison N: Ultrasound guided cannulations of the internal jugular vein. *Anesth Analg* 72:823, 1991.
165. Schwab SJ, Quarles LD, Middleton JP, et al: Hemodialysis-associated subclavian vein stenosis. *Kidney Int* 33:1156, 1988.
166. Dahlberg RJ, Falk RJ, Huffman KA: Subclavian hemodialysis catheter infections. *Am J Kidney Dis* 5:421, 1986.
167. Goldstein MB: Prevention of sepsis from central vein dialysis catheters. *Semin Dial* 5:106, 1992.
168. Vascular Access Work Group: NKF-KDOQI clinical practice guidelines for vascular access: an update. In: *Kidney Dialysis Outcomes Quality Initiative*, Philadelphia, National Kidney Foundation, 2000.
169. Cimochowski G, Sartan J, Worley E, et al: Clear superiority of internal jugular access route over the subclavian vein for temporary access: an angiographic study in 52 patients with 102 venograms. *Kidney Int* 31:230, 1987.
170. Ash S, Daugirdas J: Peritoneal access devices. In Daugirda J, Black P, Ing T. (eds): *Handbook of Dialysis*, 3rd ed. Philadelphia, Lippincott, Williams & Wilkins, 2001, p 309.
171. Strippoli P, Pilolli D, Dimgrone G, et al: A hemostasis study in CAPD patients during fibrinolytic intraperitoneal therapy with urokinase (UK). *Adv Perit Dial* 5:97, 1989.
172. Lazarus JM, Owen WF: Role of biocompatibility in dialysis morbidity and mortality. *Am J Kidney Dis* 24:1019, 1994.
173. Hakim R, Wingrad RL, Parker RA: Effect of dialysis membrane in the treatment of patients with ARF. *N Engl J Med* 331:1336, 1994.
174. Henderson LW, Koch KM, Dinarello CA, Shaldon S: Hemodialysis hypotension: the interleukin hypothesis. *Blood Purif* 1:3, 1983.
175. Dinarello CA, Koch KM, Shaldon S: Interleukin-1 and its relevance to patients treated with hemodialysis. *Kidney Int* 33(suppl 24):S-21, 1988.
176. Tetta C, David S, Biancone L, et al: Role of platelet activating factor in hemodialysis. *Kidney Int* 43(suppl 39):S-154, 1993.
177. Ing TS, Wong FK, Cheng YL, Potempa LD: The first-use syndrome revisited: a dialysis center's perspective. *Nephrol Dial Transplant* 10(suppl 10):39, 1995.
178. Roccatello D, Mazzucco G, Coppo R, et al: Functional changes of monocytes due to dialysis membranes. *Kidney Int* 32:84, 1989.
179. Vanholder R, Ringoir S, Dhondt A, Hakim R: Phagocytosis in uremic and hemodialysis patients: a prospective and cross sectional study. *Kidney Int* 39:320, 1991.
180. Vanholder R, Ringoir S: Polymorphonuclear cell function and infection in dialysis. *Kidney Int* 42(suppl 38):S-91, 1992.
181. Gutierrez A: Protein catabolism in maintenance hemodialysis: the influence of the dialysis membrane. *Nephrol Dial Transplant* 11(suppl 2):108, 1996.
182. Koch KM: Dialysis-related amyloidosis (clinical conference). *Kidney Int* 41:1416, 1992.
183. Seres DS, Strain GW, Levin NW, et al: Improvement of plasma lipoprotein profiles during high flux dialysis. *J Am Soc Nephrol* 3:1409, 1993.
184. Hakim RM: Recent advances in the biocompatibility of hemodialysis membranes. *Nephrol Dial Transplant* 10(suppl 10):7, 1995.
185. Aranout A, Hakim RM, Todd R, et al: Increased expression of an adhesion-promoting surface glycoprotein in the granulocytopenia of hemodialysis. *N Engl J Med* 312:457, 1985.
186. Himmelfarb J, Zaoui P, Hakim R: Modulation of granulocyte LAM-1 and MAC-1 during dialysis. A prospective, randomized controlled trial. *Kidney Int* 41:388, 1992.
187. Himmelfarb J, Ault KA, Holbrook D, et al: Intradialytic granulocyte reactive oxygen species production: a prospective, crossover trial. *J Am Soc Nephrol* 4:178, 1993.
188. Ward RA: Effects of hemodialysis on coagulation and platelets: are we measuring membrane biocompatibility? *Nephrol Dial Transplant* 10(suppl 10):12, 1995.
189. Schulman G, Hakim R, Arias R, et al: Bradykinin generation by dialysis membranes: possible role in anaphylactic reaction. *J Am Soc Nephrol* 3:1563, 1993.
190. Shaldon S, Lonnemann G, Koch KM: Cytokine relevance in biocompatibility. *Contrib Nephrol* 79:227, 1989.
191. Schindler R, Lonnemann G, Shaldon S, et al: Transcription, not synthesis, of interleukin-1 and tumor necrosis factor by complement. *Kidney Int* 37:85, 1990.
192. Pertosa G, Gesualdo L, Tarantino EA, et al: Influence of hemodialysis on interleukin-6 production and gene expression by peripheral blood mononuclear cells. *Kidney Int* 43(suppl 39):S-149, 1993.
193. Zaoui P, Green W, Hakim RM: Hemodialysis with cuprophan membrane modulates interleukin-2 receptor expression. *Kidney Int* 39:1020, 1991.
194. Zaoui P, Hakim RM: Natural killer-cell function in hemodialysis patients: effect of the dialysis membrane. *Kidney Int* 43:1298, 1993.
195. Pascual M, Schifferli JA: Adsorption of complement factor D by polyacrylonitrile dialysis membranes. *Kidney Int* 43:903, 1993.
196. Pascual M, Tolkoff-Rubin N, Schifferli JA: Is adsorption an important characteristic of dialysis membranes? *Kidney Int* 49:311, 1996.
197. Locatelli F: Influence of membranes on mortality. *Nephrol Dial Transplant* 11(suppl 2):116, 1996.
198. Himmelfarb J, Hakim R: The use of biocompatible dialysis membranes in acute renal failure. *Adv Ren Replace Ther* 4(suppl 1):72, 1997.
199. Karsou SA, Jaber BL, Pereira BJG. Impact of intermittent hemodialysis variables on clinical outcomes in acute renal failure. *Am J Kidney Dis* 35(5):980, 2000.
200. Schulman G, Fogo A, Gung A, et al: Complement activation retards resolution of acute ischaemic renal failure in the rat. *Kidney Int* 40:1069, 1991.
201. Schiffl LA, Lang SM, Konig A, et al: Biocompatible membrane in ARF: prospective case control study. *Lancet* 344:570, 1994.
202. Alkhunaizi A, Schrier R: Management of acute renal failure: new perspectives. *Am J Kidney Dis* 28:315, 1996.
203. Liano F, Pascual J: Epidemiology of acute renal failure: a prospective, multicenter, community-based study. Madrid Acute Renal Failure Study Group. *Kidney Int* 50:811, 1996.
204. Consentino F, Chaff C, Piedmonte M: Risk factors influencing survival in ICU acute renal failure. *Nephrol Dial Transplant* 9(suppl 4):179, 1994.
205. Jorres A, Gahl GM, Dobis C, et al: Hemodialysis-membrane biocompatibility and mortality of patients with dialysis-dependent acute renal failure: a prospective randomised multicenter trial. *Lancet* 354:1337, 1999.
206. Bergamo Collaborative Dialysis Study Group: Acute intradialytic well-being: results of a clinical trial comparing polysulfone and cuprophane. *Kidney Int* 40:714, 1991.
207. Parker TF, Wingard RL, Husni L, et al: Effect of the membrane biocompatibility on nutritional parameters in chronic hemodialysis patients. *Kidney Int* 49:551, 1996.
208. Krazlin B, Reuss A, Gretz N, et al: Recovery from ischaemic renal failure: independence from dialysis membrane type. *Nephron* 73:644, 1996.
209. Jacobs C: Membrane biocompatibilty in the treatment of acute renal failure: what is the evidence in 1996? *Nephrol Dial Transplant* 12:38, 1997.

210. Mehta R, McDonald B, Gabbai F, et al: Effect of biocompatible membranes on outcomes from acute renal failure in the ICU. *J Am Soc Nephrol* 7:1457, 1996.

211. Hakim RM, Breyer J, Ismail N, Schulman G: Effects of dose of dialysis on morbidity and mortality. *Am J Kidney Dis* 23:661, 1994.

212. Owen WF, Lew NL, Liu YL, et al: The urea reduction ratio and serum albumin concentration as predictors of mortality in patients undergoing hemodialysis. *N Engl J Med* 329:1001, 1993.

213. Hemodialysis Adequacy Work Group: NKF-KDOQI clinical practice guidelines for hemodialysis: an update. In: *Kidney Dialysis Outcomes Quality Initiative*. Philadelphia, National Kidney Foundation, 2000.

214. Bellomo R, Ronco C: Nutritional management of ARF in the critically ill patients. *Am J Kidney Dis* 28(suppl 3):S58, 1996.

215. Bellomo R, Ronco C: ARF in the intensive care unit: adequacy of dialysis and the case for continuous therapies. *Nephrol Dial Transplant* 11:424, 1996.

216. Paganini EP, Taployai M, Goormastic M, et al: Establishing a dialysis/patient outcome link in intensive care unit acute dialysis for patients with acute renal failure. *Am J Kidney Dis* 28(suppl 3):S81, 1996.

217. Frankenfeld DC, Reynolds HN, Wiles CE, et al: Urea removal during continuous hemofiltration of conventional dialytic therapy and acute continuous hemodialfiltration in the management of ARF in the critically ill. *Renal Fail* 15:595, 1993.

218. Clark WR, Mueller BA, Alaka KJ, Macias WL: A comparison of metabolic control by continuous and intermittent therapies in ARF. *J Am Soc Nephrol* 4:1413, 1994.

219. Billiau A, Vandekerckhove F: Cytokines and their interactions with other inflammatory mediators in the pathogenesis of sepsis and septic shock. *Eur J Clin Invest* 21:559, 1991.

220. Parillo JE: Pathogenetic mechanisms of septic shock. *N Engl J Med* 328:1471, 1993.

221. Bellomo R, Tipping P, Boyce N: CVVH with dialysis removes cytokines from the circulation of septic patients. *Crit Care Med* 21:522, 1993.

222. Ronco C, Tetta C, Lupi H, et al: Removal of platelet activating factors in experimental CAVH. *Crit Care Med* 23:99, 1995.

223. Jakob SM, Frey PJ, Uehlinger DE: Does CRRT favourably influence the outcome of the patients? *Nephrol Dial Transplant* 11:1250, 1996.

224. Misset B, Trinsit JF, Chevret S, et al: A randomized cross-over comparison of the hemodynamic response to intermittent HD and continuous hemofiltration in ICU patients with ARF. *Intensive Care Med* 22:742, 1996.

225. Mehta RL, McDonald B, Pahl M, et al: Continuous versus intermittent dialysis for acute renal failure in the ICU: results from a randomized multicenter trial. *J Am Soc Nephrol* 7:1456, 1996.

226. Sandy D, Moreno L, Lee JC, Paganini EP. A randomized stratified, dose equivalent comparison of continuous veno-venous hemodialysis vs intermittent hemodialysis support in ICU acute renal failure patients. *J Am Soc Nephrol* 9:225A, 1998(abstr).

227. Journois D, Silvester W: Continuous hemofiltration in patients with sepsis or multiorgan failure. *Semin Dial* 9:175, 1996.

228. Lowrie EG, Lew NL: Death risk in hemodialysis patients: the predictive value of commonly measured variables and an evaluation of death risk differences between facilities. *Am J Kidney Dis* 15:458, 1990.

229. NKF-K/DQOI: *Clinical Practice Guidelines for Nutrition in Chronic Renal Failure*. New York, National Kidney Foundation, 2001.

230. Chertow G, Bullard A, Lazarus JM: Nutrition and dialysis prescription. *Am J Nephrol* 16:79, 1996.

231. Chima CS, Meyer L, Hummell AC, et al: Protein catabolic rate in patients with acute renal failure on continuous arteriovenous hemofiltration and total parenteral nutrition. *J Am Soc Nephrol* 3:1516, 1993.

232. Renal Physicians Association and American Society of Nephrology: *Shared Decision Making in the Appropriate Initiation and Withdrawal from Dialysis. Clinical Practice Guideline Number 2*. Rockville, MD, RPA, 2000.

233. Mehta RL: Renal replacement therapy for acute renal failure: matching the method to the patient. *Semin Dial* 6:253, 1993.

234. Lazarus JM: Which dialytic therapy is best for the patient with an unstable cardiovascular system? Hemodialysis is the optimal therapy. *Semin Dial* 5:208, 1992.

235. Yoshida S, Tajika T, Yamasaki N, et al: Dialysis dysequilibrium syndrome in neurosurgical patients. *Neurosurgery* 20:716, 1987.

236. Krane NK: Intracranial pressure measurement in a patient undergoing hemodialysis and peritoneal dialysis. *Am J Kidney Dis* 13:336, 1989.

237. Lazarus JM: Complications in hemodialysis. An overview. *Kidney Int* 18:783, 1980.

238. Hegbrant J, Thysell H, Martensson L, et al: Change in plasma levels of vasoactive peptides during standard bicarbonate hemodialysis. *Nephron* 63:303, 1993.

239. Sherman RA: The pathophysiologic basis for hemodialysis-related hypotension. *Semin Dial* 1:136, 1988.

240. Travis M, Henrich WL: Autonomic nervous system and hemodialysis hypotension. *Semin Dial* 2:158, 1989.

241. Leunissen KM, Kooman JP, van Kuijk W, et al: Preventing hemodynamic instability in patients at risk for intradialytic hypotension. *Nephrol Dial Transplant* 11(suppl 2):11, 1996.

242. Levy FL, Grayburn PA, Henrich WL, et al: Improved left ventricular contractility with cool temperature hemodialysis. *Kidney Int* 41:961, 1992.

243. Agarwal R, Jost C, Henrich WL, et al: Thirty five degree Celsius dialysis increases periphery resistance and improves hemodynamic stability of patients. *J Am Soc Nephrol* 3:351, 1992.

244. Gong R, Lindberg J, Abrams J, et al: Comparison of hypertonic saline solutions and dextran in dialysis-induced hypotension. *J Am Soc Nephrol* 3:1808, 1993.

245. Rombola G, Colussi G, De FM, et al: Cardiac arrhythmias and electrolyte changes during hemodialysis. *Nephrol Dial Transplant* 7:318, 1992.

246. Silver SM, Sterns RH, Halperin ML: Brain swelling after dialysis: old urea or new osmoles? *Am J Kidney Dis* 28:1, 1996.

247. Arieff AI, Massry SG, Barrientos A, Kleeman CR: Brain water and electrolyte metabolism in uremia: effects of slow and rapid hemodialysis. *Kidney Int* 4:177, 1973.

248. Basile C, Miller JD, Koles ZJ, et al: The effects of dialysis on brain water and EEG in stable chronic uremia. *Am J Kidney Dis* 9:462, 1987.

249. Silver SM, DeSimone JA Jr, Smith DA, Sterns RH: Dialysis dysequilibrium syndrome in the rat: role of the reverse urea effect. *Kidney Int* 42:161, 1992.

250. Gullans SR, Verbalis JG: Control of brain volume during hyper- and hypoosmolar conditions. *Annu Rev Med* 44:289, 1993.

251. Arieff AI: Dialysis dysequilibrium syndrome: current concepts on pathogenesis. *Controv Nephrol* 4:367, 1982.

252. Aurigemma NM, Feldman NT, Gottlieb M, et al: Arterial oxygenation during hemodialysis. *N Engl J Med* 297:871, 1977.

253. De Broe ME: Hemodialysis-induced hypoxemia. *Nephrol Dial Transplant* 9(suppl 2):173, 1994.

254. Arnout MA, Hakim RM, Todd RF, et al: Increased expression of an adhesion promoting surface glycoprotein in the granulocytopenia of hemodialysis. *N Engl J Med* 312:457, 1985.

255. Bland LA, Favero MS, Arduino MJ: Should hemodialysis fluid be sterile? *Semin Dial* 6:34, 1993.

256. Traneus A, Heimburger O, Lindholm B: Peritonitis in chronic ambulatory peritoneal dialysis (CAPD): diagnostic findings, therapeutic outcome and complications. *Perit Dial Int* 9:179, 1989.

257. Port FK, Held PJ, Nolph KD, et al: Risk of peritonitis and technique failure by CAPD connection technique: a national study. *Kidney Int* 42:967, 1992.

258. Holley JL, Bernardini J, Piraino B: Polymicrobial peritonitis on continuous peritoneal dialysis. *Am J Kidney Dis* 19:162, 1992.

259. Keane WF, Alexander SR, Gokal R, et al: Peritoneal dialysis-related peritonitis treatment recommendations. 1996 update. *Perit Dial Int* 16:557, 1996.

260. Nomoto Y, Suga T, Nakajima K, et al: Acute hydrothorax in CAPD—a collaborative study of 161 centers. *Am J Nephrol* 9:363, 1989.

Index

Index

Page numbers followed by *f* indicate figures; page numbers followed by *t* indicate tables.